2

D1633995

Integrative Functions
of the
Autonomic Nervous System

Integrative Functions of the Autonomic Nervous System

An Analysis of the Interrelationships and Interactions of the
Sympathetic and Parasympathetic Divisions of the Autonomic
System in the Control of Body Function

Edited by

Chandler McC. Brooks

Kiyomi Koizumi

Akio Sato

UNIVERSITY OF TOKYO PRESS

ELSEVIER / NORTH-HOLLAND BIOMEDICAL PRESS

© UNIVERSITY OF TOKYO PRESS, 1979
UTP 3047–68951–5149

Library of Congress Cataloging in Publication Data
Main entry under title:

Integrative functions of the autonomic nervous system.

    Includes indexes.
    1. Nervous system, Autonomic—Congresses.
2. Biological control systems—Congresses. I. Brooks,
Chandler McC. II. Koizumi, Kiyomi, 1924–
III. Sato, Akio. [DNLM: 1. Autonomic nervous
system—Physiology. WL600 I61]
QP368.I56 1979 599′.01′88 79–16051
ISBN 0–444–80140–5

Published jointly by
UNIVERSITY OF TOKYO PRESS
and
ELSEVIER/NORTH-HOLLAND BIOMEDICAL PRESS

Sole distributors outside Japan, Asia and Australasia
Elsevier/North-Holland Biomedical Press
335 Jan van Galenstraat
P.O. Box 211, Amsterdam, The Netherlands

Sole distributors for the United States and Canada
Elsevier/North-Holland Inc.
52 Vanderbilt Avenue
New York, New York 10017
U.S.A.

Printed in Japan

CONTENTS

PREFACE

This book is a concrete expression of a newly developing interest in the autonomic nervous system and its functions. At present the genesis of new concepts is comparable to that which occurred in America and abroad during the 1920's and 1930's. The flood of new observations now being reported concerning this complex exceeds anything experienced previously. It seemed appropriate therefore that an analytical review be made of past attainments, that the present state of our knowledge be discussed, and that some consideration be devoted to the identification of future progressions. This publication should provide a new perspective for those now working in this field and a viable foundation for those just beginning studies of the autonomic nervous system.

The stimulus and opportunity for the discussions basic to this present work were provided by two international symposia. The first was held in Tokyo in 1974 (*Brain Research*, Vol. 87, April 1975, Elsevier Scientific Publishing Co., Amsterdam). It dealt primarily with somato-autonomic, viscero-autonomic reflexes, the regional organization of the system, and the characteristics of central neurons and centers controlling the complex. The second symposium, held March 14–18, 1978, in New York, continued this analysis but dealt principally with the integrative function of the autonomic system. There was discussion of sympathetic-parasympathetic interactions occurring in brain and spinal centers as well as within peripheral ganglia and plexuses in the course of regulating organ and tissue function.

The contributors endeavored to review the subject assigned to them as well as report the results of their own work. One of the unique features of the latter symposium was a consideration of the old and new methods used and the concepts now held relative to the conditioning of autonomic system function. Thus this book contains information of interest to behaviorists as well as analytically oriented neuroscientists and integrative physiologists.

Our hope is that this volume will provide some impetus to future study. To some degree this objective has already been attained in that these symposia and this group effort has resulted in the launching of a new jounral, *The Journal of the Autonomic Nervous System*. The first volume should appear in July 1979. It is thought that this publication will provide a means whereby those interested in the autonomic nervous system can not only publish their contributions but also maintain an awareness of future progress in the numerous aspects of autonomic system anatomy, pharmacology, and physiology.

DEDICATION

to

PHILIP BARD
1898–1977

It is appropriate that this book should be dedicated to Philip Bard because of his interests in and contributions to the study of the autonomic nervous system. As one of Walter B. Cannon's most distinguished students he pursued throughout his career interests he acquired while in Cannon's laboratory. Chief among these was the role of the hypothalamus in the organizing and control of emotional expression and the functional activities of the autonomic nervous system. His first major publication was entitled "A diencephalic mechanism for the expression of rage with special reference to the sympathetic nervous system" (*Amer. J. Physiol.*, 84 (1928) 490–515). His interest in the autonomic system and emotions was further indicated by papers published in *Psychological Review* in 1934, Vol. 41, "On emotional expression after decortication with some remarks on certain theoretical views"—Parts I and II. He also wrote a chapter for *A Handbook of General Experimental Psychology* (Clark Univ. Press, Worcester, 1934, pp. 264–311) entitled "Emotion: I. The neuro-humoral basis of emotional reactions". In 1939 he wrote a review article, "Central nervous mechanisms for emotional behavioral patterns in animals", for the Association for Nervous and Mental Disease (*Research Publications*, 19: 190–218).

Another early paper that we of the younger generation interested in the autonomic system read most carefully was "The central representation of the sympathetic system" (*Arch. Neurol. & Psychiat.*, 20 (1929) 230–246). He retained his interest in this topic throughout his life. For example, in 1960 he helped organize a symposium on cardiovascular and respiratory control mechanisms. His contribution was a paper dealing with the "Anatomical organization of the central nervous system in relation to the control of heart and blood vessels" (*Physiol. Rev.*, 40 (1960) 3–26).

The procedures generally followed by Dr. Bard in his research were to ablate various brain parts and then observe very carefully behavior change and changes in reactions induced thereby during recovery and after the animals reached a chronic state. He studied somatic as well as autonomic reactions. He is known for his studies of the cortical control of hopping and placing reactions ("Studies of the cerebral cortex 1. Localized control of placing and hopping reactions in the cat and their normal management by small cortical remnants". *Arch. Neurol. & Psychiat.*, 30 (1933) 40–74). I had cooperated with him in work reported previously ("Localized cortical control of some postural reactions in the cat and rat together with evidence that small cortical remnants may function normally", Philip Bard and C. McC. Brooks, *Res. Publ. Ass. nerv. ment. Dis.*, 13 (1932) 107–157). It is of interest that in studying a center of control he not only tried to determine the effects of its destruction but also to see what it could do in "isolation" from surrounding tissues. As stated previously, not only did he study somatic deficiencies following central nervous system ablations but also autonomic reactions and abilities to maintain homeostasis ("The responses to changes in environmental temperature after removal of portions of the forebrain"—with J. O. Pinkston and D. McK. Reach, 1937, 60: 73–147, and "The hypothalamus and sexual behavior"—*Res. Publ. Ass. nerv. ment. Dis.*, 20 (1940) 551–579).

During the second World War Bard spent some time, as did Cannon in World War I, studying traumatic shock and blood volume homeostasis. More unique were his studies of how motion affected gastrointestinal system reactions and vomiting and what CNS centers were responsible ("Motion sickness" with D. B. Tyler—*Physiol. Rev.*, 29 (1949) 311–369). Bard was initially involved in the use of evoked potentials in determining cortical sensory-motor localizations working with C. N. Woolsey and W. H. Marshall ("Studies on the cortical representation of somatic sensibility"—Harvey Lecture, 1937–38).

In my opinion one of the most impressive pieces of work he did in his later years, while still Professor of Physiology at the Johns Hopkins University Medical School, was the preparation of a hypothalamic island. He was able to maintain such animals for relatively long periods of time and found that this hypothalamic-hypophyseal complex even in isolation from neural connections could still maintain many essential states. Endocrinologists now frequently cut fibers leading into the hypothalamus in their studies of neuroendocrine control systems.

Philip Bard's role in maintaining interest and advancing knowledge of autonomic system physiology cannot be judged from his research alone. He was purely an American-trained physiologist and he played a major role in the conduct of the affairs of the American Physiological Society in his time. He was for many years editor of that major textbook "Medical Physiology", published by C. V. Mosby Co. He wrote the chapters dealing with the hypothalamus and autonomic nervous system, thus setting the level of knowledge American students were expected to attain. As President and Trustee of the International Foundation, he participated in providing educational and medical aid for many peoples. The International Foundation has sought to honor him by making possible publication of this volume which deals with the integrative function of the autonomic nervous system—a phenomenon which interested him greatly throughout his career.

Chandler McC. Brooks

ACKNOWLEDGMENTS

The U.S. and Japanese committees which organized two symposia on autonomic nervous system function express their appreciation for the opportunity granted by the U.S.-Japan Cooperative Science Program. In addition to support granted by the Japan Society for the Promotion of Science and the National Science Foundation of the United States, financial assistance was provided by The Research Foundation of the State University of New York, The Kroc Foundation for the Advancement of Medical Science, and The Edmond De Rothschild Foundation. We particularly appreciate the assistance of Mr. Mort Grant, Dr. Robert Kroc and Mr. George Shapiro relative to these grants. Publication of this book was made possible by a grant from the International Foundation as a commemorative act to honor Philip Bard, as a former trustee of the Foundation and as one who made significant contributions to our knowledge of autonomic system function.

We wish to thank Chancellor C. R. Wharton of the State University of New York for encouragement and for permitting us to identify this University as our host for the second of the two symposia, at which the papers in this volume were originally presented.

Mrs. Ruth Danziger, as secretary, bookkeeper and general coordinator of symposium affairs and editorial work, has been an indispensable associate. We wish to thank her and Nelle Graham Brooks for providing hospitality and any assistance needed by symposium participants and the editors of this publication. We were pleased by the friendliness and efficiency of the staff of the Roosevelt Hotel where our meetings were held.

Finally, we thank the representatives of the University of Tokyo Press for their helpful advice and the numerous members of the Tokyo Metropolitan Institute of Gerontology for their assistance in the final phases of the required editorial work. Cooperation by all concerned assured the success of the symposium and publication of this book which we trust will be helpful to many.

The Japanese Committee:
 Koji Uchizono, Chairman,
  Director of the National Institute of Physiology;
 Masami Iriki,
  Director of the Department of Physiology, Tokyo Metropolitan Institute of Gerontology;
 Akio Sato—Editor,
  Head of the Second Department of Physiology, Tokyo Metropolitan Institute of Gerontology.

The U.S.A. Committee:

    Chandler McC. Brooks, Chairman—Editor,
        Distinguished Professor of the State University of New York;
    William C. de Groat,
        Professor of Pharmacology, University of Pittsburgh, School of Medicine;
    Kiyomi Koizumi—Editor,
        Professor of Physiology, State University of New York, Downstate Medical
        Center.

SECTION   I

THE CONTROL OF ORGANS BY THE AUTONOMIC SYSTEM

Maintenance of essential body states and required behavioral activities are made possible by cooperative functioning of organ systems. The autonomic nerves are involved at three levels as they act upon organ complexes: 1) They affect the basic functional activities of cells and basic cellular states. These cellular activities occur within the units comprising an organ and are peculiar thereto; 2) The nerves act upon the several cell types and their unique processes but also unify or correlate tissue actions in such a way that the organ and organ system can meet inherent responsibilities; 3) The autonomic nerves under the direction of control centers organize the activities of organ systems. Cells are the basic units of organs but organs are the basic units of function.

The autonomic system, with its ability to deliver excitation and inhibition within the viscera, organizes support for somatic system function. It, however, is a modulator of cell and organ functions rather than being causative of most activities. The chapters of this section will deal with how autonomic nerves affect basic processes and cell action as well as the ultimate functions of special organs. They will emphasize what organ systems do and how they are controlled by nerves.

It is appropriate to begin a consideration of autonomic system control of organs by dealing with the salivary glands, which are organs but are also a part of the digestive system complex. Studies of the salivary glands reveal in miniature the total scope of autonomic nerve activity; these nerves can affect synthesis of special compounds, secretory processes, ion transport, muscle contraction and fluid movement. Salivary glands are indicators of water balance; they are affected by emotional states; they participate in digestive functions. Their reactions are unconditioned and conditioned. In the cephalic phase of digestion their action is highly related to what is externally sensed, to body need and to past experience; there is also a correlation with anticipatory gastric secretory and motor activity. Salivary gland action is integrated by higher centers acting through autonomic efferents with gastrointestinal tract function. The primary question is how the sympathetic and parasympathetic nerves act to influence the formulation and the secretion of saliva.

The initial step in salivary production is the secretion of precursor fluid by acinar cells. As this fluid passes through the salivary ducts its composition is changed. Both sympathetic and parasympathetic nerves affect the synthesis and the ionic fluxes involved. These processes are adequately described in the following chapters, as are the effects of the autonomic nerves on salivary gland development and growth. Denervation causes regression.

Autonomic nerves also control the mechanical activities of the digestive tract and modulate its secretory processes. The sympathetic and parasympathetic outflows tend to be opposed in their actions on intestinal walls and sphincters. It is of considerable interest that the secretory action of the vagus on gastric glands has not been challenged. Vagus action in liberating the gastrointestinal hormone gastrin has been more controversial. There are many more questions about the actions and interactions of autonomic nerves on the organs comprising the gastrointestinal tract than can be answered in one chapter, but new information has been contributed.

The sacral parasympathetic and lower lumbar outflow of the sympathetic system innervate the lower extremities of the gastrointestinal system and the bladder, thus controlling the eliminatory component of excretory function. This autonomic complex is also important to reproductive action. Its unique features are: 1) complex interactions between sympathetic and parasympathetic outflows in ganglia, plexuses and on effectors; 2) considerable differences in the central control of bladder and rectum; 3) an intimate relationship with the somatic or volitional control system in that sphincter reactions are associated with visceral control at both spinal and higher brain levels of integration. Higher centers are much more vital to normality of bladder function than they are to the emptying of the colon and rectum. These latter processes are managed quite well at a lower spinal level. This, however, does not indicate absence of a higher control and interaction between centers controlling micturition and defecation.

Digestive system function is not separable from metabolism, which, in turn, is affected by hormones released not only from the gut but also from the endocrine glands. The liver stands in a unique position. It stores and releases carbohydrates, it metabolizes, detoxifies, synthesizes compounds and participates in maintenance of homeostasis. It plays important roles in several compensatory reactions, for example, to hemorrhage by participating in blood clotting, manufacture of lost plasma proteins and other components of the blood. Apparently, there are sensors of body or blood states in the hepatic portal system. It reacts to changes in plasma levels of certain blood components although it is, to a degree, under nerve control, but hormones from the endocrine glands are the most important control agents. These are released by nerve action in many instances. Thus, the liver is directly and indirectly influenced by the autonomic system.

Practically every endocrine and hormone affects carbohydrate mobilization and metabolism. The gland, however, which seems to be primarily paired with the liver in maintaining carbohydrate metabolism and blood sugar homeostasis is the pancreas. The islets which secrete insulin and those that produce glucagon are controlled by multiple factors: hormones from the gut, plasma glucose levels and the nerves and transmitters of the autonomic system. The pancreas is dually innervated and the story of the reciprocal actions which occur centrally and peripherally in controlling insulin and glucagon secretion are interesting indeed. Much new information is being obtained, as has been indicated here.

It is obvious that the gastric system cannot serve the metabolic needs of the body without the cooperation of the cardiovascular and respiratory system organs. The integration of the functions of the three is largely managed by the autonomic system under control of sensors. Sensory receptors located throughout the body can initiate changes in respiratory and cardiovascular reactions; there are some which are of major importance to the integration of the actions of these visceral systems.

The receptors of the pulmonary circuit are treated here and in most studies as entities quite separate from the sensors located within heart tissues and adjacent to the coronary arteries. Possibly, afferents of the pulmonary vascular bed should be compared with those of the systemic circuit but it is important to ask what are their relationships relative to cardiac receptors as well as to those of the aorta and carotid arteries. Should they be regarded as related to the whole or a part of the total vascular system and how diverse are they in function? The major question is not so much what they can do as it is how their functions relate pulmonary and overall vasomotor and cardiac control. It is suggested that Chapter 7 and the subsequent Chapter 8 on receptors in the heart and cardiac reflexes be considered together as analyses of what we know at present concerning visceral afferents and their control of blood pressure and blood flow in organs and the body as a whole.

The salivary glands, the heart and the gastrointestinal tract present quite different pictures of the interactions between the sympathetic and parasympathetic systems. The eye is also an organ innervated by the autonomic system. It certainly is not a visceral organ in the usual sense but pupillary reactions are integrated with body states and behavior. Unquestionably, the autonomic system plays a diversity of roles in control of the eye. Certainly, both parasympathetic and sympathetic outflows participate and for the most part their actions are antagonistic. They are affected reciprocally in reflexes and generalized body responses. They are not essential to vision but denervation certainly impairs visual acuities and adjustments. It is known that autonomic nerves act on other receptors to affect their functions, but the eye presents the best example of the system's action on receptors in execution of its integrative activities. Pathways involved in pupillary dilator and constrictor reactions are still being identified. This is a preliminary requirement for analysis of central interactions. What happens in the ganglia and peripherally between the two outflows requires additional study.

The chapters of this first section contribute much to our knowledge of how the autonomic system controls organ systems and integrates their function.

CHAPTER 1

INTERACTIONS BETWEEN SYMPATHETIC AND PARASYMPATHETIC NERVES IN CONTROL OF THE SALIVARY GLANDS

Nils Emmelin

Institute of Physiology and Biophysics, University of Lund, Lund, Sweden

INTRODUCTION

Salivary glands are well supplied with nerves from both divisions of the autonomic nervous system. The secretory innervation was discovered in 1850 by Carl Ludwig[38], who found that saliva flowed from the submaxillary gland of the dog when he stimulated nerves, which later were called parasympathetic and sympathetic. Shortly afterwards Claude Bernard[2], studying the flow of blood from this gland, not only observed the vasoconstrictor effect of sympathetic stimulation which he had seen earlier in the ear of the rabbit but also described a new category of nerves, the vasodilator fibers. Later, the existence of these parasympathetic vasodilator nerves was questioned, particularly after the discovery of the vasodilator bradykinin mechanism[31], but it is now known that cholinergic fibers surround the vessels of the glands[22] and physiological evidence indicates that these nerves act as vasodilators[27,33].

It was early assumed that some contractile mechanism may cause saliva to flow from the glands; in the seventeenth century that opinion was held for instance by Stensen, the discoverer of the parotid duct. Ludwig[38] pointed out, however, that there are no muscle cells in salivary glands (except in the blood vessels), and he attributed the salivary flow and the marked pressure rise in the submaxillary duct which he obtained on nerve stimulation to activity exclusively in the secretory cells. Eckhard[7] made similar experiments on the parotid gland of the sheep, which he interpreted somewhat differently. When he connected the salivary duct to a manometer he found the pressure to rise slowly and continuously even when no nerves were stimulated. He discovered that in this particular gland, contrary to what is the case in the submaxillary gland of the dog, the secretory cells are constantly discharging saliva even in the absence of extraneous stimuli; they secrete spontaneously (see Babkin[1]). This caused the slow rise in pressure. When the sympathetic trunk in the neck was excited for a moment the pressure rose steeply and afterwards it returned almost to its starting level, to then resume its slow rise. Eckhard explained the steep pressure increase as due to contraction, and the subsequent fall to relaxation of some contractile mechanism, activated by sympathetic impulses. Interestingly, he argued that the gland may contain contractile elements other than muscle cells, and in 1881 Unna[54] suggested that these elements might be the basket cells, surrounding the acini and later called myoepithelial cells, which in salivary glands had been described by Krause[34] in 1865. There is also evidence to show that the salivary myoepithelial cells can be contracted by impulses in parasympathetic nerves[17].

Hence, the various effector cells of the salivary glands, the secretory cells, the smooth muscles of the blood vessels and the myoepithelial cells all seem to have a dual innervation. It is further obvious that antagonism between the two sets of nerves exists only in the blood vessels, whereas secretory and myoepithelial cells can be activated by both sympathetic and parasympathetic nerves. It should be stressed, however, that this does not apply to all salivary glands. Species differences are remarkably great in these glands; this is true for innervation also. For instance, there are glands in which the acinar secretory cells lack a sympathetic nerve supply, and very likely the myoepithelial cells of some glands receive motor fibers only from one division of the autonomic nervous system, although our information here is imperfect.

The picture has been further complicated as our knowledge of the secretory processes in the glands has increased. According to present opinion[49] saliva is formed in the acini as a precursor fluid, which in tonicity and content of some electrolytes resembles plasma. This is true whether secretion is evoked by parasympathetic or sympathetic nerve impulses; the difference is mainly in the flow rate, acetylcholine being a much more powerful stimulant of acinar secretion than noradrenaline. The volumes secreted are little changed when this primary saliva passes through the duct system, owing to low water permeability of the ducts, but the composition of the fluid is modified, because, for instance, sodium is absorbed and potassium secreted. Organic components such as amylase from the acinar cells are added to the primary saliva, and probably some other compounds from the duct cells. For the moment it seems reasonable to discuss separately the nervous control of acinar fluid secretion, of amylase secretion and of the events in the ducts.

Interactions in salivary glands can obviously occur when nerves activate different effectors simultaneously. A brisk salivation evoked by parasympathetic impulses is greatly reduced if sympathetic vasoconstrictor activity diminishes the blood supply of the gland[11]. It is conceivable that the secretory and absorptive processes in the ducts may be affected if the time of contact between the fluid and the duct cells is shortened because myoepithelial contraction accelerates the salivary flow. Interactions of this type may belong to a physiological pattern but are particularly likely to complicate the experiment when the efferent nerves are stimulated electrically, since the nerve trunk contains fibers for several kinds of effector. The present paper will deal mainly with interactions between sympathetic and parasympathetic nerves in one and the same type of effector, but in the case of the two processes to which particular attention will be paid, myoepithelial contraction and acinar fluid secretion, the interplay between motor and secretory events will often be referred to. It is sometimes extremely difficult to decide in the experiment whether flow of saliva obtained on nerve stimulation is due to myoepithelial contraction or acinar fluid secretion or to both. Historically, this is illustrated in the discussion of the old phenomenon of "augmented salivary secretion".

AUGMENTED SECRETION OF SALIVA

The salivary flow response to sympathetic stimulation is very variable, between species, between different glands of the same species and even in the same experiment on a single gland. Compared with the response to parasympathetic stimulation it is generally small, appears only after a long latency and requires a high frequency of stimulation; it often decreases while stimulation is going on. Langley[35] observed, however, that the effect was greatly enhanced if sympathetic stimulation was preceded by brief parasympathetic stimulation, and he named this phenomenon "augmented secretion". His explanation was that the first stimulation left the secretory cells for some time in a state of heightened excitability, so that the subsequent sympathetic stimulation could elicit an augmented response. He regarded the sympathetic nerves as purely secretory and did not consider any motor effects. Mathews[40] expressed a different opinion; he concluded that the flow of saliva obtained on sympathetic stimulation is due exclusively to contraction of muscle cells within the glands, which expels saliva present in the alveoli and ducts. His main arguments were that the flow was particularly rapid in the beginning of the stimulation period and that it decreased when sympathetic stimulation was repeated but could be restored by filling the duct system in advance. This was achieved by injecting some fluid through the duct in a retrograde direction or by brief parasympathetic stimulation; by this latter experiment his views on sympathetic innervation entered into the discussion of augmented secretion. In a series of investigations Babkin and co-workers (see Babkin[1]) came to the conclusion that the mechanisms proposed by Langley and Mathews could both operate to augment the sympathetic flow: sympathetic motor fibers, contracting myoepithelial cells expel saliva accumulated during the preceding parasympathetic stimulation; sympathetic secretory fibers act on secretory cells in a state of raised excitability, causing a "true augmented secretion". Discrepancies in the literature regarding the mechanism of augmented secretion may partly be due to species differences; furthermore, vasoconstriction during sympathetic stimulation may greatly interfere with secretory and motor effects and obscure the interpretation of the observations. There is a great need for methods by which motor, secretory and vasomotor effects of nerve stimulation can be separated in salivary glands. To some extent this is possible in the submaxillary gland of the dog with regard to its sympathetic innervation. In this gland sympathetic secretory impulses seem to be mediated by β-adrenoceptors and motor impulses by α-adrenoceptors[14]. By using the appropriate agonists or antagonists it is therefore possible to study motor and secretory effects of sympathetic stimulation separately. For instance, after administration of an α-blocking agent, sympathetic stimulation will cause secretion from this gland uncomplicated by myoepithelial contraction and vasoconstriction. This will facilitate studies of sympathetic and parasympathetic interactions on the secretory cells and of the role played by the secretory component in augmented secretion. Conversely, flow of saliva on sympathetic stimulation is likely to be due to myoepithelial contraction if obtained in the presence of a β-blocking drug.

Experiments on the submaxillary gland of the dog using such methods have supported the view that salivary myoepithelial cells may receive motor fibers from the sympathetic system, which has not always been recognized[12]. Further, experience gained in these experiments could be applied to work on parasympathetic motor innervation, and on interactions between the two sets of nerves on myoepithelial cells.

THE MYOEPITHELIAL CELLS

Contractions of salivary myoepithelial cells have not been observed directly, under the microscope, as in mammary glands[37] and sweat glands[32]. Contractility of the salivary myoepithelial cells is assumed from analogy with the cells of these other glands, from the presence of actin and myosin (which, however, have now been detected in secretory cells also[6]) and of filaments passing through the cell body out into the processes, and from the general arrangement of these star-shaped cells, enclosing the acini. Indirect methods have to be resorted to in order to detect activity in these cells, by action on the flow of saliva or on the pressure in the salivary duct, as has been done already in the early investigations quoted above.

Sympathetic Motor Nerves

By stimulating the vago-sympathetic trunk in the neck at a high frequency a prolonged slow flow of saliva can be evoked from the submaxillary gland of the dog; it can be maintained for a long time and is therefore attributed to secretion. This response can be imitated by injecting isoprenaline and it can be abolished by β-blocking drugs[14]. However, if the luminal system is filled in advance, by injection of some fluid up the duct, the picture is somewhat changed. The slow flow on sympathetic stimulation is now preceded by a phase of rapid outflow, and this part of the response, which is not seen when isoprenaline is given, persists after β-block but can be abolished by α-blocking drugs. The initial, shortlasting, rapid outflow can be mimicked by injecting the α-adrenoceptor stimulating drug phenylephrine, provided the luminal system has been filled, and when both this drug and isoprenaline are given the whole sympathetic response can be reproduced[14]. These observations indicate that the first response to sympathetic stimulation is a motor effect, presumably exerted by myoepithelial cells. Incidentally, they suggest that one function of these cells is to quicken the outflow of saliva into the mouth, which may be of importance for the protective tasks of saliva.

A biphasic response to sympathetic stimulation can also be obtained when the pressure in the duct system is recorded with a small basal pressure filling the system[14]. This is shown in Fig. 1. First, the pressure rises steeply, then follows a phase of more gradual, slow rise. The first phase, ascribed to myoepithelial contraction, can be imitated with phenylephrine. It is abolished by α-blocking drugs and the only effect remaining is a late, slow rise, similar to that obtained with isoprenaline. An interesting feature is that in this phase, produced by isoprenaline or by sympathetic stimulation after α-block and ascribed to secretion, the pressure levels are much lower than those reached in the secondary phase when the sympathetic is stimulated in the absence of α-block, or when isoprenaline is combined with phenylephrine. It seems as if outflow

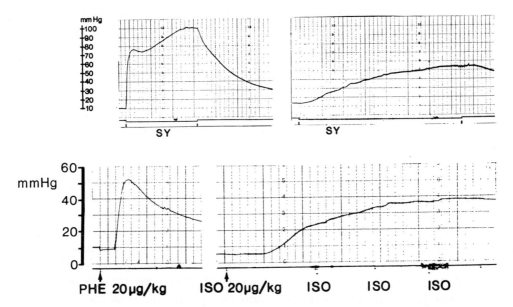

Fig. 1. Pressure in the submaxillary ducts of dogs. Upper experiment: SY=stimulation of the vagosympathetic nerve at 20 Hz before (left section) and after intravenous injection of dihydroergotamine, 0.4 mg/kg (right section). Lower experiment: intravenous injections of phenylephrine (PHE) and isoprenaline (ISO). Modified from Emmelin and Gjörstrup[14].

of saliva is more easily counterbalanced by inflow of fluid from the luminal system into the glandular tissues when the secretory cells are not supported by contraction of myo-epithelial cells, and other observations support this hypothesis[13]. An important function of the myoepithelial cells seems to be to promote the flow of the often highly viscous saliva through narrow channels, reducing back flow of fluid into the tissues.

Under physiological conditions there is always some salivary secretion to moisten the oral mucosa, at least in the waking state. Spontaneous activity in some glands may somewhat contribute to this flow, but mainly it is elicited reflexly via the parasympa-thetic pathway. In the anaesthetized animal it can be imitated by stimulating the parasympathetic nerve at a low frequency. Sympathetic stimulation superimposed on a parasympathetically-induced secretion is usually reported to inhibit the flow, an effect generally attributed to sympathetic vasoconstriction[11]. However, this effect of vasocon-striction can be largely avoided if the sympathetic nerve is excited for a few seconds only[14]. If, in the submaxillary gland of the dog, sympathetic secretion is at the same time prevented using a β-blocking drug, sympathetic stimulation will have a charac-teristic effect: It will accelerate the salivary flow, and afterwards there is a period of compensatory retardation of the flow. Both these effects are abolished by α-blocking drugs and it seems reasonable to attribute them to mechanical actions on the flow when myoepithelial cells temporarily contract and then relax. By providing a back-ground of continuous slow secretion it is thus possible to demonstrate, under these conditions, a pure motor effect of sympathetic stimulation. The experiment gives an example of an interaction between parasympathetically-evoked secretion and sympathetically-induced myoepithelial contraction. If the term "augmented salivary secretion" is extended to the situation in which the two nerves are activated simultaneously and not in succession, as has been proposed[16], the experiment also illustrates the motor component of this phenomenon.

Parasympathetic Motor Nerves

In similar flow and pressure experiments on the submaxillary gland of the dog a parasympathetic motor innervation has been demonstrated[17]. In this case conditions are less favorable, because we have no drug which strictly separates motor and secretory effects. Furthermore, the parasympathetic secretory effect is so very marked that it tends to conceal motor effects. In pressure experiments the secretory effect was reduced by stimulating the parasympathetic nerve at a low frequency. The two experiments shown in Fig. 2 may serve to illustrate this. A biphasic pressure curve could then be obtained, resembling that seen on sympathetic stimulation with an early, steep rise and a subsequent, more gradual increase of the pressure. When stimulation was discontinued, there was a biphasic pressure fall, first a steep fall, reminiscent of the initial steep rise, and then a more gradual fall. When the pressure was instead raised passively, by injecting some fluid into the system, the subsequent fall of the pressure occurred along a smooth curve. The longer the stimulation was carried out, the higher was the pressure reached in the second phase of rise, but for a certain frequency of stimulation the initial rise was the same, and so was the initial fall, whether it started from a high or from a low pressure level. On the other hand, with increasing frequency not only was the initial rise larger (and soon merged with the second phase), but also the initial fall, independently of the level reached when stimulation ceased. These various observations were taken as evidence to show that the parasympathetic stimulation activated motor fibers, causing the early, steep pressure rise; afterwards, relaxation of the myoepithelial cells gave the initial, steep fall of the pressure. The

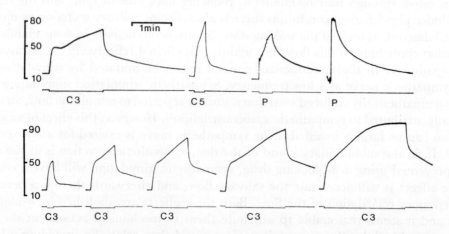

Fig. 2.   Pressure in the submaxillary ducts of dogs. Stimulation of the chorda-lingual nerve (C) at 3 Hz for increasing time periods in the lower experiment, at 3 and 5 Hz in the upper experiment. At P fluid was injected into the system. From Emmelin, Gjörstrup and Thesleff[17].

second phase of rise was explained as due to secretion, and the second phase of fall to backflow of fluid into the glandular tissues.

Flow experiments also supported the view that the gland receives parasympathetic motor nerves[17]. When a slow background secretion had been established, a brief period of parasympathetic stimulation at high frequency greatly accelerated the flow. This was no doubt mainly due to an increased secretory effect, but often a small temporary retardation could be discerned, suggesting that myoepithelial contraction had contributed to increase the flow rate and decreased it for a moment while the cells relaxed. However, a marked and only gradually vanishing after-secretion following high frequency stimulation tended to counteract the decelerating effect of myoepithelial relaxation. The outflow level of the saliva from the gland was then raised, in order to distend and increase the capacity of the luminal system, and now the poststimulatory retardation was marked and regularly obtained. It was seen independently of the mechanism by which the background secretion was elicited, by parasympathetic stimulation at low frequency, by isoprenaline injection or by sympathetic stimulation in the presence of an α-receptor blocking drug. This seems to speak in favor of the explanation that there was a simple mechanical component in the response when the parasympathetic nerve was briefly excited. The experiment offers an example of interaction between parasympathetic motor and sympathetic secretory effects.

Relationship between the Two Sets of Motor Nerves

From the previous discussion it is obvious that it is difficult to isolate the motor effects of nerve stimulation, particularly where the parasympathetic nerves are concerned. It is therefore not surprising that little work has been done on the action on the myoepithelial cells under combined sympathetic and parasympathetic stimulation. The experiment shown in Fig. 3 may give some information about the relation between the different motor nerves in the submaxillary gland of the dog[17]. Recording the pressure in the salivary duct the parasympathetic nerve was stimulated at a high frequency, at which the two phases of pressure rise could barely be distinguished. The steep initial fall, occurring when stimulation ceased and attributed to myoepithelial relaxation is evident. The sympathetic was then stimulated using a high frequency to produce a maximal pressure response. Since the experiment was carried out in the presence of a β-blocking drug abolishing sympathetic secretion, the pressure rise was

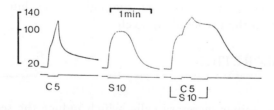

Fig. 3.   Pressure in the submaxillary duct of a dog. Stimulation of the chorda-lingual nerve at 5 Hz (C5) and of the vago-sympathetic nerve at 10 Hz (S 10). In the section to the right chorda-lingual was superimposed on sympathetic stimulation. Practolol, 2 mg/kg, had been given intravenously before the record starts. From Emmelin, Gjörstrup and Thesleff[17].

assumed to be due wholly to myoepithelial contraction. The sympathetic stimulation was repeated, and when its maximum had been reached a brief period of parasympathetic stimulation was added. The additional pressure rise obtained was thought to be caused by parasympathetic secretion and not by further myoepithelial contraction. This conclusion was based on the fact that the pressure fall when parasympathetic stimulation ceased (but sympathetic stimulation continued) was very slow, as contrasted with the fall earlier ascribed to myoepithelial relaxation. Considering the high pressure level from which it started the fall was remarkably slow, but this is in agreement with the finding mentioned previously that contracted myoepithelial cells counteract backflow of fluid into the glandular tissues[13], and in this case the maximal sympathetic contraction was maintained. The conclusion which can be drawn at least tentatively from this type of experiment is that the two sets of nerves converge on the same myoepithelial cells and that parasympathetic motor impulses cannot increase the contraction of cells already activated to the sympathetic maximum. It would obviously be of interest to study the combined motor effect when the two nerves were stimulated submaximally at the same time, but such experiments have not been carried out.

In all the experiments so far described the efferent nerves were excited electrically. It is not known whether myoepithelial cells are activated in the course of physiological events, to promote the outflow of saliva and support the secreting cells, let alone whether there is then any interaction between sympathetic and parasympathetic nerves. It does not seem unreasonable to suppose that central mechanisms activate the myoepithelial cells at the same time as the secretory cells. Such a view is at least easy to accept if it is true that the single axon can contact, *en passant*, different types of effectors in the glands. Some indirect evidence to show that the central nervous system physiologically exerts an action on the myoepithelial cells derives from denervation experiments[19]. Disconnected from the central nervous system the cells develop the supersensitivity to chemical stimuli which was so extensively studied by Cannon[4] in other neuro-effector systems. It can be shown, for instance, that the pressure-raising effects of drugs are greatly increased in the submaxillary gland of the dog some weeks after section of the preganglionic parasympathetic nerves. By analogy from other denervation experiments[10] it can be assumed that this is the result of loss of impulses from the central nervous system to the myoepithelial cells. Interestingly, the supersensitivity develops not only to acetylcholine and related agents but also to sympathomimetic drugs acting on α-receptors, suggesting some kind of interaction between the two systems in the myoepithelial cell.

ACINAR FLUID SECRETION

The Nerves

The nerves of the acinar secretory cells, which induce the secretion of primary saliva and thus determine the volumes of saliva formed, are much better known than the motor nerves. This is especially true for the powerful parasympathetic nerves, which seem to be able to activate the acini to maximal secretion of fluid. Whereas there apparently is little convergence in the parasympathetic ganglion[8,36], as usual in this division of the autonomic nervous system, convergence is very pronounced in the neuroglandular area. This opinion is founded particularly on physiological experiments[8,39]. In view of the recent finding that coupling between adjacent acinar cells is extensive[30] the "functional" convergence may be even more marked than indicated by anatomical observations. In most salivary glands the acini receive sympathetic fibers also. An intracellular electrode records "secretory potentials" from an acinar cell both on sympathetic and parasympathetic stimulation, suggesting that these nerves converge on the same cells[39], at least in a functional sense. In the submaxillary gland of the cat, which possesses two different kinds of acinar cells, early experiments demonstrated that histological changes appeared particularly in one cell type on parasympathetic, and in the other on sympathetic stimulation[1]. Recently Garrett and Kidd[26] showed that peroxidase, which is present in the demilunar cells, is secreted predominantly on sympathetic stimulation, and acid phosphatase from the central acinar cells especially on parasympathetic stimulation; there was some overlap, and it was concluded that both sets of nerves probably affect both sets of cells. This overlap seems to be more pronounced in the case of fluid secretion, for when the parasympathetic nerves are stimulated to produce their maximal flow rate, the secretion cannot be further increased by stimulating the sympathetic fibers as well, although such stimulation alone can evoke a rapid secretion from this particular gland, the submaxillary gland of the cat[11]; when sympathetic stimulation is added, the flow rate remains constant for a while and then it decreases gradually because of sympathetic vasoconstriction. Such a convergence on the acinar cells of sympathetic and parasympathetic nerves causing fluid transport has been found in other glands also, the submaxillary gland of the dog[11] and the rat[42], and can be assumed to be the prerequisite for interactions between the two sets of nerves in acinar fluid secretion.

Interactions between the Nerves

During a very brief period of sympathetic stimulation superimposed on a slow parasympathetic background secretion the flow accelerates and a subsequent short-lasting retardation reveals that myoepithelial contraction had transiently increased the outflow of saliva from the submaxillary gland of the dog[14]. After injection of an α-blocking drug to prevent this mechanical component, sympathetic stimulation still accelerates the flow, although less than before. A β-blocking drug abolishes this remaining response, suggesting that it was due to sympathetically-evoked secretion. This secretory response, obtained even when the sympathetic nerve is excited for some few seconds only is surprising, considering the remarkably long latency of sympathetic secretion when the nerve is activated in the absence of a secretory background.

Since the α-blocking drug has the additional advantage of counteracting sympathetic vasoconstriction, the relation between the secretory effects of the two autonomic nerves can be studied without interference from a restricted blood supply, and experiments of the type shown in Fig. 4 can be made[16]. It can be seen that even after α-block, the secretory response to sympathetic stimulation is poor. It takes a long time to start, in fact even longer than before the blocking drug was given, because myoepithelial contraction is lacking; the flow is slow, and tends to become even slower while stimulation is going on; and a fairly high frequency of stimulation is necessary to evoke any

14   N. Emmelin

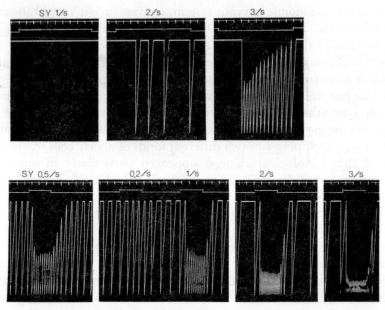

Fig. 4. Secretion from the submaxillary gland of the dog, recorded by an ordinate writer,
         recording the time interval between two drops of saliva. Records from above: minute
         marks: signal for stimulation of the vago-sympathetic nerve (SY); salivary secretion.
         In the upper row the nerve was stimulated for 10 min at the frequencies given in the
         Fig. Lower row: vago-sympathetic stimulation during 3 min superimposed on con-
         tinuous chorda-lingual stimulation at 0.2 Hz. Before the experiment started, dihydro-
         ergotamine, 0.5 mg/kg, had been given intravenously. From Emmelin and Gjörstrup[16].

secretion. Vasoconstriction is obviously not the reason why sympathetic secretion is
so relatively small in this gland, even if it may further decrease it when persisting for a
long time. Quite a different picture is obtained when a slow parasympathetic background secretion is provided. Superimposed sympathetic stimulation now quickly
accelerates the flow; the effect is marked even at low frequencies and is maintained
as long as stimulation continues. In a series of experiments the mean sympathetic
threshold frequency was lowered about ten times by the background activity. The
phenomenon corresponds to the "true augmented secretion" as described by Babkin[1]
for successive stimulations of the nerves.

This facilitating effect is even more striking in the parotid gland of the dog. In
most dogs sympathetic stimulation alone causes no secretion at all, even when vasoconstriction has been abolished; this, in spite of the fact that adrenergic fibers are present in contact with the acini[25]. However, a slow secretion elicited by the parasympathetic nerve is greatly increased by a simultaneous sympathetic stimulation at low
frequencies[16]. This latent secretory effect of the sympathetic nerve is obviously
mediated by β-adrenoceptors, for it is abolished by drugs such as propranolol. Interesting observations can also be made on the glands of cats[15]. Here the secretory responses
of the parotid gland to sympathetic stimulation are very small and elicited mainly
via β-adrenoceptors; as in the glands of the dog they can be greatly augmented by
stimulating the parasympathetic nerve at the same time. On the submaxillary gland,

on the other hand, the sympathetic nerve has a marked secretory effect, which is abolished by α-blocking agents. This secretion is further enhanced in a parasympathetic secretion, but after α-block some secretory effect of the sympathetic nerve is found to persist, and this cannot be abolished by raising the dose of the drug but disappears when a β-blocking drug is given. Small doses of isoprenaline also accelerate the parasympathetic flow, whereas very large doses of isoprenaline are needed to evoke even a small secretion from the quiescent gland[15]. The experiments thus reveal a β-mediated sympathetic secretion in this gland, which may be a normal effect of the nerve since the presence of a small amount of parasympathetic activity can be taken for granted under physiological conditions. In rabbits the parotid gland responds with secretion to sympathetic stimulation, and the effect is mediated mainly by α-, but to some extent also by β-receptors[41]; it increases when the parasympathetic nerves are stimulated as well[28]. The spontaneous secretion characteristic of the submaxillary gland of this species[41,51] is scarcely or not at all increased by stimulating the sympathetic nerve; the response when obtained is β-mediated [28,51]. No augmentation of this effect can be produced by supplying a parasympathetic secretion, even if sympathetic vasoconstriction, which in this gland seems to be very effective, is prevented using an α-blocking drug[28]. This lack of secretory interaction may be partly due simply to the fact that the acini of this gland seem to be much less well supplied with sympathetic fibers than was earlier thought[23]; a corresponding example would be the sublingual gland of the rat, where there are very few if any adrenergic nerves to the acini and

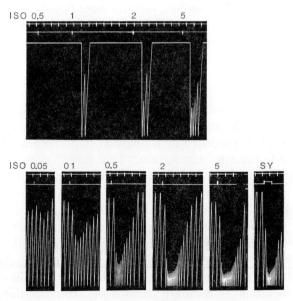

Fig. 5.   Secretion from the submaxillary gland of the dog. Records as in Fig. 4. Secretion caused by intravenous isoprenaline (ISO) in doses in μg/kg given in the Fig. In the upper tracings isoprenaline was given alone, in the lower tracings while the chorda-lingual nerve was stimulated at 0.4 Hz. SY: stimulation of the vago-sympathetic nerve at 10 Hz after injection of dihydroergotamine, 0.5 mg/kg. From Emmelin and Gjörstrup[16].

where scarcely any sympathetic secretory effect can be demonstrated, without or with concomitant parasympathetic stimulation[52]. It is also possible that the adrenergic fibers present round the acini of the submaxillary gland of the rabbit are concerned mainly with secretion of proteins and not much with the transport of fluid[28].

As the single acinar cell of most glands seems to have a dual secretory innervation, at least from a functional point of view, it is reasonable to assume that the secretory interactions now described take place in the neuro-glandular region or within the glands. Since similar interactions can be demonstrated if parasympathetic stimulation is replaced by pilocarpine injection, or sympathetic stimulation by the appropriate sympathomimetic drug (Fig. 5), the facilitation seems to be localized to postjunctional structures, concerning the effects rather than the release of the neurotransmitters[15,16]. It is probably premature to speculate on whether the action is on the permeability of the cell membrane, on mechanisms involving the calcium ion, the cyclic AMP or GMP systems or on some other point. The role of these systems in salivary secretion is far from clear and probably species differences are considerable.

In some other connections observations have been made suggestive of an interaction between adrenergic and cholinergic mechanisms in salivary glands. For instance, the secretory effect of sympathetic stimulation is reduced by atropine and pharmacologically related drugs[11]. This effect is particularly noticeable when the sympathetic is stimulated at a fairly low frequency, near the threshold frequency, and increasing the dose of the atropine-like drug does not diminish the response below a certain level. A reasonable hypothesis could be that the atropine-like agent interfered with transmission through the sympathetic ganglion, but this does not seem to be the explanation, for the effect is the same when the atropinization is restricted to the gland, by injecting the drug into it through the duct. A hypothesis suggested to explain this phenomenon is that the atropine-like drug abolishes a facilitatory action of the acetylcholine, which is known to be randomly released in subsecretory amounts from the postganglionic parasympathetic nerves[10].

The following might be related to this phenomenon[53]. Using intracellular recording in parotid acini of cats it can be shown that sympathetic stimulation has a depolarizing action. Often this is preceded by a phase of hyperpolarization, resembling that obtained on parasympathetic stimulation. This initial sympathetic phase can be abolished not only by guanethidine, which in addition prevents subsequent depolarization; atropine also abolishes the sympathetic (and the parasympathetic) hyperpolarization and it acts when given through the duct into the gland. Denervation experiments may also be quoted to suggest that there is some kind of relationship between sympathetic and parasympathetic nerves at the glandular level. For instance, degenerative section of the preganglionic parasympathetic nerve results in a very marked supersensitivity to catecholamines, which under certain conditions may give rise to "paralytic secretion"[11]. Similarly, prolonged atropinization, lasting for a week or more, sensitizes the gland to catecholamines[10]. Supersensitivity to adrenaline, created by parasympathetic decentralization is abolished by pilocarpine or eserine injections repeated over a few days[10]. Sympathetic denervation sensitizes the gland to parasympathomimetic agents. It also increases the effect of stimulation of the parasympathetic nerve[21], and conversely parasympathetic denervation produces a supersensitivity to sympathetic nerve impulses.

Physiological Significance of the Interaction

It has already been pointed out that a slow, parasympathetically-induced secretion is usually present under normal conditions. Furthermore, to abolish sympathetic vasoconstriction, as was done in most of the experiments described above, will also serve to bring the experiment closer to physiological situations, for there is scarcely reason to believe that the central nervous system, activating sympathetic secretory fibers to promote the flow of saliva, would simultaneously elicit vasoconstriction in the gland. Experimental evidence shows that at a central level sympathetic secretory and vasoconstrictor effects can be separated, as could be expected; during bleeding there is a marked vasoconstriction in the salivary gland but no secretion, whereas stimulation of the sympathetic trunk to produce an equivalent vasoconstriction causes a lively flow of saliva[11]. It seems more likely that myoepithelial contraction belongs to a physiological pattern in which sympathetic secretory fibers are stimulated, and in that case this part of the response is lost because of the α-blocking agent given. However, as shown earlier, secretion obviously can occur even if not accompanied by myoepithelial contraction; besides, it is possible that parasympathetic impulses caused some motor effect, although in the experiment the synchronized impulses were of such a low frequency as to produce scarcely any sustained myoepithelial contraction. The important question, however, seems to be whether the sympathetic impulse flow, which according to the experiment can markedly and well within the physiological frequency range increase secretion, really occurs in the course of physiological events. There is some reason to doubt this. Classical experiments on dogs report that there is no salivation on feeding after section of the parasympathetic pathway or injection of atropine[1], and this has been taken as evidence that sympathetic secretory fibers do not play any role in the secretion of fluid. Similarly, the secretion which can be elicited by afferent stimulation of glossopharyngeal or lingual fibers in anaesthetized cats is abolished by parasympathetic denervation or administration of atropine[9]. However these procedures, nerve section or atropine injection, of course deprived the glands of the parasympathetic background activity, in the absence of which sympathetic secretory impulses seem to have little effect, at least at low stimulation frequencies. In rats conditions for demonstrating a secretory effect of sympathetic impulses seem more favorable. Feeding elicits a flow of saliva, which is reduced but not abolished by section of the parasympathetic nerves; the remaining response disappears on interrupting the sympathetic pathway[43]. In cats afferent stimulation of the sciatic nerve was found to elicit a flow of submaxillary saliva, some of which remained after parasympathetic decentralization and exclusion of the adrenal glands; this remaining flow was abolished by sympathectomy[11]. This may reflect a physiological activation of the sympathetic secretory nerves; however, if this be the case, it might be part of an emergency reaction and it could be suspected that under such conditions central inhibition might abolish any facilitating parasympathetic secretion. It still seems an open question whether in general sympathetic impulses normally contribute, in cooperation with parasympathetic impulses, to the secretion of fluid when saliva is needed in the mouth for digestive and protective purposes.

SECRETION OF AMYLASE

Nervous control of the secretion of proteins into the saliva is best known in the case of amylase. Consequently, the experiments discussed in this section have been made mainly on glands rich in amylase, such as parotid glands of rats and rabbits, whereas previous sections have centered on glands of dogs and cats containing none, or very little of this enzyme. There seems to be general agreement that amylase secretion is chiefly elicited by sympathetic nerves. The role of sympathetic innervation in this respect has been studied not only by stimulating the efferent nerves electrically, but also in feeding experiments [3,24,46]. Sympathetic impulses acting on β-adrenoceptors cause degranulation of the acinar cells and extrusion of large amounts of amylase into the primary saliva [44,50]. In addition there is some secretion of fluid in the parotid glands of rats and rabbits when the sympathetic nerve is stimulated, partly via β-adrenoceptors but mainly by way of α-adrenoceptors. Conversely, α-stimulation causes some small secretion of amylase. In saliva secreted in response to parasympathetic impulses the concentration of amylase is low but the total output can be considerable since the flow rate is usually high; degranulation does not seem to be conspicuous in this case.

As the volumes of fluid secreted via β-receptors are very small, the production, under physiological conditions, of saliva rich in amylase obviously depends on cooperation between impulses acting on β-receptors to release amylase and impulses activating cholinergic receptors, and to some extent α-receptors, to provide the fluid transporting the amylase. Since parasympathetic impulses can also release amylase into the primary fluid, an interaction in amylase secretion between the two divisions of the autonomic nervous system at some other level is conceivable. In the parotid gland of the rabbit sympathetic impulses cause an output of amylase at much lower frequencies when a slow parasympathetic background secretion is supplied than when the sympathetic nerve is excited alone[29]. The following may be a related observation. While postganglionic nerves are degenerating there is a period in which the neurotransmitter is released in quantities which may be sufficient to activate the effector cells[20]. The "degeneration secretion" from the parotid gland of the rat, obtained from anaesthetized animals between 12 and 24 hours after excision of the superior cervical ganglion, is very small[5]. In contrast, the degranulation of the acinar cells seen 24 hours after sympathectomy is extensive, as if the sympathetic nerve had been stimulated at a high frequency for a long time[24]. In this instance the rats were awake during the period of "degeneration secretion". It can be assumed that in that period the parotid gland was exposed not only to the sympathetic transmitter from the degenerating nerves but also to reflexly set up parasympathetic impulses; this was not the case in the anaesthetized rat. The parasympathetic impulses might have greatly increased the degranulating effect of sympathetic "degeneration activity"[24]. The interdependence between the two nerves may also be illustrated by the fact that the secretion of amylase caused by parasympathetic stimulation can be markedly augmented by removing the sympathetic ganglion some days in advance[24].

In experiments *in vitro* on slices of the parotid glands of rabbits two observations have been made which may be examples of interactions between sympathetic and parasympathetic impulses[55]. First, it was noticed that α-adrenergic stimulation by incubation with methoxamine caused some output of amylase, which could be abolished not only with phenoxybenzamine but also with atropine. Secondly, combined effects of carbachol and isoprenaline on amylase secretion seemed to be greater than the added effects produced by each agent when given alone.

NERVOUS CONTROL OF THE DUCTS

Cholinergic and adrenergic nerves have been found close to the duct cells[24], and early papers describe histological[1] and electrical[39] changes in the duct cells when autonomic nerves were stimulated. Drugs such as carbachol and isoprenaline have been found to affect absorption and secretion of ions in the ducts[49]. In recent papers by Leon Schneyer[47,48] the discovery that stimulation of sympathetic and parasympathetic nerves can influence these events in the ducts was reported. These important findings are described in a separate chapter of this book. It still seems too early to speculate on the relationship between the two sets of nerves in these processes.

In the ducts proteins are also added to the saliva. One of the macromolecules present in granules in duct cells seems to be kallikrein, at least in some species[24,45]. Both sympathetic and parasympathetic nerves are apparently of importance for kallikrein but in somewhat different capacities. Secretion of kallikrein into the saliva occurs particularly when the sympathetic nerve is stimulated, and this may greatly reduce the kallikrein content of the gland; on the other hand, the gland can be depleted of the enzyme following parasympathetic decentralization[18,24,45].

INTERACTIONS BETWEEN THE VASOMOTOR NERVES

The existence of a sympathetic vasoconstrictor tone in salivary glands is evident from the fact that glandular blood flow increases when the sympathetic trunk is cut in the neck, as shown first by Claude Bernard[2]. This sympathetic vasoconstrictor effect is easily overcome by parasympathetic stimulation, which, as is well known, very considerably increases the blood flow through the gland. Since the vasodilatation at least initially must be due to impulses in vasodilator nerves[33], this seems to offer an important example of an antagonistic interaction between sympathetic and parasympathetic nerves, occurring each time the gland enters into secretory activity. The vasodilator effect is very powerful; in fact, a single shock applied to the parasympathetic nerve markedly increases the flow of blood through the gland[12].

When the sympathetic nerve is stimulated at a much higher frequency than that needed to restore the vascular effect of section of the cervical sympathetic trunk, salivary flow evoked by parasympathetic stimulation gradually decreases[11]. Under these conditions sympathetic vasoconstriction can apparently get the upper hand even in the presence of parasympathetic vasodilator activity. It seems doubtful whether this reflects a physiological situation; emotional dryness of the mouth is very likely due to central inhibition of the secretory mechanisms rather than to sympathetic vasoconstriction in the salivary glands.

CONCLUSIONS

The salivary glands are very much dependent on their nerves, more perhaps than most other organs innervated by the autonomic nervous system. Some salivary glands secrete spontaneously, even in the absence of extraneous stimuli, and in those the nerves increase the salivary flow rate. In most of the glands, however, there is no secretion under physiological conditions unless nerves excite the glands. The various effector cells of the glands, the smooth muscles of the blood vessels, the myoepithelial cells and the different secretory cells of acini and ducts engaged in the elaboration of the saliva receive autonomic nerves. Often both divisions of the autonomic nervous system are represented, but it should be emphasized that there are considerable variations among species and also between the different glands of the same species. The two systems act antagonistically only in the case of those parts of the vascular bed which are supplied not only with sympathetic but also with parasympathetic fibers. In secretory and myoepithelial cells both sets of nerves seem to have an excitatory function, cooperating in the production and discharge of saliva. The function of sympathetic innervation, which except in the case of vasoconstriction has been far from clear, becomes more obvious when studied in experiments where the para-sympathetic nerves are activated. In most glands, for instance, sympathetic stimula-tion causes very little secretion of fluid, in some none at all, but the effect usually be-comes marked when a slow background secretion is elicited by stimulation of the parasympathetic nerve. The pronounced effect of sympathetic impulses on the secretion of proteins in acini and ducts is easier to detect when fluid for the transport of the products is provided via the parasympathetic nervous system. In addition, the sympathetic system supplies motor nerves for the myoepithelial cells; these seem to lack inhibitory nerves. The physiological role played by sympathetic and parasym-pathetic nerves in modulating the ionic composition of the saliva passing the ducts remains to be discovered.

This article is based on a lecture dedicated to the memory of Professor L. H. Schneyer, who had been invited to take part in this conference but died October 23, 1976. Through Leon Schneyer's work over the years much fundamental knowledge of the secretory process and of the innervation of salivary glands had been gained. During his last year he was engaged in experiments in a new and fascinating field, concerning the regulatory effects of the autonomic nerves on the transport of ions in the salivary ducts, and his publication "Parasympathetic control of Na, K transport in perfused submaxillary duct of the rat" appeared in 1977 in the July issue of the *American Journal of Physiology*. His death meant a great loss to physiology and to those who had the privilege of being his friends.

REFERENCES

1 Babkin, B. P., *Secretory Mechanism of the Digestive Glands*, 2nd Ed., Hoeber, New York, 1950.
2 Bernard, C., De l'influence de deux ordres de nerfs qui déterminent les variations de couleur du sang veineux dans les organes glandulaires, *Compt. Rend.*, 47 (1858) 245–253.

3 Bennett, H., Hodgson, C. and Speirs, R. L., The influence of preganglionic cervical sympathectomy on the amylase concentration of reflexly produced parotid saliva in the rat, *J. Physiol.* (Lond.), 242 (1974) 145–147 P.

4 Cannon, W. B. and Rosenblueth, A., *The Supersensitivity of Denervated Structures*, Macmillan, New York, 1949.

5 Delfs, U. and Emmelin, N., Degeneration secretion of saliva in the rat following sympathectomy, *J. Physiol.* (Lond.), 239 (1974) 623–630.

6 Drenckhahn, D., Gröschel-Stewart, U. and Unsicker, K., Immunofluorescence-microscopic demonstration of myosin and actin in salivary glands and exocrine pancreas of the rat, *Cell Tiss. Research*, 183 (1977) 273–279.

7 Eckhard, C., Der Sympathicus in seiner Stellung zur Secretion in der Parotis des Schafes. In: C. Eckhard, *Beiträge zur Anatomie und Physiologie* IV, 1869, pp. 52–68.

8 Ekström, J. and Emmelin, N., The functional organization of the parasympathetic secretory innervation of the submandibular gland, *J. Physiol.* (Lond.), 213 (1971) 727–740.

9 Ekström, J. and Emmelin, N., The secretory innervation of the parotid gland of the cat: An unexpected component, *Q. J. exp. Physiol.*, 59 (1974) 11–17.

10 Emmelin, N., Action of transmitters on the responsiveness of effector cells, *Experientia*, 21 (1965) 57–65.

11 Emmelin, N., Nervous control of salivary glands. In: *Handbook of Physiology*, Section 6, Alimentary Canal II, American Physiological Society, Washington, D. C., 1967, pp. 595–632.

12 Emmelin, N., Garrett, J. R. and Ohlin, P., Neural control of salivary myoepithelial cells, *J. Physiol.* (Lond.), 196 (1968) 381–396.

13 Emmelin, N., Garrett, J. R. and Gjörstrup, P., Supporting effects of myoepithelial cells in submandibular glands of dogs when acting against increased intraluminal pressure, *J. Physiol.* (Lond.), 268 (1977) 73–85.

14 Emmelin, N. and Gjörstrup, P., The physiology of salivary myoepithelial cells. In: N. A. Thorn and O. H. Petersen (Eds.), *Secretory Mechanisms of Exocrine Glands*. Alfred Benzon Symp. VII, Munksgaard, Copenhagen, 1974, pp. 29–41.

15 Emmelin, N. and Gjörstrup, P., Secretory responses to sympathetic stimulation of the cat's salivary glands in a state of resting secretion, *Q. J. exp. Physiol.*, 60 (1975) 325–332.

16 Emmelin, N. and Gjörstrup, P., Interaction between sympathetic and parasympathetic salivary nerves in anaesthetized dogs, *Archs. Oral Biol.*, 21 (1976) 27–32.

17 Emmelin, N., Gjörstrup, P. and Thesleff, P., On the existence of parasympathetic motor nerves to the submaxillary gland of the dog, *Q. J. exp. Physiol.*, 62 (1977) 27–40.

18 Emmelin, N. and Henriksson, K. G., Depressor activity of saliva after section of the chorda tympani, *Acta physiol. scand.*, 30, Supp. 111 (1953) 75–82.

19 Emmelin, N. and Thulin, A., Action of drugs on denervated myoepithelial cells of salivary glands, *Br. J. Pharmac. Chemother.*, 48 (1973) 73–79.

20 Emmelin, N. and Trendelenburg, U., Degeneration activity after parasympathetic or sympathetic denervation, *Ergebn. Physiol.*, 66 (1972) 147–211.

21 Fleming, A. J. and MacIntosh, F. C., The effect of sympathetic stimulation and of autonomic drugs on the paralytic submaxillary gland of the cat, *Q. J. exp. Physiol.*, 25 (1935) 207–212.

22 Garrett, J. R., *Innervation of Salivary Glands*. (Thesis), London University, London, 1965, pp. 1–170.

23 Garrett, J. R., The autonomic innervation of rabbit salivary glands studied electron microscopically after 5-hydroxydopamine administration, *Cell Tiss. Research*, 178 (1977) 551–562.

24 Garrett, J. R., Harrop, T. J., Kidd, A. and Thulin, A., Nerve-induced secretory changes in salivary glands. In: F. P. Brooks and P. W. Evers (Eds.), *Nerves and the Gut*, C. B. Slack, Thorofare, 1977, pp. 14–39.

25 Garrett, J. R. and Holmberg, J., Effects of surgical denervations on the autonomic nerves in parotid glands of dogs, *Z. Zellforsch.*, 131 (1972) 451–462.

26 Garrett, J. R. and Kidd, A., Effects of secretory nerve stimulation on acid phosphatase and peroxidase in submandibular saliva and acini in cats, *Histochem. J.*, 9 (1977) 435–451.

27 Gautvik, K., *Studies on Vasodilator Mechanisms in the Submandibular Salivary Gland in Cats*. (Thesis), Universitetsforlaget, Oslo, 1970.

28 Gjörstrup, P., Effects of sympathetic nerve stimulation in the presence of a slow parasympathetic secretion in the parotid and submaxillary glands of the rabbit, *Acta physiol. scand.*, 101 (1977) 211–218.

29 Gjörstrup, P., Salivary amylase secretion when stimulating the sympathetic nerves during slow parasympathetic secretion, *J. Physiol.* (Lond.), 282 (1978) 10 P.

30 Hammer, M. G. and Sheridan, J. D., Electrical coupling and dye transfer between acinar cells in rat salivary glands, *J. Physiol.* (Lond.), 275 (1978) 495–505.

31 Hilton, S. M. and Lewis, G. P., The cause of the vasodilatation accompanying activity in the submandibular salivary gland, *J. Physiol.* (Lond), 128 (1955) 235–248.

32 Hurley, H. J. and Shelley, W. B., The role of the myoepithelium in the human apocrine sweat gland, *J. invest. Derm.*, 22 (1954) 143–155.

33 Karpinski, E., Barton, S. and Schachter, M., Vasodilator nerve fibres to the submaxillary gland of the cat, *Nature* (Lond.), 232 (1971) 122–124.

34 Krause, W., Ueber die Drüsennerven, *Z. Rat. Med.*, 23 (1865) 46–62.

35 Langley, J. N., The salivary glands. In: E. A. Schäfer (Ed.) *Textbook of Physiology*, Vol. 1, Pentland, Edinburgh, 1898, pp. 475–530.

36 Lichtman, J. W., The reorganization of synaptic connexions in the rat submandibular ganglion during post-natal development, *J. Physiol.* (Lond.), 273 (1977) 155–177.

37 Linzell, J. L., Some observations on the contractile tissue of the mammary glands, *J. Physiol.* (Lond.), 130 (1955) 257–267.

38 Ludwig, C., Neue Versuche über die Beihülfe der Nerven zu der Speichelsekretion, *Mittheilungen der naturforschenden Gesellschaft in Zürich*, 53–54 (1850) 210–239.

39 Lundberg, A., Electrophysiology of salivary glands, *Physiol. Rev.*, 38 (1958) 21–40.

40 Mathews, A., The physiology of secretion, *Ann. N. Y. Acad. Sci.*, 11 (1898) 293–368.

41 Nordenfelt, I. and Ohlin, P., Supersensitivity of salivary glands of rabbits, *Acta physiol. scand.*, 41 (1957) 12–17.

42 Ohlin, P., *Nervous and Hormonal Control of Salivary Glands in Rats*. (Thesis). *Acta Univ. Lund.* Sectio II, No. 7, 1966, pp. 1–21.

43 Ohlin, P., Sympathetic secretory innervation of the rat's submaxillary gland, *Q. J. exp. Physiol.*, 53 (1968) 19–22.

44 Petersen, O. H., Stimulus-secretion coupling of salivary acinar cells: The role of membrane permeability change, Ca^{2+} and cyclic AMP. In: R. M. Case and H. Goebell (Eds.), *Stimulus-Secretion Coupling in the Gastrointestinal Tract*, MTP Press Ltd., Lancester, 1976, pp. 281–302.

45 Schachter, M., Barton, S., Uddin, M., Karpinski, E. and Sanders, E. J., Effect of nerve stimulation, denervation, and duct ligation on kallikrein content and duct cell granules of the cat's submandibular gland, *Experientia*, 33 (1977) 746–748.

46 Schneyer, C. A., Role of sympathetic pathway in secretory activity induced in rat parotid by feeding, *Proc. Soc. exp. Biol. Med.*, 147 (1974) 314–317.

47 Schneyer, L. H., Sympathetic control of Na, K transport in perfused submaxillary main duct of rat, *Amer. J. Physiol.*, 230 (1976) 341–345.

48 Schneyer, L. H., Parasympathetic control of Na, K transport in perfused submaxillary duct of the rat, *Amer. J. Physiol.*, 233 (1977) F22–F28.

49 Schneyer, L. H., Young, J. A. and Schneyer, C. A., Salivary secretion of electrolytes, *Physiol. Rev.*, 52 (1972) 720–777.

50 Schramm, M. and Selinger, Z., Neurotransmitters, receptors, second messengers and responses in parotid gland and pancreas. In: R. M. Case and H. Goebell (Eds.), *Stimulus-Secretion Coupling in the Gastrointestinal Tract*, MTP Press Ltd., Lancester, 1976, pp. 49–64.

51 Smaje, L. H., Spontaneous secretion in the rabbit submaxillary gland. In: N. A. Thorn and O. H. Petersen (Eds.), *Secretory Mechanisms of Exocrine Glands*. Alfred Benzon Symp. VII, Munksgaard, Copenhagen, 1974, pp. 608–625.

52 Templeton, D. and Thulin, A., Secretory, motor and vascular effects in the sublingual gland of the rat caused by autonomic nerve stimulation, *Q. J. exp. Physiol.*, 63 (1978) 59–66.

53 Thesleff, P., Emmelin, N. and Grampp, W., Secretory potentials evoked by sympathetic stimulation of the parotid gland of cat, *Acta physiol. scand.*, 102 (1978) 16–17A.

54 Unna, P. G., Zur Theorie der Drüsensecretion, insbesondere des Speichels, *Centralblatt med. Wissenschaften*, XIX (1881) 257–263.

55 Wojcik, J. D., Grand, R. J. and Kimberg, D. V., Amylase secretion by rabbit parotid gland. Role of cyclic AMP and GMP, *Biochim. Biophys. Acta*, 411 (1975) 250–262.

In Memory of
LEON H. SCHNEYER
1919–1976

Leon H. Schneyer (1919–1976), a graduate of New York University's Dental School (1943), continued his studies at New York University in the field of enzyme physiology and soon became interested in the salivary gland. His first paper, published in 1951, dealt with the effect of temperature on salivary amylase activity. He next determined the effects of various agents, radioactive compounds in particular, on this enzyme and the glands themselves. In 1955 he devised a method for separate collection of submaxillary and sublingual salivas in humans. From then on his interests in the salivary glands and their secretions became very general; 97 of the 102 papers he published dealt with some aspect of their function. He studied flow, composition, electrolyte secretion, synthesis of proteins by the gland, salivary secretion in sleep, membrane and secretory potentials, factors influencing gland activity and the comparative physiology of different types of glands in humans and other species. He invented a means of collecting saliva from rats and did much of his work on that species. In 1968 he began to study the functions of salivary ducts and in that year published a paper on the secretory processes in the perfused excretory duct of the rat submaxillary gland. It was Dr. Schneyer's interest in the sympathetic and parasympathetic control of ion transport in salivary ducts which led us to invite him to participate in this study of autonomic system function and interaction of sympathetic and parasympathetic nerves in the control of tissues. Two of his papers were particularly appropriate to our interests: "Sympathetic control of Na, K transport in perfused submaxillary main duct of rat" (*Amer. J. Physiol.*, 230 (1976) 341–345) and "Parasympathetic control of Na, K transport in perfused submaxillary duct of the rat" (*Amer. J. Physiol.*, 233 (1977) F22–28).

We greatly regret that we were deprived of the privilege of meeting Leon Schneyer, hearing his discussion of our theme and expressing personally our respect for his contributions. The following paper submitted by his wife and associate does contain a summary of his recent thoughts. We thank Mrs. Charlotte Alper Schneyer for her generosity in preparing it for us.

Editors

CHAPTER 2

PARASYMPATHETIC AND SYMPATHETIC CONTROL OF DUCTAL TRANSPORT OF ELECTROLYTES AND OF SALIVARY GLAND DEVELOPMENT AND GROWTH

Leon H. Schneyer and Charlotte A. Schneyer

Department of Physiology and Biophysics, University of Alabama in Birmingham, Birmingham, Alabama, USA

INTRODUCTION

Secretory activity of salivary glands is generally elicited by stimulation of the autonomic pathways to these organs. While both parasympathetic and sympathetic innervation of the glands cause secretion, it is the parasympathetic that is responsible for elaboration of copious quantities of a watery fluid and it is therefore considered to be the physiologically important pathway controlling saliva production[3,4]. Recently, however, an important role of the sympathetic pathway in regulating release of intrinsic proteins (such as amylase and glycoproteins) has been uncovered[2,14,36]. The fact that sympathetic secretomotor nerves are not ubiquitous, however, also indicates that this branch is generally less important.

The glands themselves are morphologically heterogeneous, and the secretory unit itself (the salivon) is composed of a number of morphologically and physiologically distinct cellular elements, with the whole gland being a mosaic of secretory units. The secretory unit consists of acinar cells proximally and a ductal complex distally[4]. The presence of vascular elements as well as myoepithelial cells contributes to the general complexity of the gland, especially since the neural regulation of the diverse units has until recently been very controversial[3].

The final fluid produced by this complex array of parts is in fact greatly influenced by the mode of autonomic stimulation used to evoke the secretion and the characteristics of parasympathetically-evoked saliva are very different from those of sympathetically-evoked saliva. For example, parasympathetic saliva is lower in organic content and content of certain inorganic ions than that of sympathetically-evoked saliva[30].

Much has been written about the control of salivary flow and composition, the effects of drugs, the actions of cholinergic and adrenergic transmitters as well as α and β receptors of these glands[4,12,13,30,34,36]. Our commission, however, is to deal with ion transport, function of the duct system and factors affecting the growth or development of these glands. We will begin by reviewing some facts concerning control of the ion content of saliva.

DUCTAL TRANSPORT

Several ions (K, Ca, HCO_3) are usually present in higher concentration in sympathetically-evoked saliva than they are in parasympathetically-evoked saliva. However, with rat parotid it was found that calcium concentration of saliva evoked by stimulation of the auriculotemporal nerve was very high (about 11 mEq/1), and even higher than levels found in saliva evoked by stimulation of the sympathetic nerve (10 mEq/1)[21] (Fig. 1). Furthermore, while amylase and calcium have been described as being packaged and secreted together (from observations in *in vitro* parotid slices where epinephrine was used to stimulate secretion)[1,35], this relationship does not appear under all conditions of stimulation, especially those involving direct stimulation of the nerves *in vivo*[21]. In fact, until recently the relationship between secretion of calcium and secretion of amylase had not been examined under *in vivo* conditions, and especially not under conditions of direct stimulation of the innervation to the gland. It was shown for example that when stimulation of the sympathetic innervation to rat parotid was employed, concentrations of amylase and calcium in the evoked saliva were initially high, with Ca^{++} at about 10 mEq/1 and amylase at 600 mg/mg. The course

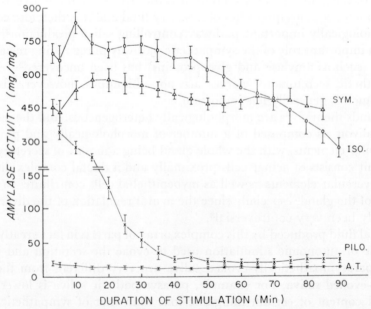

Fig. 1.   Changes in calcium concentration of parotid saliva during prolonged stimulation by various modes: ISO., isoproterenol; SYM., sympathetic nerve; A. T., auriculotemporal nerve; PILO., pilocarpine. Duration of stimulation, on the abscissa, denotes the duration of the period which followed after stimulation was started. (Taken from reference 21.)

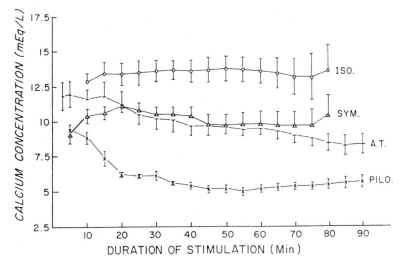

Fig. 2.　Time course of change in amylase activity of parotid saliva in response to various modes of stimulation (ISO., isoproterenol; SYM., sympathetic nerve; PILO., pilocarpine; A. T., auriculotemporal nerve). Duration of stimulation, on the abscissa, denotes the duration of the period which followed after stimulation started. (Taken from reference 21.)

of secretion of these two moieties with time proceeds in parallel for at least 60 minutes of stimulation[21] (Figs. 1 and 2).

With stimulation of the parasympathetic innervation to the gland, Ca^{++} concentration was not only higher than that in the sympathetically-evoked saliva, but amylase was only about one-twentieth to one-fortieth that of sympathetic levels, and remained at the same low level (about 20 mg/mg) throughout the period of stimulation. Ca^{++} concentration decreased about 30% during this interval and the non-parallel nature of these events was striking[21] (Figs. 1 and 2).

K is another ion which is present in saliva in very high concentrations when sympathetic stimulation is used to evoke secretion, but regardless of the mode of stimulation used, it is always unusually high. When high doses of isoproterenol are used, [K] can reach intracellular levels of 150 mEq/1, but even with cholinergic nerve stimulation, it can be as high as 40–60 mEq/1. These concentrations are generally uniformly observed at all flow rates.

In early attempts to discover the source of this high [K], and to understand the mechanisms underlying its secretion, the role of acinar cells in production of the saliva with its high concentration of K was examined[27]. One approach to delineation of transport activity at the acinar level was study of the transmembrane potentials of acinar cells. It was shown, e.g., that although acinar cells of rat submaxillary gland develop postnatally from precursor cells of the terminal tubules, resting membrane potentials of terminal tubules and of acinar cells are similar (approximately 20 mV, inside of cell is negative)[29]. Hence, even at an early stage in gland development, the most proximal secretory elements (terminal tubule or acinar cell) show characteristic and similar functional attributes, including an identical transmembrane potential[29,32]. It appears that more than one ionic shift occurs across the cell membranes of rat acinar cells during secretion, and that the form of the potential depends on the algebraic balance of ionic movements at any particular time.

Effects of stimulation on ion movements were also investigated using slice preparations from rat submaxillary gland[28]. It was established, e.g., that in slices from whole submaxillary gland, there was an active transport of potassium into cells. Stimulation *in vitro* by pilocarpine caused a reduction in net accumulation of K; this was assumed to be due to an increased permeability of cells (mainly acinar) to potassium. Such an increase in permeability appears to be an important factor in mediating release of K, a distinguishing early ("transient") phase of secretion after start of stimulation.

The main impetus, however, to understanding mechanisms of salivary secretion came with the introduction of methods whereby transport capabilities of specific glandular units could be determined; these included micropuncture and microperfusion techniques. From analysis of fluid (so-called precursor fluid) obtained from the acinar-intercalated duct complex, it was found that the electrolyte composition from the most proximal unit of the gland resembled that of an ultrafiltrate of plasma[9]. Micropuncture studies of the more distal ducts revealed modifications in Na and K content and ratios so that the composition of the fluid no longer resembled that of the precursor fluid. These observations, when combined with microperfusion studies of the luminally-perfused main duct of submaxillary gland modified current thinking concerning mechanisms of salivary secretion and established the sites where electrolyte transport occurs[9,11]. Figure 3 is a diagram of how an isolated duct is perfused; this is an especially useful technique since it permits measurement of the transport capabili-

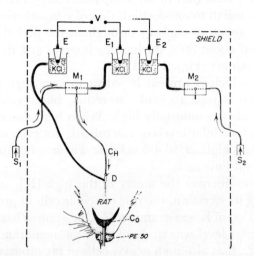

Fig. 3.   Experimental system: Rat submaxillary main excretory duct, perfused through its lumen. Perfusion medium is pumped from a syringe (S) to a manifold (M), and then through a hilar cannula (C_H) to the lumen of the duct (D) and oral cannula (C_O), into collecting tubing (PE 50). Transductal PD is recorded by voltmeter (V) from calomel electrodes (E) in electrical contact with the duct surfaces. (Taken from reference 22.)

ties of ductal elements in a gland. It was found that, in the main perfused duct, Na absorption and K secretion occur to a significant degree[38]. Vascular supply to the perfused segment of the excretory duct was examined and found to be adequate even after insertion of a perfusion catheter[11,22,31]. When net fluxes of Na, K and Cl and transductal potential were measured in the luminally-perfused excretory duct, they were found to be stable for at least five hours. Thus mechanisms of Na and K transport by ductal cells were determined, and the active transfer of Na out and of K into the duct lumen was demonstrated [22,23,38]. This recent work permits a more complete view of how saliva is elaborated. It is apparent that the mode of stimulation affects the final composition of saliva[27,37], but the composition of the precursor fluid (that obtained by micropuncture from acinar-intercalated duct regions) is independent of what stimuli act upon the glands[39]. The rate of precursor fluid production, however, is not independent of the mode of stimulation. The volume produced by parasympathetic stimulation is eight times that produced by sympathetic stimulation[9,39]. According to the modified view, elaboration of saliva occurs as a two-step process: The first step involves an active process whereby ions are secreted and water follows to form a "precursor fluid" at the acinar-intercalated duct level. There is little reabsorption or additional secretion of water by more distal elements of the gland. In the second stage, the primary fluid, with concentrations of Na, K and Cl very similar to those of serum, is delivered to the duct system of the gland where sodium is reabsorbed by a mechanism having a maximum transport capacity, the rate of which is uninfluenced by gland stimulation. Thus, with increasing gland stimulation, increasing loads of Na-rich primary secretion are delivered to the Tm-limited ductal reabsorptive mechanism with the result that saliva collected at low flow rates would be relatively Na-free, whereas with increased flow rate, the reabsorptive mechanism becomes saturated and the salivary [Na] would rise[34].

Na and Cl reabsorption occur in the distal duct system. Additionally, K and HCO_3 are secreted. Because in the ducts reabsorption ordinarily occurs at a faster rate than secretion, and because ductal permeability to water is low, final saliva is hypotonic[34].

Secretion of potassium by ductal epithelial cells is of particular interest since potassium is often the predominant ion of saliva. Active processes are involved in the secretion of K in the main duct, and the active transport is probably located at the contraluminal surface[23]; however, even at the luminal border transfer of K is evidently mainly carrier-mediated[23,34]. Secretion of K does not ordinarily generate any significant PD; hence transport across the luminal membrane probably occurs in conjunction with transport of another ion. Sodium and hydrogen ion have been suggested as two possibilities[22,38]. Using amiloride at the luminal surface, it has been shown[24] that changes in uni-directional movements of Na and K are consistent with carrier-mediated exchange of Na and K at the luminal border. This work indicates that secretion of K is not tightly, or completely, linked to absorption of sodium in the salivary duct system and may involve paired transport with a different ion.

While ductal secretory events have been greatly clarified in recent years, the mechanism by which these events are regulated still requires elucidation. The initial work on autonomic regulation of electrolyte transport in the main duct was done with

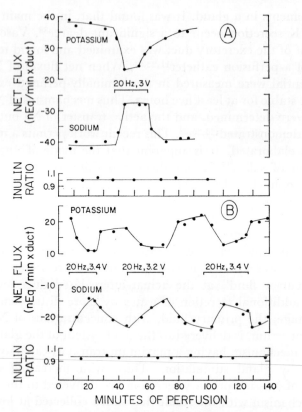

Fig. 4.   Changes in net fluxes of potassium and sodium, and inulin ratio in luminally-perfused
main excretory duct, during periods of electrical stimulation of cervical sympathetic
nerve (two representative experiments). Negative values for the net flux indicate
absorption from lumen; positive values indicate secretion into lumen. (Taken from
reference 25.)

drugs, rather than direct stimulation of the glandular innervation. In brief summary
of the findings[31,33,40] it can be said that the use of isoproterenol and other compounds
indicated the presence of β receptors in duct cells. It became more important, therefore, to determine the action of nerves on duct function. This was attempted using the
perfused duct technique and it was found that when the cervical sympathetic trunk
was stimulated during perfusion of the main duct segment with isotonic NaCl there
was a decrease in Na net flux from, and of K net flux to, the lumen[25]. Net flux of water
was unaffected. Transductal PD decreased by about 30% during supramaximal
stimulation of the sympathetic innervation. Changes in PD and net cation fluxes
were reversible upon cessation of stimulation. These points are supported by the type
of data in Figs. 4 and 5. Inhibition of Na and K fluxes was apparent immediately after
3.5 minutes of supramaximal stimulation of the cervical sympathetic nerve trunk
and reached a peak by six–20 minutes. This inhibition was sustained during the entire
period of stimulation and was rapidly reversed with cessation of stimulation. When
steady values were reached, the magnitude of the inhibition of net flux was between

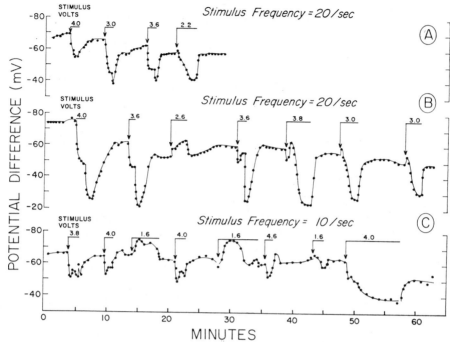

Fig. 5.   Changes in transductal PD of perfused main excretory duct, in response to stimulation of cervical sympathetic nerve trunk (three representative experiments). Start of stimulation is denoted by head of each arrow, while duration of stimulation is given by length of its horizontal limb. Sign of potential is with regard to interstitial side. (Taken from reference 25.)

30–40% for both Na and K (Figs. 4 and 5). The inulin ratio, however, was unchanged during stimulation, indicating that transductal net movement of water, which was small in control rats, was not affected by stimulation of the sympathetic nerve.

There was also a rapid decrease in transductal PD with stimulation of the sympathetic innervation. The decrease appeared rapidly, reached its maximum within two to four min, and remained near this maximum for as long as stimulation continued. The magnitude of the maximal decrease was 17.6 ± 1.9 mV. This represented about a 30% change from the unstimulated control level. The PD rose upon cessation of stimulation, usually to the pre-stimulation level (Fig. 5).

Both α and β adrenergic antagonists phenoxybenzamine and propranolol were administered but only phenoxybenzamine gave consistent results. A decrease in mean transductal PD was observed if phenoxybenzamine was administered prior to stimulation of the sympathetic nerve[25]. Even though the difference was small (only about 6 mV), it was statistically significant ($P < 0.01$).

The effects on Na, K and PD caused by sympathetic nerve stimulation resembled those produced by administration of large doses of isoproterenol[34]. However, the mechanisms underlying these effects have so far not been delineated. They probably are not primarily related to accompanying vascular changes for two reasons. First, while vasoconstriction does result from stimulation of the glandular sympathetic inner-

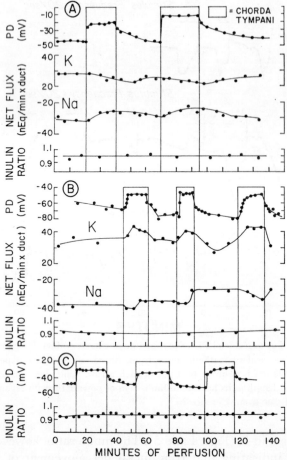

Fig. 6.　Changes in transductal net fluxes of K and Na, inulin ratio and PD during maximal stimulation of chorda tympani nerve in typical experiments. Negative sign for Na flux indicates absorption. Ducts were perfused throughout with isotonic medium containing (in mM) 140 Na, 4K, 124 CL, 20 HCO_3. A) Note that Na, K fluxes were increased slightly during stimulation, while in B) fluxes were slightly reduced. Flux changes were not significant. (Taken from reference 26.)

vation, its effect on secretory activity seems to require appreciable delay[25], whereas changes in transductal PD at least, occur very rapidly after the start of sympathetic stimulation. Second, the decrease in transductal PD which characteristically accompanies sympathetic, or sympathomimetic, stimulation has also been observed after addition of isoproterenol to ducts perfused *in vitro*[25,34] and in these conditions vascular changes could not greatly affect the cellular responses.

The evidence thus suggests that while β receptor activity can modify transport in the main duct (since isoproterenol affects this), α receptors are the important mediators of changes, at least in transductal PD, when the ducts are stimulated through their sympathetic innervation[25].

In contrast to these effects of sympathetic nerve stimulation, stimulation of the parasympathetic innervation affected transductal PD but not net flux of Na or K. The decrease in PD that occurred during perfusion of the submaxillary main duct when the chorda was stimulated appeared rapidly, was sustained for the entire period of stimulation (even as long as 20 min), and was immediately reversed when stimulation was halted (Figs. 5 and 6). The chorda-induced decrease in PD could be suppressed by i.p. administration of atropine during nerve stimulation but not by phenoxybenzamine and propranolol. Thus, the effects did not involve mediation by adrenergic nerves, either directly or by current spread.

Since a decrease in net flux of sodium has been reported with high doses of carbachol[8,40], and low concentrations of acetylcholine[10], and since Na conductance at the luminal membrane decreased, it was surprising that a change in net flux of sodium did not occur during chorda stimulation[26]. The possibility had to be considered that sodium flux from the lumen was actually reduced by chorda stimulation, and that net Na flux remained unchanged because of a similar reduction in backflux to the lumen. This possibility was tested by adding ^{22}Na to the luminal perfusion medium and measuring sodium flux from the lumen. It was found to be unchanged during chorda stimulation. Consequently, it seemed unlikely that a decrease in sodium conductance of the luminal membrane was important in mediating the change in PD observed during stimulation.

This matter was studied further and various possibilities were tested[26]. The results available at present provide evidence that parasympathetic cholinergic fibers innervate ductal epithelial cells and also clarify several inconsistencies between present findings with cholinergic nerve stimulation and earlier findings using cholinergic drugs. For example, the discrepancy between effects of chorda and carbachol stimulation *in vivo* on K, but not Na, transport may be spurious since the inhibitory effects of carbachol have not been observed with ducts perfused *in vitro*[8,40]. Field and Young[5] have suggested that the inhibitory effects observed *in vivo* with higher doses of carbachol are actually the indirect artifactual effects of sympathetic involvement.

Net transport of Na and K are unaffected but transductal PD is consistently reduced with chorda stimulation of the perfused duct, and the reduction is blocked by atropine. Since one-way flux of Na from the lumen was not changed during chorda stimulation, the effect of stimulation on PD is not likely due to changes at the luminal border of the ductal cells[26]. Studies of occurrences at the contraluminal border are required to elucidate these points further.

SALIVARY GLAND DEVELOPMENT

Another matter of interest to those concerned with autonomic system function is the effect of these nerves on the development and morphological state of the salivary glands. The structural integrity of these glands is definitely affected by autonomic nerve activity. In the absence of secretomotor activity over a prolonged period of time (one–three weeks), gland weights decrease and glandular elements (especially acini) are reduced in size[6,12,34]. Conversely, excessive autonomically-induced activity of the gland leads to an increase in size of the gland and constituent cells[12]. In each of these contrasting situations, the effects are neurally mediated through either branch of the innervation. However, it appears that, just as in elaboration of saliva, the parasympathetic innervation also has the principal role in mediation of structural changes in the gland[13]. The effects mentioned have usually been examined following surgical or chemical denervation, or introduction over an extended period of time of excessive amounts of neurotransmitter-like substances. More recently, the same effects have been examined under more physiological conditions. It has been shown that substitution of an all-liquid diet for the normal chow diet results in a decrease in the size of parotid gland and its acinar cells that is maximal (35–40% decrease)[7] within four days after the dietary substitution. Gland size of animals on liquid diet can be restored to normal by re-introduction of solid chow; a marked burst of mitosis (18–45 mitotic figures/ 1000 acinar cells in contrast to a normal level of .02–.05) is observed, and cell size returns to normal within two days. The increase in size of glands of rats on bulk diet is also accompanied by an increase in mitotic activity two days after introduction of bulk or solid diet, DNA increases, and cell size and RNA increase markedly[13]. In all of these conditions it appears that the change from one level of reflexly-mediated activity to a higher one results in increased size of the gland. Furthermore, mitotic increases always accompany these changes. In the absence of the parasympathetic innervation, the effects usually produced with liquid or bulk diet do not occur. These findings constitute evidence of a primary role of the parasympathetic innervation in regulation of mitotic activity as well as in salivary gland size[19]. Functional activity of the "atrophic" gland (i.e., animals on liquid diet) is also altered and amylase is decreased and salivary flow diminished. This is the case for both rats or humans[13].

The autonomic innervation to the glands also plays an important role in their postnatal development. At birth, salivary glands are incompletely developed, and growth and differentiation continue for at least six weeks postnatally. Changes can be divided into two periods, an early preweanling period that is characterized by marked proliferative activity, but by little change in size or degree of differentiation of acinar cells. After weaning, cell size and maturation change markedly and the mitotic rate drops precipitously[17]. The parotid of the immature gland also shows lack of functional differentiation, and electrolyte concentration, amylase concentration and volume of fluid elaborated by parotid of 16–21-day-old rats is markedly different from that of adults.

Morphologically, the postnatal development of salivary glands can be accelerated by administration of large doses of isoproterenol. Cell size is greatly increased within a few days, and by eight to nine days of age, a gland resembling that of an adult can be recognized morphologically. Functional changes in secretion of electrolytes are not seen but amylase levels are altered[12,20], and other biochemical changes accompany the size increase. The effects however are not permanent and are reversed upon cessation of drug administration.

These are rather drastic measures to employ, however; recently, it has been shown that deprivation of parasympathetically-mediated glandular activity (induced by surgical denervation) modifies the changes that usually accompany postnatal development. Size of acinar cells as well as number are reduced, with total DNA about one-half that of control litter mates. The effects of denervation are not conspicuous if the end point for observation of changes precedes weaning[16]. Increased neurally-mediated activity appears associated with the increase in masticatory activity provided by the change from milk to solid chow diet[18,19]. The sympathetic innervation exerts some role, especially on amylase development, but little on size and number of the cells[15].

SUMMARY

Use of the perfused rat submaxillary duct has permitted analysis of the duct's role in determining the composition of saliva, in particular ion transport and the effects of autonomic nerves thereon. With passage of precursor fluid from the acinar cells into the main duct, absorption of Na from and secretion of K into the ductal lumen occurs; the transductal potential is -70 mV. Isoproterenol and carbachol have been shown to reduce transductal potential (PD) and to inhibit Na and K fluxes. In very low doses isoproterenol increases Na absorption from the duct lumen. The duct receives both a sympathetic and parasympathetic innervation; stimulation of these nerves affects PD and ion fluxes. Sympathetic nerve action decreases Na absorption and increases K secretion (30–40% changes are produced). Parasympathetic nerve stimulation has no effect on ion fluxes but reduced PD by 30%. These effects are in addition to nerve control of amylase and calcium secretion. With sympathetic nerve stimulation there is a parallelism in effect on amylase and calcium. Autonomic nerves, the parasympathetic in particular, can affect the development and hypertrophy of the salivary glands. Denervation causes regression.

Leon H. Schneyer held the National Institute of Health Research Career Award (5-KO6-DE 3341) until his death.

REFERENCES

1   Batzri, S. and Selinger, Z., Enzyme secretion mediated by the epinephrine β-receptor in rat parotid slices, *J. Biol. Chem.*, 248 (1973) 356–360.
2   Dische, Z., Kahn, N., Rotheschild, C., Danilchenko, A., Licking, J. and Wang, S. C., Glycoproteins of submaxillary saliva of the cat: Differences in composition produced by sympathetic and parasympathetic nerve stimulation, *J. Neurochem.*, 17 (1970) 649–658.
3   Emmelin, N. and Gjorstrup, P., The physiology of salivary myoepithelial cells. In: N. A. Thorn and O. H. Petersen (Eds.), *Secretory Mechanisms of Exocrine Glands*, Munksgaard, Copenhagen, 1974, pp. 29–41.
4   Emmelin, N., Schneyer, C. A. and Schneyer, L. H., The Pharmacology of salivary secretion. In: P. Holton (Ed.), *Pharmacology of Gastro-intestinal Motility and Secretion. International Encyclopedia of Pharmacology and Therapeutics*, Vol. 1, Sect. 39A, Pergamon, Oxford, 1973, pp. 1–39.
5   Field, M. J. and Young, J. A., Kinetics of Na transport in the rat submaxillary main duct perfused *in vitro*, *Pflügers Arch.*, 345 (1973) 207–220.
6   Garrett, J. R. and Thulin, A., Changes in parotid acinar cells accompanying salivary secretion in rats on sympathetic or parasympathetic nerve stimulation, *Cell Tiss. Res.*, 159 (1975) 179–193.
7   Hall, H. D. and Schneyer, C. A., Salivary gland atrophy in rat induced by liquid diet, *Proc. Soc. exp. Biol. Med.*, 117 (1964) 789–793.
8   Martin, C. J., Fromter, E., Gebler, B., Knauf, H. and Young, J. A., The effects of

carbachol on water and electrolyte fluxes and transepithelial potential differences of the rabbit submaxillary main duct perfused *in vitro*, *Pflügers Arch.*, 341 (1973) 131–142.

9 Martin, C. J. and Young, J. A., Electrolyte concentrations in primary and final saliva of the rat sublingual gland studied by micropuncture and catheterization techniques, *Pflügers Arch.*, 324 (1971) 344–360.

10 Martin, C. J. and Young, J. A., A microperfusion investigation of the effects of a sympathomimetic and parasympathomimetic drug on water and electrolyte fluxes in the main duct of the rat submixillary gland, *Pflügers Arch.*, 327 (1971) 303–323.

11 Martinez, J. R., Holzgreve, H. and Frick, A., Micropuncture study of submaxillary glands of adult rats, *Pflügers Arch.*, 290 (1966) 124–133.

12 Schneyer, C. A., Regulation of salivary gland growth. In: R. Goss (Ed.), *Regulation of Organ and Tissue Growth*, Academic Press, N. Y., 1972, pp. 211–232.

13 Schneyer, C. A., Autonomic regulation of secretory activity and growth responses of rat parotid gland. In: N. A. Thorn and O. H. Petersen (Eds.), *Secretory Mechanisms of Exocrine Glands*, Munksgaard, Copenhagen, 1974a, pp. 42–67.

14 Schneyer, C. A., Role of sympathetic pathway in secretory activity induced in rat parotid by feeding, *Proc. Soc. exp. Biol. Med.*, 147 (1974b) 314–317.

15 Schneyer, C. A. and Hall, H. D., Effects of denervation on development of function and structure of immature rat parotid, *Amer. J. Physiol.*, 212 (1967) 871–876.

16 Schneyer, C. A. and Hall, H. D., Time course and autonomic regulation of development of secretory function of rat parotid, *Amer. J. Physiol.*, 214 (1968) 808–813.

17 Schneyer, C. A. and Hall, H. D., Growth pattern of postnatally developing rat parotid gland, *Proc. Soc. exp. Biol. Med.*, 130 (1969) 603–607.

18 Schneyer, C. A. and Hall, H. D., Autonomic regulation of postnatal changes in cell number and size of rat parotid, *Amer. J. Physiol.*, 219 (1970) 1268–1272.

19 Schneyer, C. A. and Hall, H. D. Parasympathetic regulation of mitosis induced in rat parotid by dietary change, *Amer. J. Physiol.*, 229 (1975) 1614–1617.

20 Schneyer, C. A. and Shackleford, J. M., Accelerated development of salivary glands of early postnatal rats following isoproterenol, *Proc. Soc. exp. Biol. Med.*, 112 (1963) 320–324.

21 Schneyer, C. A., Sucanthapree, C. and Schneyer, L. H., Neural regulation of calcium and amylase of rat parotid saliva, *Proc. Soc. exp. Biol. Med.*, 156 (1977) 132–135.

22 Schneyer, L. H., Secretory processes in perfused excretory duct of rat submaxillary gland, *Amer. J. Physiol.*, 215 (1968) 664–670.

23 Schneyer, L. H., Secretion of potassium by perfused excretory duct of rat submaxillary gland, *Amer. J. Physiol.*, 217 (1969) 1324–1329.

24 Schneyer, L. H., Amiloride inhibition of ion transport in perfused excretory duct of rat submaxillary gland, *Amer. J. Physiol.*, 219 (1970) 1050–1055.

25 Schneyer, L. H., Sympathetic control of Na, K transport in perfused submaxillary main duct of rat, *Amer. J. Physiol.*, 230 (1976) 341–345.

26 Schneyer, L. H., Parasympathetic control of Na, K transport in perfused submaxillary duct of the rat, *Amer. J. Physiol.*, 233 (1977) F22–F28.

27 Schneyer, L. H. and Emmelin, N., Salivary secretion. In: E. D. Jacobson and L. L. Shanbour (Eds.), *Gastrointestinal Physiology. MTP International Review of Science*, Vol. 4, Ser. 1, Butterworths, London, 1974, pp. 183–226.

28 Schneyer, L. H. and Schneyer, C. A., Effects of pilocarpine on exchange of K^{42} in slices of submaxillary gland, *Proc. Soc. exp. Biol. Med.*, 116 (1964) 813–817.

29 Schneyer, L. H. and Schneyer, C. A., Membrane potentials of salivary gland cells of rat, *Amer. J. Physiol.*, 209 (1965) 1304–1310.

30 Schneyer, L. H. and Schneyer, C. A., Inorganic composition of saliva. In: C. F. Code

(Ed.), *Handbook of Physiology. Alimentary Canal*, Vol. 2, Sect. 6, American Physiological Society, Washington, D. C., 1967, pp. 497–530.

31 Schneyer, L. H. and Schneyer, C. A., Responses of perfused main duct of rat submaxillary gland to pharmacological agents. In: N. Emmelin and Y. Zotterman (Eds.), *Oral Physiology*, Pergamon, Oxford, 1972, pp. 61–72.

32 Schneyer, L. H., Schneyer, C. A. and Yoshida, Y., Membrane potentials of developing cells in immature rat submaxillary gland, *Amer. J. Physiol.*, 215 (1968) 1146–1150.

33 Schneyer, L. H. and Thavornthon, T., Isoproterenol-induced stimulation of sodium absorption in perfused salivary duct, *Amer. J. Physiol.*, 224 (1973) 136–139.

34 Schneyer, L. H., Young, J. A. and Schneyer, C. A., Salivary secretion of electrolytes, *Physiol. Rev.*, 52 (1972) 720–777.

35 Schramm, M., Secretion of enzymes and other macromolecules, *Ann. Rev. Biochem.*, 36 (1967) 307–320.

36 Speirs, R. L. and Hodgson C., Control of amylase secretion in the rat parotid gland during feeding, *Arch. Oral Biol.*, 21 (1976) 539–544.

37 Yoshida, Y., Sprecher, R. L., Schneyer, C. A. and Schneyer, L. H., Role of β-receptors in sympathetic regulation of electrolytes in rat submaxillary saliva, *Proc. Soc. exp. Biol. Med.*, 126 (1967) 912–916.

38 Young, J. A., Fromter, E., Schogel, E. and Hamann, K. F., A micro-perfusion investigation of sodium resorption and potassium secretion by the main excretory duct of the rat submaxillary gland, *Pflügers Arch.*, 295 (1967) 157–172.

39 Young, J. A. and Martin, C. J., The effect of a sympatho- and a para-sympathomimetic drug on the electrolyte concentrations of primary and final saliva of the rat submaxillary gland, *Pflügers Arch.*, 327 (1971) 284–302.

40 Young, J. A., Martin, C. J., Asz, M. and Weber, F. D., A microperfusion investigation of bicarbonate secretion by the rat submaxillary gland. The action of a parasympathomimetic drug on electrolyte transport, *Pflügers Arch.*, 319 (1970) 185–199.

CHAPTER 3

NEURAL CONTROL OF GASTRIC MOTILITY
WITH SPECIAL REFERENCE TO
CUTANEO-GASTRIC REFLEXES

Y. Aihara*, H. Nakamura*, A. Sato* and A. Simpson**

*2nd Department of Physiology, Tokyo Metropolitan Institute of Gerontology, Tokyo, Japan, and
**Department of Physiology, Showa University, Tokyo, Japan

INTRODUCTION

The purpose of this chapter is to discuss the extrinsic innervation of the stomach, the nerve fiber types and the neural interconnections which are involved in reflex gastric motility responses to somatic afferent stimulation.

The stomach is essentially a sack made up of three layers of smooth muscle with a lining of secretory cells, and with intrinsic nerve plexuses lying between the layers. Anatomically it is divided into the cardiac region where food enters, and the fundus, corpus, antrum and pylorus in sequence from the proximal to the distal end. The stomach has three functions: it has a storage capacity, it secretes, and it mixes and propels its contents toward the pyloric sphincter. It is a rather ideal reservoir since it readily adapts to large volume with relatively slight pressure increase and yet just as readily contracts when the volume diminishes. From the parietal cells in the lining, it secretes HCl which activates the pepsinogen secreted from chief cells into pepsin to digest proteins. It also secretes small quantities of other enzymes to begin the digestion of other foods. Mucus is secreted from mucous neck cells to protect the inner wall, and other factors are secreted which are essential to digestion and absorption. Secretion is not the primary topic of this chapter so further discussion of this subject will be left to others[7]. As the third gastric function, the stomach churns and mixes the food, and propels it in appropriate quantities into the duodenum. This gastric motility is provided by the layers of smooth muscle: the internal oblique layer, the middle circular layer, and the external longitudinal layer.

Secretion and motility, being functions of secretory and smooth muscle cells, are subject to the inherent characteristics of these cells. In addition these functions are controlled by hormones produced both locally and remotely, and by an intrinsic and extrinsic innervation.

The intrinsic nervous system consists of the myenteric plexus (Auerbach's plexus) between the longitudinal and circular muscle layers and the submucous plexus

(Meisner's plexus) between the circular muscle layer and the mucosa. These intrinsic plexuses interact with cells in the stomach wall, with each other[40] and with the extrinsic nerves.

The extrinsic innervation, which will be discussed in detail, consists of the sympathetic and parasympathetic systems. These two systems connect with the intrinsic gastric neurons to modulate stomach activity, and the sympathetic system also has some terminations on muscle and secretory cells to exert direct control. Each of the extrinsic systems includes both afferent and efferent nerves in their gastric branches[41].

Some afferent signals generated in the stomach are carried directly to the brain stem through the vagi. Some of these vagal afferents make interconnection with vagal motoneurons in the brain stem, and some ascend to the hypothalamus and to the limbic system directly or indirectly. Within the brain stem, there are probably synaptic connections to descending fibers within the spinal cord which could in turn influence the functioning of sympathetic preganglionic neurons. Because there has not yet been enough investigation, questions about the physiological significance of these known and possible connections still await answers in detail[37].

The second pathway for gastric afferent signals is through the gastric sympathetic nerves. A few synapses in this path occur at the celiac ganglion. These form the shortest possible reflex arcs, ganglionic reflexes. Most synapses occur after entrance of the splanchnic afferent nerves into the spinal cord through dorsal roots. Within the spinal cord some splanchnic afferent nerves interconnect with preganglionic splanchnic efferent nerves (gastro-gastric spinal reflexes), while others ascend to the brain stem or beyond (for example, to the somatosensory cortex) where they may in turn influence extrinsic neural gastric controls[37]. Gastric afferents which reach the level of the hypothalamus probably contribute to the sensations of satiation and hunger.

Vagal efferents include both excitatory and inhibitory fibers[41]. These efferent fibers synapse with the intrinsic neurons. How the excitatory and inhibitory efferent fibers synapse with intrinsic neurons to effect gastric smooth muscle, is not really understood in detail. Functions of the intrinsic neurons will be discussed by Wood. The excitatory transmitters are believed to be mostly cholinergic although a few noncholinergic agents have been reported. The nature of the inhibitory transmitters is unknown, but they are considered to be noncholinergic and nonadrenergic. Knowledge of transmitters has advanced rapidly, and discussion of that subject will also be left to others. In 1931 McSwiney[25] reported that excitatory fibers were more active when gastric tonus was low while high gastric tonus increased inhibitory effects. It has been shown histologically and neurophysiologically that the gastric vagal branch contains both myelinated and unmyelinated fibers[26]. It has been assumed since Martinson's experiment[24], that type and degree of motility are related to intensity of stimulation of the different fiber types. During weak stimulation of the vagus, excitation alone occurs; while inhibition also appears when the stimulation is more intense. This assumption has recently been substantiated by experiments which will be discussed in more detail in RESULTS in this chapter.

Splanchnic efferent nerve functions, like the vagal efferent functions, are both inhibitory and excitatory[41]. However, unlike the vagus, the splanchnic efferent nerves innervate the gastric muscle directly as well as through the intrinsic plexuses. As with the vagus, the nature of the contributions by the different splanchnic nerve fiber types has, until recently, been surmised but not proven. The proof, presented by Aihara et al.[1], will be discussed later.

The physiological significance and neural mechanisms of vagal and sympathetic efferent effects on gastric motility have been studied in detail by stimulation of various central regions and different visceral afferents. Central stimulation effects on gastric motility have been investigated, for example, for the following regions: limbic system[2,3,4,9,15,18,35,36]; thalamus[9]; hypothalamus[8,10,11,12,19,36] and medulla oblongata[10,33,34]. Viscero-gastric reactions have been reported for: gastric afferents[6]; intestinal afferents[38,39]; and rectum afferents[42].

Influence on gastrointestinal motility by somatic afferent stimuli has been reported for dogs[3,22,23], cats [14,16,17], monkeys[27] and for humans[13,29]. However, the neural control mechanisms of these somato-gastrointestinal motility reflexes were not analyzed in detail until recently when the neural mechanisms of cutaneo-visceral reflexes for gastric functions were investigated[30] as an extension of general neurophysiological studies of the somato-sympathetic reflex[32]. It was found that gastric motility could be affected by stimulation of the skin anywhere over the entire surface of the body of anesthetized rats. The nature of the response, whether facilitation or inhibition, was related to the stimulated area: Abdominal stimulation produced strong inhibition and paw stimulation produced facilitation[21]. The neural mechanisms of reflex facilitation and inhibition of gastric motility in response to skin stimulation have recently been analyzed[20].

RECENT RESULTS

All results reported in the remaining part of this chapter were obtained from chloralose-urethane anesthetized rats. Other conditions and techniques (respiration, blood pressure body temperature recording and maintenance, noxious mechanical stimulation of the skin by pinching, balloon method for measuring stomach pressure, recording evoked potentials and counting efferent sympathetic and vagal discharge activity, vagal and splanchnic preparation, stimulation) were as described by Sato et al.[30] and Aihara et al.[1].

Gastric Motility and Associated Nerve Fibers

Gastric motility changes and evoked mass potentials in response to electrical stimulation of autonomic nerves were investigated by Aihara et al. in 1978[1]. A representative example of the results of vagus stimulation is presented in Fig. 1. The insets in Fig. 1A are specimen records of gastric motility responses to 20 sec stimulation of the peripheral cut end of the left cervical vagus. Deviation limits of the dashed midlines shown in the insets were used to determine the magnitude of motility response change (facilitation, up; inhibition, down) from the prestimulus level. The upper record shows a transient small initial decrease followed by a large increase in gastric motility, while the lower record shows a small increase only. The graph in Fig. 1A shows the initial inhibition (open circles) and strong facilitation (filled circles) which were produced by stimulus intensities above 1.5 V at a frequency of 10 Hz. This initial inhibition increased with stimulus intensity to a maximum at about 3–4 V, and maximum facilita-

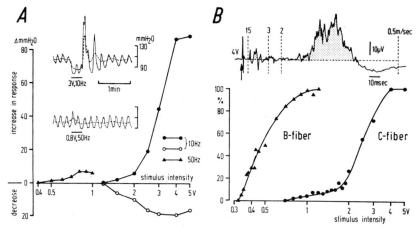

Fig. 1.   Vagus stimulation: effect on gastric motility, and evoked potentials. A: graph of facilitation in gastric motility (▲) by B fibers stimulated by 0.5 msec pulses at 50 Hz for 20 sec; facilitation (●) and inhibition (○) of C fibers stimulated by 0.5 msec pulses at 10 Hz for 20 sec. Abscissa: stimulus intensity in volts. Ordinate: increase (up) and decrease (down) of luminal pressure in mm H_2O (changes from prestimulus control value depicted by dashed midlines in inset recordings). Insets: specimen records of gastric motility responses. Stimulus parameters as shown. B: top, mass potentials evoked by single 0.5 msec stimulus pulses (4 V at arrow for this example), computer average of 16 sweeps. Conduction velocities indicated at top ends of vertical dashed lines. Nerve length, 71 mm. Shaded sectors show areas used to compute relative response magnitudes. Graph: B (▲) and C (●) fiber responses to stimulus intensity. Abscissa: stimulus intensity in volts. Ordinate: response magnitude in percent of maximum response (100%) of each fiber type. (Taken from ref. 1.)

tion was reached at intensities of about 4–5 V. Stimulation at 50 Hz (triangles) produced weak facilitation of gastric motility which increased with stimulus intensity from 0.5 V to 0.8 V, and then decreased slightly at 1.0 V. Prominent bradycardia and hypotension precluded use of stimulus intensities above 1.0 V at 50 Hz. Small initial facilitation instead of inhibition was observed during 20 sec stimulation in some cases. In all cases, marked facilitation was observed for 10–50 sec after termination of the stimulation.

Figure 1B, top, shows an example of evoked volleys recorded from the isolated gastric vagus branch after the data for Fig. 1A was obtained. The example shows evoked mass potentials of the B (15–3 m/sec) and C (2–0.5 m/sec) fibers produced by stimulating the left vagus with 4.0 V (arrow) at the cervical level. Fig. 1B bottom, is a graph of the relations between stimulus intensity (abscissa) and magnitude of evoked nerve volleys (ordinate) of the vagal B (triangles) and C (circles) fibers. The shaded areas under the curve (Fig. 1B, top) were used as a measure of the magnitude which is expressed as percentage of the maximum value of the B or C volley. Thresholds were 0.34 V for the B and 0.8 V for the C volleys. Maximum responses occurred at 1.0 V for the B and 4.0 V for the C volleys. The observations include efferent B and C, some afferent Aδ (30–12 m/sec) and afferent C potentials. Afferent Aα and β (120–30 m/sec) potentials are not discussed in this report.

Comparison of the graph of Fig. 1A with that of Fig. 1B indicates that the slight facilitation of gastric motility (Fig. 1A, lower inset) evoked by low intensity, 50 Hz stimulation of the vagus (such as 0.5–0.8 V in Fig. 1) was caused by excitation of B fibers only. High intensity, 10 Hz stimulation (such as 1.5–5 V in Fig. 1) elicited initial inhibition followed by strong facilitation (Fig. 1A, upper inset), probably due primarily to excitation of C fibers. After atropinization (0.5–1.0 mg/kg, i. v.), gastric inhibition became more dominant and the stimulus threshold decreased slightly to a value which was still within the range of C fiber excitation (1.5 V to 1.2 V). Thus, facilitatory and inhibitory effects must be acting simultaneously during stimulation of 20 sec. This investigation did not disclose whether the effect of vagal C fiber stimulation on gastric motility was due to orthodromic transmission from efferent fibers or antidromic signals from afferent C fibers.

Typical gastric motility resulting from splanchnic nerve stimulation is shown in Fig. 2. Four specimen records of inhibitory gastric motility responses to 20 sec stimulation of the splanchnic nerve, with the stimulus parameters indicated, are shown in Fig. 2A. Relations between stimulus intensity (abscissa) and magnitude of gastric motility response (ordinate) are summarized for 10 Hz (circles) and 50 Hz (triangles) in the graphs in Fig. 2A. Stimulation at 1 Hz was ineffective (not shown). As with the vagus, splanchnic nerve volleys shown in the specimen record in Fig. 2B were recorded after the motility measurements. Thresholds were 0.3 V for the B volleys and 0.6 V for the C volleys, and the respective maxima occurred at around 1.2 V and 4 V (Fig. 2B).

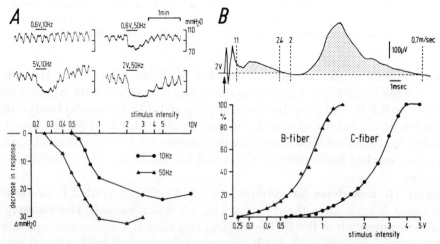

Fig. 2. Splanchnic nerve stimulation: effect on gastric motility and evoked potentials. A: top, specimen records of inhibition in gastric motility in response to 10 Hz (left) and 50 Hz (right) at voltage indicated, for 20 sec (time shown by overbar); bottom, graphs of motility inhibition by 0.5 msec pulses at 50 Hz (▲) and 10 Hz (●) applied for 20 sec. Abscissa: stimulus intensity in volts. Ordinate: decrease in luminal pressure from control level (change measured as described for Fig. 1A). B: top, mass potentials evoked by single 0.5 msec stimulus pulses (2 V at arrow for this example), computer average of 16 sweeps. Vertical dashed lines as in Fig. 1B. Nerve length, 12 mm. Graph: B and C fiber response to stimulus intensity. Other descriptions as for Fig. 1B. (Taken from ref. 1.)

The B fiber conduction velocities illustrated were 11–2.4 m/sec, and the C fiber conduction velocities were 2–0.7 m/sec. Reversal of the stimulating and recording electrodes did not change the results, so the volleys recorded were not transmitted across synapses.

Low accuracy over the short measurement path used in these experiments prevented consideration of signals having velocities faster than 15 m/sec, (sometimes 11 m/sec) which include Aα, β and δ afferent fibers. In all splanchnic nerve stimulation tests, the adrenal branch of the splanchnic nerve was crushed to eliminate humoral contributions to gastric motility changes.

Contrary to a previous report of facilitation of gastric motility by splanchnic nerve stimulation[5], such facilitation was not observed in these experiments. The inhibitory effect of 50 Hz stimulation of the B fibers (which C fibers cannot follow well) was greater than that of 10 Hz stimulation of both B and C fibers, and inhibition increase was only slight for 10 Hz stimulation above the C fiber threshold. This indicates that most of the motility-inhibiting efferents are B fibers.

Cutaneo-gastric Reflex

Relations between stimulation site and gastric motility reflex response to nociceptive skin stimulation were investigated by Kametani et al.[21]. When the pressure in an intragastric balloon was increased from 0 to about 100 mm H_2O by expanding the volume of the balloon with water, rhythmic contraction waves of five to six per min, corresponding to peristaltic movements, could be observed and continuously recorded. Figure 3A–F shows specimen records of gastric motility reflex responses elicited by pinching the various skin areas indicated in G for 20 sec. The responses in A, B, E and F represent reflex facilitation; Those in C and D represent reflex inhibition. The criteria for reflex facilitation was increased amplitude of gastric contraction and/or increased gastric tone; while reflex inhibition decreased in those measurements. Both reflex facilitation and inhibition of gastric motility began one to five sec after the onset of pinching, reached a maximum within 10–30 sec and returned to normal within an additional 20–60 sec.

Figure 3G and H summarizes the results of pinching different skin areas in rats for 20 sec every two to three min (a minimum of three times) and calculating the mean response magnitude which was measured as indicated in Fig. 3J. The response magnitudes, indicated by open circle (facilitation) and filled circle (inhibition) size, were expressed as percentages (Fig. 3K) of the maximum mean response elicited by each rat at one site. Pinching of the abdominal skin produced strong inhibition; pinching of the middle and caudal ventral and the dorsal thorax produced moderate or weak inhibition; pinching of the paws, nose, forearms and tail produced medium facilitation; and pinching of the face, ears, neck, legs and sacral area produced weak facilitation.

Experiments were performed by Kametani et al.[20] to determine the mechanisms of extrinsic gastric autonomic control of facilitation and inhibition of gastric motility when stimulating the skin. Based on the above results[21], the hind paw and abdomen were selected as representative sites for producing the gastric motility facilitation and inhibition to be investigated. In these experiments, care was taken to eliminate visible somatic motor reflexes and possible pressure accumulation which might be caused by secondary effects of skeletal muscle contractions when the abdomen or a hind paw

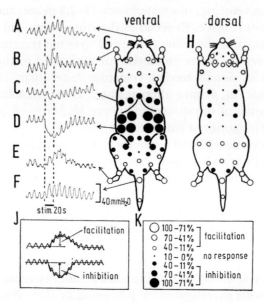

Fig. 3.   Effect on gastric motility of pinching various skin areas in rats. A–F: specimen
records of gastric motility. Bar and vertical dotted lines: 20 sec duration pinch.
Upward direction, gastric contraction; downward direction, gastric relaxation.
G and H: schematic diagrams relating skin areas pinched to reflex changes in gastric
motility. J: model illustrating method of estimating magnitude of reflex response.
Midline for each wave was drawn and maximum shift of this line from prestimulus
level was magnitude of reflex response. Largest mean absolute value in each rat
taken as 100%; all other mean reflex responses in same rat expressed as percent
of this value. K: open circles, facilitation; filled circles, inhibition; circle size, relative
magnitude. (Taken from ref. 21.)

was pinched. Gallamine (20 mg/kg), when used to eliminate skeletal muscle contraction, did not affect reflex inhibition of gastric motility caused by pinching abdominal
skin, or reflex amplitude produced by pinching a hind paw, but it did prolong onset
and peak latencies in the latter case. Thus, the reflex inhibition and facilitation of
gastric motility which were reported were substantially independent of skeletal muscle
contraction and relaxation.

Bilateral splanchnic section completely abolished reflex inhibition of gastric
motility caused by pinching the abdominal skin, but it did not abolish the reflex facilitation produced by pinching a hind paw. The results indicate that the splanchnic
nerves are essential for reflex inhibition of the gastric motility produced by pinching
the abdominal skin, but not for the reflex facilitation produced by pinching a hind paw.
The results also suggest that the gastric vagus nerves mediate the reflex facilitation of
gastric motility.

In order to verify vagal contributions to reflex gastric motility changes, reflex
changes before and after bilateral vagotomy at the cervical level were compared. In
the absence of vagal innervation, pinching the abdominal skin still produced significant reflex inhibition of gastric motility while pinching a hind paw produced occa-

sional slight inhibition. These results verified the splanchnic nerve and vagus contributions to the reflex gastric motility responses produced by pinching the abdominal skin and a hind paw.

Efferent activity from the proximal cut end of the gastric vagal branch near the stomach surface was recorded and counted. Figure 4 shows the increased gastric vagal efferent activity produced by pinching a hind paw (B), and the absence of significant effect when pinching the abdomen (A). Usually, vagal activity increased with a latency of less than one sec, reached a maximum within five sec, then gradually decreased to the control level within 30 sec. Since sympathetic nerves on their way to the stomach join the vagal nerves around the esophagus at the level of the thorax and abdomen, all sympathetic nerve branches joining the vagus in this region were carefully dissected and sectioned for this experiment.

Figure 5 shows sample records of gastric sympathetic efferent activity changes produced by pinching the abdominal skin (A), and a hind paw (B). Pinching the abdominal skin substantially increased the activity, while pinching a hind paw was either ineffective or produced a slight increase in activity. The latency of the increase in sympathetic activity after the onset of pinching was usually about one sec. The vagus

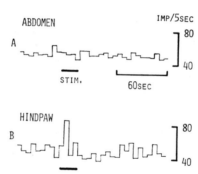

Fig. 4.   Evoked vagal reflex activity. Gastric efferent response to pinching abdominal skin (A) and hind paw (B). A, B: Specimen records of mass discharge rate of gastric vagal efferent activity. Count: Impulses per 5 sec. Under bars: 20 sec pinch. All data from same rat. Sympathetic nerves were cut. (Modified from ref. 20.)

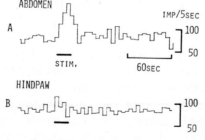

Fig. 5.   Evoked splanchnic nerve reflex activity. Gastric efferent response to pinching abdominal skin (A) and hind paw (B). A–B: Specimen records of mass discharge rate of activity of gastric postganglionic sympathetic branch of celiac ganglion. Count: Impulses per 5 sec. Under bars: 20 sec pinch. All data from same rat. Vagi were cut. (Modified from ref. 20.)

was always severed bilaterally at the cervical level to avoid contamination of gastric sympathetic activity by vagal reflex components in these experiments.

After spinal transection at the cervical level, effects on gastric motility response to pinching the abdominal skin or a hind paw were examined. Special care was exercised to maintain blood pressure above 90 mmHg after spinal transection by administration of Macrodex-D and 5% glucose solution, as needed. Substantial reflex inhibition of gastric motility was produced by pinching the abdominal skin, and slight reflex inhibition of gastric motility was obtained by pinching a hind paw.

Interactions, if any, between the opposed gastric reflexes which have been discussed might disclose some interesting and important facts about the relative populations of the various fiber types, sympathetic parasympathetic interactions and possibly some synaptic information. The combined motility responses to simultaneous stimulation of the abdominal skin and hind paws were examined, and reflex inhibition was always obtained when both skin areas were pinched simultaneously, although the amplitude and duration were somewhat reduced.

The classical concept that the vagus stimulates and the sympathetic system inhibits gastric motility is still generally true in rats. No gastric facilitation was seen when the splanchnic nerve was stimulated in rats, and although an initial transient inhibitory component was produced by vagal stimulation it was overwhelmed by the excitatory component of gastric motility[1]. Nociceptive abdominal skin stimulation evoked marked splanchnic efferent nerve discharges and strong gastric inhibition, but no vagal efferent activity. It can thus be concluded that the cutaneo-gastric reflex path from the abdomen is primarily, if not totally, through gastric sympathetic efferent (possibly inhibitory) nerves. Hind paw stimulation, on the other hand, while evoking some splanchnic nerve activity, produced a greater change in gastric vagal efferent fiber activity (possibly excitatory) and facilitated gastric motility. Forepaw stimulation also facilitated gastric motility. It is thus apparent that the vagus is the main efferent pathway of the cutaneo-gastric reflex from the paws. There appears to be a clear topography of cutaneous afferents to vagal motoneurons within the brain stem which could be a counterpart of the somatosensory map in the sensory cortex[28].

The inhibitory effect of abdominal skin stimulation on gastric motility is graded from highest for a mid-abdominal segment to lower values for both rostral and caudal. This might be explained by segmental organization in the spinal cord which is analogous to that found by Sato and Schmidt[31,32] when sympathetic reflex discharges were evoked from the thoracolumbar white rami by electrical stimulation of spinal somatic afferents at various spinal segments. They found that the reflex sympathetic discharge intensity was directly related to the proximity of the segments from which the somatic and sympathetic nerves emanated.

The physiological significance of the cutaneo-gastric reflex control of gastric motility is obscure. It might be noted, on the one hand, that the simple act of walking or running stimulates the feet and hence stimulates gastric motility. On the other hand, nociceptive stimulation of the abdomen, which inhibits motility, could conceivably be associated with serious circumstances in which the discomfort might be less if gastric motility were decreased.

The observations of cutaneo-gastric reflexes emphasize the importance of cutaneous afferents which modulate the autonomic control of visceral organs. The effect of somatic muscular afferent stimulation was not discussed here, but it is quite probable that stimulation of muscle afferents would influence gastric motility[16,17]. These factors of somatic (both cutaneous and muscular) afferent stimulation should not be ignored in the search for better understanding of autonomic contributions to homeostasis and function of the organism.

SUMMARY

1. A brief, general review of extrinsic nervous control of gastric motility was presented.

2. Recent experiments with rats by Aihara et al.[1], using electrical stimulation of vagal and splanchnic B and C fibers, showed that gastric motility was slightly facilitated by repetitive stimulation of vagal B fibers and was greatly facilitated by repetitive stimulation of vagal C fibers. Vagal C fiber stimulation also evoked an initial inhibition of motility. Splanchnic C fiber stimulation inhibited gastric motility, but the splanchnic B fiber contribution to inhibition was much greater.

3. Kametani, et al.[21] observed decreased gastric motility and/or gastric muscle tonus when abdominal, middle and caudal ventral thorax and dorsal thorax skin areas were pinched, and increased gastric motility and/or gastric muscle tonus while pinching the skin of nose, face, ears, neck, arms, legs, paws, sacral area or tail.

4. Kametani, et al.[20] reported that hind paw stimulation markedly increased efferent activity of the gastric vagal nerve while only slightly affecting gastric sympathetic afferent activity, and produced moderate reflex facilitation of gastric motility. Abdominal skin stimulation greatly increased efferent gastric sympathetic nerve activity without affecting gastric vagal efferent activity, and caused pronounced reflex inhibition of gastric motility. It was concluded that those extrinsic nerve fibers which are involved in cutaneo-gastric facilitatory and inhibitory motility reflexes are the gastric vagal excitatory efferents and the gastric sympathetic inhibitory efferents, respectively. The gastric vagal excitatory and sympathetic inhibitory contributions to the gastric motility change produced by simultaneous stimulation of the hind paw and abdominal skin were shown to interact at the peripheral level.

This work was supported by grants from the Ministry of Education of Japan and Daiwa Health Foundation (to A. Sato).

REFERENCES

1 Aihara, Y., Nakamura, H., Sato, A. and Simpson, A., Relations between various fiber groups of vagal and splanchnic nerves and gastric motility in rats, *Neuroscience Letters*, 10 (1978) 281–286.

2 Babkin, B. P., The cerebral cortex and gastric motility, *Gastroenterology*, 14 (1950) 479–484.

3 Babkin, B. P. and Kite, W. C., Jr., Central and reflex regulation of motility of pyloric antrum, *J. Neurophysiol.*, 13 (1950) 321–334.

4 Bailey, P. and Sweet, W. H., Effects on respiration, blood pressure and gastric motility of stimulation of orbital surface of frontal lobe, *J. Neurophysiol.*, 3 (1940) 276–281.

5 Brown, G. L., McSwiney, B. A. and Wadge, W. J., The sympathetic innervation of the stomach. I. The effect on the stomach of stimulation of the thoracic sympathetic trunk, *J. Physiol.* (Lond.), 70 (1930) 253–260.

6 Cannon, W. B. and Murphy, F. T., The movements of the stomach and intestine in some surgical conditions, *Ann. Surg.*, 43 (1906) 512–536.

7 Code, C. F., *Handbook of Physiology, Sect. 6, Alimentary Canal, Vol. II, Secretion*, Amer. Physiol. Society, Washington, D. C., 1967.

8 Delgado, J. M. R. and Anand, B. K., Increase of food intake induced by electrical stimulation of the lateral hypothalamus, *Amer. J. Physiol.*, 172 (1953) 162–168.

9 Eliasson, S., Cerebral influences on gastric motility in the cat, *Acta physiol. scand.*, 26, Suppl. 95 (1952) 1–70.

10 Eliasson, S., Activation of gastric motility from the brain stem of the cat, *Acta physiol scand.*, 30 (1953–1954) 199–214.

11 Folkow, B. and Rubinstein, E. H., Behavioral and gastrointestinal changes (motility and bloodflow) induced by electrical stimulation of the lateral hypothalamus in cats, *Acta physiol. scand.*, 59, Suppl. 213 (1963) 44.

12 Folkow, B. and Rubinstein, E. H., Behavioral and autonomic patterns evoked by stimulation of the lateral hypothalamic area in cats, *Acta physiol. scand.*, 65 (1965) 292–299.

13 Freude, V. E., Der experimentelle Nachweis des thermischen Haut-Eingeweidereflexes, *Münch. Med. Woch.*, 52 (1927) 2211–2212.

14 Hodes, R., Reciprocal innervation in the small intestine, *Amer. J. Physiol.*, 130 (1940) 642–650.

15 Hoffman, B. L. and Rasmussen, T., Stimulation studies of insular cortex of Macaca mulatta, *J. Neurophysiol.*, 16 (1953) 343–351.

16 Jansson, G., Extrinsic nervous control of gastric motility, *Acta physiol. scand.*, Suppl. 326 (1969a) 1–42.

17 Jansson, G., Effect of reflexes of somatic afferents of the adrenergic outflow to the stomach in the cat, *Acta physiol. scand.*, 77 (1969b) 17–22.

18 Kaada, B., Somato-motor, autonomic and electro-corticographic responses to electrical stimulation of rhinencephalic and other structures in primates, cat, and dog, *Acta physiol. scand.*, 24, Suppl. 83 (1951) 1–285.

19 Kabat, H., Anson, B. J., Magoun, H. W. and Ranson, S. W., Stimulation of the hypothalamus with special reference to its effect on gastrointestinal motility, *Amer. J. Physiol.*, 112 (1935) 214–226.

20 Kametani, H., Sato, A., Sato, Y. and Simpson, A., Neural mechanisms of reflex excitation and inhibition of gastric motility due to stimulation of various skin areas in rats, *J. Physiol.* (Lond.), in press (1979).

21 Kametani, H., Sato, A., Sato, Y. and Ueki, K., Reflex facilitation and inhibition of gastric motility from various skin areas in rats. In: M. Ito (Ed.), *Integrative Control Functions of the Brain*, Vol. I, Kodansha Scientific, Tokyo, 1978, 336–338.

22 Kehl, H., Studies of reflex communications between dermatomes and jejunum, *J. Am. Osteopath. Assoc.*, 74 (1975) 667–669.

23 Lehman, A. V., Studien über reflektorishe Darmbewegungen beim Hunde, *Pflügers Arch.*, 149 (1913) 413–433.

24 Martinson, J., Studies on the efferent vagal control of the stomach, *Acta physiol. scand.*, 65, Suppl. 255 (1965) 1–24.

25 McSwiney, B. A., Innervation of the stomach. *Physiol. Rev.*, 11 (1931) 479–514.

26 Paintal, A. S., Vagal afferent fibres, *Ergebn. Physiol.*, 52 (1963) 24–156.

27 Patterson, T. L. and Rubright, L. W., The influence of tonal conditions on the muscular response of the monkey's stomach, *Q. J. exp. Physiol.*, 24 (1934) 3–21.

28 Penfield, W. and Rasmussen, T., *The Cerebral Cortex of Man*, Macmillian, New York, 1950.

29 Ruhmann, W., Örtliche Hautreizbehandlung des Magens und ihre physiologischen Grundlagen, *Arch. f. Verdauungskr.*, 41 (1927) 336–350.

30 Sato, A., Sato, Y., Shimada, F. and Torigata, Y., Changes in gastric motility produced by nociceptive stimulation of the skin in rats, *Brain Res.*, 87 (1975) 151–159.

31 Sato, A. and Schmidt, R. F., Spinal and supraspinal components of the reflex discharges into lumbar and thoracic white rami, *J. Physiol. (Lond.)*, 212 (1971) 839–850.

32 Sato, A. and Schmidt, R. F., Somatosympathetic reflexes: Afferent fibers, central pathways, discharge characteristics, *Physiol. Rev.*, 54 (1973) 916–947.

33 Semba, T., Fujii, K. and Kimura, N., The vagal inhibitory response of the stomach to stimulation of the dog's medulla oblongata, *Nō To Shihkei*, 17 (1965) 485–489.

34 Semba, T., Noda, H. and Fujii, K., On splanchnic motor responses of stomach movements produced by stimulation of the medulla oblongata and spinal cord. *Jap. J. Physiol.*, 13 (1963) 466–478.

35 Shealy, C. N. and Peele, T. L., Studies on amygdaloid nucleus of cat, *J. Neurophysiol.*, 20 (1957) 125–139.

36 Ström, G. and Uvnäs, B., Motor responses of gastrointestinal tract and bladder to topical stimulation of the frontal lobe, basal ganglia and hypothalamus in the cat. *Acta physiol. scand.*, 21 (1950) 90–104.

37 Thomas, J. E. and Baldwin, M. V., Pathways and mechanisms of regulation of gastric motility. In: C. F. Code (Ed.), *Handbook of Physiology, Sect. 6, Alimentary Canal, Vol. IV., Motility*, Amer. Physiol. Society, Washington, D. C., 1968, 1937–1968.

38 Thomas, J. E. and Crider, J. O., Inhibition of gastric motility associated with the presence of products of protein hydrolysis in the upper small intestine, *Amer. J. Physiol.*, 126 (1939) 28–38.

39 Thomas, J. E., Crider, J. O. and Mogan, C. J., A study of reflexes involving the pyloric sphincter and antrum and their role in gastric evacuation, *Amer. J. Physiol.*, 108 (1934) 683–700.

40 Wood, J. D., Neurophysiology of Auerbach's plexus and control of intestinal motility, *Physiol. Rev.*, 55 (1975) 307–324.

41 Youmans, W. B., Innervation of the gastrointestinal tract. In: C. F. Code (Ed.), *Handbook of Physiology, Sect. 6, Alimentary Canal, Vol. IV, Motility*, Amer. Physiol. Society, Washington, D. C., 1968, 1655–1663.

42 Youmans, W., B. and Meek, W. J., Gastrointestinal inhibition in unanesthetized dogs during rectal stimulation, *Amer. J. Physiol.*, 120 (1937) 750–760.

CHAPTER 4

NEURAL CONTROL OF THE URINARY BLADDER
AND LARGE INTESTINE

W. C. de Groat, A. M. Booth, J. Krier, R. J. Milne, C. Morgan and I. Nadelhaft

Department of Pharmacology, Medical School, University of
Pittsburgh, Pittsburgh, Pennsylvania, USA

INTRODUCTION

The lower urinary tract and distal segments of the large intestine are responsible for the storage and periodic elimination of body wastes. The performance of these functions requires complex neural control systems which coordinate the activities of a variety of effector organs, including smooth muscles of the urinary bladder and large intestine and smooth and striated muscles of the urethral and anal sphincters[3,10,11,36,39,44].

Three sets of peripheral nerves are involved in the regulation of excretory function: (1) sacral parasympathetic, (2) thoracolumbar sympathetic and (3) sacral somatic nerves (primarily the pudendal). Sacral parasympathetic preganglionic fibers, which travel in the pelvic nerve, provide the major excitatory input to the urinary bladder and large intestine[42]. Preganglionic axons project to ganglion cells on the surface of the organs[20,42] and presumably to nerve cells in the myenteric plexus[6,53]. Parasympathetic ganglion cells in the bladder provide an excitatory input to the detrusor smooth muscle via the release of either acetylcholine or a purinergic transmitter[6], whereas in the intestine parasympathetic excitatory neurons are primarily cholinergic. Parasympathetic preganglionic axons may also synapse in the myenteric plexus with purinergic neurons which produce inhibition of rectal and colonic smooth muscle[6,37].

Sympathetic pathways which originate in the thoraco-lumbar segments of the spinal cord provide an inhibitory input to the colon and detrusor region of the bladder and an excitatory input to trigone and smooth muscle of the urethral and anal sphincters[36,39]. Striated sphincter muscles receive an excitatory innervation via the pudendal nerves.

Afferent activity arising in the bladder and large intestine is conveyed to the central nervous system over both sets of autonomic nerves. Mechanoreceptor afferents which evoke reflex contractions and excretory responses travel in the pelvic nerve to the sacral cord[36,39,44]. On the other hand, mechanoreceptors and nociceptive fibers contained in sympathetic nerves elicit vasomotor and inhibitory reflexes to the intestine. These reflexes seem to be routed through prevertebral sympathetic ganglia[8,54,55] as well as through the spinal cord[32,37,38]. The effect of sympathetic afferent activity on bladder function is not known.

Similar patterns of reflex responses occur during micturition and defecation. The primary stimulus for micturition is bladder distension, which leads to reflex activation of the parasympathetic pathway[3,39,44], depression of the sympathetic inhibitory pathway[23,30] and depression of the somatic efferent input to the external urethral sphincter, allowing the sphincter to relax[39,44]. Secondary reflexes elicited by the passage of urine through the urethra may reinforce these primary reflexes and facilitate complete emptying of the bladder[3]. The stimulus for defecation is the movement of feces into the rectum. This initiates afferent firing in pelvic nerves and in turn a reflex discharge in parasympathetic excitatory pathways and an inhibition of the tonic efferent discharge to the external anal sphincter[11,36]. In the cat the sympathetic outflow to the intestine does not appear to be depressed during defecation[22].

The relative importance of these pathways is obvious from lesion experiments. For example, interruption of sympathetic innervation produces rather transient and minor alterations in bladder and intestinal function, whereas destruction of the sacral parasympathetic pathways markedly depresses the activity of these organs, the bladder being more severely affected[10,11,39,43]. The greater sensitivity of the bladder to decentralization does not appear to be related to differences in the intrinsic properties of the bladder and intestinal smooth muscle, since both organs are composed of single-unit smooth muscle which exhibits slow waves and spontaneous activity in the absence of a neural input. Rather it is probably attributable to the existence in the intestine, but not in the bladder, of an intramural plexus which can coordinate propulsive movements following decentralization. When the intramural plexus is damaged, as in Hirschsprung's disease, then intestinal transport is also severely compromised.

The central mechanisms controlling micturition and defecation also seemed to be organized differently and to vary considerably in sensitivity to lesions of the spinal cord or brain. The early studies of Barrington[1,2] in the cat indicated that micturition was mediated by a spino-bulbospinal pathway through a center in the rostral pons, whereas the investigations of Garry[34,36] showed that the defecation reflex in the cat was organized in the sacral spinal cord. Micturition reflexes are severely depressed by damage to bulbospinal pathways or lesions in the pontine region, whereas defecation reflexes persist in acute spinal animals.

Recent electrophysiological and neuroanatomical studies in our laboratory have confirmed and extended these observations and have demonstrated numerous other differences in the reflex pathways underlying micturition and defecation. This paper will review certain aspects of these studies.

METHODS

Experiments were performed on cats anesthetized with chloralose (50–60 mg/kg i.v.). Sympathetic (hypogastric and lumbar colonic nerves) and parasympathetic (pelvic nerve) extrinsic nerves to the urinary bladder and large intestine were exposed through a midline abdominal incision and isolated for stimulation or recording. Post-ganglionic nerves arising from ganglia on the surface of the bladder and distal colon were sectioned and prepared for monophasic recording. Postganglionic action potentials were recorded with standard techniques and averaged with a digital computer.

The technique for locating and recording from sacral preganglionic neurons and for the iontophoretic application of drugs has been described in previous papers[12,25]. Preganglionic cells were identified by antidromic invasion in response to stimulation of the ventral roots or the pelvic nerve. Extracellular action potentials were recorded with single micropipettes or the center barrel of five-barrel micropipettes.

Bladder and intestinal intraluminal pressures were measured with water-filled rubber condoms or open-ended cannulae which were inserted, respectively, through an incision in the fundus of the bladder and through the urethra or the anal canal.

Preganglionic neurons and visceral afferent input to the sacral cord were labelled with horseradish peroxidase (HRP) by immersing the central stump of the sectioned pelvic nerve or branches of the nerve to the bladder or colon in a 25% solution of HRP for four to six hours. After allowing sufficient time (30–60 hours) for transport of HRP from the periphery to the cord, the animal was perfused with fixative, the cord was sectioned serially on a freezing microtome and sections were processed using the benzidine method for HRP. Supraspinal projections to the region of the sacral autonomic nucleus were studied with the same technique. Small quantities of HRP (0.5 μl) were injected into the spinal autonomic area and after two to three days transport time the brain stem was removed, serially sectioned and processed for HRP.

RESULTS

Sacral Efferent and Afferent Pathways to the Urinary Bladder and Large Intestine

Electrophysiological experiments revealed that the sacral preganglionic pathways to the bladder and large intestine have different properties. Preganglionic axons to the bladder are primarily myelinated with conduction velocities between 2–15 m/sec, whereas preganglionic axons to the large intestine are unmyelinated and conduct at 0.5–1.4 m/sec[19,20,25].

These two preganglionic pathways also rise from different locations in the spinal cord. It was shown with HRP tracing techniques that the sacral autonomic nucleus extends eight to ten mm along the length of the spinal cord with the majority of cells in the S_2 segment[46,47,48]. In the transverse plane the nucleus has the shape of an inverse "L", composed of a lateral band of cells along the edge of the intermediate grey matter and a dorsal band of cells along the inferior edge of the dorsal horn (Fig. 1B). When HRP was applied to nerves innervating the bladder, cells in the lateral band were labelled, whereas application of HRP to nerves on the surface of the colon labelled cells in the dorsal band (Fig. 1C). A large proportion of cells in both areas were spindle shaped, however the dorsally-located cells were on the average smaller (12.7×31 μm) than cells in the lateral region (17×36.6 μm). In addition, the orientation of the cells and their dendrites in the two regions was different (Fig. 1B). Cells in the dorsal band were commonly oriented with their long axes in the mediolateral direction and with dendrites projecting within the nucleus toward the midline and

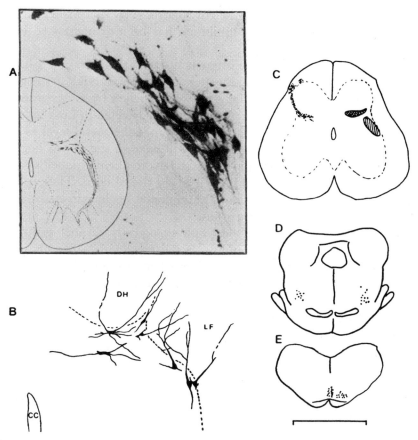

Fig. 1. A: Brightfield photomicrograph of HRP-labelled cells in the lateral band of the
sacral parasympathetic nucleus (SPN). The insert shows the position of these cells
in the mid-S_2 cord as well as their axonal path along the lateral edge of the grey
matter. B: a composite camera lucida drawing showing the dendrites of dorsal
band cells projecting medially toward the central canal (CC) and dorsolaterally
along the lateral edge of the dorsal horn (DH). The lateral band cells also project
to the lateral edge of the DH and to the dorsolateral funiculus (LF). C: the area
occupied by the SPN at the mid-S_2 level is shown in the right side of the drawing.
Colon cells occupy the dorsal, cross-hatched area; and bladder cells, the lateral-
shaded area. The distribution of primary afferent projections from the pelvic nerve
(left side) is primarily along the lateral DH. D and E are representative composite
sections of brain stem where HRP-labelled cells (dots) were found after injection of
HRP into the region of the left sacral autonomic nucleus. D: cells located bilaterally
in pontine reticular formation. E: cells are in medullary raphe pallidus and ipsilateral
ventral reticular formation. Bar represents 85 μm in A; 0.5 mm in B; 2 mm in C;
6.2 mm in D; 10 mm in E.

toward and along the lateral edge of the dorsal horn. Cells in the lateral group were
oriented dorsoventrally and sent dendrites into the dorsolateral funiculus and dorsally
and ventrally within the nucleus. Both groups of cells sent dendrites into the marginal
zone (lamina I) of the dorsal horn. The axons of both groups of cells passed into the

ventral horn along the lateral edge of the gray matter (Fig. 1A). Axon collaterals could not be detected, although recurrent inhibition has been demonstrated in the sacral autonomic nucleus[15,26].

The termination of pelvic nerve afferent fibers in the sacral cord has also been studied with the HRP technique[46]. Following application of HRP to the pelvic nerve, afferent axons and/or terminals in the cord were labelled by anterograde transport. As illustrated in Fig. 1C, HRP reaction product was detected in Lissauer's tract along a considerable length of the lumbosacral cord and at the sacral level as fine lines of granules in the marginal layer along the lateral edge of the dorsal horn extending into the dorsal part of the autonomic nucleus. Less frequently, labelling occurred in the lateral region of the nucleus and medial to the dorsal horn. Thus, it appears that visceral primary afferents enter the sacral autonomic nucleus to make contact with preganglionic neurons and/or interneurons.

At least two functionally and electrophysiologically distinct groups of pelvic nerve afferents are involved in excretion. Small myelinated afferents ($A\gamma\delta$) to the urinary bladder initiate the micturition reflex whereas unmyelinated afferents from the rectum and distal colon elicit the defecation reflex[21,27].

Parasympathetic Reflex Pathways

Large intestine. When sacral parasympathetic efferent firing and colonic motility were monitored simultaneously in the cat an enhancement of neural activity was noted prior to the occurrence of spontaneous or afferent-evoked propulsive waves in the colon (Fig. 2C)[21]. The propulsive waves were associated with the appearance of a tonic constriction ring in the mid-proximal colon, contraction of the longitudinal muscle as evidenced by shortening of the entire colon and aboral movements of colonic contents. Neural and effector organ responses were abolished by transection of the sacral dorsal or ventral roots indicating that they were reflex in origin. Propulsive waves were characterized by their large amplitude (40–80 cm H_2O), long duration (six to eight min) and by their occurrence simultaneously over considerable lengths of the large intestine, i.e., from the proximal colon to the rectum. Their amplitude, however, varied in different regions. Significantly higher pressures were generated in the proximal colon than in the distal colon and rectum. This data suggests that during defecation an oral to aboral pressure gradient develops which could promote the aboral movement of colonic contents. This pattern of activity must be dependent on parasympathetic pathways since it is unlikely that a peripheral mechanism such as peristalsis, which has a slow conduction velocity, could mediate the simultaneous activation of large segments of bowel.

The sacral outflow may also regulate other intestinal activity. Parasympathetic efferent firing increased during the occurrence of smaller amplitude slow rhythmic pressure waves which probably reflect segmental contractions (Fig. 2A). These waves correlated with rhythmic contractions of circular muscle and were peripheral in origin since they occurred in decentralized preparations. They were abolished by the administration of atropine or ganglionic blocking agents, indicating that they were produced by neurons in the intrinsic plexus, however under certain conditions these waves appeared to be facilitated by a central outflow. Also a low level of spontaneous

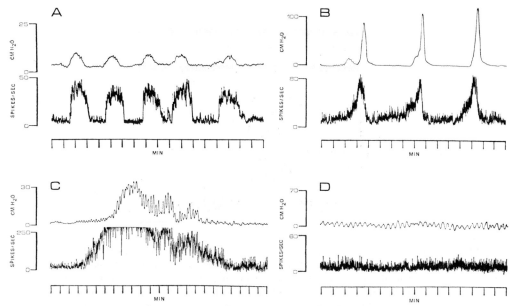

Fig. 2. Relationship between efferent firing recorded in parasympathetic postganglionic
nerves to the colon and spontaneous colonic (A–C) and rectal (D) motility. The
upper traces in records A–D represent intraluminal pressures in four different cats
from distal (A), proximal (B), mid colon (C) and rectum (D), while the lower
traces in each record represent the integration of the neural discharge. Record A
depicts slow pressure waves and neural discharge in a cat anaesthetized with pentobarbitone, while records B, C and D represent slow, tonic and fast pressure waves,
respectively, and neural activity recorded in chloralose anaesthetized cats. Vertical
calibrations are equal to the intraluminal pressures, in cm H_2O and efferent discharge
in spikes/sec. Reproduced with permission from the *Journal of Physiology*[21].

parasympathetic efferent firing was observed when the colon was completely empty.
While the function of this activity is unknown, it is possible that it could reflect: (1) a
tonic control over basal smooth muscle activity, (2) regulation of secretion or ion
transport[5] or (3) firing in the proposed sacral inhibitory outflow to the intestine[37].
Recordings from single preganglionic neurons in the sacral spinal cord also revealed a
tonic discharge in the absence of intestinal distension (Fig. 3). It is assumed that these
preganglionic neurons provided an efferent input to the intestine since they were
located in the dorsal band of the autonomic nucleus, had axons that conducted at C
fiber velocities, were inhibited by distension of the urinary bladder and were activated
during a defecation reflex elicited by mechanical stimulation of the anal canal (Fig. 3).
The sacral parasympathetic reflexes to the large intestine must be organized entirely
within the sacral cord since transection of the spinal cord above the sacral level did not
block propulsive waves and associated efferent firing[21].

More detailed information about the reflex pathway was obtained by studying
synchronous postganglionic reflexes elicited by electrical stimulation of intestinal
afferents[21]. Evoked discharges occurred at relatively long latencies (mean 210 msec).
However, a considerable part of the latency was attributable to slow conduction

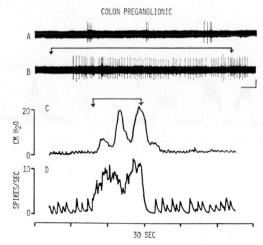

Fig. 3. Discharge of a preganglionic neuron in the dorsal part of the sacral autonomic
nucleus. A: spontaneous firing; B: firing evoked by mechanical stimulation (indicated by the arrows) of the rectum-anal canal. C and D: simultaneous recording
of intraluminal pressure (cm H_2O) in the midcolon and firing of a sacral preganglionic neuron during stimulation of rectum-anal canal (between arrows). Horizontal
and vertical calibrations in B represent 1 sec and 250 μV, respectively.

velocity in unmyelinated afferent and preganglionic efferent limbs of the reflex. The
estimated central delay for the reflex was very long (45–60 msec) for a spinal pathway.
The reflex was similar in chronic spinal animals but was depressed in acute spinal
preparations, indicating that it might be facilitated by a bulbospinal pathway.

Urinary bladder. In contrast to the defecation reflex which is organized at the
spinal level, the parasympathetic component of the micturition reflex is dependent
upon a supraspinal pathway originating in the rostral pons (Fig. 5). Barrington[1,2]
showed that micturition could be elicited in cats decerebrated at the intercollicular
level, but that micturition was abolished by transection of the neuraxis at any point
below the inferior colliculus. Electrical stimulation in the brain stem in the region of
the dorsolateral pontine reticular formation elicited contractions of the urinary
bladder, whereas lesions placed in the same region produced irreversible depression
of bladder reflexes. As noted by other investigators[39], areas of the brain rostral to the
pons also have excitatory and inhibitory influences on bladder activity. These suprapontine centers are believed to have a modulating action on the basic reflex pathway.

Electrophysiological studies have confirmed the supraspinal organization of
bladder reflexes. The reflex firing of sacral preganglionic neurons innervating the
bladder occurred at a long latency (80–120 msec) following stimulation of bladder
afferents in the pelvic nerve. The reflexes were present in decerebrated animals with
an intact central nervous system, but were absent in acute spinal animals. Intracellular
recording revealed that pelvic afferent stimulation evoked EPSP's at 65–100 msec
latency. Short-latency EPSP's and reflex firing were not observed.

Recently the location of supraspinal centers involved in micturition has been
studied in our laboratory with electrical stimulation and HRP tracing techniques.

SACRAL INTERNEURON

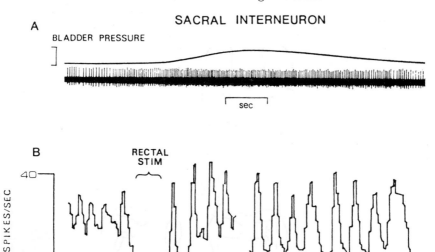

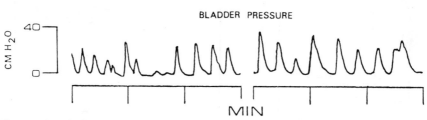

Fig. 4. Correlation between bladder contractions and the discharge of an interneuron in
the sacral autonomic nucleus. A: top trace, intravesical pressure and bottom trace,
neuronal firing. Vertical calibration represents 30 cm H_2O pressure. B: simultaneous
recording of spontaneous firing (upper trace) and intravesical pressure (lower trace)
in the absence of and during mechanical stimulation of the rectum-anal canal.
Bladder was distended with 20 ml of saline and maintained under constant volume
conditions. Vertical calibrations, average rate of firing of cells in spikes/sec obtained
with a ratemeter and intravesical pressure in cm H_2O.

It was observed that electrical stimulation at various points in the brain stem of cats
produced firing of sacral preganglionic neurons and contractions of the bladder[14,41].
However, the shortest latency responses (latencies of 45–60 msec) occurred following
stimulation in the lateral pontine reticular formation at the level of the locus coeruleus
and in the same general area designated by Barrington as the "pontine micturition
center". Stimulation of afferents in the pelvic nerve evoked negative field potentials
in the same area at latencies of 30–40 msec. The sum of the two latencies approximated
the central delay for the micturition reflex.

  Injection of small quantities (0.5 μl of a 10% solution) of HRP into the sacral
spinal cord in the region of the autonomic nucleus labelled neurons in the lateral
pontine reticular formation (Fig. 1D) as well as at other sites throughout the brain
stem including the raphe pallidus (Fig. 1E), nucleus reticularis ventralis (Fig. 1E),
nucleus reticularis gigantocellularis, red nucleus, nucleus gracilis and nucleus tractus
solitarius. Since a similar distribution of labelled cells has been reported following

BLADDER   COLON

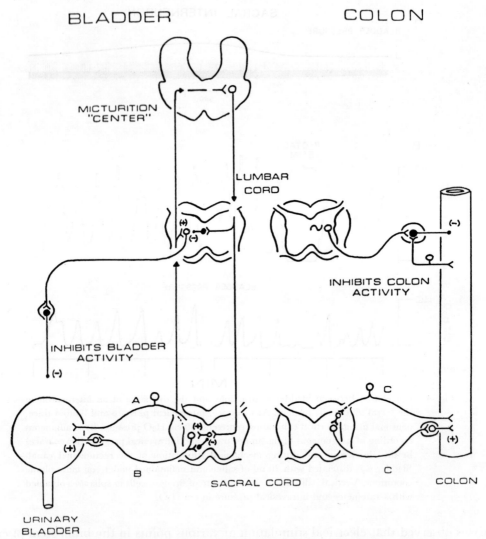

Fig. 5.   Diagram of the parasympathetic and sympathetic reflex pathways to the urinary
          bladder and colon of the cat. Plus and minus signs indicate excitatory and inhibitory
          synapses, respectively. In the lumbar cord the sine wave indicates the oscillator cir-
          cuit for generation of sympathetic firing. See text for further description.

injections of HRP into other levels of the spinal cord[4,7,40] the importance of these nuclei
in the regulation of bladder activity is uncertain. However, the experiments did establish the existence of direct neuronal connections from the region of the pontine
micturition center to the sacral spinal cord. Assuming a conduction distance from the
pons to the sacral level of 40 cm and that micturition reflexes occur over such a direct
pathway, it would appear that the bulbospinal fibers involved in micturition have peak
conduction velocities of 6–9 m/sec.

It is not known whether the descending fibers make synaptic connections directly with the preganglionic neurons or with interneurons in the sacral cord. As shown in Fig. 4, interneurons (i. e., cells that were not antidromically activated by stimulation of preganglionic axons) exhibiting firing correlated with bladder activity were encountered in the region of the sacral autonomic nucleus. With the bladder empty these neurons maintained a slow rhythmic pattern of firing while preganglionic neurons under the same conditions were quiescent. As the bladder was distended, interneuronal firing increased linearly with bladder pressure, reaching maximum frequencies of 10–20 Hz[45]. With the bladder distended and held at constant volume, preganglionic neurons and interneurons fired prior to and during rhythmic bladder contractions (Fig. 4). This observation suggests that both types of neurons are on the micturition reflex pathway and that the interneurons may provide a synaptic link between bulbospinal axons and the preganglionic cells.

Although spino-bulbospinal reflexes mediate micturition in adult cats with an intact neuraxis, spinal reflexes are important in producing micturition under other conditions, e.g., chronic spinal cats[25] and neonatal kittens[18]. In adult cats transection of the spinal cord initially blocks the micturition reflex; however, within several weeks after transection micturition recovers. As in normal animals, distension of the bladder evokes firing in the sacral parasympathetic pathways, relaxation of the urethral sphincters and elimination of urine, however micturition is generally less efficient and the bladder never empties completely. In these preparations long latency excitatory reflexes to sacral parasympathetic neurons could not be demonstrated, but short-latency EPSP's (3–5 msec) and firing (7–25 msec) were elicited by pelvic afferent stimulation[25]. It is not known whether the appearance of a short latency spinal reflex is due to formation of new pathways by axonal sprouting or to the unmasking of an existing pathway after the removal of bulbospinal inhibitory controls.

Transection of the spinal cord in cats also unmasks or facilitates an excitatory somatovesical reflex pathway which can initiate micturition in response to tactile stimulation of the perineal region. A similar reflex (i.e., the "mass" reflex) is observed in chronic spinal humans[10] and neonatal kittens[18]. In kittens and in neonates of many other species, micturition as well as defecation are elicited when the mother cat licks the perineal region[31]. In kittens the micturition response is very prominent during the first four postnatal weeks after which the latency for the response progressively increases[18]. In most kittens the reflex disappears by the age of seven to eight weeks, which is the approximate age of weaning. Although micturition to perineal stimulation does not occur in adult animals, remnants of the excitatory reflex can be demonstrated under certain conditions (e.g., when bladder pressure was below the micturition threshold), and with more sensitive techniques (e.g., recording bladder pressure or parasympathetic efferent firing)[13,16,18,52]. In adult cats perineal stimulation also produces an inhibition of bladder activity[13,27,52]. This will be discussed below.

Transection of the spinal cord at the thoracic level in older kittens (eight to ten weeks) causes the reemergence of the perineal-induced micturition reflex. This process usually requires one week (range three to twelve days). In some spinal animals the reflex latencies are initially prolonged (30–60 sec) but two to three weeks after spinalization all animals respond at latencies (three to ten sec) equivalent to those of the newborn animals.

At the time when a micturition response to perineal stimulation develops in chronic spinal cats electrophysiological studies revealed that stimulation of afferent fibers from the perineal region elicited short-latency EPSPs and firing (three to five msec) in sacral preganglionic neurons. On the other hand, in adult animals with an intact spinal cord, stimulation of the same afferents produced short-latency IPSPs (five msec) followed by longer latency (60–80 msec) EPSPs and firing[27]. These observations provide further evidence for reorganization of bladder reflexes in chronic spinal animals.

The sacral parasympathetic outflow to the bladder is subject to several types of inhibitory inputs, including recurrent inhibition and inhibition from sacral visceral and somatic afferents. The presence of a recurrent inhibitory pathway was first suggested by the finding that bladder activity and firing of sacral preganglionic neurons could be depressed by electrical stimulation (10–20 Hz) of the central end of a transected sacral ventral root[26]. The inhibition only occurred with stimulation of ventral roots containing preganglionic axons and only at intensities of stimulation above the threshold for activating these axons. The inhibition exhibited a number of important differences from recurrent inhibition of motoneurons, most notably its strong contralateral as well as ipsilateral distribution. The inhibition was blocked by intravenous administration of strychnine, suggesting that glycine might be the transmitter in the inhibitory pathway. Interneurons were encountered in the region of the sacral autonomic nucleus which were excited synaptically by antidromic volleys in the ventral roots. The synaptic responses of these cells had characteristics which clearly distinguished them from Renshaw cells. Since the firing of these presumed inhibitory cells and the intensity of recurrent inhibition were reduced at high bladder pressures, it was proposed that the recurrent inhibitory pathway was depressed during micturition, thereby facilitating the parasympathetic outflow to the bladder.

Recent studies[15,16] on the central mechanism of recurrent inhibition indicate that the inhibition does not occur directly on the preganglionic neurons but at some point earlier on the micturition pathway. It was shown that ventral root stimulation depressed the spontaneous firing of parasympathetic preganglionic neurons but did not depress the firing elicited by directly activating the cells with an excitant amino acid (DL-homocysteic acid). Further, it was observed that while intravenously-administered strychnine blocked recurrent inhibition, locally-applied strychnine did not modify recurrent inhibition although it did block the effects of glycine. Both of these observations indicate that recurrent inhibition of parasympathetic neurons is related to disfacilitation, (i.e., an inhibition of interneurons on the excitatory pathway to the parasympathetic neurons) and not to postsynaptic inhibition of the parasympathetic neurons (Fig. 5). This view is supported by the finding that interneurons in the sacral autonomic nucleus exhibiting firing correlated with bladder activity are inhibited by antidromic activation of the sacral ventral roots.

A similar mechanism must underlie the inhibition of bladder reflexes produced by cutaneous afferent input from the perineal region. As mentioned above, in adult cats perineal stimulation blocked the reflex firing of sacral preganglionic neurons in response to bladder distension. However, perineal stimulation did not block the firing elicited by the iontophoretic administration of excitant amino acid[13,16]. It is reasonable to conclude, therefore, that this inhibition also occurred by disfacilitation.

On the other hand, distension of the rectum or mechanical stimulation of the anal canal inhibited micturition and firing of preganglionic neurons elicited reflexly or by the administration of an excitant amino acid. Thus this inhibition must be mediated at least in part by a direct depression of the preganglionic cells as well as at interneuronal sites (Fig. 4). The significance of anal- and perineal-induced inhibition is uncertain; however, it is tempting to speculate that the former may contribute to the reciprocal inhibition that occurs between urinary bladder and distal bowel and that the latter may be involved in the inhibition of bladder activity during copulation.

Sympathetic Reflex Pathways

Large intestine. Transection of the sympathetic innervation to the large intestine enhances spontaneous and neurally evoked intestinal motility, thus indicating that the intestine is subject to a tonic sympathetic inhibition[22,35,43,49]. The inhibition is related to a direct depression of smooth muscle as well as depression of synaptic transmission within the myenteric plexus[32]. Firing in sympathetic inhibitory fibers is generated in part by the central nervous system[22,35,49] and in part via peripheral reflex pathways in prevertebral ganglia[54,55].

Sympathetic inhibitory outflow from the spinal cord to the large intestine could be produced by several different mechanisms including: (1) reflexes initiated by afferent input from the gastrointestinal tract or other viscera, (2) local circuits at supraspinal centers analogous to the "medullary cardiovascular center", (3) local circuits within the spinal cord.

These possibilities were studied in the cat by simultaneously recording colonic motility and sympathetic efferent activity in the lumbar colonic nerves before and after lesions at various levels of the neuraxis. It was noted that spinal transection at the cervical level or isolation of the upper lumbar segments of the spinal cord by cord transection at T_{12} and L_5 coupled with transection of the lumbar dorsal roots bilaterally did not alter neural or intestinal activity[22]. However, destruction of the lumbar ventral roots or removal of the isolated segment of lumbar cord markedly reduced the sympathetic efferent discharge and enhanced colonic motility. These findings indicate that neither supraspinal mechanisms nor spinal afferent input are essential for the generation of the inhibitory outflow. By exclusion it must be related to existence of endogenous oscillator circuits in the lumbar cord. These pathways presumably can be modulated by afferent input from the small intestine or proximal colon and descending pathways from various areas in the brain[32,37,38,50].

Urinary bladder. Interruption of the sympathetic input to the urinary bladder by pharmacological agents or by transection of the hypogastric nerves enhances spontaneous and reflexly-evoked bladder contractions[29] and decreases the tone of the urethral sphincter[44]. These observations led to the proposal that sympathetic fibers provide a tonic inhibitory control over detrusor activity and an excitatory input to the urethra.

Various evidence indicates that these responses are generated reflexly by afferent activity arising in the bladder[23,28,29,44]. It has been shown that electrical stimulation of vesical afferents ($A\gamma\delta$) entering the sacral spinal cord or physiological activation of afferents by bladder distension evokes reflex firing in postganglionic sympathetic fibers in the hypogastric nerve and in nerves on the surface of the urinary bladder[28,29].

The responses were mediated by an intersegmental spinal pathway since they persisted following transection of the spinal cord at the lower thoracic level, but were abolished by bilateral lesions in the dorsolateral quadrants of the spinal cord at L_4–L_5. Reflex firing in postganglionic sympathetic fibers on the surface of the urinary bladder occurred at long latency (100–160 msec) following stimulation of vesical afferents. A major part of this latency represented conduction time in the peripheral efferent pathway, whereas the central delay for the reflex was relatively short ranging from 10–25 msec. The reflex was facilitated by distending the bladder with intravesical pressures below the threshold for inducing micturition; however, when bladder pressure was artifically raised above the micturition threshold the reflex was inhibited. This inhibition was abolished by transecting the spinal cord at a lower thoracic level[23], indicating that the inhibition originated at a supraspinal site, possibly the "pontine micturition center" (Fig. 5).

Activation of vesical afferents also evoked effector organ responses that could be attributed to sympathetic reflex firing[28]. Repetitive stimulation (one to 15 Hz) of afferents produced reflex inhibition of detrusor contractions, depression of transmission in vesical parasympathetic ganglia and a contraction of the trigonal region of the bladder. These responses mimicked the effects of stimulation of sympathetic efferents in the hypogastric nerve and were blocked by transection of the hypogastric nerves. The inhibitory responses were also abolished after the administration of adrenergic blocking agents.

Thus vesico-sympathetic reflexes have the potential for exerting an important regulatory influence on bladder activity. The pathway represents a negative feedback system whereby an increase in bladder pressure tends to increase inhibitory input to vesical ganglia and smooth muscle, thus allowing the bladder to accommodate to larger volumes. Increased sympathetic firing to the trigone would complement these mechanisms by increasing the tone of the bladder neck (internal urethral sphincter). During micturition these reflexes are probably depressed by supraspinal controls thereby allowing micturition to proceed uninhibited and the bladder to empty completely.

Role of the Monoamines in the Lumbosacral Reflex Pathways to the Urinary Bladder and Colon

Since autonomic nuclei in the spinal cord contain dense accumulations of monoaminergic terminals[9] there is considerable interest in the role of monoamines as transmitters in central autonomic pathways. Our studies of the sacral outflow indicate that the monoamines may have an inhibitory function. Norepinephrine and 5-hydroxytryptamine administered iontophoretically to sacral preganglionic neurons inhibited synaptic- and amino acid-evoked firing[51]. Furthermore the administration of 5-hydroxytryptophan (5-HTP), the precursor of 5-hydroxytryptamine, in a dose of 15–30 mg/kg i.v. depressed reflex firing in parasympathetic postganglionic fibers to the urinary bladder and colon as well as the reflex contractions of these organs[17]. The effects were not blocked by a peripherally-acting 1-amino acid decarboxylase inhibitor (MK 486), but were blocked by a centrally acting inhibitor (RO 4–4602), demonstrating that the conversion of 5-HTP to 5-hydroxytryptamine was necessary for the inhibitory effect. The depressant effects of 5-HTP on the bladder were observed in intact as well as chronic spinal animals, indicating that the site of action was at the spinal level.

The intravenous administration of clonidine, an agent which supposedly mimics the central actions of norepinephrine, had relatively weak depressant effects on parasympathetic reflexes but markedly depressed sympathetic reflexes to the bladder. On the other hand 5-HTP had weak facilitatory effects on vesico-sympathetic firing. These observations are consistent with the report that 5-hydroxytryptamine and norepinephrine, have excitatory and inhibitory effects, respectively, on sympathetic preganglionic neurons[24]. It is interesting however, that neither 5-HTP nor clonidine altered the lumbar sympathetic outflow to the colon.

These pharmacological data raise the possibility that bulbospinal serotonergic pathways exert an inhibitory influence on the sacral autonomic outflow to the urinary bladder and colon. On the other hand, descending noradrenergic pathways may inhibit lumbar sympathetic reflexes to the bladder.

SUMMARY

As indicated in Fig. 5 there are numerous differences in the organization of the lumbosacral reflex pathways to the urinary bladder and large intestine. Sympathetic inhibitory outflow to the bladder is initiated by vesical afferent activity via an inter-segmental spinal reflex, whereas sympathetic inhibitory input to the intestine is generated by peripheral reflexes in prevertebral ganglia and by endogenous oscillator circuits in the lumbar cord. Sympathetic reflexes to the bladder are inhibited by supraspinal mechanisms during micturition, whereas the inhibitory input to the colon seems to be unaltered during defecation.

Parasympathetic reflexes to these organs also differ, at least in cats with an intact neuraxis. Reflexes to the bladder are mediated by a supraspinal pathway which is activated only when bladder pressure exceeds the micturition threshold. This pathway is essentially involved in only one function: the elimination of urine. After destruction of bulbospinal pathways, micturition can be initiated by spinal reflexes. The mechanism underlying the emergence of these reflexes is not known.

In contrast to the sacral outflow to the bladder, the sacral parasympathetic reflex pathway to the large intestine is organized within the sacral spinal cord and may subserve various functions. This pathway is responsible for coordinating large amplitude, sustained, propulsive contractions which occur during defecation. In addition it seems to be involved in the regulation of nonpropulsive or segmental colonic activity and possibly the control of secretion or ion transport[5,38] and the modulation of myenteric inhibitory pathways to the rectum and colon[6,33]. The existence of a tonic discharge in intestinal sacral preganglionic neurons unrelated to excretory reflexes and the absence of such a discharge in bladder preganglionic neurons further underscores the difference in function of these two systems.

Information regarding interneuronal inputs to sacral preganglionic neurons is still very preliminary. Various indirect evidence indicates that both spinal and supraspinal reflex pathways to bladder and intestine are mediated by sacral inter-neurons and that these interneurons may be the locus for certain spinal inhibitions (Fig. 5). However, it is noteworthy that HRP tracing techniques show extensive dendritic processes extending from preganglionic neurons in both the colon and bladder part of the autonomic nucleus to a region of the dorsal horn (lamina 1) which contains axonal processes from primary afferents in the pelvic nerve[46]. These observations raise the possibility of direct synaptic contacts between visceral primary afferents and preganglionic neurons. Spinal reflexes to the intestine occur with a considerable central delay (45–60 msec) and therefore are unlikely to be monosynaptic; however, reflexes to bladder preganglionic neurons in chronic spinal animals occur with a very short latency (three to five msec) that more closely approaches the latency expected for a monosynaptic pathway.

In animals with an intact neuraxis the latencies for the micturition and defecation reflexes (i.e., time from afferent stimulation to postganglionic firing) are both very long. However, the micturition reflex which occurs over a much longer conduction distance surprisingly has a shorter latency (80–120 msec) than that of the defecation reflex (180–260 msec). This difference reflects in part the slow conduction velocity in the peripheral innervation to the intestine. It is also interesting that afferent and preganglionic efferent components in each reflex are matched according to conduction velocity and seem to complement the organization of the central pathways. For example, faster conducting fibers (A and B) are associated with the long spinobulbospinal micturition reflex and slower conducting fibers (C) are involved with the short spinal defecation reflex. The significance of these differences is uncertain, however it does appear that in contrast to bladder reflexes, intestinal reflexes are more primitive in their organization, probably subserve multiple functions and are appropriately designed for the regulation of a slowly-responding effector organ.

This research was supported in part by a NINDS grant NB 07923 and fellowships from Benevolent Foundation of Scottish Rites Freemasonry and the NIH.

REFERENCES

1   Barrington, F. J. F., The relation of the hindbrain to micturition, *Brain*, 44 (1921) 23–53.
2   Barrington, F. J. F., The effect of lesion of the hind- and midbrain on micturition in the cat, *Q. J. exp. Physiol.*, 15 (1925) 81–102.
3   Barrington, F. J. F., The component reflexes of micturition in the cat, Parts I and II, *Brain*, 54 (1931) 177–188.
4   Basbaum, A. I. and Fields, H. L., The dorsolateral funiculus of the spinal cord: A major route for descending brain stem control. *Society for Neuroscience Abstracts*, 3 (1977) 499.
5   Browning, J. G., Hardcastle, J., Hardcastle, P. T. and Sanford, P. A., The role of acetylcholine in the regulation of ion transport by rat colon mucosa, *J. Physiol* (Lond.), 272 (1977) 737–754.
6   Burnstock, G., Purinergic transmission. In: L. Iversen, S. Iversen and S. Snyder (Eds.), *Handbook of Psychopharmacology*, New York, Plenum Publishing 5, 1975, pp. 131–194.
7   Burton, H. and Lowey, A. D., Projections to the spinal cord from medullary somatosensory relay nuclei, *J. comp. Neurol.*, 173 (1977) 773–792.
8   Crowcroft, P. J., Holman, M. E. and Szurszewski, J. H., Excitatory input from the distal colon to the inferior mesenteric ganglion in the guinea-pig, *J. Physiol.* (Lond.), 219 (1971) 443–461.
9   Dahlstrom, A. and Fuxe, K., The distribution of monoamine terminals in the central nervous system. II. Experimentally induced changes in the interneuronal amine levels

of bulbospinal neuron systems, *Acta physiol. scand.*, 64, Suppl. 274 (1965) 1–36.

10 Denny-Brown, D. and Robertson, E. G., On the physiology of nervous control of defecation, *Brain*, 56 (1933) 149–190.

11 Denny-Brown, D. and Robertson, E. G., An investigation of the nervous control of defecation, *Brain*, 58 (1935) 256–310.

12 de Groat, W. C., The effects of glycine, GABA and strychnine on sacral parasympathetic preganglionic neurons, *Brain Res.*, 18 (1970) 542–544.

13 de Groat, W. C., Excitation and inhibition of sacral parasympathetic neurons by visceral and cutaneous stimuli in the cat, *Brain Res.*, 33 (1971) 499–503.

14 de Groat, W. C., Nervous control of the urinary bladder of the cat, *Brain Res.*, 87 (1975) 201–211.

15 de Groat, W. C., Mechanisms underlying recurrent inhibition in the sacral parasympathetic outflow to the urinary bladder, *J. Physiol.* (Lond.), 257 (1976) 503–513.

16 de Groat, W. C., Inhibitory mechanisms in the sacral reflex pathways to the urinary bladder. In: R. W. Ryall and J. S. Kelly (Eds.), *Iontophoresis and Transmitter Mechanisms in the Mammalian Central Nervous System.* Elsevier, Holland, 1978, pp. 366–368.

17 de Groat, W. C. and Douglas, J. W., The effects of L-5-hydroxytryptophan (5-HTP) and clonidine on central sympathetic and parasympathetic reflex pathways to the urinary bladder of the cat, *Fed. Proc.*, 34 (1975) 795.

18 de Groat, W. C., Douglas, J. W., Glass, J., Simonds, W., Weimer, B. and Werner, P., Changes in somato-vesical reflexes during postnatal development in the kitten, *Brain Res.*, 94 (1975) 150–154.

19 de Groat, W. C. and Krier, J., Preganglionic C-fibers: A major component of the sacral autonomic outflow to the colon of the cat, *Pflügers Arch.*, 359 (1975) 171–176.

20 de Groat, W. C. and Krier, J., An electrophysiological study of the sacral parasympathetic pathway to the colon of the cat, *J. Physiol.* (Lond.), 260 (1976) 425–445.

21 de Groat, W. C. and Krier, J., The sacral parasympathetic reflex pathway regulating colonic motility and defecation in the cat, *J. Physiol.* (Lond.), 276 (1978) 481–500.

22 de Groat, W. C. and Krier, J., The central control of the lumbar sympathetic pathway to the large intestine of the cat, *J. Physiol.* (Lond.), 289 (1979) n. pag.

23 de Groat, W. C. and Lalley, P. M., Reflex firing in the lumbar sympathetic outflow to activation of vesical afferent fibres, *J. Physiol.* (Lond.), 226 (1972) 289–309.

24 de Groat, W. C. and Ryall, R. W., An excitatory action of 5-hydroxytryptamine on sympathetic preganglionic neurones, *Exp. Brain Res.*, 3 (1967) 299–305.

25 de Groat, W. C. and Ryall, R. W., The identification and characteristics of sacral parasympathetic preganglionic neurones, *J. Physiol.* (Lond.), 196 (1968) 563–577.

26 de Groat, W. C. and Ryall, R. W., Recurrent inhibition in sacral parasympathetic pathways to the bladder, *J. Physiol.* (Lond.), 196 (1968) 579–591.

27 de Groat, W. C. and Ryall, R. W., Reflexes to sacral parasympathetic neurones concerned with micturition in the cat, *J. Physiol.* (Lond.), 200 (1969) 87–108.

28 de Groat, W. C. and Theobald, R. J., Sympathetic inhibitory reflexes to the urinary bladder and bladder ganglia evoked by electrical stimulation of vesical afferents, *J. Physiol.* (Lond.), 259, (1976) 223–237.

29 Edvardsen, P., Nervous control of urinary bladder in cats. I. The collecting phase, *Acta physiol. scand.*, 72 (1968) 157–171.

30 Edvardsen, P., Nervous control of urinary bladder in cats. II. The expulsion phase, *Acta physiol. scand.*, 72 (1968) 172–182.

31 Fox, M. W., Reflex development and behavioral organization. In: W. A. Himwich (Ed.), *Developmental Neurobiol.*, Thomas, Springfield, Ill., 1970, pp. 553–580.

32 Furness, J. B. and Costa, M., The adrenergic innervation of the gastrointestinal tract, *Ergebn. Physiol.*, 69 (1973) 1–52.

33 Gardette, B. and Gonella, J., Etude electromyographique *in vivo* de la commande nerveuse orthosympathique du colon chez le chat, *J. Physiol.* (Paris), 68 (1974) 671–692.

34 Garry, R. C., The responses to stimulation of the caudal end of the large bowel in the cat, *J. Physiol.* (Lond.), 78 (1933) 208–224.

35 Garry, R. C., The nervous control of the caudal region of the large bowel, *J. Physiol.* (Lond.), 77 (1933) 422–431.

36 Garry, R. C., The movements of the large intestine, *Physiol. Rev.*, 14 (1934) 103–132.

37 Gonella, J. and Gardette, B., Etude electromyographique *in vivo* de la commande nerveuse extrinseque parasympathique du colon, *J. Physiol.* (Paris), 68 (1974) 395–413.

38 Hulten, L., Extrinsic nervous control of colonic motility and blood flow, *Acta physiol. scand. suppl.* 335 (1969) 1–111.

39 Kuru, M., Nervous control of micturition, *Physiol. Rev.*, 45 (1965) 425–494.

40 Kypers, H., G. J. M. and Maiskey, V. A., Retrograde axonal transport of horseradish peroxidase from spinal cord to brain stem cell groups in the cat, *Neuroscience Letters*, 1 (1975) 9–14.

41 Lalley, P. M., de Groat, W. C. and McLain, P. L., Activation of the sacral parasympathetic pathway to the urinary bladder by brainstem stimulation, *Fed. Proc.*, 31 (1972) 386.

42 Langley, J. N. and Anderson, H. K., The innervation of the pelvic and adjoining viscera. Part II. The bladder, *J. Physiol.* (Lond.), 19 (1895) 71–84.

43 Learmonth, J. R. and Markowitz, J., Studies of the function of the lumbar sympathetic outflow, *Amer. J. Physiol.*, 89 (1929) 686–691.

44 Mahony, D. T., Laferte, R. O. and Blais, D. J., Integral storage and voiding reflexes, neurophysiologic concept of continence and micturition, *Urology*, 9 (1977) 95–106.

45 Milne, R. J., Booth, A. M. and de Groat, W. C., Firing patterns of preganglionic neurons and interneurons in the sacral autonomic nucleus of the cat, *Society for Neuroscience Abstracts*, 4 (1978) 22.

46 Morgan, C., de Groat, W. C. and Nadelhaft, I., Identification of visceral afferents to the sacral cord of the cat using horseradish peroxidase, *Society for Neuroscience*, 4 (1978) 23.

47 Nadelhaft, I., Morgan, C., Schauble, T. and de Groat, W. C., Localization of the sacral autonomic (parasympathetic) nucleus in the spinal cord of cat and monkey by the horseradish peroxidase technique, *Society for Neuroscience Abstracts*, 3 (1977) 75.

48 Nadelhaft, I., Morgan, C. W. and de Groat, W. C., Localization of the sacral autonomic nucleus in the spinal cord of the cat by the horseradish peroxidase technique, *J. comp. Neurol.*, submitted.

49 Rostad, H., Colonic motility in the cat. II. Extrinsic nervous control, *Acta physiol. scand.*, 89 (1973) 91–103.

50 Rostad, H., Colonic motility in the cat. IV. Peripheral pathways mediating the effects induced by hypothalamic and mesencephalic stimulation, *Acta physiol. scand.*, 89 (1973) 154–168.

51 Ryall, R. W. and de Groat, W. C., The microelectrophoretic administration of noradrenaline, 5-hydroxytryptamine, acetylcholine and glycine to sacral parasympathetic preganglionic neurones, *Brain Res.*, 37 (1972) 345–348.

52 Sato, A., Sato, Y., Sugimoto, H. and Terui, N., Reflex changes in the urinary bladder after mechanical and thermal stimulation of the skin at various segmental levels in cats, *Neuroscience*, 2 (1977) 111–117.

53 Schofield, G. C., Experimental studies of the myenteric plexus in mammals, *J. comp. Neurol.*, 119 (1962) 159–179.

54 Szurszewski, J. H. and Weems, W. A., Control of gastrointestinal motility by prevertebral ganglia. In: E. Bülbring and M. F. Shuba (Eds.), *Physiology of Smooth Muscle*, 1976, pp. 313–319.

55 Weems, W. A. and Szurszewski, J. H., Modulation of colonic motility by peripheral neural inputs to neurons of the inferior mesenteric ganglion, *Gastroenterology*, 73 (1977) 273–278.

CHAPTER 5

CONTROL OF LIVER FUNCTION AND NEUROENDOCRINE REGULATION OF BLOOD GLUCOSE LEVELS

A. Niijima

Department of Physiology, Niigata University School of Medicine, Niigata, Japan

INTRODUCTION

It is well known that blood glucose is a major source of energy for cellular activities and the liver is an important organ for the storage of glucose in the form of glycogen. It is generally recognized that the maintenance of blood glucose levels is relatively constant, and catecholamines (epinephrine and norepinephrine) released from the adrenal gland and insulin and glucagon released from the pancreas play important roles in the regulation of these levels. Insulin is a key substance in controlling the entry of glucose into the cell and the utilization of glucose in the cell. Another insulin effect is to increase the storage of glycogen in the liver and other tissues. These actions of insulin result in a fall in blood glucose levels. Glucagon, epinephrine and norepinephrine cause the release of glucose from the liver into the circulating blood by stimulating hepatic glycogenolysis. It is known that during starvation an increase in the rate of secretion of glucagon and epinephrine and norepinephrine occurs which causes a facilitation of release of glucose from the liver and plays an important role in the maintenance of blood glucose concentration above the lower limit of the physiological range. This is an important factor, guaranteeing a reasonable utilization of glucose by the body and brain cells. It can be stated that insulin is an indispensable hormone for the utilization of glucose, and epinephrine, norepinephrine and glucagon are the hormones which raise and maintain the glucose levels in order to support the utilization of blood glucose. It has been reported that sympathetic nerve stimulation to the adrenal medullae causes release of epinephrine and norepinephrine into the circulating blood, which results in release of glucose from the liver. Although it is mainly stated that the glucose concentration of blood plasma has a direct effect on the islet of Langerhans in the pancreas in controlling the rate of insulin and glucagon secretion, the existence of an autonomic neural control mechanism for regulating the rate of secretion of these substances is strongly suggested.

Recently, it has been reported by many workers, as described below, that electrical stimulation of the vagus nerve or splanchnic nerve causes a change in insulin and glucagon outputs from the pancreas.

Frohman[15] and other workers[21] reported an increase in plasma insulin concentration in response to stimulation of the peripheral end of the vagus nerve in the dog; Daniel and Henderson[9] observed a similar response in the baboon. Insulin release occurred in response to vagal stimulation in the isolated perfused pancreas[14] and the effect could be mimicked by acetylcholine[20] *in vivo* and *in vitro*[18] showing that it is a direct response to stimulation of parasympathetic fibers innervating the pancreas. Stimulation of efferent vagal fibers also caused release of pancreatic glucagon in the dog[22] and the calf[7]. Release of glucagon by the vagus seems to be due to stimulation of acetylcholine receptors within the islets since the effect could be reproduced by administration of acetylcholine[18,20,22].

Edwards and Bloom reported[5] that stimulation of the peripheral ends of the splanchnic nerves invariably caused a profound inhibition of insulin release in adrenalectomized animals of various species. These reports are in accord with those of Miller[25] and Girardier[16], and Seydoux and Campfield. Inhibition of insulin release during sympathetic stimulation was first demonstrated by Porte[35]. He reported that it is due to the activation of α-receptors. Recently it has been stated by Smith and Porte[44] that the activation of β-receptors of B cells in the islet provides a tonic stimulation of insulin release.

Stimulation of the splanchnic innervation to the pancreas has been shown to cause release of pancreatic glucagon in cats, dogs, calves and sheep[5,6,13,16,19]. A review of neural control of endocrine pancrease was recently published by Woods and Porte[47].

It has been reported by Edwards, Silver and other workers[12,41] that stimulation of the peripheral end of the splanchnic nerve rapidly depletes glycogen reserves in the liver and raises the concentration of glucose in the circulatory plasma with both adrenal glands removed. They mentioned that the response is due to the activation of sympathetic nerve branches innervating the liver. Shimazu and Amakawa[41,42] have shown that maximal splanchnic nerve stimulation in the rabbit causes activation of the two glycogenolytic enzymes, phosphorylase and glucose-6-phosphatase, in the liver. Furthermore, the results these workers obtained show that enzyme activation in response to nerve stimulation reaches a maximum within 30 sec, and they concluded that the sympathetic innervation represents a more rapid means of controlling the activity of the hepatic glycogenolytic enzymes than catecholamines released from the adrenal medulla. Shimazu[40] further reported that electrical stimulation of the vagus nerve in the pancreatectomized rabbit resulted in a marked increase in the total activity of liver glycogen synthetase. These results suggest that vagal stimulation results directly in acceleration of glycogenesis in the liver and decrease in blood glucose.

Anand[1], Oomura and other workers[32,33] proved the existence of glucose-sensitive nerve cells in the hypothalamic region by means of an electrophysiological technique. It might be expected that these glucose sensitive nerve cells send signals to the adrenal medullae to release epinephrine and norepinephrine, and to the pancreas to release insulin and glucagon.

Besides these glucose-sensitive neurons in the hypothalamic region, Russek[36] suggested the existence of glucoreceptors in the liver which send signals through the vagus nerve to the central nervous system. He mentioned that these receptors monitor the blood glucose levels of the portal venous blood, and that signals from these glucoreceptors play a role in the regulation of glucose levels in the systemic blood. These receptors may have the reflex effect of controlling activity in adrenal and pancreatic nerves.

It has been shown in several species that there is a cephalic phase of insulin secretion that occurs within a few minutes after the onset of a meal. This rapid secretion of insulin is believed to precede absorption of glucose into the blood and is attributed to increased neural input to the pancreas. Woods[48] described in his paper how this contention is supported by the observation that the cephalic phase of insulin secretion occurs when animals are sham fed, that it occurs when animals eat nonnutritive substances and that it is eliminated by removal of the vagal input to the pancreas via vagotomy. Steffens[45] observed in rats that during a meal insulin and glucagon levels rise during the first minute. He mentioned that these early rises in insulin and glucagon levels are caused by receptors in the oral cavity and it is tempting to conclude that the ventromedial hypothalamus is part of a reflex arc mediating insulin and glucagon release. It is also reported that sensory input from oropharyngeal receptors can be traced into the hypothalamus[24,38]. Stomach and gut wall receptors send information to the hypothalamus through the vagus nerve[39]. Mei, Boyer and Arlhac[23] recorded unitary discharges from the nodose ganglion cells of the cat induced by intestinal perfusion with glucose solution. They reported that stimulation of these intestinal glucoreceptors produces an enhancement of the insulin release via the vagus nerve. Studies of the innervation of endocrine pancreas and the liver reported here present information about the nervous regulatory mechanism of blood glucose levels. These studies can be classified following four categories: 1) studies on the relationship between blood glucose levels and pancreatic and adrenal nerve activities; 2) innervation of the liver and its role in the regulation of blood glucose levels; 3) glucose-sensitive afferent nerve fibers in the liver and regulation of blood glucose; 4) oral and gastrointestinal inputs for the regulation of blood glucose levels.

This paper will deal with our work on these four subjects in connection with the neural regulatory mechanism of blood glucose levels.

METHODS AND RESULTS

Studies of the Relationship between Blood Glucose Levels and Pancreatic and Adrenal Nerve Activities

Adult rabbits of both sexes were used for the recording of efferent nerve discharges. The animals were anesthetized by intravenous (i.v.) injection of pentobarbitone (25–35 mg/kg), and the trachea intubated. Glucose and other test solutions were injected through a catheter placed in the cranial end of the carotid artery or the cardiac side of the jugular vein. Before intra-arterial injection, both depressor nerves were cut and the sinus nerves were severed bilaterally by pinching with a pair of forceps to eliminate the effect of baroreceptor reflex following injection. Samples of arterial blood were withdrawn from a catheter inserted into the cardiac side of the carotid artery for estimation of glucose content. Efferent discharges were mainly recorded from fine filaments dissected from splanchnic nerve branches innervating the left adrenal gland (adrenal nerve) and vagal nerve branches innervating the pancreas. Dissections were made under a binocular microscope ($\times 16$). The discharge was amplified by means of a condenser-coupled amplifier, monitored by an oscilloscope and stored on magnetic tape. All analyses of nervous activity were performed after conversion of raw data to standard pulses by a window discriminator, which picked out discharge from background noise. The standard pulses were then fed to a rate-meter with a reset time of five or ten sec for studying the time course of discharge rate. The discharge rate was displayed on a polygraph record along with the signals indicating injections.

Recordings were made on multi-unit nerve preparations in most of the experiments. Following i.a. injection of 3 ml of 10% D-glucose solution, a decrease in discharge rate was observed in the adrenal nerve filament. Injection of the same amount of D-mannose solution and physiological saline were without effect[27]. An i.a. injection of 3 ml of 10% D-glucose solution, caused an increase in discharge rate in the pancreatic (coeliac) branch of the vagus nerve. The same amount of 10% D-mannose solution and physiological saline showed no effect.

In the next experiment, 1.5 ml 5% D-mannose solution (isotonic) was mixed with 1.5 ml physiological saline. The isotonic mixed solution contained 75 mg mannose in 3 ml. The injection of this solution into the carotid artery caused no change in the firing rate of the adrenal nerve or that of the pancreatic branch of the vagus nerve. An injection of 3 ml isotonic glucose solution, which was made by 1.5 ml 5% D-glucose solution (isotonic) mixed with 1.5 ml physiological saline and contains 75 mg glucose, caused a remarkable decrease in the firing rate of adrenal nerve and an increase in the activity of pancreatic branch of the vagus nerve.

In the third experiment, the effects of injection of glucose into the carotid artery and jugular vein on the rate of single unit discharge in the adrenal nerve filament were compared. An i.a. injection of 0.1 ml of 10 mg/kg D-glucose dissolved in physiological saline caused a slight decrease in firing rate after the injection. A more remarkable depression in firing rate was followed by an i.a. injection of 25 mg/kg D-glucose solution (0.25 ml). However, little change in activity was observed after i.v. injection of the same dose of glucose (Fig. 1A). Also, i.a. injection of glucose was much more effective than i.v. injection in increasing the discharge rate of the pancreatic branch of the vagus nerve.

These results can be summarized as follows. First, injection of glucose into the carotid artery caused a decrease in the firing rate of efferent fibers in the adrenal nerve and an increase of firing rate in the pancreatic branch of the vagus nerve; however, mannose showed no effects. Second, it is unlikely that hypertonicity of the solution injected into the carotid artery caused these responses. Third, injection of glucose into the carotid artery was much more effective than injections made into the jugular vein. It is concluded from these observations that glucose itself has, but mannose does not have, the effect of decreasing activity of the adrenal nerve and increasing it in the pancreatic branch of the vagus nerve. An associated suggestion is that the glucose-sensitive area in the brain probably plays a major role in changing activity of these two nerve bundles.

It is recognized that there are two centers in the hypothalamus regulating food intake, designated as a feeding center in the lateral hypothalamus (LHA) and a satiety center in the ventromedial hypothalamus (VMH)[2,3]. It has been reported that systemic

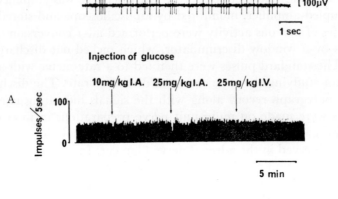

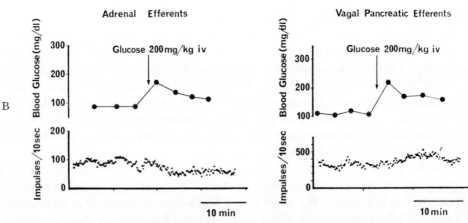

Fig. 1. A: Single unit discharge recorded from a fine filament of the adrenal nerve and
effect of glucose on the discharge rate. Upper trace shows single unit discharge.
Lower trace shows the time course of discharge rate. B: Effect of i. v. injection of
glucose on the blood glucose levels and efferent discharge rate.

administration, as well as direct application of glucose, increases the discharge rate of
VMH neurons and decreases that of LHA neurons[1,8,32]. The depressive effect of glucose
infusion on the activity of the adrenal nerve might be initiated in these hypothalamic
neurons and mediated through a pathway to the adrenal nerve cells in the spinal cord,
since transection of the spinal cord abolished the depressive effect of glucose[28]. Activity
of the pancreatic branch of the vagus nerve was drastically decreased after bilateral
section of the cervical vagus. The activating effect of glucose on the pancreatic branch
of the vagus nerve was abolished after vagotomy. These observations suggest that the
activation of the pancreatic branch of the vagus nerve following infusion of glucose
might originate in the glucose-sensitive LHA and VMH neurons of the hypothalamus.

It has been reported that the administration of 2-deoxy-D-glucose (2-DG), an
analogue of glucose, increase feeding in response to decreased glucose utilization[43] and
that the hypothalamus is sensitive to this substance[4]. For this reason we can expect
that this substance may have effects similar to those of hypoglycemia on the activity

of glucose-sensitive hypothalamic neurons. Increased epinephrine production, following administration of 2-DG has also been reported[17]. In our experiments after injection of 250 mg/kg 2-DG a remarkable increase in discharge rate of adrenal filament was observed. An increase in epinephrine production and a rise in blood glucose level following 2-DG administration can be explained in this light. In the pancreatic branch of the vagus nerve i.v. injection of the same amount of 2-DG caused a decrease in discharge rate.

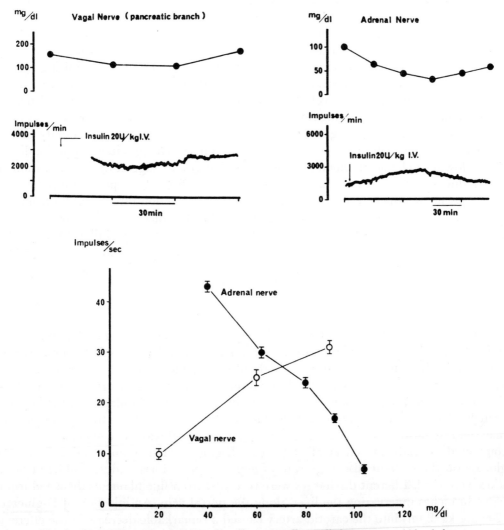

Fig. 2.   Top: Effect of i. v. infusion of insulin on the efferent discharge rate and blood glucose levels. Left, time course of the discharge rate of pancreatic branch of the vagus nerve. Right, time course of the discharge rate of the adrenal nerve. Bottom: Relationship between glucose concentration in the arterial blood and efferent discharge rate. Full circles, discharge rate of adrenal nerve with standard errors. Open circles, discharge rate of pancreatic branch of the vagus nerve with standard errors.

The next experiments show the relationship between glucose content in arterial blood and efferent discharge rate in the adrenal nerve and pancreatic branch of the vagus nerve. It was observed that an elevation of blood glucose levels following i.v. injection of D-glucose 200 mg/kg accompanied a decrease in discharge rate in the adrenal nerve and an increase of it in the pancreatic branch of the vagus nerve (Fig. 1B).

A decrease in blood glucose concentration following i.v. injection of regular insulin (20 U/kg), which lasted about two-and-one-half hours caused an increase in discharge rate in the adrenal nerve[27]. The lowest value of blood glucose concentration coincided with the peak of the discharge rate. A decrease in blood glucose levels after i.v. administration of the same amount of insulin accompanied a decrease in efferent discharge rate in the pancreatic branch of the vagus nerve[27] (Fig. 2, top). Figure 2 (bottom) shows the relationship between glucose content in the arterial blood and firing rate of efferent fibers in the adrenal nerve and pancreatic branch of the vagus nerve. It shows that the higher the glucose level, the lower the discharge rate in the adrenal nerve. On the contrary, a higher firing rate was observed at higher blood glucose levels in the pancreatic branch of the vague nerve[27]. These results show that the activity of the adrenal nerve and pancreatic branch of the vagus nerve changes in an opposite direction following a change in blood glucose levels. The results suggest that an elevation of blood glucose levels causes an increase in nerve signals from the hypothalamus through the vagus nerve which results in an increase in the secretion rate of insulin from the islet of Langerhans in the pancreas. A fall in blood glucose levels causes activation of the nerve pathway from the hypothalamus to adrenal medullae through the splanchnic nerve which results in an increase in the rate of secretion of epinephrine and norepinephrine. The former response supports the utilization of glucose and the latter response guarantees a lower level of blood glucose.

Innervation of the Liver and Its Role in the Regulation of Blood Glucose Levels

There are reports of a hyperglycemic response and depletion of glycogen reserves in the liver following stimulation of the peripheral cut end of the splanchnic nerve in calves and other animal species with both adrenal glands removed[10,11,12]. It was observed in the isolated liver of the toad that a remarkable increase in glucose concentration occurred in the perfusate from the liver in response to stimulation of the hepatic branch of the splanchnic nerve[30]. The glucose-sensitive neurons in the hypothalamus may send signals to the liver through the splanchnic pathway. The experiments were conducted to study the effect of D-glucose, L-glucose, D-mannose and 2-deoxy-D-glucose on the efferent discharge rate of hepatic nerve fibers. Adult rabbits of both sexes were used. Efferent discharges were recorded from fine filaments dissected from nerve branches innervating the liver along the portal vein. An injection of D-glucose (200 mg/kg, 2 ml) into the carotid artery caused a remarkable decrease in the efferent discharge rate of the hepatic nerve which lasted about three min. An intra-arterial injection of L-glucose and D-mannose (200 mg/kg, 2 ml, each) showed no decrease in firing rate (Fig. 3A, upper trace). An i.v. injection of the same amount of D-glucose showed a smaller effect on firing rates. An i.v. injection of 2-deoxy-D-glucose caused a remarkable increase in firing rates which lasted longer than three hours (Fig. 3A,

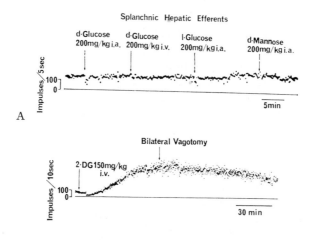

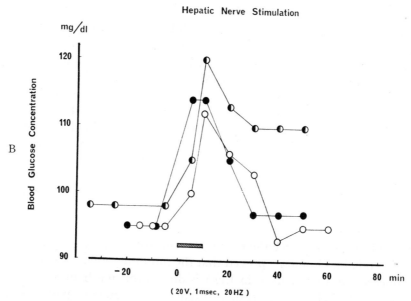

Fig. 3. A: Time course of the discharge rate of sympathetic efferents in the hepatic branch of the splanchnic nerve. Upper trace, effect of injection of glucose and mannose. Lower trace, effect of i. v. injection of 2-DG. B: Effect of repetitive stimulation of the peripheral end of hepatic branch of the splanchnic nerve on blood glucose concentration. Condition of stimulation, 20 V, one msec, 20 Hz for 10 min.

lower trace). Bilateral vagotomy, indicated by an arrow, made no change in firing rate, indicating that the nerve signals are not mediated by the vagus nerve but through the splanchnic nerve.

In the next experiments the relationship between glucose content in arterial blood and efferent discharge rate in the hepatic nerve was studied. A gradual decrease in blood glucose concentration from 130 mg/dl to 110 mg/dl following i.v. injection of regular insulin (Novo, 40 U/kg) caused a gradual increase in discharge rate. These results show that the increase in glucose levels in carotid arterial blood causes the decrease, and the decrease in glucose levels results in an increase in the efferent discharge rate in the hepatic branch of the splanchnic nerve. The existence of a nerve pathway from glucose-sensitive nerve cells in the hypothalamus to the liver through the hepatic branch of the splanchnic nerve is suggested by these results. As shown in Fig. 3B, repetitive stimulation of the cut end of the hepatic branch of the splanchnic nerve results in an increase in blood glucose levels indicating the activation of this system plays a role in the release of glucose from the liver.

Glucose Sensitive Afferent Nerve Fibers in the Liver and Regulation of Blood Glucose

Besides the regulation of blood glucose levels through nerve loops connecting glucose-sensitive neurons in the hypothalamic region and adrenal medulla and islet of Langerhans, a reflex control of blood glucose by the glucose-sensitive afferents in the liver will be considered. The existence of glucoreceptors in the liver was pointed out of Russek[36]. Electrophysiological observations of these afferents were made in perfused liver preparations in the guinea pig[26]. Afferent discharge in the hepatic branch of the vagus nerve showed a decrease in the firing rate following administration of glucose through the portal vein to the liver. In the next step of these studies, experiments were made in the guinea pig *in vivo*. Accompanying a gradual increase in glucose content in the portal venous blood which followed intraduodenal infusion of 5% glucose (5 ml) a decrease in afferent discharge rates of hepatic efferents was observed (Fig. 4B). These observations demonstrated that an increase in glucose concentration in portal venous blood results in a decrease in the rate of signals from the liver to the central nervous system, perhaps to the hypothalamic region through the vagus nerve.

It was also confirmed that after infusion of 15 μg ouabain into the portal vein, an injection of D-glucose made no change in the firing rate. The decrease in the firing rate of the hepatic afferents by glucose seems to be due to the activation of the energy-dependent sodium pump, since the reaction is effectively blocked by a cardiac glycoside such as ouabain. Oomura[24] proved that the inhibitory effect of glucose on the activity of glucose-sensitive neurons in LHA is due to this mechanism.

A report by Schmitt[37] suggests the existence of a splanchnic pathway of hepatic-portal glucose-sensitive afferents which runs to the LHA neurons in the hypothalamus; this was supported by recording of single cell activity by microelectrodes.

To study the reflex effect of these glucose-sensitive afferents in the liver on the activity of adrenal nerve and pancreatic branch of the vagus nerve, we performed a number of experiments on rabbits. A catheter was inserted into the portal vein and another catheter was placed in the left jugular vein for glucose infusion. The mean discharge rates of these two nerves before and after injection of glucose were compared. To calculate the mean discharge rate, the number of spikes in a five-sec period was averaged over 50 sec in the adrenal nerve, and over 100 sec in the pancreatic branch of the vagus nerve. As seen in Fig. 4A, the results show that i.v. infusion of D-glucose 25 mg/kg caused no significant difference in the mean discharge rate of the adrenal nerve and pancreatic branch of the vagus nerve after the infusion.

However, i.p.v. infusion of the same amount of glucose resulted in a significant

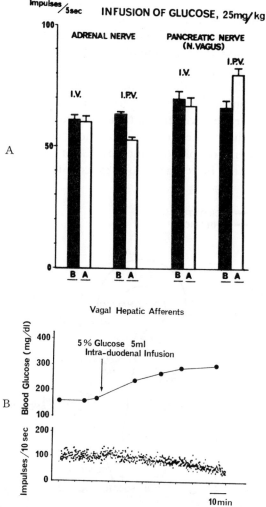

Fig. 4. A: Reflex effect of infusion of glucose (25 mg/kg) on the efferent discharge rate of the adrenal nerve and pancreatic branch of the vagus nerve. *A*, before infusion of glucose. *B*, after infusion. Each column shows mean±S. E. (N=10, adrenal nerve and N=20, pancreatic branch of the vagus nerve).

B: Effect of intraduodenal infusion of glucose on the glucose content of portal venous blood and firing rate of glucose-sensitive afferents from the liver.

decrease in the mean discharge rate in the adrenal nerve after the infusion (p<0.01). The i.p.v. infusion of glucose also caused a significant increase in the discharge rate of pancreatic branch of the vagus nerve after the infusion (0.01<p<0.02).

These results mean that an increase in glucose concentration in the portal venous blood causes a reflex inhibition of adrenal nerve activity and reflex activation of pancreatic nerve firing. The reflex change in activities of these two nerves may cause a change in the rate of secretion of epinephrine and insulin, presumably a decrease in epinephrine secretion and an increase in insulin secretion. Our studies on these three subjects demonstrated that there is a nervous control of the secretion of insulin, epinephrine and norepinephrine. The pathway controlling insulin secretion is from the hypothalamus to the B cells in the islet of Langerhans via the pancreatic branch of the vagus nerve. The pathway for epinephrine secretion is from hypothalamus to the adrenal medulla via the splanchnic nerve. The pathway of direct sympathetic innervation of the liver cells is via the hepatic branch of the splanchnic nerve. Norepinephrine might be a substance released from the nerve terminal of this system. Hyperglycemia following repetitive stimulation of hepatic branch of the splanchnic nerve is likely due to the direct effect of this substance on liver cells. Vasoconstriction in the liver following liberation of norepinephrine from the sympathetic nerve terminals may play a role in the increase of blood glucose levels by squeezing out portal

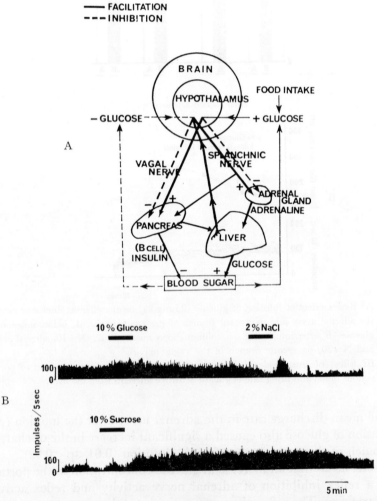

Fig. 5.   A: Block diagram of humoral and nervous network for the regulation of blood glucose levels. B: Effect of application of glucose, sucrose and NaCl solution to the tongue surface on the efferent discharge rate of coeliac branch of the vagus nerve.

venous blood, which contains a large amount of glucose, into the systemic circulations. There might be two other pathways, via vagus and splanchnic nerves from hypothalamus to A cells in the islet of Langerhans. These systems might work through control of the secretion of glucagon. Still another possible pathway, which is suggested by Shimazu[40] and Szabo[46], is from hypothalamus to the liver through the vagus nerve. Electrophysiological observations should be employed to study the possible function of these last three systems.

Results of the above-described experiments show that activity of efferent nerves from the hypothalamus to the endocrine pancreas, liver and adrenal medulla are not only directly controlled by blood glucose levels but also controlled by ascending nerve signals from the glucose-sensitive afferents in the liver. A schematic block diagram of these nervous networks is shown in Fig. 5A.

Oral and Gastro-intestinal Inputs as Regulatory Mechanisms Governing Blood Glucose Levels

Steffens observed a rise of plasma insulin in the rat during the first minute of a meal which preceded the second well-recognized rise of insulin level coincident with the increase in blood glucose level. He named this phenomenon the early rise in insulin (EIR)[45]. He indicated that the oral cavity plays a major role in bringing about EIR. Since an increase in activity of taste and smell receptors can be followed into the VMH, this area may be a candidate for mediating the EIR. It is known that the VMH projects to the nuclei of the autonomic system, which plays an important role in the release of insulin[47].

Experiments were conducted in the rat to study the EIR by means of electro-physiological techniques. Under anesthesia with urethane (1 g/kg, i.p. injection) efferent discharges were recorded from the central cut end of the coeliac nerve branch, which contains the efferent nerve fibers to the pancreas, from the vagus nerve. A ratemeter was used to observe the time course of the discharge. As shown in Fig. 5B an application of 10% D-glucose to the tongue, which was washed away about five min after application, caused an abrupt increase in discharge rate that lasted about 30 min. An application of 10% sucrose caused a stronger and longer increase in firing rate; this lasted about 50 min. On the contrary, an application of 2% NaCl solution caused a drastic decrease in the firing rate.

It is likely that the taste of sweetness causes an increase in the efferent activity of the coeliac branch of the vagus nerve, which in turn possibly increases the rate of secretion of insulin from the pancreas. The observations made by Steffens can be explained in this light.

In electrophysiological studies of the glucoreceptors in the gastrointestinal canal we observed an increase in afferent discharge rate recorded from the peripheral cut end of the coeliac branch of the vagus nerve during perfusion of 10% D-glucose solution through the duodeno-intestinal canal. Although this result suggests the existence of glucoreceptors in the wall of the duodeno-intestinal canal, further carefully performed studies should be attempted relative to this subject.

DISCUSSION

Experiments were conducted on four subjects which were described as the four main categories of interest relative to the control of liver function and neuroendocrine regulation of blood glucose levels. These were as follows: 1) studies of the relationship between blood glucose levels and pancreatic and adrenal nerve activities; 2) innervation of the liver and its role in the regulation of blood glucose levels; 3) glucose-sensitive afferent nerve fibers in the liver and regulation of blood glucose thereby; 4) oral and gastrointestinal inputs possibly involved in the regulatory mechanism controlling blood glucose levels.

With respect to the first subject, the results showed that an increase in the blood glucose content causes an increase in the activity of the pancreatic branch of the vagus nerve and causes a decrease in the activity of the adrenal nerve. The results further demonstrated that a decrease in blood glucose activated the sympatho-adrenal system and suppressed the vago-pancreatic system. It is rational that these responses should be involved in the maintenance of blood glucose levels. Studies on the second subject have clarified the conclusion that sympathetic innervation of the liver may play a direct role in providing for a prompt hyperglycemic response through the liberation of norepinephrine from the nerve terminals to the liver cells. The experiments conducted relative to the third subject have indicated that the role of the glucose-sensitive afferents in the liver is to initiate a reflex control of the blood glucose levels. With respect to the fourth subject it can now be stated that the concept of an EIR response, reported by Steffens, is supported by our electrophysiological observations.

From these experimental results a block diagram of the nervous and humoral networks involved in the regulation of the blood glucose levels has been devised (Fig. 5A).

SUMMARY

Intra-arterial injection into the carotid artery and i.v. injection of glucose caused a decrease in efferent discharge rate of the adrenal nerve and an increase in discharge rate of the pancreatic branch of the vagus nerve. It is likely that these responses are due to the increase in blood glucose content. Decrease in blood glucose levels following injection of insulin increased adrenal nerve activity and caused a decrease in the activity of the pancreatic branch of the vagus nerve. Administration of 2-DG resulted in an increase in adrenal nerve activity and a decrease in pancreatic nerve activity. The results suggest the existence of a nervous regulatory mechanism of blood glucose levels. A reflex mechanism from the glucose-sensitive afferents in the liver for the regulation of the blood glucose levels was also investigated and found present. It was further observed that an oral application of glucose or sucrose increased the efferent discharge rate of the coeliac branch of the vagus nerve and an application of 2% NaCl solution suppressed the firing rate. This response might be related to the early rise in insulin levels during meals.

REFERENCES

1 Anand, B. K., Chhina, G. S., Sharma, K. N., Dus, S. and Singh, B., Activity of single neurons in the hypothalamic feeding centers: Effect of glucose, *Amer. J. Physiol.*, 207 (1964) 1146–1154.

2 Anand, B. K., Nervous regulation of food intake, *Physiol. Rev.*, 41 (1961) 677–708.

3 Anand, B. K., Dua, S. and Shoenberg, K., Hypothalamic control of food intake in cats and monkeys, *J. Physiol.* (Lond.), 127 (1955) 143–152.

4 Balagura, S. and Kanner, M., Hypothalamic sensitivity to 2-deoxy-d-glucose and glucose effect on feeding behavior, *Physiol. Behav.*, 7 (1971) 251–255.

5 Bloom, S. R. and Edwards, A. V., The release of pancreatic glucagon and inhibition of insulin in response to stimulation of the sympathetic innervation, *J. Physiol.* (Lond.), 253 (1975) 157–173.

6 Bloom, S. R., Edwards, A. V. and Vaughan, N. J. A., The role of the sympathetic innervation in the control of plasma glucagon concentration in the calf, *J. Physiol.* (Lond.), 233 (1973) 457–466.

7 Bloom, S. R., Edwards, A. V. and Vaughan, N. J. A., The role of the autonomic innervation in the control of plasma glucagon concentration in the calf, *J. Physiol.* (Lond.), 236 (1974) 611–623.

8 Brown, K. A. and Melzack, R., Effect of glucose on multi-unit activity in the hypothalamus, *Exp. Neurol*, 24 (1969) 363–373.

9 Daniel, P. M. and Henderson, J. R., The effect of vagal stimulation on plasma insulin and glucose levels in the baboon, *J. Physiol.* (Lond.), 192 (1967) 317–326.

10 Edwards, A. V., The glycogenolytic response to stimulation of the splanchnic nerves in adrenalectomized calves, sheep, dogs, cats and pigs, *J. Physiol.* (Lond.), 213 (1971) 741–759.

11 Edwards, A. V., The hyperglycaemic response to stimulation of the hepatic sympathetic innervation in adrenalectomized cats and dogs, *J. Physiol.* (Lond.), 220 (1972) 697–716.

12 Edwards, A. V. and Silver, M., The glycogenolytic response to stimulation of the splanchnic nerves in adrenalectomized calves, *J. Physiol.* (Lond.), 211 (1970) 109–124.

13 Esterhuizen, A. C. and Howell, S. L., Ultrastructure of the A-cells of cat islets of Langerhans following sympathetic stimulation of glucagon secretion, *J. Cell Biology*, 46 (1970) 593–631.

14 Findlay, J. A., Gill, J. R., Lever, J. D., Randle, P. J. and Springgs, T. L. B., Increased insulin output following stimulation of the vagal supply to the perfused rabbit pancreas, *J. Anat.*, 104 (1969) 580.

15 Frohman, L. A., Ezdinli, E. Z. and Javid, R., Effect of vagotomy and vagal stimulation on insulin secretion, *Diabetes*, 16 (1967) 443–448.

16 Girardier, L., Seydoux, J. and Campfield, L. A., Control of A and B cells *in vivo* by sympathetic nervous input and selective hyper- or hypo-glycemia in dog pancreas, *J. Physiol.* (Paris), 72 (1976) 801–814.

17 Hokfelt, B. and Bydgeman, S., Increased adrenaline production following administration of 2-deoxy-d-glucose in the rat, *Proc. Soc. exp. Biol. Med.*, 106 (1961) 537–539.

18 Iversen, J., Effect of acetylcholine on the secretion of glucagon and insulin, from the isolated perfused canine pancreas, *Diabetes*, 22 (1973) 381–387.

19 Kaneto, A., Kajinuma, H. and Kosaka, K., Effect of splanchnic nerve stimulation on glucagon and insulin output in the dog, *Ednocrinology*, 96 (1975) 143–150.

20   Kaneto, A. and Kosaka, K., Stimulation of glucagon and insulin secretion by acetylcho-
     line infused intrapancreatically, *Endocrinology*, 95 (1974) 676–681.

21   Kaneto, A., Kosaka, K. and Nakao, K., Effects of stimulation of the vagus nerve on
     insulin secretion, *Endocrinology*, 80 (1967) 530–536.

22   Kaneto, A., Miki, E. and Kosaka, K., Effects of vagal stimulation on glucagon and
     insulin secretion, *Endocrinology*, 95 (1974) 1005–1010.

23   Mei, N., Boyer, A. and Arlhac, A., Activite unitaire des glucidorecepteurs vagaux de
     l'intestin. Relation avec la glycemie, *J. Physiol.* (Paris), 67 (1973) 294 A.

24   Miller, J. J., Mogenson, G. J. and Stavaraky, G. W., Effects of stimulation of the
     septum, sciatic nerve, and olfactory bulb on lateral hypothalamic neurons, *Fed. Proc.*,
     29 (1970) 837.

25   Miller, R. E., Neural inhibition of insulin secretion from the isolated canine pancreas,
     Amer. J. Physiol., 229 (1975) 144–149.

26   Niijima, A., Afferent impulse discharges from glucoreceptors in the liver of the guinea
     pig, *Ann. N. Y. Acad. Sci.*, 157 (1969) 690–700.

27   Niijima, A., An electrophysiological study on the regulatory mechanism of blood sugar
     level in the rabbit, *Brain Res.*, 87 (1975) 195–199.

28   Niijima, A., The effect of 2-deoxy-d-glucose and d-glucose on the efferent discharge rate
     of sympathetic nerves, *J. Physiol.* (Lond.), 251 (1975) 231–243.

29   Niijima, A., The effect of glucose on the activity of the adrenal nerve and pancreatic
     branch of the vagus nerve in the rabbit, *Neuroscience Letters*, 1 (1975) 159–162.

30   Niijima, A. and Fukuda, A., Release of glucose from perfused liver preparation in
     response to stimulation of the splanchnic nerves in the toad, *Jap. J. Physiol.*, 23 (1973)
     497–508.

31   Niijima, A., Nervous regulatory mechanism of blood glucose levels. In: Y. Katsuki, M.
     Sato, S. F. Takagi and Y. Oomura (Eds.), *Food Intake and Chemical Senses*, Japan Sci.
     Soc. Press, Tokyo, 1977, pp. 413–426.

32   Oomura, Y., Kimura, K., Ooyama, H., Maeo, T., Iki, M. and Kuniyoshi, N., Reci-
     procal activities of the ventromedial and lateral hypothalamic areas of cats, *Science*, 143
     (1964) 484–485.

33   Oomura, Y., Ooyama, H., Yamamoto, T., Ono, T. and Kobayashi, N., Behavior of
     hypothalamic unit activity during electrophoretic application of drugs, *Ann. N. Y. Acad.
     Sci.*, 157 (1969) 642–665.

34   Oomura, Y., Ooyama, H., Sugimori, M., Nakamura, T. and Yamada, Y., Glucose
     inhibition of glucose-sensitive neurone in the rat lateral hypothalamus, *Nature*, 247
     (1974) 284–286.

35   Porte, D., Jr., A receptor mechanism for the inhibition of insulin release by epinephrine
     in man, *J. clin. Invest.*, 46 (1967) 86–94.

36   Russek, M., Participation of hepatic glucoreceptors in the control of intake of food,
     Nature, 197 (1963) 79–80.

37   Schmitt, M., Influence of hepatic portal receptors on hypothalamic feeding and satiety
     centers, *Amer. J. Physiol.*, 225 (1973) 1089.

38   Scott, J. W. and Pfaffmann, C., Characteristics of responses of lateral hypothalamic
     neurons to stimulation of the olfactory system, *Brain Res.*, 48 (1970) 251–264.

39   Sharma, K. N., Receptor mechanisms in the alimentary tract: Their excitations and
     functions. In: C. F. Code (Ed.), *Control of Food and Water Intake, Handbook of Physiology*,
     Sec. 6, Vol. 1, American Physiological Society, Washington, D. C., 1967, pp. 225–239.

40   Shimazu, T., Glycogen synthetase activity in liver: Regulation by autonomic nerves,
     Science, 156 (1967) 1256–1257.

41 Shimazu, T. and Amakawa, A., Regulation of glycogen metabolism in liver by the autonomic nervous system. 2. Neural control of glycogenolytic enzymes, *Biochim. Biophys. Acta*, 165 (1968) 335–348.

42 Shimazu, T. and Amakawa, A., Regulation of glycogen metabolism in liver by the autonomic nervous system. 3. Differential effects of sympathetic nerve stimulation and catecholamines on liver phosphorylase, *Biochim. Biophys. Acta*, 165 (1968) 349–356.

43 Smith, G. P. and Epstein, A. N., Increased feeding in response to decreased glucose utilization in the rat and monkey, *Amer. J. Physiol.*, 217 (1969) 1083–1087.

44 Smith, P. H., Woods, S. C. and Porte, D., Jr., Cotrol of the endocrine pancreas by the autonomic nervous system and related neural factors. This volume, pp. 84–97.

45 Steffens, A. B., The relation between the hypothalamus, the islet of Langerhans, and the regulation of food intake. In: Y. Katsuki, M. Sato, S. F. Takagi and Y. Oomura (Eds.), *Food Intake and Chemical Senses*, Japan Sci. Soc. Press, Tokyo, 1977, pp. 367–381.

46 Szabo, J. A. and Szabo, O., Influence of the insulin-sensitive central nervous system glucoregulator receptor on hepatic glucose metabolism, *J. Physiol.* (Lond.), 253 (1975) 121–133.

47 Woods, S. C. and Porte, D., Jr., Neural control of endocrine pancreas, *Physiol. Rev.*, 54 (1974) 596–619.

48 Woods, S. C., Conditioned insulin secretion. In: Y. Katsuki, M. Sato, S. F. Takagi and Y. Oomura (Eds.), *Food Intake and Chemical Senses*, Japan Sci. Soc. Press, Tokyo, 1977, pp. 357–365.

CHAPTER 6

CONTROL OF THE ENDOCRINE PANCREAS BY THE AUTONOMIC NERVOUS SYSTEM AND RELATED NEURAL FACTORS

Phillip H. Smith*, Stephen C. Woods** and Daniel Porte, Jr.***

*Department of Anatomy, Upstate Medical Center, State University of New York, Syracuse, New York, USA, **The Department of Psychology and Medicine, University of Washington, Seattle, and ***The Department of Medicine, University of Washington and the Division of Endocrinology and Metabolism, Veterans Administration Hospital, Seattle, Washington, USA

INTRODUCTION

Insulin and glucagon are the primary hormones produced by the pancreatic islets. The generally opposing actions of these hormones are responsible to a large degree for the regulation of plasma levels of metabolic fuels. As might be expected, substrates such as glucose, amino acids and free fatty acids play a major role in the control of islet hormone secretion. This interaction between substrate levels and islet hormone release has led, therefore, to the widely-held concept that control of the endocrine pancreas is solely within the domain of substrate-mediated signals. However, the primacy of substrate control has been challenged by numerous studies showing that extrapancreatic hormones and neural factors exert a significant influence upon the secretion of insulin and glucagon. Thus, in the past few years, it has become necessary to consider that there are a number of modulating control systems which change how the pancreatic islets respond to plasma substrate levels.

This chapter will focus on the role of the autonomic nervous system in the regulation of insulin and glucagon secretion. In doing so, we shall examine the influence of endogenous neurally-related factors such as acetycholine, catecholamines, serotonin, prostaglandins and somatostatin upon pancreatic islet function. Most of our discussion will be limited to normal physiology; however, where appropriate we will briefly illustrate the importance of these factors in pathophysiologic states. Since information concerning the role of substrates and extrapancreatic hormones in the control of islet function is available in several reviews[23,41,76], in-depth coverage of those topics will not be presented here.

RESULTS AND DISCUSSION

The Central Nervous System and Islet Function

Twenty years prior to the discovery of the pancreatic islets, Claude Bernard (1849)[4] reported that dogs became diabetic following puncture of the floor of the fourth cerebral ventricle. That observation has been followed by other findings showing that nearly all areas of the central nervous system can be implicated in the control of metabolic homeostasis. However, the major emphasis of research in this field has been directed toward the ventral hypothalamus, as it has been found to be the area most closely linked to neural control of blood glucose levels. This may be due to a number of reasons related to the anatomy of this region. First of all, this area of the brain forms part of the lateral and ventral surfaces of the third cerebral ventricle. Thus, in addition to its rich vascular supply[68], the ventral hypothalamus also can be influenced by the contents of the cerebrospinal fluid. Another important reason is the association of this region with the dorsal motor nucleus of the vagus and the sympathetic areas of the spinal cord. Finally, the ventral hypothalamus receives a variety of metabolically-related inputs from other areas of the brain[56], and is closely linked to the regulation of anterior pituitary function.

Electrical stimulation of the ventrolateral hypothalamic area (VLH) elicits an increase of insulin secretion and a decrease of plasma glucose[36,82]. In some experiments this effect has been blocked by subdiaphramatic vagotomy. Since electrical stimulation of the vagus nerves increases insulin release[82], and in some species glucagon release as well[5], the VLH has been implicated as a parasympathetic center of the hypothalamus. Further evidence for the role of the VLH in the control of islet function comes from lesioning experiments. Bilateral stereotaxic destruction of the VLH results in a decrease of insulin levels in rats[69] and genetically obese mice[16]. In humans, sectioning of the vagus nerves may result in the impairment of both insulin and glucagon secretion[6,65]. Studies involving rats have shown that vagotomy prevents conditioned insulin secretion[81] and also leads to a decrease of pancreatic islet mass[71].

The most studied area, however, is the ventromedial hypothalamic area (VMH) Electrical stimulation of the VMH area produces a decrease of insulin and a concomitant increase of glucagon levels[20]. Because these changes of islet hormone levels also occur during stimulation of the splanchnic nerves[54,82], the VMH has frequently been considered to be a sympathetic center in the hypothalamus. Some of the most dramatic changes of pancreatic islet biology occur following bilateral destruction of the VMH[57,82]. Typically, the syndrome includes hyperinsulinemia, hypertrophy of the islets, obesity and hyperphagia. Recent evidence suggests that animals with VMH lesions also display decreased levels of circulating glucagon[31] and a reduction of pancreatic somatostatin[83], a neurohormone involved in the local control of insulin and glucagon secretion. The effects of VMH destruction involve both parasympathetic and sympathetic components. Hyperinsulinemia and obesity resulting from VMH lesions are reversed by vagotomy[57,82]. Thus, these effects illustrate the parasympathetic action of the ventral hypothalamus totally unopposed by the counter-regulatory influence of sympathetic outflow. On the other hand, the decrease of circulating glucagon and the reduction of salivary gland size[31] suggest the simultaneous decrease of sympathetic-like signals following VMH lesioning.

When considering the sympathetic- and parasympathetic-like changes observed following experimental manipulations of the ventral hypothalamus, it is important to keep in mind that such alterations may not necessarily originate in the anatomically designated nuclei (VMH or VLH). Recent studies indicate that many of the functions attributed to the VMH are more correctly associated with axons of distant neurons that are passing through or near this nucleus. Specifically, in this case, noradrenergic and serotonergic neurons from the lower brain stem appear to mediate some of the VMH effects[1,17]. Similarly, cell bodies located in the substantia nigra that are dopaminergic may be responsible for some of the effects observed following stimulation or destruction of the VLH[76]. For example, stimulation of the VLH *per se* elicits increased insulin secretion only in the face of elevated plasma glucose. Conversely, stimulation of the area just posterior to the VLH results in enhanced insulin release that is independent of glucose levels[70]. The important fact, however, is that the ventral hypothalamus contains neurons—regardless of their origin—that possess the ability to alter the sympathetic and parasympathetic input to the endocrine pancreas and other metabolically important organs.

Innervation of the Pancreatic Islets

In his now classic study, Langerhans (1869)[37] was the first to recognize the presence of nerves in the pancreatic islets. Since that time numerous reports have demonstrated that with few exceptions, the endocrine pancreas of most vertebrates contains an abundant nerve supply[71,82]. The islets of some species have been found to contain intrinsic neurons[29,82], in addition to axons and their terminals. It is possible that these intrinsic neurons are postganglionic, parasympathetic nerves[10], but their identification as such has not been determined precisely. Far more information is available regarding the morphology and functional significance of the extrinsic islet nerves.

In most species, axons from the vagi and splanchnic trunks enter the pancreas as a mixed nerve and innervate islets, ducts, acini and blood vessels. Afferent fibers from the pancreas that follow the splanchnic nerves to the spinal cord also have been identified[74]. Presumably these axons mediate pain due to distension; however, little is known as to whether or not some of the afferents might originate within the islets themselves.

Investigations based on the use of light and/or electron microscopic (EM) methods have demonstrated the presence of three basic types of axon terminals within the endocrine pancreas. Parasympathetic terminals stain positively for cholinesterase[19], and by EM are found to display typical agranular synaptic vesicles of 30–50 nm in diameter[59]. Terminals of the sympathetic neurons also contain synaptic vesicles of 30–50 nm[59], but these vesicles contain "dense-cored" granules, providing a means of distinguishing between sympathetic and parasympathetic terminals. A more positive method for demonstrating sympathetic fibers is the fluorescent technique of Falk-Hillarp. Using this technique numerous investigators[14,71,82] have demonstrated the presence of axons containing primary catecholamines (dopamine and norepinephrine) in the islets of various species including humans. A third type of nerve ending containing large opaque vesicles 60–200 nm in diameter has been found in the islets of certain lower vertebrates[9]. Since these vesicles resemble those of the purinergic nerves described by Burnstock[11,12], it is possible that these terminals release ATP as a neurotransmitter substance. Similar terminals have not been reported in mammalian islets, but recent immunohistochemical studies indicate that a small number of axons in the islets of some species contain vasoactive intestinal polypeptide (VIP)[38] and some vagal fibers contain somatostatin[77]. Thus, there is evidence for both aminergic and peptidergic terminals in the endocrine pancreas of mammals. In the case of lower vertebrates there is some evidence for the presence of purinergic islet nerves, as well as the other two types.

The relationship of the nerve terminals to the various hormone-producing cells of the islet is quite variable. In some species nerve fibers enter the islet and arborize to form a so-called peri-insular plexus; but in others the nerves may be distributed as an intra-insular plexus at the more central regions of the islet[71,82]. While there are frequently different ratios of cholinergic to adrenergic terminals in the islets of various species, there appears to be no preferential association of one type of nerve ending to a particular kind of islet cell. In fact, some islet cells are innervated by several terminals of each type, while other endocrine cells appear to be some distance from the closest nerve ending[19,35]. Classic pre- and post-synaptic complexes are found between nerve endings and islet cells in teleosts[9] and reptiles[71]. However, in the islets of mammals most of the nerve terminals end blindly 10–20 nm from the cell membrane of the endocrine cells. This suggests that when neurotransmitters are released they may diffuse through the extracellular space and affect several islet cells simultaneously.

Recent electron microscopic studies combining freeze-fracture and heavy metal tracer techniques have shown the presence of gap-junctions between various cell types in the islets[48], and between nerve endings and some of the endocrine cells[49]. Because gap-junctions are areas of low electrical resistance between cells that also permit the passage of small molecules, these observations suggest additional mechanisms for the neural control of islet function. It is possible that an electrical and/or chemical signal could be transmitted from nerve to islet cell—and then throughout the islet parenchyma by means of gap-junction connections. This type of signal transfer allows one to consider the islet as a "functional syncytium" capable of responding rapidly to neural stimulation from one or more axons. Support for such a concept can be drawn additionally from electrophysiological studies showing that islet cells are electrically active and display synchronization of this activity between cells from different areas within the same islet[47].

Functional Aspects of the Intra-islet Nerves

As mentioned previously, electrical stimulation of the vagus nerves produces, in most species, an increase of circulating insulin[3] and glucagon[5] simultaneously. This effect also occurs following stimulation of the mixed pancreatic nerve in the presence of appropriate adrenergic blocking agents (see below). In either case there is an interaction between the neural signals to the islet and the circulating levels of glucose. Insulin release during nerve stimulation is small or absent in the presence of normo- or hypoglycemia. However, when glucose levels are slightly elevated there is a marked potentiation of insulin secretion by vagal stimulation. On the other hand, increased glucagon release due to vagal stimulation appears to be relatively independent of plasma glucose levels.

The administration of acetylcholine[34] or other parasympathomimetic drugs[71] produces a prompt and concurrent increase in insulin and glucagon secretion. These effects are blocked by prior treatment with atropine[3,82], suggesting that parasympathetic stimulation of islet function is mediated by muscarinic receptors. Atropine also blocks conditioned insulin release in rats[81], illustrating the role of endogenous parasympathetic signals in the control of islet function.

Electrical stimulation of the splanchnic nerves, or the mixed pancreatic nerve in atropinized animals, results in an increase of glucagon[46] release but a decrease of insulin secretion[54]. These effects are also influenced by the level of circulating glucose. Hyperglycemia decreases the release of glucagon normally observed during sympathetic stimulation. Under these conditions, however, insulin secretion is inhibited independently of the glucose level.

Since direct sympathetic stimulation is frequently difficult for technical reasons, or impossible in the case of clinical investigation, much of our current knowledge of how adrenergic agents affect islet function is derived from the study of drug actions. In humans, for example, infusions of epinephrine or norepinephrine produce a prompt inhibition of glucose-induced insulin secretion and a decline in basal insulin levels[23,71,82]. If these infusions are continued for sufficient periods of time there is a seemingly paradoxical increase of insulin with a continued inhibition of glucose-mediated insulin release. Studies using adrenergic blocking drugs have shown that this complex effect is due to the simultaneous but differing activities of the α- and β-adrenergic receptors[55,71]. Prior treatment with phentolamine, an α-adrenergic blocker, prevents the inhibitory effect of epinephrine upon glucose-stimulated insulin release. Thus, the inhibitory action of catecholamines is mediated by α-adrenergic activity. Phentolamine also produces an increase of basal insulin levels, suggesting that under normal conditions there is a tonic α-adrenergically mediated suppression of insulin release[64]. On the other hand, the administration of propranolol, a β-adrenergic antagonist, produces a suppression of basal insulin levels and prevents the late rise in insulin during epinephrine infusion. This observation indicates that β-receptors mediate the stimulation of insulin secretion during a catecholamine infusion and normally provide for a tonic stimulation of insulin secretion. Therefore, when one considers the action of the sympathetic nervous system in the control of insulin release there are simultaneous inhibitory (α) and stimulatory (β) components[21,55,71,82].

In terms of the pathophysiology of insulin release it is relatively easy to imagine that an imbalance of this push-pull system might exist. This may be the case in diabetes mellitus. Insulin release to glucose is absent in diabetic patients, although in many instances they have normal or slightly elevated basal insulin levels. This situation is remarkably similar to the experimental findings in normal volunteers given infusions of epinephrine[63]. It is possible, therefore, that part of the problem in diabetes is an oversensitivity to circulating catecholamines and/or abnormal α-adrenergic tone. In fact, several investigations tend to confirm this hypothesis. Treatment of hyperglycemic, adult-onset diabetics with phentolamine has been shown to improve glucose-induced insulin secretion[55,63]. Further study has revealed that the levels of circulating catecholamines are abnormally increased in these individuals. Appropriate clinical management of the diabetic condition in these patients results in a decrease of catecholamines[25]. Therefore, some of the islet dysfunction known to occur in human diabetes appears related to an increase of sympathetic signals to the endocrine pancreas.

In comparison to their effects upon insulin secretion, the role of α-and β-adrenergic receptors in the control of glucagon release is less clear-cut. Stimulation of glucagon secretion observed following the administration of catecholamines to most species has been found to be a function of β-receptor activation and is blocked by propranolol[23,71]. However, some reports indicate that stimulation of glucagon is also associated with the activity of α-receptors. In one study of rats forced to swim[26], the stress-related increase of glucagon release was blocked by phentolamine, implicating α-receptors as the mediator of hyperglucagonemia. However, results from another laboratory have demonstrated that, under similar experimental conditions, stress-induced glucagon secretion in adrenomedullated rats is blocked only by the β-antagonist propranolol[43]. In humans, some investigators have found no ability to alter gucagon levels by catecholamine infusions[79] whereas in others, β-adrenergic stimulation clearly increased glucagon levels. There is even one report that methoxamine, a relatively specific α-adrenergic agonist, decreases glucagon release in humans[23]. Thus, there is evidence that both α- and β-adrenergic receptors play a role in the stimulation of glucagon secretion, but this appears to be species- and experimental protocol-dependent. The findings that α-receptor activation stimulates glucagon release in some species and decreases in another, or that the increase is β-adrenergically mediated under slightly different experimental situations, suggests that the receptors of the islet A-cell are less well defined or are more easily modulated in their activity, than those on the B-cell.

The Role of Other Neural Factors in Islet Physiology

In addition to the presence of amines within nerve terminals of the islets, histochemical studies have also demonstrated the existence of serotonin (5-hydroxytryptamine) and/or dopamine in endocrine cells of the pancreas[14,50]. These amines are generally more abundant in islet cells of younger animals than in those of older ones. Islet cells of albino strains normally lack serotonin or dopamine, but these amines are synthesized after the administration of appropriate precursors (5-hydroxytryptophan or dihydroxyphenylalanine, respectively). For this reason, islet cells have been classified as members of the APUD series because of their properties of amine precursor uptake and decarboxylation. APUD cells, as described in more detail by Pearse[52], are believed to be derived from the neuroectoderm, suggesting an additional link between the nervous system and the endocrine pancreas.

The precise role of intracellular serotonin and dopamine in the regulation of insulin and glucagon secretion is unclear because of conflicting conclusions. Part of the reason for this controversy lies in the fact that some investigators have approached the study of serotonin and dopamine from the point of view that they are either extracellular or intracellular regulators of endocrine pancreatic function. It is perhaps more correct to assume that these amines exert two different actions and that their intracellular effects are probably quite distinct from their extracellular actions.

Reports concerning both actions of serotonin and/or dopamine upon insulin secretion have reached the general conclusion that these amines are inhibitory in terms of B-cell function[45,50,80]. Again, there are certain areas of conflict and complexity. This has been due largely to the use of blockers of serotonin and dopamine action whose modes of action are not completely specific. As an example, methysergide—a drug known to block serotonin action—decreases the inhibition of insulin secretion observed following the administration of 5-hydroxytryptophan[80]. Presumably, methysergide acts as an antagonist of intracellular serotonin. However, methysergide is also an antagonist of α-adrenergic activity and thus alters the effect of extracellular cate-cholamines on insulin secretion. In some studies the degradation of intracellular serotonin has been blocked using inhibitors of the enzyme monoamine oxidase (MAO). At high doses many of the MAO blockers produce other toxic side effects and an inhibi-tion of insulin release. While lower doses of these same drugs frequently elicit an increase of insulin secretion[2], this is not universal. In addition to effects related to the concentration of these drugs, some MAO inhibitors have been found to produce hypoglycemia unrelated to the secretion of insulin[42] which itself alters insulin responses to challenge. While it seems reasonable to conclude that intracellular serotonin and dopamine are inhibitors of insulin release, the various interactions between these amines and other factors make conclusions very tentative at this time.

As extracellular agents, serotonin and dopamine have been found to stimu-late[21,22,40], inhibit[21,40,44] or have no effect[40,45] on insulin and glucagon secretion. The mixed action of these two amines can be related to a variety of factors. Serotonin appears to have a direct inhibitory effect upon insulin release under certain condi-tions[62], but it may also influence islet hormone release indirectly by altering blood flow to the pancreas or by enhancing the local release of catecholamines[58]. With regard to this latter point, there is recent evidence that the mixed action of dopamine on insulin secretion may be due to its metabolism to norepinephrine[22], rather than via a direct interaction with dopaminergic receptors of the islet cells. Since catecholamines have been implicated in both the extracellular and intracellular action of serotonin and dopamine, it will be necessary to gain further information about the individual effects of these latter amines before a complete understanding of aminergic control of islet function can be reached.

The prostaglandins (PGs), a family of 20 carbon fatty acids, also have been im-plicated as mixed regulators of insulin and glucagon secretion. Although PGs counter-regulate neurotransmitters in some systems[27], their role as controllers of intra-islet acetylcholine and norepinephrine release has not been investigated fully. There is evidence both for and against an interaction between PGs and neurotransmitters in the control of islet function. Studies involving mice[8] *in vivo* have shown that PGE_1 stimu-lates insulin release. This effect was reversed by treatment with propranolol, suggest-ing that the observed increase of insulin was related to β-adrenergic stimulation. In contrast, administration of PGE_1 to anesthetized dogs produces an inhibition of insulin release that is not reversed by phentolamine[62]. This latter finding suggests that inhibi-tion of insulin release by PGE_1 is unrelated to the α-adrenergic action of catechola-mines. PGE_1 or E_2 has been found to stimulation glucagon release *in vitro*[53] and *in vivo*[66]. It is likely that this effect is due to a direct action because sympathectomy or β-blockade using propranolol does not alter the *in vivo* response of glucagon secretion following PGE₁ administration[66]. On the other hand, some interaction between PGs, substrates and catecholamines would not be totally unexpected. In an interesting series of experiments Burr and Sharp[13] reported that PGE₁ stimulated insulin release *in vitro* of the glucose concentration in the medium was low; however, PGE₁ inhibited insulin secretion when the glucose levels were raised. In these same experiments, the combination of PGE₁ and epinephrine stimulated insulin release to high glucose concentrations. This paradoxical effect (i.e., either agent would normally inhibit insulin release) suggests that PGs and catecholamines may interact in complex ways to alter the sensitivity of the islet cells to substrate-mediated signals.

The recent demonstration that PGE₂ inhibits insulin release in humans[60] has led to the concept that PGs may play a role in the pathophysiology of diabetes mellitus. Using normal volunteers, it has been shown that the effect of PGE₂ is glucose-specific and is not reversed by phentolamine. Thus, PGE₂ mimics the effect of catecholamines, but does not inhibit the secretion of insulin via activation of α-adrenergic receptors. Further evidence for the role of PGs as controllers of human islet function has been found using sodium salicylate, an inhibitor of endogenous PG synthesis. Infusions of sodium salicylate in normal volunteers results in an augmentation of glucose-stimulated insulin release. More importantly, however, this same treatment in diabetic patients[15] partially restores the acute release of insulin to glucose and also improves glucose tolerance. These latter findings raise the interesting possibility that some of the abnormalities of islet function in diabetes are related to an oversensitivity to PGs —just as some of these problems may involve an oversensitivity to catecholamines.

Somatostatin is another neural agent known to play an important role in the control of insulin and glucagon secretion. This polypeptide was first isolated from the hypothalamus, and was so named because of its inhibition of somatotropin release[7]. Numerous investigations have demonstrated that somatostatin blocks the release of a wide variety of polypeptide hormones[24], including the secretion of insulin and glucagon to nearly all known secretogogues. This rather dramatic effect upon islet hormone release has gained considerable attention due to the fact that prior to the discovery of somatostatin no agent was known to simultaneously inhibit the secretion of both insulin and glucagon. For a short time the action of somatostatin, in terms of islet function, was viewed as simply a new pharmacologic tool. However, immunohistochemical[28] and radioimmunoassay[78] studies have demonstrated the presence of considerable amounts of somatostatin within the pancreas. Specifically, this polypeptide, or an immunologically similar substance, has been localized to the D-cells of the endocrine pancreas. These newer findings, therefore, indicate that somatostatin may be an important local regulator of insulin and glucagon secretion.

Very little is currently known about how the secretion of pancreatic somatostatin is regulated. Preliminary studies[34,51] suggest that substrates and gastrointestinal hormones stimulate the release of somatostatin. This increase of somatostatin may, in turn, act to counterregulate the stimulatory effect of substrate and intestinal hormones on insulin and glucagon secretion. Infusions of acetylcholine appear to inhibit somatostatin release from the islet, whereas β-adrenergic stimulation using isoproterenol enhances the release of this D-cell hormone[67]. The parasympathetic stimulation of insulin and glucagon release, therefore, seems likely to be modulated by a change in somatostatin secretion. The influence of sympathetic β-adrenergic signals on somatostatin secretion adds additional complexity to the role of catecholamines upon insulin and glucagon secretion. For example, recent studies in our laboratory[72,73] have shown that the inhibitory effect of somatostatin on insulin and glucagon release *in vivo* can be reversed by α-adrenergic blockade. Although somatostatin does not appear to act directly as an α-receptor agonist[18], its action is apparently modulated by the net sympathetic tone of the islets. Thus, even an apparently "universal" inhibitor of insulin and glucagon secretion is influenced by ongoing neural signals, and presumably by a number of factors not yet recognized.

SUMMARY

As discussed in the preceding sections, the importance of the autonomic nervous system and neurally-related substances in the regulation of insulin and glucagon secretion has been demonstrated by various techniques. Stimulation or destruction of specific areas of the central nervous system produced alterations in the balance of parasympathetic and sympathetic signals to the islets. Similar changes of autonomic tone can be demonstrated by stimulation or sectioning of the nerves to the pancreas. All of these effects have been confirmed by the administration of appropriate neurotransmitters. Further, the application of specific precursors has been shown to alter islet function due to the appearance of certain amines within the endocrine cells themselves. Therefore, mechanisms for the neural control of the endocrine pancreas are present at different levels ranging from the brain to intracellular events within the islet cells.

It is not possible, however, to consider the nervous system as a controller of islet function apart from its interaction with extrapancreatic hormones and metabolic substrates. In fact, as we have pointed out, in several instances the alterations of islet function due to neural signals are generally dependent upon the level of circulating glucose. It is also important to keep in mind that changes of autonomic tone affect the release of several gastrointestinal hormones that may act directly as stimulators of insulin and/or glucagon release—depending, of course, on the substrate levels.

How, then, is it possible to develop a coherent working hypothesis for the role of the many neural factors in controlling insulin and glucagon secretion? Any attempt at forming such a general hypothesis is speculative at best. Nonetheless, we believe that all of the neural factors previously discussed can be divided into three categories. Acetylcholine is an example of a neural factor that possesses only stimulatory properties. In contrast, somatostatin exhibits only inhibitory effects upon insulin and glucagon secretion. The other neurally-related substances (i.e., serotonin, dopamine, epinephrine, norpinephrine and prostaglandins) are mixed controllers of islet function. These latter factors may stimulate or inhibit the secretion of insulin and/or glucagon depending upon the net effect of all signals impinging upon the islet cells. In an overall sense, these three types of neuroregulators operate in concert with hormones to integrate endogenous metabolic events with meal-related exogenous substrates (glucose, amino acids and fat) to provide for both the short- and long-term control of metabolic homeostasis through the coordinated release of insulin and glucagon.

This chapter was written with the support of funds from the National Institutes of Health (AM25325, AM12829, AM17047), the University of Washington Diabetes Center and the Medical Research Service of the Veterans Administration. We wish to thank our colleagues Drs. Jeffrey B. Halter, R. Paul Robertson, Stewart Metz and Jerry P. Palmer for their stimulating discussions.

REFERENCES

1   Ahlskog, J. E. and Hoebel, B. G., Overeating and obesity from damage to a noradrenergic system in the brain, *Science*, 182 (1973) 166–169.

2   Aleyassine, H. and Gardiner, R. J., Dual action of antidepressant drugs (MAO inhibitors) on insulin release, *Endocrinology*, 96 (1975) 702–710.

3   Bergman, R. N. and Miller, R. E., Direct enhancement of insulin secretion by vagal stimulation of the isolated pancreas, *Amer. J. Physiol.*, 225 (1973) 481–486.

4   Bernard C., Chiens rendus diabetiques, *Compt. Rend. Soc. Biol.*, 1 (1849) 60.

5   Bloom, S. R., Edwards, A. V. and Vaughn, N. J. A., The role of the autonomic innervation in the control of glucagon release during hypoglycemia in the calf, *J. Physiol.* (Lond.), 236 (1974) 611–623.

6   Bloom, S. R., Vaughn, N. J. A. and Russell, R. C. G., Vagal control of glucagon release in man, *Lancet*, 2 (1974) 546–549.

7   Brazeau, P., Vale, W., Burgus, R., Ling, N., Butcher, M., Rivier, J. and Guillemin, R., Hypothalamic polypeptide that inhibits the secretion of immunoreactive pituitary growth hormone, *Science*, 179 (1973) 77–79.

8   Bressler, R., Vargas-Condon, M. and Lebovitz, H. E., Tranylcypromine: A potent insulin secretogogue and hypoglycemic agent, *Diabetes*, 17 (1968) 617–624.

9   Brinn, J. E., Pancreatic islet cytology of Ictaluridae (Teleostei), *Cell Tiss. Res.*, 162 (1975) 357–365.

10 Brinn, J. E., Burden, H. W. and Schweisthal, M. R., Innervation of the cultured fetal rat pancreas, *Cell Tiss. Res.*, 182 (1977) 133–138.

11 Burnstock, G., Purinergic Nerves, *Pharmacol. Rev.*, 24 (1972) 509–581.

12 Burnstock, G., Comparative studies of purinergic nerves, *J. exp. Zool.*, 194 (1975) 103–134.

13 Burr, I. M. and Sharp, R., Effects of prostaglandin E_1 and of epinephrine on the dynamics of insulin release *in vitro*, *Endocrinology*, 94 (1974) 835–839.

14 Cegrell, L., Adrenergic nerves and monoamine containing cells in the mammalian endocrine pancreas, *Acta physiol. scand.*, Suppl. 314 (1968) 1–60.

15 Chen, M. and Robertson, R. P., Restoration of the acute insulin response by sodium salicylate, *Diabetes*, 27 (1978) 750–756.

16 Chlouverakis, C. and Bernardis, L. L., Ventrolateral hypothalamic lesions in obese hyperglycemic mice (ob/ob), *Diabetologia*, 8 (1972) 179–184.

17 Coscina, D. V. and Stancer, H. C., Selective blockade of hypothalamic hyperphagia and obesity in rats by serotonin-depleting midbrain lesions, *Science*, 195 (1977) 416–418.

18 Efendic, S. and Luft, R., Studies on the mechanism of somatostatin action on insulin release in man. Effect of blockade of α-adrenergic receptors, *Acta Endocrinol.*, 78 (1975) 516–523.

19 Esterhuizen, A. C., Spriggs, T. L. B. and Lever, J. D., Nature of islet-cell innervation in the cat pancreas, *Diabetes*, 17 (1968) 33–36.

20 Frohman, L. A. and Bernardis, L. L., Effect of hypothalamic stimulation on plasma glucose, insulin, and glucagon levels, *Amer. J. Physiol.*, 221 (1971) 1596–1603.

21 Gagliardino, J. J., Nierle, C. and Pfeiffer, E. F., The effect of serotonin on *in vitro* insulin secretion and biosynthesis in mice, *Diabetologia*, 10 (1974) 411–414.

22 George, D. T. and Bailey, P. T., The effect of adrenergic and ganglionic blockers upon the L-dopa-stimulated release of glucagon in the rat, *Proc. Soc. exp. Biol. Med.*, 157 (1978) 1–4.

23 Gerich, J. E., Charles, M. A. and Grodsky, G. M., Regulation of pancreatic insulin and glucagon secretion, *Ann. Rev. Physiol.*, 38 (1976) 353–388.

24 Guillemin, R. and Gerich J. E., Somatostatin: Physiological and clinical significance, *Ann. Rev. Med.*, 27 (1976) 379–388.

25 Halter, J. and Porte, D., Jr., Increased adrenergic activity in diabetes mellitus: Response to therapy and pharmacologic stimulation, *Clin. Res.*, 25 (1977) 160A.

26 Harvey, W. D., Faloona, G. R. and Unger, R. H., The effect of adrenergic blockade on exercise-induced hyperglucagonemia, *Endocrinology*, 94 (1974) 1254–1258.

27 Hedqvist, P., Basic mechanisms of prostaglandin action on autonomic neurotransmission, *Ann. Rev. Pharm. Toxicol.*, 17 (1977) 259–280.

28 Hökfelt, T., Efendic, S., Hellerström, C., Johansson, O., Luft, R. and Arimura, A., Cellular localization of somatostatin in endocrine-like cells and neurons of the rat with special reference to the A_1-cells of the pancreatic islets and to the hypothalamus, *Acta Endocrinol.*, Suppl. 200 (1975) 1–41.

29 Honjin, R., The innervation of the pancreas of the mouse with special reference to the structure of the peripheral extension of the vegetative nervous system, *J. Comp. Neurol.*, 104 (1956) 331–371.

30 Inoue, S. and Bray, G. A., The effects of subdiaphragmatic vagotomy in rats with ventromedial hypothalamic obesity, *Endocrinology*, 100 (1977) 108–114.

31 Inoue, S. Campfield, L. A. and Bray, G. A., Comparison of metabolic alterations in hypothalamic and high fat diet-induced obesity, *Amer. J. Physiol.*, 233 (1977) R162–R168.

32 Ipp, E., Dobbs, R. E., Harris, V., Arimura, A., Vale, W. and Unger, R. H., The effects of gastrin, gastric inhibitory polypeptide, secretion, and the octapeptide of cholecystokinin upon immunoreactive somatostatin release by the perfused canine pancreas, *J. clin. Invest.*, 60 (1977) 1216–1219.

33 Iversen, J., Adrenergic receptors and the secretion of insulin and glucagon from the isolated, perfused canine pancreas, *J. clin. Invest.*, 52 (1973) 2102–2116.

34 Iversen, J., Effect of acetylcholine on the secretion of glucagon and insulin from the isolated, perfused canine pancreas, *Diabetes*, 22 (1973) 381–387.

35 Kobayashi, S. and Fujita, T., Fine structure of mammalian and avian pancreatic islets with special reference to D cells and nervous elements, *Z. Zellforsch.*, 100 (1969) 340–363.

36 Kuzuya, T., Regulation of insulin secretion by the central nervous system. II. The role of the hypothalamus and the pituitary gland upon insulin secretion, *J. Japan. Soc. int. Med.*, 51 (1962) 65–74.

37 Langerhans, P., *Contributions to the Microscopic Anatomy of the Pancreas*, Thesis, Berlin, 1869, Translated by H. Morrison, The Johns Hopkins Press, Baltimore, MD, 1937.

38 Larsson, L.-I., Fahrenkrug, J., Schaffalitzky de Muckadell, O., Sundler, F., Håkanson, R. and Rehfield, J. F., Localization of vasoactive intestinal polypeptide (VIP) to central and peripheral neurons, *Proc. nat. Acad. Sci.* (USA), 73 (1976) 3197–3200.

39 Lebovtiz, H. E. and Feldman, J. M., Pancreatic biogenic amines and insulin secretion in health and disease, *Fed. Proc.*, 32 (1973) 1797–1802.

40 Lechin, F., Coll-Garcia, E., Van der Dijs, B., Pena, F., Bentolila, A. and Rivas, C., The

effect of serotonin (5-HT) on insulin secretion, *Acta physiol. lantinoam.*, 25 (1975) 339–346.

41 Lefebvre, P. J. and Unger, R. H., *Glucagon, Molecular Physiology, Clinical and Therapeutic Implications*, Pergammon Press, Oxford, 1972.

42 Lundquist, I., Ekholm, R. and Erickson, L. E., Monoamines in the pancreatic islets of the mouse, *Diabetologia*, 7 (1971) 414–422.

43 Luyckx, A. S., Dresse, A., Cassion-Fossion, A. and Lefebvre, P. J., Catecholamines and exercise-induced glucagon and fatty acid mobilization in the rat, *Amer. J. Physiol.*, 229 (1975) 376–383.

44 Marco, J., Hedo, J. E., Martinell, J., Calle, C. and Villanneva, M. L., Potentiation of glucagon secretion by serotonin antagonists in man, *J. clin. Endocr. Metab.*, 42 (1976) 215–221.

45 Marco, J., Hedo, J. A. and Villanneva, M. L., Inhibition of glucagon release by serotonin in mouse, *Diabetologia*, 13 (1977) 585–588.

46 Marliss, E. B., Girardier, L., Seydoux, J., Wollheim, E. B., Kanazawa, Y., Orci, L., Renould, A. E. and Porte, D., Jr., Glucagon release induced by pancreatic nerve stimulation in the dog, *J. clin. Invest.*, 52 (1973) 1246–1259.

47 Meissner, H. P., Electrophysiological evidence for coupling between β-cells of pancreatic islets, *Nature*, 262 (1976) 502–504.

48 Orci, L., Malaisse-Lagae, F., Ravazzola, M., Rouiller, D., Renould, A. E., Perrelet, A. and Unger, R. H., A morphological basis for intercellular communication between α- and β-cells in the endocrine pancreas, *J. clin. Invest.*, 56 (1975) 1066–1070.

49 Orci, L., Perrelet, A., Ravazzola, M., Malaisse-Lagae, F. and Renould, A. E., A special membrane junction between nerve endings and B-cells in islets of Langerhans, *Europ. J. clin. Invest.*, 3 (1973) 443–445.

50 Owman, C., Håkansen, R. and Sundler, F., Occurrence and function of amines in endocrine cells producing polypeptide hormones, *Fed. Proc.*, 32 (1973) 1785–1791.

51 Patton, G. S., Ipp, E., Dobbs, R. E., Orci, L., Vale, W. and Unger, R. H., Pancreatic immunoreactive somatostatin release, *Proc. nat. Acad. Sci.* (USA), 74 (1977) 2140–2143.

52 Pearse, A. G. E., The cytochemistry and ultrastructure of polypeptide hormone-producing cells of the APUD series and the embryologic, physiologic and pathologic implications of the concept, *J. Histochem. Cytochem.*, 17 (1969) 303–313.

53 Pek, S., Tai, T.-Y., Elsten, A. and Fajans, S. S., Stimulation by prostaglandin E_2 of glucagon and insulin release from isolated rat pancreas, *Prostaglandins*, 10 (1975) 493–502.

54 Porte, D., Jr., Girardier, L., Seydoux, J., Kanazawa, Y. and Posternak, J., Neural regulation of insulin secretion in the dog, *J. clin. Invest.*, 52 (1973) 210–214.

55 Porte, D., Jr. and Robertson, R. P., Control of insulin secretion by catecholamines, stress and the sympathetic nervous system, *Fed. Proc.*, 32 (1973) 1792–1796.

56 Powley, T. L., The ventromedial hypothalamic syndrome, satiety, and a cephalic phase hypothesis, *Psychol. Rev.*, 84 (1977) 89–126.

57 Powley, T. L. and Opsahl, C. A., Autonomic components of the hypothalamic feeding syndromes. In: D. Novin, W. Wyrwicka, and G. Bray (Eds.), *Hunger: Basic Mechanisms and Clinical Implications*, Raven Press, New York, 1976, pp. 313–326.

58 Quickel, K. E., Feldman, J. M. and Lebovitz, H. E., Inhibition of insulin secretion by serotonin and dopamine: Species variation, *Endocrinology*, 89 (1971) 1295–1302.

59 Richardson, K. C., The fine structure of the albino rat iris with special reference to the identification of adrenergic and cholinergic nerves and nerve endings in its intrinsic muscles, *Amer. J. Anat.*, 114 (1964) 173–205.

60 Robertson, R. P. and Chen, M., A role of prostaglandin E in defective insulin secretion

and carbohydrate intolerance in diabetes mellitus, *J. clin. Invest.*, 60 (1977) 747–753.

61 Robertson, R. P., Gavareski, D. J., Porte, D., Jr. and Bierman, E. L., Inhibition of *in vivo* insulin secretion by prostaglandin E₁, *J. clin. Invest.*, 54 (1974) 310–315.

62 Robertson, R. P. and Guest, R. J., Reversal by methysergide of inhibition of insulin secretion by prostaglandin E, *J. clin. Invest.*, 62 (1978) 1014–1019.

63 Robertson, R. P., Halter, J. B. and Porte, D., Jr., A role for alpha-adrenergic receptors in abnormal insulin secretion in diabetes mellitus, *J. clin. Invest.*, 57 (1976) 791–795.

64 Robertson, R. P. and Porte, D., Jr., Adrenergic modulation of insulin secretion in man, *Diabetes*, 22 (1973) 1–8.

65 Russell, R. C. G., Thompson, J. P. S. and Bloom, S. R., The effect of truncal and selective vagotomy on the release of pancreatic glucagon, insulin and enteroglucagon, *Brit. J. Surg.*, 61 (1974) 821–824.

66 Sacca, L. and Perez, G., Influence of prostaglandins on plasma glucagon levels in the rat, *Metabolism*, 25 (1976) 127–130.

67 Samols, E., Weir, G. C., Patel, T. C., Loo, S. W. and Gabbay, K. H., Autonomic control of somatostatin and pancreatic peptide secretion by the isolated perfused canine pancreas, *Clin. Res.*, 25 (1977) 499A.

68 Scremin, O. U., The vascular anatomy of the rat's hypothalamus in stereotaxic coordinates, *J. comp. Neurol.*, 139 (1965) 31–52.

69 Steffens, A. B., Mogenson, G. J. and Stevenson, J. A. F., Blood glucose, insulin and free fatty acids after stimulation and lesions of the hypothalamus, *Amer. J. Physiol.*, 222 (1972) 1446–1452.

70 Stephens, D. N. and Morrissey, S. M., Hypothalamic stimulation induces acid secretion, hypoglycemia, and hyperinsulinemia, *Amer. J. Physiol.*, 228 (1975) 1206–1209.

71 Smith, P. H. and Porte, D., Jr., Neuropharmacology of the pancreatic islets, *Ann. Rev. Pharm. Toxicol.*, 16 (1976) 269–285.

72 Smith, P. H., Woods, S. C., Ensinck, J. W. and Porte, D., Jr., Phentolamine prevents the somatostatin-mediated inhibition of pancreatic glucagon secretion, *Metabolism*, 26 (1977) 841–845.

73 Smith, P. H., Woods, S. C. and Porte, D., Jr., Phentolamine blocks the somatostatin-mediated inhibition of insulin secretion, *Endocrinology*, 98 (1976) 1073–1076.

74 Tiscornia, O. M., The neural control of exocrine and endocrine pancreas, *Amer. J. Gastroent.*, 67 (1977) 541–560.

75 Unger, R. H., Alpha- and beta-cell interrelationships in health and disease, *Metabolism*, 23 (1974) 581–593.

76 Ungerstedt, U., Stereotaxic mapping of the monoamine pathways in the rat brain, *Acta physiol. scand.*, Suppl. 367 (1971) 1–48.

77 Ünvas-Wallensten, K., Efendic, S. and Luft, R., The occurrence of somatostatin-like immunoreactivity in the vagal nerves, *Acta physiol. scand.*, 102 (1978) 248–250.

78 Vale, W., Ling, N., Rivier, J., Villarreal, J., Rivier, C., Douglas, C. and Brown, M., Anatomic and phylogenetic distribution of somatostatin, *Metabolism*, 25 (1976) 1491–1494.

79 Walter, R. M., Dudl, R. J., Palmer, J. P. and Ensinck, J. W., The effect of adrenergic blockade on the glucagon response to starvation and hypoglycemia in man, *J. clin. Invest.*, 54 (1974) 1214–1220.

80 Wilson, J. P., Downs, R. W., Feldman, J. M. and Lebovitz, H. E., Beta cell monoamines: Further evidence for their role in modulating insulin secretion, *Amer. J. Physiol.*, 227 (1974) 305–311.

81 Woods, S. C., Conditioned hypoglycemia: Effect of vagotomy and pharmacological blockade, *Amer. J. Physiol.*, 223 (1972) 1424–1427.

82 Woods, S. C. and Porte, D., Jr., Neural control of the endocrine pancreas, *Physiol. Rev.*, 54 (1974) 596–619.

83 Woods, S. C., West, D. B., Ensinck, J. W. and Smith, P. H., Ventral hypothalamic (VMH) lesions reduce pancreatic somatostatin (SRIF) content, *Diabetes*, 27 (1978) 441.

CHAPTER 7

AFFERENTS OF THE PULMONARY VASCULAR BED
AND THEIR ROLE

H. M. Coleridge and J. C. G. Coleridge

*Cardiovascular Research Institute and Department of Physiology, University of California
San Francisco, San Francisco, California, USA*

INTRODUCTION

The beat-to-beat regulation of autonomic outflow to the cardiovascular system is largely determined by activity in afferent pathways from specialized vasosensory areas. In this symposium Drs. Nishi and Brooks will discuss the afferent pathways that arise from the heart itself, and we propose to give a brief account of those originating in the pulmonary vascular bed. Writers of textbooks and reviews are usually careful to avoid the label 'autonomic' for these visceral afferent pathways, although Langley[23] himself was the originator of the convenient term 'afferent sympathetic fiber'. Instead, writers generally adhere to Langley's subsequent definition of the autonomic nervous system as a purely efferent one. Nevertheless, both Langley[23] and Gaskell[19] regarded a reflex arc that included the central nervous system as the functional unit of autonomic activity, for, to quote Gaskell, "The evidence indicates that the involuntary nervous system is built up on the same plan as the voluntary nervous system, with receptor, connector and excitor elements". There is little doubt that both authors recognized that information, transmitted along afferent pathways to connector neurons, is an essential element in determining the pattern of autonomic outflow, and we firmly believe that if present knowledge and techniques had been available to them, they would have included these afferent pathways, as well as the 'autonomic centers' of the brain and spinal cord, in a broader definition of the system.

Investigators who wish to manipulate autonomic efferent traffic to the cardiovascular system commonly make use of the two afferent pathways from the carotid baroreceptors and chemoreceptors. This is largely a matter of convenience, for the autonomic inputs from this restricted vasosensory region are unusually easy to isolate, and their impulse traffic can be controlled without directly producing changes in the variables to be studied. Using these inputs, investigators have been able to establish the general principles governing reflex cardiovascular regulation. By contrast, the inputs accessible from the 'lesser circulation' cannot be isolated so easily, and to control them experimentally without producing changes in cardiac output and in arterial gas tensions may require major surgical interference. Much information about the functional characteristics of afferent fibers arising from the pulmonary circulation, particularly of those that travel in the vagus nerves, has been obtained from studies of their reflex effects and from records of impulse activity in individual units. The reflex cardiovascular changes that occur when the lungs are inflated or the lesser circulation is distended are not wholly abolished by vagotomy, however; some part of the afferent input travels in sympathetic branches, a component that has been relatively neglected until recently.

What sort of information is conveyed to the central nervous system in these autonomic afferent fibers from the pulmonary vascular bed? There are three major categories of vagal afferent ending to be considered: namely, conventional baroreceptors that signal pressure changes in the major arterial branches, slowly adapting stretch receptors that signal changes in transpulmonary pressure and C fiber endings that signal pressure changes downstream to the pulmonary resistance vessels. Vagal C fibers also supply the larger pulmonary arteries; their function is uncertain. No vagal nerve endings have been found that are pulmonary chemoreceptors in the sense of being associated with specialized cells, and of responding to changes in P_{O_2}, P_{CO_2} and pH in pulmonary arterial blood. A search for an afferent machanism of this sort has been a recurrent theme of reflex studies, however, for many of the changes that occur so promptly with the onset of exercise could be readily explained by the existence of an afferent mechanism capable of responding to the metabolic consequences of exercise, that is, one able to 'taste' mixed venous blood. In the fetus, small groups of chemoreceptor cells, identical in structure with the cells of the carotid body, are supplied by a branch of the pulmonary artery, but after birth this vessel disappears, and thereafter the chemoreceptor cells are supplied with systemic arterial blood[8]. Pulmonary stretch receptors in mammals are chemosensitive in the sense that their activity is modified by changes in alveolar CO_2, but the range of CO_2 over which these effects occur does not suggest that these afferents have a reflex role in exercise. Vagal C fibers with endings close to the pulmonary capillaries[11,28] are strongly stimulated by certain exotic chemicals, and also by endogenous substances such as the prostaglandins, that may be formed and released in the lung[7], but they are unaffected by changes in P_{O_2} and P_{CO_2}. As for sympathetic afferent fibers arising from the pulmonary circulation, so far only those with endings in the pulmonary arteries and veins outside the lungs have been examined systematically; there is little information about fibers that supply structures within the lung. The endings do not appear to differ from sympathetic afferent endings found elsewhere in the great vessels and in the heart, and although they function as mechanoreceptors, and under certain conditions fire with each pressure pulse, their response is so different from that of the vagal mechanoreceptors that they do not appear to be well suited to participate in the beat-to-beat regulation of the cardiovascular system.

PULMONARY ARTERIAL BARORECEPTORS

Pulmonary arterial baroreceptors, whose impulse activity has been recorded in both dogs and cats, have a firing pattern closely resembling that of the carotid and aortic baroreceptors (for references, see 14). They are active at normal pulmonary arterial pressures, and their discharge reaches a maximum of 20–30 impulses/cycle at pressures of 45–50/20–25 mm Hg. They are supplied by Aδ vagal fibers, and their terminals appear on histological examination to be similar to those of baroreceptors elsewhere. They are concentrated in the main branches of the pulmonary artery outside the lungs; there are very few in the main pulmonary trunk. Nerve endings that fire with a similar pattern of discharge have also been located within the lungs[13].

Investigating the reflex properties of these pulmonary baroreceptors in dogs, Coleridge and Kidd[15] converted the main right pulmonary artery into a closed sac, which was distended with blood under pulsatile pressure. In about half the experiments, distension with pressures around a mean of 20–40 mm Hg caused a decrease in systemic arterial pressure, sometimes accompanied by bradycardia (Fig. 1). Depressor effects were larger, and were obtained more frequently, if the buffering influence of the sinus and aortic nerves was first eliminated. Effects were abolished by vagotomy.

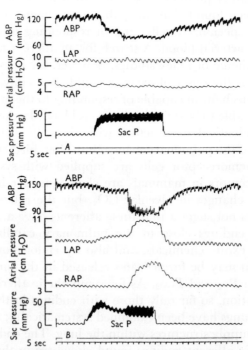

Fig. 1.   Reflex depressor effects evoked in dogs by distending the right pulmonary artery, which (with its nerve supply intact) had been converted into a closed sac. Only the left lung was ventilated and it received the whole output of the right ventricle. Experiments A and B were in different dogs. ABP, arterial blood pressure; LAP, RAP, left and right atrial pressure, respectively. Sac P, pressure in right pulmonary arterial sac. In A, arterial blood pressure decreased by about 40 mm Hg when the sac was distended; heart rate was unchanged. In B, reflex effects of distension were small until pulse pressure in the sac was increased further, when blood pressure decreased from 135 to 90 mm Hg, and heart rate fell from 170 to 60 beats/min. Reflex depressor effects in A and B were abolished by vagotomy. (From Coleridge and Kidd[15].)

Such results confirmed the conclusions of early investigators[16], as well as the more recent ones of Lloyd[25], that there are within the pulmonary vascular tree receptors that share the reflex function of the sino-aortic baroreceptors, and are capable of inhibiting sympathetic cardiovascular neurons and of exciting the vagal cardiac center. Coleridge and Kidd[15] found, however, that effects were reversed when the sac was distended with high pressures (mean 80–100 mm Hg), i.e., pressures higher than those required for maximum engagement of baroreceptors: arterial pressure increased and vigorous breathing movements occurred. Cooling the vagus nerves to 7–8°C blocked the depressor effects of low sac pressures, but the excitatory effects of high sac pressures could still be obtained. Since both reflexes were abolished by vagotomy, Coleridge and Kidd concluded that the pressor response was due to some powerful overriding vagal reflex mechanism with afferent endings either in the pulmonary arterial wall, or closely adjacent to it.

Recently, Ledsome and Kan[24] have come to quite different conclusions about the reflex properties of receptors in the pulmonary artery. In their experiments, also in dogs, the right ventricle was bypassed and venous return was pumped directly to the lungs; the main pulmonary trunk and the extrapulmonary part of both right and left pulmonary arteries were distended with steady pressures. Stepwise distension of the pulmonary arteries over the physiological range caused progressive increases in hind limb vascular resistance and phrenic nerve activity which were abolished by vagotomy; renal vascular resistance was unaffected. When the fluid in the vascular segment was cooled, peripheral resistance decreased. Ledsome and Kan concluded that receptors in or near the pulmonary artery generate sympathetic vasoconstrictor tone and excite the respiratory center.

In seeking to explain the reflex effects of distending the pulmonary artery, one must recognize that endings other than baroreceptors may be excited. For example, vagal C fibers have afferent endings in the pulmonary arterial wall that are often silent under control conditions, but may be stimulated when pulmonary arterial pressure is greatly increased (Fig. 2A). Although insensitive to hypoxia, they are vigorously stimulated by low concentrations of chemicals such as phenyl diguanide and capsaicin. They are part of a widespread system of vagal C fiber endings supplying the heart and vessels, whose functional significance has still to be defined[6], so that their reflex role, if any, in experiments involving pulmonary arterial distension must remain uncertain.

Another complication is the presence of small clusters of chemoreceptor cells lying between the pulmonary artery and the aorta. Many of these are actually embedded in the pulmonary arterial adventitia, and Krahl[22] believed that a particular aggregation of these cells, that he termed the 'glomus pulmonale', received a direct blood supply from the pulmonary artery in adult animals, and functioned as a mixed venous chemoreceptor. Repeated attempts to confirm Krahl's theory have failed. The cell mass he described appears to be merely one of the many scattered groups of chemoreceptor cells that comprise the aortic bodies, the thoracic analogs of the more compact carotid bodies. The aortic bodies are supplied with blood by descending branches of the aorta and by ascending branches from the left coronary artery, which anastomose in the pulmonary arterial adventitia and supply vasa vasorum to the

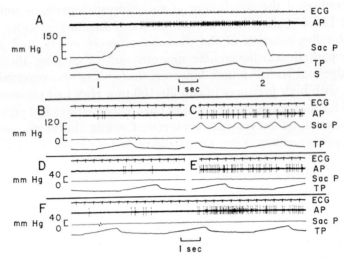

Fig. 2.   Afferent vagal endings stimulated by distending the right pulmonary artery which
had been converted into a closed sac (see legend, Fig. 1). E. C. G., electrocardiogram;
AP, action potentials (right vagus nerve); Sac P, pressure in pulmonary arterial
sac; TP, tracheal pressure (upstroke represents inflation); S, signal. A, dog; open
chest; vagal C fiber ending in the wall of the right pulmonary arterial sac (fiber
conduction velocity, 1.3 m/sec). Sac distended between 1 and 2. The ending was
not stimulated when the lungs were ventilated with 5% O_2 in N_2. B–F, dog; open
chest; impulses from a group 4 aortic body chemoreceptor lying between the pulmonary artery and the aorta. B, before, and C, during distension of the sac (lungs
ventilated with air). D, E, lungs ventilated with air, and with 5% O_2 in N_2, respectively. F, 100 μg NaCN injected into the left atrium 6 sec before the beginning of
the record (lungs ventilated with air). (Fig. 2A from Coleridge et al.[6], by permission of the American Heart Association, Inc.)

wall[8,9]. We have direct electrophysiological evidence that at least some of these aortic
chemoreceptors are stimulated when the pulmonary artery is distended by pulsatile
pressures exceeding 80 mm Hg (Fig. 2B and C). Probably such distension restricts
blood flow in the fine vasa vasorum of the pulmonary arterial wall, causing stagnant
hypoxia of the glomus cells[6]. It is conceivable that in the preparation used by Ledsome
and Kan[24], aortic chemoreceptors were stimulated by sac pressures within the physiological range, because distending pressures were steady and were applied over a
wider region. If, in their preparation, aortic chemoreceptor activity was initially high
because of interference with blood supply, cooling the fluid that perfused the proximal
part of the pulmonary arterial tree might decrease chemoreceptor discharge and
cause depressor effects. Nevertheless, Ledsome and Kan do not believe that their results
can be explained on this basis, because renal vasoconstriction, an important component
of the reflex effects of chemoreceptor stimulation, was never observed in their experiments. Clearly the afferent innervation of the pulmonary artery will continue to be a
focus of investigation for some time.

SLOWLY ADAPTING PULMONARY STRETCH RECEPTORS

Although their distribution within the lung is still a matter of debate, stretch receptors clearly fall within the scope of this review, for there is good evidence that many of them are in structures directly supplied by the pulmonary circulation[2]. Their primary stimulus is stretch of the lung, but their response may be considerably modified by a number of factors, including inhalation of volatile anesthetics, lung congestion and changes in lung P_{CO_2}. This last is presently arousing considerable interest because of a possible link between pulmonary CO_2 and the regulation of breathing (for references, see 5). A fall in alveolar P_{CO_2} below the normal level sensitizes the endings to lung stretch, so that at constant tidal volume, activity increases as lung P_{CO_2} falls (Fig. 3)[5,30]. It is not necessary to postulate a special degree of CO_2 sensitivity on the part of pulmonary stretch receptors, for comparable levels of hypocapnia are well known to have prominent effects on the threshold and excitability of somatic sensory nerves. However, stimulation by hypocapnia acquires a special significance when incorporated into an inhibitory feedback loop that controls ventilation, and there are many conditions (anxiety, pain, heat, fever, hypoxia of high altitude, even exercise) in which lung P_{CO_2} falls below the resting level. There appears to be little change in the activity of pulmonary stretch receptors when P_{CO_2} increases above normal.

Pulmonary stretch receptor input has a powerful influence on cardiovascular regulation (see 17). Thus an increase in lung volume causes an increase in heart rate by inhibiting the vagal cardiac center, an effect quite independent of central inspiratory activity, and one that can be demonstrated when respiratory drive is abolished by hypocapnia[1]. The afferent input evoked by an increase in lung volume also causes a marked reduction of sympathetic vasoconstrictor outflow to the vascular bed of skeletal muscle, with lesser effects on splanchnic and cutaneous vascular beds[18]. These effects, which serve to promote an overall increase in cardiac output and to divert blood flow to skeletal muscle, assume a particular importance when ventilation increases as a result of chemoreceptor excitation, for they effectively oppose the direct circulatory effects of the chemoreceptor drive. Thus when freely-breathing animals are exposed to hypoxia, as in ascent to altitude, the primary cardiovascular effects of chemoreceptor excitation (i.e., bradycardia and vasoconstriction) are limited in proportion to the increase in pulmonary stretch receptor activity caused by hyperventilation. In the light of what we have already said about the effects of lung P_{CO_2} on pulmonary stretch receptors, it is noteworthy that in dogs hyperventilating as a result of carotid body hypoxia, both tachycardia and vasodilatation are attenuated if alveolar P_{CO_2} is prevented from falling (see 17). Gerber and Polosa[20] have shown, by direct electrophysiological recording, that inflation of the lung inhibits activity in sympathetic neurons of the cervical trunk.

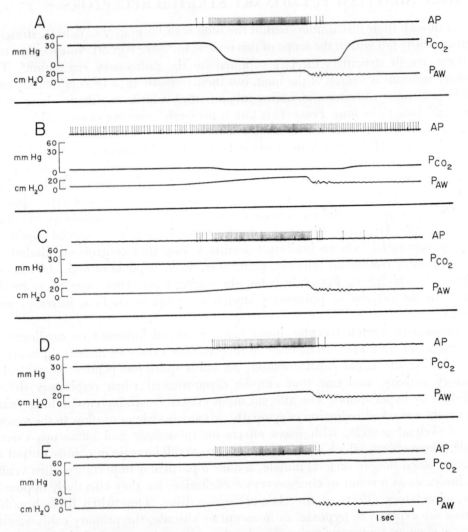

Fig. 3. Effect on a slowly-adapting pulmonary stretch receptor (in the left lung) of occluding the left pulmonary artery and of adding CO_2 to the O_2 ventilating the left
lung. (Experiment on a dog whose right and left lungs were ventilated separately
through a double-lumen endotracheal tube. When the left pulmonary artery was
occluded, left lung P_{CO_2} fell, and gas exchange was maintained with the right lung
only.) AP, action potentials (left vagal); P_{CO_2}, tidal CO_2 from the left lung; P_{AW},
airway pressure (left lung). A, left pulmonary artery patent; B–E, left pulmonary
artery occluded. The left lung was ventilated with: O_2 (A and B), and with (approximately) 3% CO_2 in O_2 (C), 4.5% CO_2 in O_2 (D), and 7% CO_2 in O_2 (E). Average
firing frequency during the ventilatory cycle: A, 19.1 impulses/sec; B, 35.2 impulses/
sec; C, 17.9 impulses/sec; D, 15.9 impulses/sec; E, 15.2 impulses/sec. (From Coleridge
et al.[5].)

PULMONARY C FIBERS

Afferent vagal C fibers greatly outnumber their myelinated counterparts in the pulmonary vagal branches. Their action potentials are small and their discharge is sparse and irregular, so that they could be easily overlooked without some artificial means of evoking an increase in their activity. They are promptly stimulated when chemicals such as capsaicin are injected into the pulmonary circulation (Fig. 4B); perhaps more important from the functional standpoint, they are sensitive to certain endogenous chemicals, the prostaglandins, that are known to be formed and released by the lung in a variety of physiological and pathological conditions[7]. They are also stimulated by pulmonary emboli, by hyperinflation of the lungs (Fig. 4A) and by high concentrations of volatile anesthetics, including ether and halothane

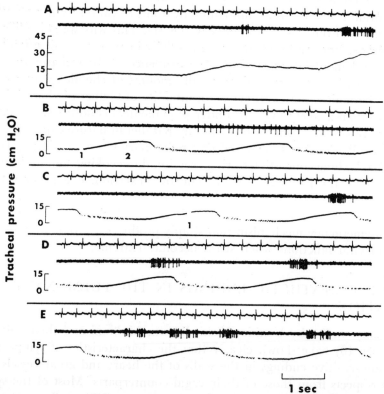

Fig. 4.   Response of a pulmonary C fiber ending to various procedures. Dog; open chest; positive pressure ventilation. From above down; ECG; afferent impulses recorded from left vagal slip; tracheal pressure. A, effect of hyperinflation; the ventilatory outlet tube was clamped so that the lungs were progressively inflated for 3 strokes of the pump. B, capsaicin (5 μg/kg) was injected into the right atrium between 1 and 2. C, D (continuous), beginning at 1, the lungs were ventilated with air which had passed over a column of trichloroethylene. E, bursts of activity produced by gently pinching the left lower lobe. (From Coleridge et al.[12].)

(Fig. 4C, D)[11,12]. Some authorities have classed them as 'alveolar nociceptors', probably because most of the above stimuli could reasonably be described as noxious, but there is little doubt that pulmonary C fiber endings are capable of responding to stimuli whose intensity is well within the physiological range. For example, a small stepwise increase in pulmonary venous pressure in dogs, produced by inflating a balloon at the mitral orifice, leads to a progressive increase in impulse activity[4]. Moreover the firing frequency of pulmonary C fiber endings is significantly higher in spontaneously-breathing dogs than in dogs with open chest and lungs ventilated at normal tidal volume and functional residual capacity[4]. This effect is probably related to the larger pulmonary blood volume in the former condition. It seems reasonable to suppose, therefore, that these endings exert some reflex influence under normal circumstances.

Pulmonary C fibers are responsible for the pulmonary chemoreflex triad of apnea, bradycardia and peripheral vasodilatation evoked by right atrial injection of capsaicin in dogs and cats[11,12], or of phenyl diguanide in cats[28], in amounts too small to affect the endings of myelinated fibers. In the last ten years this response has attracted a good deal of attention because it is accompanied by a loss of voluntary muscle tone and an inhibition of spinal reflexes (for references, see 21). This widespread reflex inhibition of somatic motor function by an increase in activity in an autonomic afferent pathway is yet another demonstration of the interdependence of the somatic and autonomic divisions of the nervous system. Even small amounts of chemicals such as capsaicin and phenyl diguanide, however, evoke an intensity of C fiber discharge that is many times greater than is likely to occur under physiological conditions, so that the question whether this reflex phenomenon has any parallel in nature can only be a matter for conjecture. Paintal[29] has suggested that pulmonary C fiber endings ('J receptors') are stimulated by lung congestion during exercise, thus evoking an inhibition of central nervous activity ('the J reflex') that prevents over-exertion. It is perhaps more likely that the total reflex response, consisting of both visceral and somatic components (hypotension, bradycardia, apnea and inhibition of somatic motor activity) represents some sort of emergency mechanism that simply produces a profound and widespread inhibition of vital functions when stress becomes extreme.

AFFERENT SYMPATHETIC ENDINGS IN THE PULMONARY CIRCULATION

The many studies by Uchida, Nishi, Brown, Malliani and their colleagues (for references, see 10) have shown clearly that the characteristics of sympathetic fibers with mechanosensitive endings in the walls of the heart and great vessels differ in a number of respects from those of their vagal counterparts. Most of the sympathetic fibers described are in the Aδ range, though some are C fibers. In contrast to vagal mechanoreceptors, whose stimulus-response characteristics are such that they can signal changes in transmural pressure or volume on either side of normal, sympathetic endings function at the lower end of their potential firing frequency, even when transmural pressures are grossly elevated. Control activity is sparse (about 0.3 impulses/sec) and irregular, and there is little in the pattern of discharge to indicate the position of an ending. However, even the lightest touch in the region of a sensitive terminal causes a brisk burst of spikes, so that the endings are easy to locate. Almost half the axons branch in their peripheral course (as do many of the afferent sympathetic fibers that supply the intestine) and may have terminals on quite separate, though often adjacent, anatomical structures (for references, see 10). Nishi et al.[27] describe the response of 'sympathetic baroreceptors' with endings in the left pulmonary artery, and draw attention to similarities with the response of cutaneous and intestinal touch receptors with multiple terminals. A sudden increase in pulmonary arterial pressure causes prominent bursts of impulses with each cardiac cycle, but these are maintained for a few seconds only, and sustained activity rarely exceeds one to two impulses/beat. The characteristics of endings in the extrapulmonary parts of the pulmonary veins, described by Lombardi et al.[26], are generally similar, although these authors emphasize that no fiber was found to have more than a single ending. This has not been our experience, and we believe that afferent sympathetic fibers that innervate the pulmonary veins are as likely to branch as those that supply other vascular structures. Fibers with endings in the left atrium, for example, often have endings in pulmonary veins also, and fibers with endings in arteries or veins at the lung root may have additional endings in neighboring bronchi or pleural folds. Endings in the pulmonary veins increase their activity to one or two impulses/cardiac cycle when blood volume is increased by intravenous infusions, although this response, also, may be transient[10]. They are also stimulated by inflation of the lungs.

Perhaps one of the most interesting features of these sympathetic afferent units, and one in which they resemble cutaneous mechanoreceptors with Aδ fibers, is their response to small amounts of algesic substances, such as bradykinin, applied locally in concentrations that are known to be present in the tissues in certain conditions. Some endings are sensitized, and begin to fire one to two impulses with each cardiac cycle, others are stimulated, and fire irregularly. Effects may last for two minutes or more. Dr. Nishi presents evidence at this symposium that this is an important feature of the response of cardiac endings. We have observed a similar response in

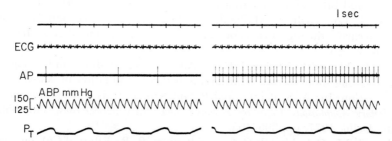

Fig. 5.   Stimulation by bradykinin of sympathetic afferent ending in a cat. ECG, electrocardiogram; AP, action potentials recorded from 3rd left thoracic sympathetic
ramus; ABP, aortic blood pressure; P$_T$, tracheal pressure (upstroke represents
inflation). The pericardial sac was opened and its edges were retracted widely. The
afferent ending was located in the ventral wall of the main pulmonary trunk; fiber
conduction velocity was 5.2 m/sec. Left panel: control (resting discharge, 0.25
impulses/sec). Right panel: 20 sec after 1 ml bradykinin solution (1 µg/ml) had been
dripped on to the main pulmonary artery inside the pericardium (discharge 3.5
impulses/sec). (By courtesy of Drs. David Baker and Tone Nerdrum.)

sympathetic fibers with mechanosensitive endings in the pulmonary arteries and veins (Fig. 5).

Although in many circumstances stimulation of afferent sympathetic fibers from the viscera may cause 'pseudo-affective' responses, there is no doubt that sympathetic input from cardiovascular endings may be increased considerably by stimuli not perceived as painful. Indeed, activity in afferent sympathetic fibers may produce reflex effects solely at the spinal level, without involving higher centers. By activating sympathetic afferent endings, intravenous infusions in cats may produce reflex tachycardia[3] and a fall in a renal vascular resistance[31]; and a sympathetic afferent input contributes to the reflex vasodilatation caused by lung inflation in dogs[17]. Since mechanosensitive endings in the pulmonary veins are stimulated by both procedures, they may contribute to the reflex effects[26]. Thus in some circumstances the sympathetic and vagal inputs can act in concert to produce tachycardia and vasodilatation. However, when stimulus intensity reaches a critical level, which probably corresponds to the pain threshold, sympathetic afferent activity has conspicuous pressor effects. The pain threshold may be reached when endings are sensitized or stimulated by local release of substances such as bradykinin, because it is only in the presence of such chemical agents that a relatively high frequency of discharge is sustained for more than a few seconds.

Original work reported here was supported by the U.S. Public Health Service Program Project Grant HL-06285 from the National Heart, Lung and Blood Institute.

REFERENCES

1   Anrep, G. V., Pascual, W. and Rossler, R., Respiratory variations of the heart rate. I. The reflex mechanism of the respiratory arrhythmia, *Proc. Roy. Soc. Lond. Ser. B.*, 119 (1936) 191–217.

2   Armstrong, D. J. and Luck, J. C., Accessibility of pulmonary stretch receptors from the pulmonary and bronchial circulations, *J. appl. Physiol.*, 36 (1974) 706–710.

3   Bishop, V. S., Lombardi, F., Malliani, A., Pagani, M. and Recordati, G., Reflex sympathetic tachycardia during intravenous infusions in chronic spinal cats, *Amer. J. Physiol.*, 230 (1976) 25–29.

4   Coleridge, H. M. and Coleridge, J. C. G., Afferent vagal C-fibers in the dog lung: Their discharge during spontaneous breathing, and their stimulation by alloxan and pulmonary congestion. In: A. S. Paintal and P. Gill-Kumar (Eds.), *Krogh Centenary Symposium on Respiratory Adaptations, Capillary Exchange and Reflex Mechanisms*, Vallabhbhai Chest Institute, Delhi, 1977, pp. 396–406.

5   Coleridge, H. M., Coleridge, J. C. G. and Banzett, R. B., Effect of CO_2 on afferent vagal endings in the canine lung, *Respir. Physiol.*, 34 (1978) 135–151.

6   Coleridge, H. M., Coleridge, J. C. G., Dangel, A., Kidd, C., Luck, J. C. and Sleight, P., Impulses in slowly conducting vagal fibers from afferent endings in the veins, atria and arteries of dogs and cats, *Circulation Res.*, 33 (1973) 87–97.

7   Coleridge, H. M., Coleridge, J. C. G., Ginzel, K. H., Baker, D. G., Banzett, R. B. and Morrison, M. A., Stimulation of 'irritant' receptors and afferent C-fibres in the lungs by prostaglandins. *Nature* (Lond.), 264 (1976) 451–453.

8   Coleridge, H. M., Coleridge, J. C. G. and Howe, A., A search for pulmonary arterial

chemoreceptors in the cat, with a comparison of the blood supply of the aortic bodies in the new-born and adult animal, *J. Physiol.* (Lond.), 191 (1967) 353–374.

9   Coleridge, H. M., Coleridge, J. C. G. and Howe, A., Thoracic chemoreceptors in the dog: A histological and electrophysiological study of the location, innervation and blood supply of the aortic bodies, *Circulation Res.*, 26 (1970) 235–247.

10   Coleridge, H. M., Coleridge, J. C. G. and Kidd, C., Afferent innervation of the heart and great vessels: A comparison of the vagal and sympathetic components, *Acta physiol. pol.*, (1978) in press.

11   Coleridge, H. M., Coleridge, J. C. G. and Luck, J. C., Pulmonary afferent fibers of small diameter stimulated by capsaicin and by hyper-inflation of the lung, *J. Physiol.* (Lond.), 179 (1965) 248–262.

12   Coleridge, H. M., Coleridge, J. C. G., Luck, J. C. and Norman, J., Effect of four volatile anaesthetic agents on the impulse activity of two types of pulmonary receptor, *Brit. J. Anaesth.*, 40 (1968) 484–492.

13   Coleridge, J. C. G. and Kidd, C., Vascular receptors in the lungs, *J. Physiol.* (Lond.), 148 (1959) 30P.

14   Coleridge, J. C. G. and Kidd, C., Relationship between pulmonary arterial pressure and impulse activity in pulmonary arterial baroreceptor fibres, *J. Physiol.* (Lond.), 158 (1961) 197–205.

15   Coleridge, J. C. G. and Kidd, C., Reflex effects of stimulating baroreceptors in the pulmonary artery, *J. Physiol.* (Lond.), 166 (1963) 197–210.

16   Daly, I. de B. and Hebb, C., *Pulmonary and Bronchial Vascular Systems*, Edward Arnold, London, 1966.

17   Daly, M. de B., Interaction of cardiovascular reflexes, *Sci. Basis Med. ann. Rev.*, (1972) 307–332.

18   Daly, M. de B and Robinson, B. H., An analysis of the reflex systemic vasodilator response elicited by lung inflation in the dog, *J. Physiol.* (Lond.), 195 (1968) 387–406.

19   Gaskell, W. H., *The Involuntary Nervous System*, Longmans, Green and Co., London, 1916.

20   Gerber, U. and Polosa, C., Effects of pulmonary stretch receptor afferent stimulation on sympathetic preganglionic neuron firing, *Can. J. Physiol. Pharmacol.*, 56 (1978) 191–198.

21   Ginzel, K. H. and Eldred, E., Reflex depression of somatic motor activity from heart, lungs and carotid sinus. In: A. S. Paintal and P. Gill-Kumar (Eds.), *Krogh Centenary Symposium on Respiratory Adaptations, Capillary Exchange and Reflex Mechanisms*, Vallabhbhai Chest Institute, Delhi, 1977, pp. 358–395.

22   Krahl, V. E., The glomus pulmonale: Its location and microscopic anatomy. In: A. V. S. Reuck and M. O'Connor (Eds.), *Ciba Foundation Symposium on Pulmonary Structure and Function*, J. and A. Churchill Ltd., London, 1962, pp. 53–69.

23   Langley, J. N., The autonomic nervous system, *Brain*, 26 (1903) 1–26.

24   Ledsome, J. R. and Kan, W.-O., Reflex changes in hind limb and renal vascular resistance in response to distension of the isolated pulmonary arteries of the dog, *Circulation Res.*, 40 (1977) 64–72.

25   Lloyd, T. C., Jr., Control of systemic vascular resistance by pulmonary and left heart baroreflexes, *Amer. J. Physiol.*, 222 (1972) 1511–1517.

26   Lombardi, F., Malliani, A. and Pagani, M., Nervous activity of afferent sympathetic fibers innervating the pulmonary veins, *Brain Res.*, 113 (1976) 197–200.

27   Nishi, K., Sakanashi, M. and Takenaka, F., Afferent fibers from pulmonary arterial baroreceptors in the left cardiac sympathetic nerve of the cat, *J. Physiol.* (Lond.), 240 (1974) 53–66.

28 Paintal, A. S., Mechanism of stimulation of type J pulmonary receptors, *J. Physiol.* (Lond.), 203 (1969) 511–532.

29 Paintal, A. S., The mechanism of stimulation of type J receptors, and the J reflex. In: R. Porter (Ed.), *Breathing: Hering-Breuer Centenary Symposium*, Ciba Foundation Symposium, Churchill, London, 1970, pp. 59–71.

30 Schoener, E. P. and Frankel, H. M., Effect of hyperthermia and $PaCO_2$ on the slowly adapting pulmonary stretch receptor, *Amer. J. Physiol.*, 222 (1972) 68–72.

31 Weaver, L. C., Cardiopulmonary sympathetic afferent influences on renal nerve activity, *Amer. J. Physiol.*, 233 (1977) H592–599.

CHAPTER 8

RECEPTORS IN THE HEART AND THE INTEGRATIVE ROLE OF CARDIAC REFLEXES

K. Nishi* and C. McC. Brooks**

*Department of Pharmacology, Kumamoto University Medical School, Kumamoto, Japan, and
**Department of Physiology, State University of New York,
Downstate Medical Center, Brooklyn, New York, USA

PREFACE

There are three closely related topics which concern those who study the autonomic system's regulation of cardiac function. These are: 1) the responses of the heart to external stimuli that evoke behavioral reactions requiring cardiac support; 2) the responses of the heart to intrinsic stimulations of intracardiac receptors, these stimuli being produced by occurrences resulting from behavioral activities or conditions within the myocardium; 3) the overall effect on the body of cardiac reflexes and signals received by the central nervous system from the heart.

The primary objectives of the present paper are to define the nature of receptors within the heart, what reactions they evoke and the total or integrative effects of the reflexes originating from within the heart. It is recognized of course that action of control centers is affected by stimuli received concurrently from the periphery as well as from the heart. The three topics mentioned can therefore not be considered completely independently.

There is another matter which should be kept in mind by those considering the autonomic system and control of the heart. It is that the autonomic system plays a modulatory role in controlling organ function; this is well illustrated by its actions on the heart. The origin of the heart beat is myogenic. The autonomic nerves can affect pacemaker action as well as other cardiac activities but they are not essential thereto. Furthermore, the heart is autoregulatory and even when denervated or isolated it can respond to forces acting upon it. Even isolated cardiac tissues respond to stretch, accommodate thereto and show reversals of action thereafter (see 7, pp. 95–96). Nerve action can affect the myogenic responses in ways quite different from those suggested by their effects on rate of beat. This concern will be discussed in connection with the consideration of reflexes since some responses of the heart to intrinsic stimuli do not involve reflexes or nerves[6].

RECEPTORS OF THE HEART (*K. Nishi*)

INTRODUCTION

For more than 20 years the cardiac receptors with their afferent fibers in the vagus nerve have been extensively studied and valuable information on their characteristics as well as functional significance has been accumulated. In the atria complex unencapsulated nerve endings with myelinated vagal afferent fibers are located predominantly at the junctions of the atrial walls with the intrapericardial portion of the system and pulmonary veins[14]. The presence of at least two types of atrial receptors, Type A and Type B receptors, has been proposed by Paintal[42,43]. Although these two types of receptors are not always clearly distinguishable, Type A receptors are activated presumably by changes in atrial volume, while Type B receptors are stimulated by atrial contraction. However, this has been questioned by other investigators, because they occasionally observed spontaneous shifts of A- to B-type discharges and vice versa[30,37]. More recent studies have shown that irrespective of the receptor type, all atrial afferent fibers appear to originate from identical mechanoreceptors in the atria[1]. Functionally, these receptors in the atria participate in the "Bainbridge Reflex"; when the atrial receptors are stimulated by distension, a reflex increase in heart rate and a small but significant decrease in vascular resistance occurs[3,12,23,40]. Furthermore, it has been suggested that the atrial receptors are involved in regulation of blood volume. Distension of the atria results in an increase in urine outflow, and an increase in water excretion; stimulation of the atrial receptors often cause an increase in sodium excretion by the kidney[13,18,24].

It is well known that in the vagus nerve afferent myelinated and unmyelinated nerve fibers originate from the subendocardium of both ventricles[15,46], the parietal pericardium[46] and in or near the left main coronary artery[8]. In most instances, the ventricular receptors with vagal myelinated fibers fire an early systolic burst of impulses before the aortic valve opens, while the receptors with nonmyelinated fibers usually have only a sparse and irregular spontaneous discharge. Both these receptors are stimulated by veratridine. The receptors in the venticle or epicardium of the ventricle, when stimulated by elevating ventricular pressure or by injecting veratridine, elicit a reflex bradycardia and a decrease in systemic vascular resistance[2,45]. Section of the vagal fibers of the cardiac plexus causes an increase in peripheral vascular resistance. Thus, the ventricular receptors play an important role in reflex regulation of the cardiovascular system, but also exert a tonic inhibition on the vasomotor center[35,41]. Recent reviews of these receptors have discussed in detail the mechanism of impulse initiation at nerve terminals, characteristics of the receptors and their functional role in circulatory control[14,42,43].

Since in 1892 Edgeworth first suggested the existence in the cardiac sympathetic nerves of afferent fibers, more complete histological and physiological evidence of the presence of the sensory nerve endings with afferent fibers in sympathetic trunks has been obtained by several investigators[16,20,21,50]. Some of these afferent fibers show a spontaneous discharge in phase with atrial or ventricular systole, and others are

activated by acute myocardial ischemia induced by coronary art
increase in the pressure in the coronary artery or by direct mech
wall of the ventricle. Mechanosensitive endings of these fibers
pathetic nerve are located in the ventricle, aorta, main coronary ar
artery[8,9,10,34,38,39,48]. Stimulation of the afferent fibers, both myeli
nated, by electrical current pulses causes a reflex increase in myoc
and in the heart rate[44]. At this moment, however it is not clear ..nether such an
excitatory reflex has any functional role in normal circulatory control. On the other
hand, it has been suggested that the afferent fibers in the cardiac sympathetic nerve
participate in transmitting impulses leading to cardiac pain in humans[33,49] and also
in experimental animals. Afferent fibers in these nerves are activated by acute myocardial ischemia, which initiate pseudo-affective reaction typically associated with
pain[9,47]. These observations lend support to the idea that some of the afferent fibers,
particularly small myelinated and unmyelinated fibers, in the cardiac sympathetic
nerve may originate from "cardiac nociceptors". However, in most instances, discharges in these fibers induced by coronary occlusion occur synchronously with
cardiac mechanical events, or when the size of the heart is increased during interruption of coronary flow[10,47]. Thus, it is unclear whether the afferent fibers respond to
myocardiac ischemia. There is, however, another possibility: The mechanically
excitable receptor may also be responsive to humoral substances, possibly produced
by myocardial ischemia[11,25]. In fact, recent studies on the afferent fibers in the cardiac
sympathetic nerve has indicated the presence of a certain number of afferent fibers
with polymodal sensitivity[39]. The main attempt of the present paper is to describe
electrophysiological as well as pharmacological characteristics of these sensory receptors in the heart and discuss the functional significance of the afferent fibers in the
cardiac sympathetic nerve.

METHODS

The methods employed in the present paper were essentially similar to those
described in previous publications[38,39]. Experiments were performed on adult cats of
either sex, weighing 1.5–3 kg, anesthetized with sodium pentobarbitone (30 mg/kg,
i.p.). The animals were ventilated artificially. The thoracic cavity was opened and the
left stellate ganglion and its branches were exposed. A suitable length of the inferior
cardiac nerve or the third left thoracic sympathetic ramus was cleaned of surrounding
connective tissue and then cut. The peripheral end of the nerve was dissected into
fine filaments containing either single or a few active units. The action potentials were
led off from the nerve with bipolar electrodes, amplified for display on an oscilloscope
and simultaneously led to an FM-data recorder for later analysis. Arterial blood pressure was recorded from a femoral artery and an ECG was also recorded. Action potentials, arterial blood pressure and ECG records were stored on different channels of
magnetic tape.

The anterior aspect of the heart was exposed by pericardiotomy and direct
mechanical probing of the wall of the heart and the pulmonary artery was perforated
by a round glass rod 1 mm in diameter, or a sharp needle. Controlled mechanical

stimuli were delivered by an electromagnet driving a fine metal probe. The electromagnet was excited by a power source of very low impedance from an electronic pulse generator. Actual displacement of the tip of the probe was not monitored, but the stimulus strength was controlled by changing the amplitude of rectangular pulses supplying the electromagnet, and thus adjusted to elicit a response in the receptors. Thermal stimuli were applied by a fine electronic cautery to the surface of the heart and the pulmonary artery after death of the animal. A probe for holding the cautery, with a tip two mm in diameter, was placed over the points most sensitive to mechanical stimuli. Cautery stimulus strength was controlled by moving the tip of the heating probe closer or farther from the surface of the heart. Temperature was monitored by a thermistor placed on the surface of heart and artery approximately five mm above the mechanosensitive spots. Chemical substances were delivered through a femoral vein. In other instances, a filter paper disc, three mm in diameter, saturated with Locke's solution containing various concentrations of the chemical substances being tested was placed on the sites sensitive to mechanical stimuli.

Approximate values for fiber conduction velocity were determined at the termination of the experiment. A pair of fine platinum electrodes, two mm apart, were placed on the spot most sensitive to mechanical stimuli, and action potentials evoked by electrical stimulation were displayed on the oscilloscope. The electrical shock applied to the surface of the heart or the pulmonary artery caused a local twitch and occasionally evoked a train of two or three action potentials of different amplitude and configuration. The action potential evoked by electrical stimulation, of which the amplitude and configuration were identical to those mechanically evoked, was used for calculation of the conduction velocity in the afferent fibers. On other occasions, the metal probe driven by the electromagnet was placed on the surface of the heart and the pulmonary artery on the spot sensitive to mechanical stimuli. The time from the start of the current pulse to the onset of the action potential thus evoked varied, depending upon the stimulus strength. Therefore, the shortest time of appearance of the action potential elicited by a stimulus of submaximal strength was used for calculation of conduction velocities.

Data analysis. Pharmacological agents such as norepinephrine or acetylcholine produce an increase in discharge frequency in some afferent fibers in cardiac sympathetic nerves[34,38]. The increase in discharge frequency following injections of chemical substances does not necessarily mean that the afferent units in question are sensitive to the agent per se; it is also possible that the fibers may be activated by mechanical changes in the myocardium following injections of the chemicals. Therefore, the relationship between occurrence of each action potential and the pulsatile pressure of arterial blood pressure was analyzed in detail. The sweep of the beam of the oscilloscope was triggered by each QRS-complex of the ECG and superimposed action potentials and pulsatile blood pressure were photographed for 10–15 QRS-complexes. In cases where discharges in the afferent fibers were elicited solely by mechanical changes in the cardiac events, most action potentials appeared at some identifiable phase of each pressure pulse and showed a clear relation to the cardiac cycle. However, in other instances, the discharges were distributed randomly without showing any particular relation to arterial blood pressure, leading to the deduction that the fiber or receptor was sensitive to the substances injected per se. The method permitted us to examine effects of chemical substances on afferent fibers in the cardiac sympathetic nerve when the heart was beating.

RESULTS

Location of Receptors

Seventy-three single afferent units in the left cardiac sympathetic nerve were identified. Among them 46 fibers were excited by direct mechanical probing of the wall of the heart and the pulmonary artery. Two had receptor fields on the left atrium, 21 on the left ventricle, 23 on the left pulmonary artery, two on the pericardium and six on the descending aorta or the dimple between the aorta and the pulmonary artery. Seventeen afferent fibers could not be excited by mechanical probing of the epicardial surface of the heart, although in 10 fibers impulses occurred in phase with an identifiable part of the cardiac cycle. In the remaining seven afferent fibers, discharges occurred irregularly without showing any particular relation to the pulsatile pressure and the activity was abolished when 0.1% procaine solution was injected

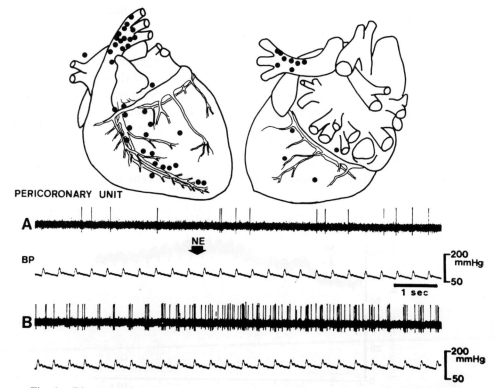

Fig. 1.   Diagrammatic representation of position of mechanosensitive spots on the wall of the heart and the pulmonary artery, and impulse discharges in a single afferent fiber with a pericoronary mechanosensitive receptor. Norepinephrine (NE) (2 μg/kg) injected intravenously at arrow. BP: arterial blood pressure. A and B: continuous record.

into the pericardial sac. Figure 1 shows a diagrammatic representation of the position of mechanosensitive spots on the wall of the heart and the pulmonary artery and an example of unitary discharges in a single afferent fiber from a ventricular receptor. Mechanical probing of the wall of the heart revealed an uneven distribution of mechanosensitive spots. The receptors in the ventricle were found to lie along the left descending coronary artery, while those in the pulmonary artery were localized in the distal region of the artery, but not on the main trunk. The stimulus strength required to elicit afferent discharges in the fibers arising from the left ventricle varied; some of the fibers were excited by light tactile stimuli, while others were activated only by pressure with a sharp needle. It was difficult to localize precise sites of the receptors while the heart was beating. Therefore, receptors were localized immediately after death of the animals (cardiac arrest). In most instances, the receptor region was found to consist of one or two point-like spots less than five mm apart. In other cases, the fibers were activated by forcible pressure or tapping an area on the wall of the ventricle with a dull-pointed probe, the mechanically sensitive region not being sharply defined.

General Characteristics of Afferent Fibers with Mechanosensitivity: Afferent Fibers with Ventricular Mechanosensitive Receptors

     Twenty-one afferent fibers arising from the ventricular mechanosensitive receptors were identified. The rate of spontaneous discharges in these fibers showed a considerable variation depending upon individual fibers. Under open chest, anesthetized conditions approximately half of the fibers did not show regular spontaneous activity. In the rest of the fibers, one or two action potentials occurred during the rising phase of each pulsatile pressure in the artery, but each cardiac cycle was not always accompanied by impulse activity as previously observed by Malliani, et al.[34]. However, in all cases, discharges increased when arterial blood pressure was raised either by intravenous injections of norepinephrine or by occlusion of the aorta. An example of elevation of arterial blood pressure by an intravenous injection of norepinephrine (NE) (2 μg/kg) and effects on discharges in a single afferent fiber arising from the

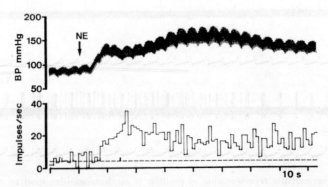

Fig. 2.   Changes in discharge frequency in a single afferent fiber with a ventricular mechano-sensitive receptor after an intravenous injection of norepinephrine (NE) (2 μg/kg). Upper record: arterial blood pressure and lower one: discharge frequency; impulses counted for one second and represented in vertical bars.

ventricle is illustrated in the lower panel of Fig. 1 and in Fig. 2. During the control period discharges were sparse, but a rhythmic burst of discharges consisting of two to four impulses appeared with each cardiac cycle after injection of the agent, but the discharge frequency did not increase further and gradually declined, even though the level of arterial blood pressure was far higher than that of the control. In most cases, continuous trains of impulse discharges were not observed even when arterial blood pressure was elevated maximally by NE or by occlusion of the aorta.

Afferent Fibers with Pulmonary Arterial Mechanosensitive Receptors
    Under artificial ventilation, spontaneous activity in these fibers was irregular and the resting rate of the discharges of different fibers ranged from 0.1 to 1.8 impulses/sec. When pulmonary arterial blood pressure was raised by an intravenous infusion of Locke's solution, a small dose of acetylcholine (Ach) or by NE, the discharges started to appear synchronously with each systolic pressure pulse in the artery. Impulse activity diminished or disappeared when pulmonary arterial blood pressure was lowered by bleeding from the femoral artery. A progressive rise in pulmonary arterial blood pressure elicited two or three impulses per cardiac cycle, but a further increase in the number of impulses for each cardiac cycle was not observed. Occlusion of the lung root, which produced a sustained rise in pulmonary arterial blood pressure, induced a burst of discharges, followed by four to six impulses per heart beat for several seconds. However, prolongation of the occlusion led to a reduction in the number of impulses per heart beat, although pulmonary arterial blood pressure remained at the same level during the occlusion. In most cases, adaptation of the receptors occurred within 20 sec after the onset of occlusion. When the receptor was stimulated by repetitive mechanical stimuli through a fine metal probe attached to an electromagnet, the impulse followed the stimuli in a one-to-one manner up to 10 sec. However, repetitive stimulation above 20 sec resulted in a progressively decreased responsiveness, so that after a number of stimuli no discharge was observed.

Effects of Pain-producing Substances on Afferent Fibers Sensitive to Mechanical Stimuli
    Bradykinin. Six afferent fibers arising from left ventricular mechanosensitive receptors were activated by bradykinin injected intravenously in doses ranging from 10 μg/kg to 50 μg/kg, or applied topically. When the agent was injected, discharges increased after a latency of seven–10 sec from the start of the injections, and the excitatory effect lasted for about 30 sec with a relatively low frequency. The discharges induced by injections of the agent occurred randomly without showing any relation to pulse pressure in the artery. Immediately after the deaths of animals, a small piece of filter paper immersed in Locke's solution containing bradykinin (80 μg/ml) placed on the mechanosensitive spots on the wall of the ventricle excited three fibers which previously had responded to the agent injected intravenously. Twelve fibers from the pulmonary arterial mechanosensitive receptors were also stimulated by bradykinin applied intravenously. The conduction velocities of four fibers from the ventricular receptor which responded to bradykinin ranged from 5.8 m/sec to 11.5 m/sec.
    5-Hydroxytryptamine. 5-Hydroxytryptamine (5-HT) was applied both intravenously and topically. Seven fibers with ventricular mechanosensitive receptors and

six fibers from pulmonary arterial mechanosensitive receptors were excited by 5-HT (2–10 μg/kg, i.v.). The injections of 5-HT induced a marked fall in arterial blood pressure, followed by a slight elevation of the pressure. The discharges in most instances started to increase 20–30 sec after the injection and the effect lasted for about 30 sec. Repeated injections of the same dose of the agent at short intervals led to a drastic decline in the sensitivity to the agent. Topical application of 5-HT (10 μg/ml) on the receptor loci also evoked discharges with a latency of about 40 sec. Analysis of the discharges in these fibers elicited by 5-HT did not reveal any relation to changes in blood pressure or cardiac mechanical events.

Histamine. Histamine was injected intravenously (2–10 μg/kg), or applied topically (100 μg/mg). Histamine induced a marked fall in arterial pressure, which lasted for two to five min. Four afferent fibers with ventricular mechanosensitive receptors and three fibers with pulmonary arterial mechanosensitive receptors responded to the agent by increasing discharge frequencies. The reaction of afferent fibers showed great variation. Usually, discharges in these fibers started to increase with a latency of about 10 sec and the excitatory effect of the agent lasted for 20–50 sec. Because of the prolonged depressive action of histamine on arterial blood pressure, a further higher dose of the agent was not applied to test the reactivity of the fibers which had not responded to previous low doses of histamine. Topical application of the agent also evoked discharged in two fibers arising from the left ventricular mechanosensitive receptors.

Acetylcholine. Four afferent fibers arising from the ventricular mechanosensitive receptors were excited by Ach injected intravenously (2–5 μg/kg). The effect of the agent in higher doses was not clear; a large dose (10–20 μg/kg, i.v.) induced a sudden cardiac arrest or marked bradycardia associated with a short-duration fall in blood pressure, during which occasional short bursts of impulses occurred. Topical application of filter paper saturated with Locke's solution containing Ach (1 mg/ml) on a left ventricular mechanosensitive spot activated three fibers. The effects of Ach on the afferent fibers innervating pulmonary arterial mechanosensitive receptors were unclear, since a small dose of the agent causes pulmonary hypertension and such hypertension of itself is associated with an increase in discharge frequency of these fibers[38]. Topical application of Ach to the pulmonary artery produced an increase in discharge frequency in three afferent fibers after a relatively short latency.

Veratridine. Veratridine (30–50 μg/kg, i.v.) induced a marked increase in discharge frequency in four ventricular mechanosensitive receptors and seven fibers from the left pulmonary arterial receptors. Five seconds after an intravenous injection of veratridine (40 μg/kg) a marked increase in the discharge frequency was observed and this excitatory effect lasted for about 30 sec; thereafter the discharge frequency returned to the control level. Several seconds after the onset of the increase in the discharge, bradycardia and a marked fall in blood pressure appeared.

Reactivity of Afferent Fibers to the Various Substances

The results thus far described suggested that chemical substances applied to the animals may excite nonspecifically the afferent fibers with mechanosensitivity included in the cardiac sympathetic nerve[36]. Therefore, the reactivity of each single unitary fiber with a mechanosensitive receptor to these substances were examined in five cats.

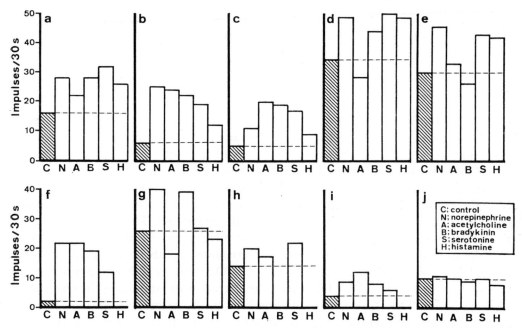

Fig. 3.   Response profile of mechanosensitive units to algesic substances. Discharges in each single fiber during the 30-sec period after intravenous injections of chemical substances were counted and represented in each column. Hatched columns indicate spontaneously occurring discharges in 30 sec during the control period. Small letters, a-j, represent different single afferent fibers in the cardiac sympathetic nerve. C: control. N: norepinephrine 2 μg/kg. A: acetylcholine 5 μg/kg. B: bradykinin 40 μg/kg. S: 5-hydroxytryptamine 10 μg/kg. H: histamine 10 μg/kg.

Results are shown in Fig. 3, in which discharges in a single afferent fiber during a 30-sec period after injections of the chemical substances were counted and represented in each column. Three afferent fibers responded to all chemical substances, and three fibers also showed sensitivity to three different substances except for norepinephrine. The remaining four responded to at least two different chemical substances, although higher doses of the agents were not applied. Thus, the results indicate that a certain population of cardiac afferent fibers with mechanosensitivity in the cardiac sympathetic nerve are nonspecifically sensitive to a certain chemical substance or substances. The conduction velocities of these fibers ranged from 2.8 m/sec to 8.4 m/sec.

Effects of Thermal Stimulation on Afferent Fibers with Mechanosensitivity

There is a possibility that the afferent fibers with mechanosensitivity in the cardiac sympathetic nerve may respond to modes of stimuli other than a mechanical one, since some of the cutaneous mechanoreceptors innervated by small myelinated or unmyelinated fibers show polymodal sensitivity[22]. Therefore, effects of thermal stimulation on mechanosensitive receptors of the ventricular wall after death of the animal were examined, since it was difficult to apply thermal stimulation to the narrow receptor area while the heart was beating. One left atrial receptor and four ventricular receptors were found to be activated by thermal stimuli. Evoked responses from these fibers started at temperatures of 40–50°C, and continued to increase in discharge frequency for several seconds after removal of thermal stimuli. Conduction velocities for five fibers ranged from 2.3 m/sec to 14.6 m/sec.

DISCUSSION

General Characteristics

The present report has shown response characteristics of mechanosensitive afferent fibers in the cardiac sympathetic nerve innervating the ventricle and the pulmonary artery. Most of the receptors in the ventricle were excited by direct mechanical probing of the epicardial surface of the ventricle; in some fibers action potentials were evoked by light tactile stimuli, while in others only mechanical displacement induced by forcible pressure was effective in eliciting impulse discharges. This is probably a reflection of the location of the nerve ending in the ventricle, since Malliani et al. have stated that the ventricular mechanosensitive fibers are more excitable to probing of the endocardial than epicardial surface of the ventricle[34]. On the basis of the approximate values for conduction velocity (2.3–14.6 m/sec), the afferent fibers supplying the receptors are likely to be small myelinated fibers falling into the Aδ category[17]. In most instances, spontaneously occurring discharges in these fibers were sparse and only a single or at most two impulses occurred during each cardiac cycle. These results are consistent with those obtained by previous investigators[34,47]. However, the response characteristics of these fibers are quite different from those of vagal afferent fibers with ventricular mechanoreceptors; in these vagal fibers a burst of discharges occurs during each cardiac cycle. The difference may be due to the transducing properties of the endings; the endings of the afferent cardiac sympathetic nerves may be diffuse and thin.

In the afferent fibers with pulmonary arterial mechanosensitive receptors, impulse discharges did not occur regularly and firing was at a low frequency during the control period. However, a slight elevation in pulmonary arterial pressure within the range of 2.5–5/0–4 mmHg (systolic/diastolic) elicited impulses synchronous with the systolic pressure pulse of the pulmonary artery, but a further elevation of the pressure did not cause a marked increase in the number of impulses per heart beat. A sustained, relatively high pressure, induced by occlusion of the lung root, led to a burst of impulse discharges followed by a progressive decrease in the discharge during each subsequent cardiac cycle. Therefore, it is likely that the afferent fibers from pulmonary arterial mechanosensitive receptors in the cardiac sympathetic nerve are not active at the pressures normally prevailing in the pulmonary arterial circuit. This is also clearly different from the functional features of the pulmonary arterial baroreceptors supplied by the vagus, in which the number of impulses per heart beat and maximum frequency of discharges showed a relatively linear relation to an increase in pressure. Thus, the functional characteristics of the afferent fibers in question show that they are excited by phasic mechanical events but also have a relatively rapid adaptation to sustained pressure. A failure to respond to repetitive mechanical stimuli of high frequency in a one-to-one manner is another characteristic of the receptors; this is similar to the behavior of cutaneous touch receptors[22] and to that of mechanoreceptors in the intestine[4].

Reactivity of Afferent Fibers with Mechanosensitive Receptors to Pain-producing Substances

Chemical substances known to produce pain in humans and pseudo-affective reactions in experimental animals induced an increase in discharge frequency in some afferent fibers of the cardiac sympathetic nerve whose endings were mechanically excitable. The possibility that the increased discharge frequency in these fibers may have been caused by mechanical displacement of the myocardium of the beating heart following intravenous injections of a chemical substance seems unlikely, since the chemically-elicited discharges did not show any particular relation to the arterial pressure of the ECG. Furthermore, topical application of chemical agents also activated these afferent fibers. With chemical stimulation, two afferent fibers of the 10 single afferent fibers systemically studied were activated by bradykinin, acetylcholine, histamine and 5-hydroxytryptamine, and seven afferent fibers responded to at least one or more of these algesic substances. The results obtained by the present author and others indicate the existence of a certain population of afferent fibers in the cardiac sympathetic nerves whose endings are activated by mechanical stimuli as well as chemical substances. The characteristics of these fibers are similar to those of cutaneous receptors and C-fiber muscle receptors; some of these sensory fibers exhibit responsiveness to both mechanical stimuli and algesic agents[11,19,29,30]. Moreover, the mechanosensitive receptors on the left ventricle and the pulmonary artery were excited by thermal stimulation, responses occurring at temperatures of 40°–50°C. The threshold temperature was uncertain, because the method of monitoring the temperature only gave an approximate value of the temperature around the receptor region. Since a considerable gradient around the thermode might be expected, the actual temperature at which the receptor was activated may have been significantly higher and produced tissue damage, thereby causing pain in humans and experimental animals. Thus, some of the receptors in the ventricle as well as the pulmonary artery exhibit characteristics similar to polymodal nociceptors in the skin and C-fiber receptors; three forms of stimulation namely, mechanical stimulation of moderate to strong intensity, noxious heating and some kinds of algesic substances, are all effective in activating this type of receptor. These observations might suggest that some afferent fibers in the cardiac sympathetic nerves are far from qualified as a highly-specific type, but remain in a primitive stage of development. In this respect, it is interesting to note that some afferent fibers with ventricular mechanosensitive receptors in the cardiac sympathetic nerve increased their frequency during acute myocardiac ischemia induced by coronary arterial occlusion[10]. One of the algesic substances examined, bradykinin, which has been shown to be capable of exciting some of the afferent fibers, has been suggested as the substance responsible for the pain in angina pectoris[11]. In fact a marked elevation of bradykinin contents in the ischemic area has been demonstrated[25], and its contents would be in the range reportedly sufficient to produce pain, or a pseudo-affective reaction in experimental animals. Therefore, it is conceivable that with the arrest of circulation liberated bradykinin may accumulate in the ischemic area and its contact with nerve endings could be sufficiently long to initiate action potentials at nerve endings possessing polymodal sensitivity.

One of the characteristics of the afferent fibers in the cardiac sympathetic nerve is that some of these afferent fibers can provide the spinal cord with information not only of mechanical changes in cardiac events, but also changes in the chemical environment of the nerve endings, possibly produced by myocardial ischemia. At present the existence of "pure mechanoreceptors or baroreceptors" or "pure cardiac nociceptors" innervated by afferent fibers in the cardiac sympathetic nerves cannot be ruled out, and remains to be explored further.

CARDIAC REFLEXES AND THEIR INTEGRATIVE EFFECTS
(C. McC. Brooks)

INTRODUCTION

There can no longer be any questioning of the fact that receptors within the heart and adjacent blood vessels can evoke reflex actions of the heart[32]. My associate in summarizing our knowledge of receptors in the heart has presented the thoughts of others relative to their roles in reflex action. It is obvious that receptors acting through afferent fibers of the vagi can play a role not only in adjusting cardiovascular function but also in the regulation of plasma volume and water balance. Other receptors, many of which have afferent connections through sympathetic trunks, can be classified as pain or nociceptive receptors. This does not mean they are not of physiological significance and do not normally participate in evoking physical and psychological reactions of the individual. In all probability they are involved when stimuli applied are very strong or when abnormal conditions such as ischemias are present.

Cardiac reflexes differ, even those evoked by distension of or stretch of the tissues of the right and left atria. Some cardiac reflexes are superimposed on myogenic effects but others are not. In the present paper only those reflexes evoked from the atria will be considered. The first statement required is that the receptors excited by the stimuli used are those which act through vagal afferents. However, very severe stretch, that exceeding the possible physiological range, does excite other sensors which feed through cardiac sympathetics and can evoke a reflex response[28].

METHODS

Most of the results to be reported were obtained from dogs anesthetized initially with i.v. thiopental sodium (Pentothal, 20–30 mg/kg) followed by intramuscular administration of morphine chloride (0.5 mg/kg); as the effect of the pentathal diminished it was replaced gradually by i.v. chloralose as needed until a total dosage of 70 mg/kg was reached. As reported in previous work[28] artificial respiration was begun and the heart was exposed; branches of cardiac sympathetic and vagal trunks were isolated and prepared for recording of efferent discharges therein. In some experiments reflexes were evoked by distending right and left atria by inflation of inserted balloons or umbrella-like devices. In the majority of experiments it was found to be equally satisfactory and preferable in many ways to attach a strong thread to the sinoatrial node region of the right atrium or to the pulmonary vein—left atrial junctional region and then to stretch these areas by attaching weights (20–150 g) to the threads which had been run over pulleys[26]. Blood pressure, heart beats and tacho-meter analyses of heart rates were continuously recorded.

Heart rate changes did provide an indication of response to stretch applied but in situations in which changes of myogenic origin were possible the only adequate criteria of reflex responses were provided by simultaneous recording of changes in rates of discharge in vagal and sympathetic cardiac efferents.

RESULTS

Reflex Actions Induced by Stretch of Right Atrial Tissues

Such stretch produces acceleration even in the denervated heart. Comparison of the response to a given stretch before and after vagal and sympathetic fibers to the

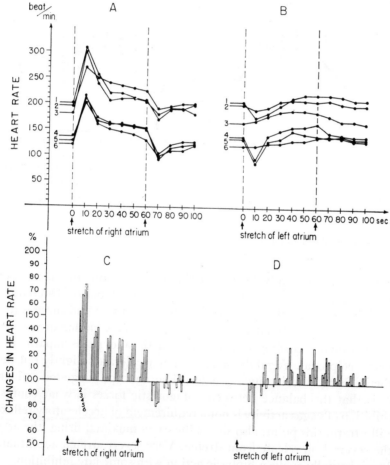

Fig. 4. Changes in heart rate evoked by stretch of the right (A and C) and the left (B and D) atria. Results from Six dogs, each indicated by number (1–6) in all figures. A and B: Changes expressed in beats/min. C and D: Percentage changes over and below prestimulus levels; each bar represents the average number of beaters in 10 sec[28].

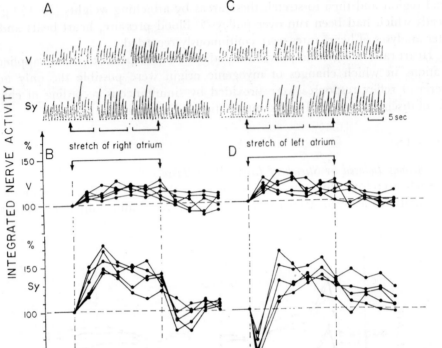

Fig. 5. Integrated records of vagal and sympathetic cardiac nerve activity and their response
to atrial stretch. A and C: responses obtained from the same dog. Vagal (V) and
sympathetic (SY) nerve activity integrated every second. The breaks in the record
represent 19–20 sec intervals. B and D: Percentage changes in integrated nerve
activity, relative to control values, produced by stretch. Each point represents the
summed discharges in 10 sec intervals. Results from five dogs[28].

heart are cut indicates that only 20–30% of the response is due to reflex action. Neural
recordings, however, confirm the fact that a reflex does occur. Discharge and rate
response are initially large, they plateau as stimuli continue and there is frequently a
reversal when stretch is terminated (Fig. 4A). One interesting feature of the response
revealed by neuronal recording is that sympathetic and parasympathetic responses
are not always reciprocal. Vagal discharges often accelerated slightly but the increase
in sympathetic firing rate is much greater. The concept suggested, which is quite
reasonable, is that the balance between antagonistic forces is what counts in reflex
actions; inhibition of vagus activity is not a requirement of acceleratory reflexes. Figure
5A, which illustrates this point, also shows the early maximal firing, the accommodation and the reversal on release from stretch. Very severe stretch accentuates this reversal and may actually evoke a biphasic action with some late inhibition.

Reflex Actions Induced by Stretch of the Left Atrium
     Reactions induced by stretch of left atrial tissues are purely neurogenic; there is

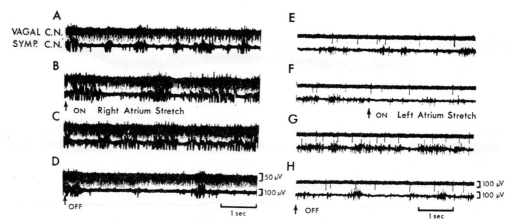

Fig. 6. Responses of vagal and sympathetic cardiac nerves, simultaneously recorded, to atrial stretch. A–D: Stretch of the right atrium applied between arrows. Strips are samples taken from moving film; records are in sequence but not continuous. Stretch applied for one minute (S↓↑). Note increase in activity in both nerves during stretch (B and C) and sudden inhibition of sympathetic activity (reversal of response) at the end of stretch (D). E–H: Records of effects of stretching the left atrium. Note the initial inhibition of sympathetic activity (F) (reciprocal action) and augmentation of discharge in both nerves (G). Reversal effect not seen after stretch[28].

no chronotropic myogenic response. This seems reasonable since pacemaker tissues are located in the right atrium. Figures 4B and 5B show that the heart rate and neural responses are biphasic and reciprocal initially. This is better seen in samples of neuron recordings (Fig. 6). The initial inhibition is very real but this is followed by a mild acceleration which diminishes and does not reverse on termination of stretch. As stated previously this reflex is evoked primarily by vagus afferents.

Generalized and Integrative Actions of These Cardiac Reflexes

1. It has not always been recognized that receptors in the right and left atria might have a different function to perform. It seems reasonable enough if one considers the emphasis in right-sided function is to receive blood and initiate appropriate heart rates. The positive or accelerator reflex and myogenic actions do seem appropriate. There is inhibitory control exerted by vagal action on the pacemaker and right atrium and even some intrinsic accommodation to diminish the response to stretch, but recent studies of actions of nerves on autoregulatory actions has revealed another phenomenon of some physiological and philosophical interest. The hyperpolarization induced by vagal inhibition which slows the heart does not abolish the myogenic acceleratory response to stretch; it augments the acceleration thus produced (Fig. 7)[6,31]. It seems as though this enables stretch to produce sufficient acceleratory action to break though inhibition if venous blood is pooled to an excessive extent in the right atrium.

Inhibition of the cardiovascular system is concentrated on the left side or in the systemic circuit. Certainly the depressor and carotid sinus reflexes originate there and it seems reasonable there should be some inhibitory reflex action possible from the

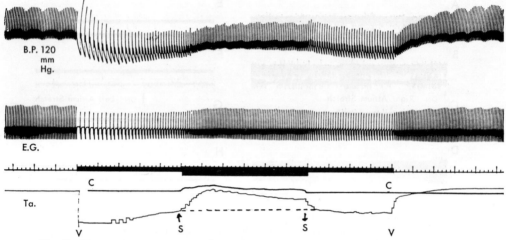

Fig. 7.   Response to same amount of stretch (50 g) of the right atrium before (C) and during
          vagus stimulation (V). Stretch applied (S↑↓). All external nerves cut. BP: Blood
          Pressure; EG: Electrogram; Ta: Tachogram. From[31].

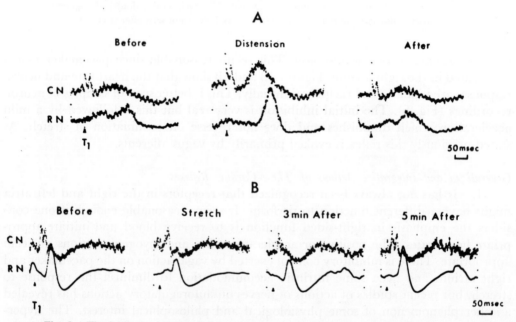

Fig. 8.   The facilitatory action of right atrial stretch on response of cardiac (CN) and renal
          nerve (RN) to stimulation of a somatosensory nerve (T₁) (A). The inhibitory effect
          of left atrial stretch on the same T₁ reflex (B)[26].

left atrium, and ventricle for that matter[5], to reduce the level of activity or keep
pressures from becoming excessive. However, the left atrium must pass on its load
and a late acceleration to distension seems physiologically reasonable.

   2.   The cardiac reflexes have a general action akin to their effects on the heart.

Stretch of the right atrium, which causes acceleration of the heart rate, facilitates autonomic reflexes evoked by stimulation of somatic afferents from skin and muscle. This is true at least for the reflex discharges to the heart and kidney. The inhibitory reflex from the left atrium has an inhibitory action on the autonomic reactions concurrently evoked from somatic sensory nerves (Fig. 8A and B). One can entertain the concept that the cardiac reflexes are of considerable significance to autonomic system responses as a whole, which means they affect many functions of the body[26].

3.   The cardiac reflexes are not insignificant, at least relative to their power to dominate. The barostatic reflexes are generally considered to be very powerful yet when, during a carotid reflex inhibition, right atrial stretch is performed the consequent accelerator action breaks through the inhibition imposed by this depressor reflex (Fig. 9). This is another example of how the stretch reaction, reflex and myogenic combined, is actually augmented by depressor effects[31].

4.   Cardiac reflexes affect body states and physiological balances. It is not demonstrated as yet that the acceleratory and facilitatory reactions from the right heart affect neuroendocrines or endocrine glands other than adrenal and possibly renin release but certainly reflexes from the left do. Stretch of the left atrium act on the supraoptic-paraventricular nuclei of the hypothalamus to inhibit their activity[27]. Such action relates to plasma volume control and control of water balance. The concurrent inhibition of renal vasoconstrictors, produced by left atrial stretch, would

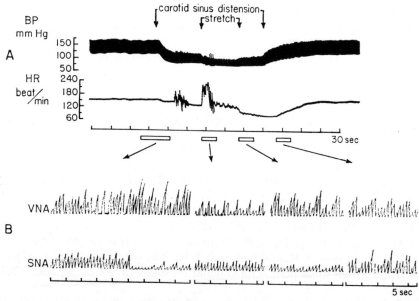

Fig. 9.   Effect of right atrial stretch applied during carotid sinus distension (depressor reflex). A: Blood pressure recorded from femoral artery (BP) and heart rate (HR) as recorded by a tachometer triggered by R wave of ECG. B: Vagal (VNA) and Sympathetic (SNA) cardiac nerve activity recorded simultaneously. Records of integrated activity of each second. The periods during which four nerve activity records of B were taken are indicated in A by white bars[28].

certainly contribute to a diuresis, a phenomenon frequently mentioned as an accompaniment of left atrial distension[13,18,24,28]. It is obvious that extension of these studies of the role of these cardiac reflexes in the control of neuroendocrine reactions should be undertaken.

CONCLUSION

Finally, I wish to suggest that just as emotional states and anticipatory reactions can affect the heart, events in the heart acting through the cardiac reflexes can affect body states. They can evoke or modify the physical, somatic, visceral and psychological states which determine the nature and quality of behavior.

Original work report here was supported by a grant from the New York Heart Association, Inc. and USPHS (NS-00847).

REFERENCES

1 Arndt, J. O., Brambring, P., Hindorf, K. and Röhnelt, M., Afferent discharge pattern of atrial mechano-receptors in the cat during sinusoidal stretch of atrial strips *in situ*, *J. Physiol.* (Lond.), 240 (1974) 33–52.

2 Aviado, D. M., Jr. and Schmidt, C. F., Cardiovascular and respiratory reflexes from the left side of the heart, *Amer. J. Physiol.*, 196 (1959) 726–730.

3 Bainbridge, F. A., The influence of venous filling upon the rate of the heart, *J. Physiol.* (Lond.), 50 (1915) 65–78.

4 Bessou, J. A. and Perl, E. R., A movement receptor of the small intestine, *J. Physiol.* (Lond.), 182 (1966) 404–426.

5 Brooks, C. McC., The autonomic system's involvement in behavior and homeostasis, *Proc. XVIII Int'l. Congr. Neurovegetative Research*, Tokyo, 1977.

6 Brooks, C. McC. and Lange, G., Interaction of myogenic and neurogenic mechanisms that control heart rate, *Proc. nat. Acad. Sci. USA*, 74 (1977) 1761–1762.

7 Brooks, C. McC. and Lu, H. H., *The Sinoatrial Pacemaker of the Heart*, Chas. C. Thomas, Springfield, 1972.

8 Brown, A. M., Mechanoreceptors in or near the coronary arteries, *J. Physiol.* (Lond.), 177 (1965) 203–214.

9 Brown, A. M., Excitation of afferent cardiac sympathetic nerve fibres during myocardiac ischemia, *J. Physiol.* (Lond.), 190 (1967) 35–53.

10 Brown, A. M. and Malliani, A., Spinal sympathetic reflexes initiated by coronary receptors, *J. Physiol.* (Lond.), 212 (1971) 685–705.

11 Burch, G. E. and DePasquale, N. P., Bradykinin, *Amer. Heart J.*, 65 (1963) 116–123.

12 Carswell, F., Hainsworth, R. and Ledsome, J. R., The effects of distension of pulmonary vein-atrial junctions upon peripheral vascular resistance, *J. Physiol.* (Lond.), 207 (1970) 1–14.

13 Carswell, F., Hainsworth, R. and Ledsome, J. R., The effects of left atrial distension upon usine flow from the isolated perfused kidney, *Q. J. exp. Physiol.*, 55 (1970) 173–182.

14 Coleridge, H. M. and Coleridge, R. C. G., Cardiovascular receptors. In: C. B. B. Downman (Ed.), *Modern Trends in Physiology*, Appleton-Century-Crofts, New York, 1972, pp. 245–267.

15 Coleridge, H. M., Coleridge, J. C. G., Dangel, A., Kidd, C., Luck, J. C. and Sleight, P., Impulses in slowly conducting vagal fibers from afferent endings in the veins, atria, and arteries of dogs and cats., *Circulation Res.*, 33 (1973) 87–97.

16 Edgeworth, F. H., On a large-fibred sensory supply of the thoracic and abdominal viscera, *J. Physiol.* (Lond.), 13 (1892) 260–271.

17 Erlanger, J. and Gasser, H. S., *Electrical Signs of Nervous Activity*, Univ. Penn Press, Philadelphia, 1937.

18 Gillespie, D. J., Sandberg, R. L. and Koike, T. I., Dual effect of left atrial receptors on excretion of sodium and water in the dog, *Amer. J. Physiol.*, 225 (1973) 706–710.

19 Handwerker, H. O., The influences of the algogenic substances serotonin and bradykinin on the discharges of unmyelinated cutaneous nerve fibres identified as nociceptors. In: *First World Congress of Pain* (abst), 1975, p. 33.

20 Hirsch, E. F. and Orme, J. F., Sensory nerves of the human heart, *Archs. Path.*, 44 (1947) 325–335.

21 Hirsh, E. F., Nigh, C. A., Kaye, M. P. and Cooper, T., Terminal innervation of the heart. II. Studies of the perimysial innervation apparatus and of the sensory receptors in the rabbit and in the dog with techniques of total extrinsic denervation, bilateral cervical vagotomy, and bilateral thoracic sympathectomy, *Archs. Path.*, 77 (1964) 172–187.

22 Hunt, C. C. and McIntyre, A. K., Properties of cutaneous touch receptors in cat, *J. Physiol.* (Lond.), 153 (1960) 88–98.

23 Kappagoda, C. T., Linden, R. L. and Snow, H. M., A reflex increase in heart rate from distension of the junction between the superior vena cava and the right atrium, *J. Physiol.* (Lond.), 220 (1972) 177–197.

24 Kappagoda, C. T., Linden, R. J., Snow, H. M. and Whitaker, E. M., Left atrial receptors and the antidiuretic hormone, *J. Physiol.* (Lond.), 237 (1974) 663–683.

25 Kimura, E., Hashimoto, K., Fukukawa, S. and Hayakawa, H., Changes in bradykinin level in coronary sinus blood after the experimental occlusion of a coronary artery, *Amer. Heart J.*, 85 (1973) 635–647.

26 Koizumi, K., Ishikawa, T., Nishino, H. and Brooks, C. McC., Cardiac and autonomic system reactions to stretch of the atria, *Brain Res.*, 87 (1975) 247–261.

27 Koizumi, K. and Yamashita, H., Influence of atrial stretch receptors on hypothalamic neurosecretory neurons, *J. Physiol.* (Lond.), in press.

28 Kollai, M., Koizumi, K., Yamashita, H. and Brooks, C. McC., Study of cardiac sympathetic and vagal efferent activity during reflex responses produced by stretch of the atria, *Brain Res.*, 150 (1978) 519–532.

29 Kumazawa, T. and Mizumura, K., The polymodal C-fiber receptor in the muscle of the dog, *Brain Res.*, 101 (1976) 589–593.

30 Landgren, D., Entlandungsmuster und allgemine Reizbedingungen von Vorhof-receptoren bei Hund und Katz, *Pflügers Arch.*, 271 (1960) 257–269.

31 Lange, G. and Brooks, C. McC., Neural influences on autoregulatory processes in the heart, *J. A. N. S.*, submitted.

32 Linden, R. J., Reflexes from the heart, *Progr. Cardiovasc. Dis.*, 18 (1975) 201–221.

33 Lindgren, I. and Olivecrona, H., Surgical treatment of angina pectoris, *J. Neurosurg.*, 4 (1947) 19–39.

34 Malliani, A., Recordati, G. and Schwartz, P. J., Nervous activity of afferent cardiac sympathetic fibres with atrial and ventricular endings, *J. Physiol.* (Lond.), 229 (1973) 457–469.

35 Mancia, G. and Donald, D. E., Demonstration that atria, ventricles, and lungs are

responsible for a tonic inhibition of the vasomotor center in the dog, *Circulation Res.*, 36 (1975) 310–318.

36 Mense, S. and Schmidt, R. F., Activation of group IV afferent units from muscle by algesic agents, *Brain Res.*, 72 (1974) 305–310.

37 Neil, E. and Joels, N., The impulse activity in cardiac afferent vagal fibres, Naunyn-Schmiedebergs, *Arch. exp. Path. Pharmak.*, 240 (1961) 453–460.

38 Nishi, K., Sakanashi, M. and Takenaka, F., Afferent fibres from pulmonary arterial baroreceptors in the left cardiac sympathetic nerve of the cat, *J. Physiol.* (Lond.), 240 (1974) 53–66.

39 Nishi, K., Sakanashi, M. and Takenaka, F., Activation of afferent cardiac sympathetic nerve fibers of the cat by pain producing substances and by noxious heat, *Pflügers Arch.*, 372 (1977) 53–61.

40 Nonidez, J. F., Identification of the receptor areas in the venae cavae and pulmonary veins which initiate reflex cardiac acceleration (Bainbridge's reflex), *Amer. J. Anat.*, 61 (1937) 203–231.

41 Öberg, B. and White, S., Circulatory effects of interruption and stimulation of cardiac vagal afferents, *Acta physiol. scand.*, 80 (1970) 383–394.

42 Paintal, A. S., Cardiovascular receptors. In: E. Neil (Ed.), *Enteroceptors, Handbook of Sensory Physiology, Vol. III*, Springer-Verlag, Berlin, Heidelberg, New York, 1972, pp. 1–45.

43 Paintal, A. S., Vagal sensory receptors and their reflex effects, *Physiol. Rev.*, 53 (1973) 159–227.

44 Peterson, D. F. and Brown, A. M., Pressor reflexes produced by stimulation of afferent fibers in the cardiac sympathetic nerves of the cat, *Circulation Res.*, 28 (1971) 605–610.

45 Ross, J., Jr., Frahm, G. J. and Braunwald, E., The influence of intracardiac baro-receptors on venous return, systemic vascular volume and peripheral resistance, *J. clin. Invest.*, 40 (1961) 563–572.

46 Sleight, P. and Widdicombe, J. G., Action potentials in fibres from receptors in the epicardium and myocardium of the dog's left ventricle, *J. Physiol.* (Lond.), 181 (1965) 235–258.

47 Uchida, Y., Kamisaka, K. and Ueda, H., Experimental studies on anginal pain mode of excitation of afferent cardiac sympathetic nerve fibers, *Jap. Circ. J.*, 35 (1971) 141–161.

48 Ueda, H., Uchida, Y. and Kamisaka, K., Distribution and responses of the cardiac sympathetic receptors to mechanically-induced circulatory changes, *Jap. Heart J.*, 10 (1969) 70–81.

49 White, J. C., Cardiac pain, *Circulation*, 16 (1957) 644–655.

50 Woollard, H. H., The innervation of the heart, *J. Anat.*, 60 (1926) 345–373.

CHAPTER 9

NEURAL REGULATION OF THE PUPIL

A. D. Loewy

Department of Anatomy and Neurobiology, Washington University
School of Medicine, St. Louis, Missouri, USA

INTRODUCTION

Despite the publication of a number of reviews[15,28,33] on the neuroanatomical organization of pupillary pathways, a considerable amount of new anatomical and electrophysiological data has been produced to merit a brief review of certain aspects of these pathways. This review will focus on new areas of information pertaining to the pupillary system. Detailed accounts of reflex (nociceptive) pupillary dilatation[33] and the role of the cerebral cortex[25] in pupillary control have already been published and, thus, will not be considered. Similarly, since relatively limited information exists concerning the central regulation of the lens and of the ocular vasculature, these subjects will not be considered.

One of the primary functions of the iris is the modification of pupillary diameter in such a way as to maximize visual acuity, particularly during accommodation. The iris functions to improve the optical resolution of the lens by setting the optimal diameter for each level of luminosity, and thereby minimizing the chromatic and spherical aberrations inherent in the optics of the eye. It can, thus, be regarded as an image quality optimizer[1,7], which is modulated by a number of different neuronal systems, some of which will be discussed below.

The pupillary light reflex is traditionally said to involve the following pathways: (1) Some as yet unidentified group of retinal ganglion cells sends its axons to the midbrain by way of the brachium of the superior colliculus; these fibers terminate in the pretectal area; (2) Certain neurons in the pretectal complex send their axons to both sides of the Edinger-Westphal nucleus, those to the contralateral side crossing in the posterior commissure; (3) Preganglionic pupilloconstrictor neurons in the Edinger-Westphal nucleus send their axons via the oculomotor nerve to the ciliary ganglion where they synapse; and (4) Postganglionic fibers arising from the neurons of the ciliary ganglion send axons via the short ciliary nerves to innervate the sphincter of the iris (see Fig. 1). However, it is becoming increasingly clear that the neural pathways involved in the pupillary light reflex are considerably more complex than has been assumed and the following review will summarize some of the more recent information bearing on this problem.

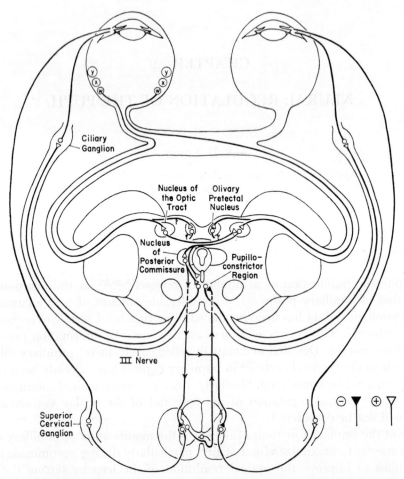

Fig. 1. The organization of the pupillomotor pathways is illustrated in diagrammatic fashion. Luminosity information from the visual fields is transmitted by W-retinal ganglion cells to the nucleus of the optic tract in the pretectum. From here, neurons project to the contralateral nucleus of the optic tract and the nucleus of the posterior commissure as well as possibly directly to the pupilloconstrictor neurons. Neurons in the nucleus of the posterior commissure may also have descending inhibitory projections to the intermediolateral cell column. This inhibition is probably mediated by an interneuron which is not illustrated in this figure. In addition, afferents from the dorsal horn are shown crossing the midline, ascending in the ventral funiculus of the spinal cord and terminating on pupilloconstrictor neurons.

RESULTS AND DISCUSSION

Retinal Ganglion Cells

In the cat, (and possibly in other mammals), there are at least three types of retinal ganglion cells (W, X, and Y-cells), which have distinctive receptive field properties, conduction velocities and morphology[5,11,22,27,32,47]. The W cells are the smallest retinal ganglion cells and appear to project to mesencephalic centers and lamina C of the lateral geniculate nucleus[52]; the X cells are medium size neurons and project predominantly to the diencephalon; and the Y cells are the largest ganglion cells and project to both the mesencephalon and the diencephalon[11,22,27]. This classification was originally introduced to describe two cell types: X cells and Y cells, on the basis of whether the cell summed the influence of the center and the surrounding regions of their receptive fields linearly (X cells) or non-linearly (Y cells)[16]. A variety of other types of retinal ganglion cell that have different receptive field properties and/ or conduction velocities have been grouped under the heading of W cells[48]. It is thought that a particular subclass of W cells that fire tonically and have on-center receptive fields may function as luminance detectors[47]. Each of these "tonic-on" W cells may monitor the luminance of a small part of the visual field and provide an afferent input for pupilloconstrictor relay neurons of the pretectum. In addition to these cells, there are other subclasses of W cells, some of which provide directional information and may function in other types of visual processing, such as in fixation and optokinetic nystagmus.

Axonal degeneration and autoradiographic studies have established that retinal ganglion cells send their axons to: (1) the dorsal lateral geniculate nucleus; (2) the ventral lateral geniculate nucleus; (3) the nucleus of the optic tract; (4) the olivary pretectal nucleus; (5) the superior colliculus; (6) the accessory optic nuclei; and (6) the suprachiasmatic nucleus[3,20,30,43]. The precise projections of each type (and subtype) of retinal ganglion cell are as yet unknown. Kelly and Gilbert[27] have analyzed the retinal projections to the superior colliculus and dorsal lateral geniculate nucleus by making injections of the histochemically demonstrable enzyme marker, horseradish peroxidase (HRP), in some of these structures and found that the W (small) and Y (large) cells projected to the superior colliculus while the X (medium) and Y (large) cells projected to the dorsal lateral geniculate nucleus. By electrophysiological techniques, it has been shown that W cells also go to the lateral geniculate nucleus[52]. Unfortunately, comparable HRP experiments have not yet been reported for the retino-pretectal projection system. On the basis of latency measurements, Cleland and Levick[11] have suggested that all three classes of ganglion cells may project to the pretectum. Whether other classes of cells, in addition to certain W cells, provide luminosity information for the pupillary reflexes remains unknown.

Pretectum. Retinal afferents involved in the light reflex reach the pretectum via the brachium of the superior colliculus. In 1935, Hare, Magoun and Ranson[19] demonstrated that electrical stimulation of the pretectal region, but not the superior colliculus, elicited pupillary constriction in the cat in which the optic nerves had been severed two to six weeks prior to the experiment. Unfortunately, these studies did not establish which subnucleus or subnuclei in the pretectum were concerned with the pupillary light reflex. Conflicting data have been published with regard to the site(s) of termination of retinal afferents in the pretectum, but Berman[3] has re-examined this problem by making intraocular injections of [3H] amino acids and then studying labeling patterns in autoradiographic preparations of the pretectum. Retinal afferents terminate bilaterally in the nucleus of the optic tract and the olivary pretectal nucleus[43]. In addition, the posterior and anterior pretectal regions may also receive retinal afferents.

The receptive field properties of neurons found in the pretectum of the cat have also been analyzed. Directionally-sensitive and luminosity-sensitive units are present in both the nucleus of the optic tract and olivary pretectal nucleus (see for example references 10, 21, 45). The nucleus of the optic tract appears to contain mainly luminosity-sensitive units and the olivary pretectal nucleus mainly directionally-sensitive units. The nucleus of the optic tract contains some units that can be excited both phasically and tonically by spots of light, and these may be concerned with the onset and maintenance of the pupillary light reflex. Other units have been identified that are tonically inhibited by light and show a sustained discharge at the end of illumination. These neurons may be involved in the active mechanism which causes pupillary dilatation during darkness. Finally, a third type of unit has been identified which responds only phasically to light and/or to darkness. Units in the olivary pretectal nucleus have very large receptive fields and fire at a constant rate that varies rather directly with the level of ambient luminosity (Berman, personal communication). The role of these cells in the neural regulation of the pupil is unknown but it should be noted that mild pupilloconstriction can be elicited from this region by electrical stimulation (see Fig. 2 of Sillito and Zbrożyna[46]). This may indicate that the olivary pretectal nucleus functions as another component of the pupillary system.

Until recently, it was thought that neurons from the pretectum project bilaterally to the Edinger-Westphal nucleus. While this view had been based on axonal degeneration studies and there are some recent anatomical studies to support it[2,8,17,24], other investigators[3,18] have not been able to find evidence for such a system of connections. Instead, the evidence suggests that the pretectal light-sensing neurons project first to the contralateral nucleus of the posterior commissure[3]. Neurons in the nucleus of the posterior commissure in turn appear to then send axons ventrally in the central gray matter to the region of the Edinger-Westphal nucleus. After HRP injections in the oculomotor complex, Graybiel and Hartwieg[18] have reported that neurons of the nucleus of the posterior commissure were labeled but none were found in the pretectal region. The significance of these recent findings is unclear and further studies will be needed to resolve the role of the nucleus of the posterior commissure in the pupillary responses to light.

Pupilloconstrictor neurons. It has generally been assumed that the neurons of the Edinger-Westphal nucleus send their axons exclusively through the oculomotor nerve to the ciliary ganglion where they synapse, and thus form the parasympathetic preganglionic outflow which mediates pupillary light and accomodation reflexes. Warwick[51] found that removal of the ciliary ganglion in the monkey results in chromatolysis in the neurons of the Edinger-Westphal nucleus. Other studies[4,6,12,31,53] indicate that the neurons in the Edinger-Westphal nucleus of other mammals (cat, rabbit and mouse) do not undergo chromatolysis after oculomotor nerve lesions. Whether this means that these cells of these other species are resistant to chromatolysis or that they do not project to the ciliary ganglion is not known. Following incubation of ciliary ganglion of the cat in an HRP solution[36], retrogradely labeled cells were found dorsal, lateral, and ventral to the Edinger-Westphal nucleus, but only a few labeled cells were found in the nucleus itself. Similarly, there is electrophysiological evidence suggesting that pupilloconstrictor neurons may lie in the ventral tegmental area and the periaqueductal gray matter, as well as within the Edinger-Westphal nucleus[46]. Sillito and Zbrożyna[46] have reported that maximal pupillary constriction is elicited by electrical stimulation of the region ventral to the Edinger-Westphal nucleus, and on stimulating the preganglionic parasympathetic fibers to the ciliary ganglion, antidromically-evoked responses could be recorded in the ventral part of the periaqueductal gray matter, the oculomotor nucleus, the ventral tegmental area, as well as the Edinger-Westphal nucleus.

Interestingly, there is now anatomical evidence which suggests that the Edinger-Westphal nucleus has more widespread projections than has been suspected. First, it was established that following injections of HRP into the spinal cord of the cat, rat and monkey neurons in the Edinger-Westphal nucleus were retrogradely labeled[42]. Retrograde cell labeling occurred even after injections of HRP in the sacral spinal cord, suggesting that this system may be involved in other functions besides pupillary control[36]. Second, in a series of studies in which ^{3}H amino acids were injected stereotaxically into the region of the Edinger-Westphal nucleus in the cat, Loewy and Saper[35] were able to trace efferent projections from this nucleus to a number of sites in the lower brain stem and spinal cord heretofore not known to receive an afferent input from the zone. Confirmatory evidence for some of these projections was obtained from a series of experiments in which a solution of HRP was injected into a number of target sites where this descending pathway traveled[35]. Apart from projecting to the ciliary ganglion, the Edinger-Westphal nucleus projects to the medial parabrachial nucleus, the subtrigeminal nucleus, the dorsal column nuclei and dorsal accessory olive. In addition, this pathway continues into the spinal cord where it appears to terminate in the marginal layer (lamina I) as well as possibly in the base of the dorsal horn (lamina V) (Fig. 2).

Sharpe, Pickworth and Martin[44] have made microinjections of various drugs into the oculomotor complex of the dog and reported that injections of cholinergic drugs cause pupillary dilatation (presumably by inhibition of the pupilloconstrictor neurons by a muscarinic effect) while similar injections of opioid, dopaminergic and adrenergic drugs cause pupilloconstriction possibly by their excitatory effects on the pupilloconstrictor neurons. The latter result correlates with the observations presented by Dahlstrom et al.[13] that the Edinger-Westphal nucleus receives an adrenergic input. Interestingly, injections of 5-hydroxytryptamine had no effect on pupil diameter, suggesting that the serotonergic neurons do not directly affect the pupilloconstrictor neurons. The respiratory rate, heart rate, and a number of other physiological parameters were examined during these experiments, and some of these, particularly respiration, paralleled the pupillary responses. Although the significance of these results must await further study because of the potential diffusion of these drugs to other sites in the central nervous system, it is not unreasonable to suggest that the Edinger-Westphal nucleus may be involved in more widespread autonomic and/or somatic functions than is usually thought.

Pupillodilator pathways. The pupillodilator preganglionic sympathetic fibers arise from the intermediolateral cell column at the C8, T1, and T2 levels of the spinal cord. The preganglionic fibers leave the spinal cord by the way of the ventral roots to reach the superior cervical ganglion where they synapse. From there postganglionic fibers

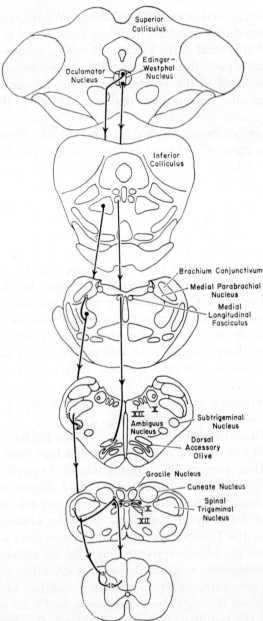

Fig. 2. A schematic drawing indicating the organization of the descending projection from
the region of the Edinger-Westphal nucleus. A lateral descending pathway projects
into the medial tegmentum and then caudally into the ventrolateral reticular formation where it appears to terminate in the medial parabrachial nucleus. Another
part of this system passes through and terminates in the subtrigeminal nucleus.
Axons from this system course along the ventral edge of the spinal trigeminal nucleus
and the dorsal horn and appear to terminate in laminae I and possibly in and near V.
Another component terminates in the dorsal column nuclei and also travels into
dorsal columns of the spinal cord. A medial pathway appears to travel in the medial
longitudinal fasciculus and terminates in the dorsal accessory olive.

travel with branches of the internal carotid artery and eventually accompany the ophthalmic branch of the trigeminal nerve into the orbit where they continue in its nasociliary division. From here fibers branch off and innervate the pupillodilator muscle.

Preganglionic sympathetic neurons receive descending inputs from a number of brain stem nuclei, including the hypothalamus. Karplus and Kreidl[26] were the first to demonstrate that electrical stimulation of the hypothalamus produced a number of autonomic effects, including retraction of the eyelids and nictitating membranes and pupillary dilatation. These investigators as well as others subsequently went on to show that this stimulation caused widespread changes in other autonomic functions (blood pressure, respiration, bladder, sweating). These studies were largely ignored until Ranson and Magoun[41] and their associates began their systematic studies of the role of the hypothalamus in autonomic control. Recently, with the introduction of more sensitive anatomical techniques, some of these descending pathways to the inter-mediolateral cell column have been analyzed[42] (see also Saper, this volume).

On the basis of stimulation techniques, a descending, excitatory pupillodilator pathway which was thought to originate in the hypothalamus was localized in the ventrolateral tegmentum and was traced at successively caudal levels in a position dorsolateral to the medial lemniscus[34]. At more caudal levels, this pathway occupies a position on the ventrolateral surface of the medulla immediately lateral to the pyramidal tract. It continues in the cervical spinal cord in a superficial position in the lateral funiculus near the insertion zone of the denticulate ligament. Loewy, Araujo and Kerr[34] demonstrated that after central tegmental lesions which destroyed the descending pupillomotor tract, axonal degeneration could be traced from the tegmentum to the region of the intermediolateral cell column. The exact site of origin of this descending pupillary pathway is not known but the subsequent studies done by Saper et al.[42] indicate that neurons in at least three hypothalamic nuclei (paraventricular, lateral and posterior) send fibers directly to the spinal cord.

In addition, pupillary dilatation can be produced by stimulation of the spino-thalamic tract and lateral part of the central gray matter but the exact pathways that mediate this response are not known.

An ascending inhibitory pathway was described by Loewy, Araujo and Kerr[34] originating from the region of the paramedian reticular formation in the medulla and this pathway was traced rostrally through the pons to a postition in the medial tegmental reticular formation immediately dorsal to the region of the medial lemniscus. At rostral levels, this system appeared to lie immediately lateral to the interpeduncular nucleus. Stimulation of this pathway caused pupillary dilatation even after the cervical sympathetic nerves were transected. The physiological significance of this pathway remains unknown, but it may be part of an ascending vestibular pathway that can modulate the ocular system.

DeSantis and Gernandt[14] and Markham, Estes and Blanks[38] studied the effects of utricle stimulation of ocular reflexes. Different pupillary responses occurred during the different phases of nystagmus[14]. During a brisk, conjugant deviation of the eyes in response to a single air puff in the utricle, pupillary constriction occurred during the fast phase of the eye movement while pupillary dilatation occurred during the slow phase of the nystagmus. Thus, vestibular nystagmus is accompanied by pupillary reactions which are in synchrony with the nystagmic beats. The neuronal circuitry that is involved in this reflex remains uncertain, but appears to involve only neuronal systems that project to the pupilloconstrictor neurons because Cl spinal cord transection or cervical sympathectomy had no effect on these reflexes. Markham and associates[38] suggested that the pathway(s) responsible for this response ascends independently from the medial longitudinal fasciculus as vestibuloreticular fibers, but the exact site of origin was not determined. However, Morrison and Pompeiano[37] have suggested that the integrity of the medial and the descending vestibular nuclei are necessary for pupillary dilatation that occurs during paradoxical sleep.

The cerebellum plays a role in a variety of autonomic functions, including the modulation of pupillomotor activity. A number of investigators have observed that electrical stimulation of certain parts of the cerebellum results in pupillary dilatation and these responses were elicited from stimulation of the fastigial nucleus[23]. The fastigial neurons appear to function by improving the frequency characteristics of the pupillary responses so that the pupil can follow changes in light stimuli. Evidence for this hypothesis comes from studies in which it was shown that lesions of the fastigial nucleus decrease the frequency response of the pupil to a sinusoidal light stimulus[23,50]. While the anatomical basis for this response is uncertain, some of the efferents from the fastigial nucleus may travel directly to the region of the pupilloconstrictor neurons[49].

Integration of Pupilloconstrictor and Pupillodilator Responses

During retinal illumination, there is concomitant inhibition of the sympathetic fibers and excitation of the parasympathetic fibers that innervate the iris[39]. The anatomical basis of this coordination between the sympathetic and parasympathetic outflow is unclear. Inhibition of the sympathetic system appears mediated by a system of fibers that arises in the midbrain and projects bilaterally to the interomediolateral cell column[40]. A likely candidate for the site of origin of the neurons that coordinate this integrative activity may be the nucleus of the posterior commissure which contains neurons that project both to the spinal cord[9] and to the region of the Edinger-Westphal nucleus[3,18] as well as receive an input from the pretectum[3]. Further anatomical and electrophysiological studies of this nucleus will be needed to resolve the anatomical basis of this integrative activity. In addition to this integration, other neuronal circuits may provide other dual inputs to sympathetic and parasympathetic preganglionic neurons. For example, ascending information from somatic and possibly autonomic centers may reach the nucleus of the posterior commissure as well as pupilloconstrictor neurons and provide further integration of this system. Kerr[29] has reported that following lesions of the ventral funiculus at the midcervical level of the spinal cord in the monkey he could trace axonal degeneration to a number of sites in the mesencephalon, including the Edinger-Westphal nucleus. Kerr has suggested that this may be one of the routes whereby reflex dilatation of the pupils occurs after noxious stimulation; alternatively, it may be part of a reciprocal autonomic system linking the parasympathetic and sympathetic preganglionic neurons for coordinated regulation of the pupil.

This review was written with the support of funds from the USPHS Grant NS 12751. The author thanks Drs. Nancy Berman, W. M. Cowan, N. W. Daw, A. L. Pearlman, C. B. Saper and L. E. Sharpe for their helpful discussions.

REFERENCES

1 Barlow, H. B., Dark and light adaptation: Psychophysics. In: D. Jameson and L. M. Hurvich (Eds.), *Visual Psychophysics*, Springer-Verlag, Berlin, 1972, pp. 1–28.

2 Benevento, L. A., Rezak, M. and Santos-Anderson, R., An autoradiographic study of the projections of the pretectum in the rhesus monkey (*Macaca mulatta*): Evidence for sensorimotor links to the thalamus and oculomotor nuclei, *Brain Res.*, 127 (1977) 197–218.

3 Berman, N., The connections of the pretectum in the cat, *J. comp. Neurol.*, 174 (1977) 227–254.

4 Biervliet, J. van., Noyau d'origine du nerf oculo-moteur common du lapin, *La Cellule*, 16 (1899) 7–33.

5 Boycott, B. B. and Wässle, H., The morphological types of ganglion cells of the domestic cat's retina, *J. Physiol.* (Lond.), 240 (1974) 397–419.

6 Cajal, S. y Ramón, *Histologie du systéme nerveux de l'homme et des vertébrés*, CSIC, Madrid, 1911, p. 240.

7 Campbell, F. W. and Gregory, A. H., Effect of size of pupil on visual activity, *Nature*, 187 (1960) 1121–1123.

8 Carpenter, M. B. and Pierson, R. J., Pretectal region and the pupillary light reflex: An anatomical analysis in the monkey, *J. comp. Neurol.*, 149 (1973) 271–300.

9 Castiglioni, A. J., Gallaway, M. C. and Coulter, J. D., Spinal projections from the midbrain in monkey, *J. comp. Neurol.*, 178 (1978) 329–346.

10 Cavaggioni, A., Madarasz, I. and Zampollo, A., Photic reflex and pretectal region, *Archs ital. Biol.*, 106 (1968) 227–242.

11 Cleland, B. G. and Levick, W. R., Brisk and sluggish concentrically organized ganglion cells in the cats regina, *J. Physiol.* (Lond.), 240 (1974) 421–456.

12 Crouch, R. L., The efferent fibers of the Edinger-Westphal nucleus, *J. comp. Neurol.*, 64 (1936) 365–373.

13 Dahlstrom, A., Fuxe, K., Hillarp, N. A. and Malmfors, I., Adrenergic mechanisms in the pupillary light-reflex path, *Acta physiol. scand.*, 62 (1964) 119–124.

14 DeSantis, M. and Gernandt, B. E., Effect of vestibular stimulation on pupillary size, *Exp. Neurol.*, 30 (1971) 60–77.

15 Duke-Elder, S. and Wybar, R. W., *System of Opthalmology*, Vol. 2, Mosby, St. Louis, Missouri, 1961, pp. 813–874.

16 Enroth-Cugell, C. and Robson, J. G., The contrast sensitivity of retinal ganglion cells of the cat, *J. Physiol.* (Lond.), 187 (1966) 517–552.

17 Graybiel, A. M., Some efferents of the pretectal region in the cat, *Anat. Rec.*, 178 (1974) 365.

18 Graybiel, A. M. and Hartweig, E., Some afferent connections of the oculomotor complex in the cat: An experimental study with tracer techniques, *Brain Res.*, 81 (1974) 543–551.

19 Hare, W. K., Magoun, H. W. and Ranson, S. W., Pathway for pupillary construction, *Archs Neurol. Psychiat.* (Chicago), 34 (1935) 1189–1194.

20 Hendrickson, A. E., Wagoner, N. and Cowan, W. M., An autoradiographic and electron microscopic study of retino-hypothalamic connections, *Z. Zellforsch.*, 135 (1972) 1–26.

21   Hoffmann, K.-P. and Schoppmann, A., Retinal input to direction selective cells in the nucleus tractus opticus of the cat, *Brain Res.*, 99 (1975) 359–366.

22   Hoffmann, K.-P. and Stone, J., Central terminations of W-, X- and Y- type ganglion cells from the cat retina, *Brain Res.*, 49 (1973) 500–501.

23   Ijichi, Y., Kiyohara, T., Hosoba, M. and Tsukahara, N., The cerebellar control of the pupillary light reflex in the cat, *Brain Res.*, 128 (1977) 69–79.

24   Itoh, K., Efferent projections of the pretectum in the cat, *Exp. Brain Res.*, 30 (1977) 89–105.

25   Jampel, R. S., Convergence, divergence, pupillary reactions and accomodations of the eye from faradic stimulation of the macaque brain, *J. comp. Neurol.*, 115 (1960) 371–399.

26   Karplus, J. P. and Kreidl, A., Gehirn und Sympathicus. I. Zwischenhirnbasis und Halssympathicus, *Pflügers Arch.*, 129 (1909) 138–144.

27   Kelly, J. P. and Gilbert, C. D., The projections of different morphological types of ganglion cells in the cat retina, *J. comp. Neurol.*, 163 (1975) 65–80.

28   Kerr, F. W. L., The pupil-functional anatomy and clinical correlation. In: J. Lawson Smith (Ed.), *Neuro-Opthalmology, Symposium of the University of Miami and the Bascom Palmer Eye Institute*, Vol. 4, Mosby, St. Louis, Missouri, 1968, pp. 49–80.

29   Kerr, F. W. L., The ventral spinothalamic tract and other ascending systems of the ventral funiculus of the spinal cord, *J. comp. Neurol.*, 159 (1975) 335–356.

30   Laties, A. M. and Sprague, J. M., The projection of optic fibers to the visual centers in the cat, *J. comp. Neurol.*, 127 (1966) 35–70.

31   Latumeten, J. A., *Over de Kernen van den Nervus Oculomotorius*, Den Boer, Utrecht, 1924.

32   Levick, W. R. and Cleland, B. G., Receptive fields of cat retinal ganglion cells have slowly conducting axons, *Brain Res.*, 74 (1974) 156–160.

33   Loewenfeld, I. E., Mechanisms of reflex dilatation of the pupil: Historical review and experimental analysis, *Docum. Ophthal.* (Den Haag), 12 (1958) 185–448.

34   Loewy, A. D., Araujo, J. C. and Kerr, F. W. L., Pupillodilator pathways in the brain stem of the cat: Anatomical and electrophysiological identification of a central autonomic pathway, *Brain Res.*, 60 (1973) 65–69.

35   Loewy, A. D. and Saper, C. B., Edinger-Westphal nucleus: Projections to the brain stem and spinal cord in the cat, *Brain Res.*, 150 (1978) 1–27.

36   Loewy, A. D., Saper, C. B. and Yamodis, N. D., Re-evaluation of the efferent projections of the Edinger-Westphal nucleus, *Brain Res.*, 141 (1978) 153–159.

37   Morrison, A. R. and Pompeiano, O., Vestibular influences during sleep. VI. Vestibular control of autonomic functions during the rapid eye movements of desynchronized sleep, *Archs ital. Biol.*, 108 (1970) 154–180.

38   Markham, C. H., Estes, M. S. and Blanks, R. H. I., Vestibular influences on ocular accommodation in cats, *Equilibrium Res.*, 3 (1973) 101–115.

39   Nisida, I., Okada, H. and Nakano, O., The activity of the ciliospinal centres and their inhibition in pupillary light reflex, *Jap. J. Physiol.*, 10 (1960) 73–84.

40   Okada, H., Nakano, O., Okamoto, K., Nakayama, R. and Nisida, I., The central path of the light reflex via the sympathetic nerve in the cat, *Jap. J. Physiol.*, 10 (1960) 646–658.

41   Ranson, S. W. and Magoun, H. W., Respiratory and pupillary reactions induced by electrical stimulation of the hypothalamus, *Archs Neurol. Psychiat.* (Chicago), 29 (1933) 1179–1194.

42   Saper, C. B., Loewy, A. D., Swanson, L. W. and Cowan, W. M., Direct hypothalamo-autonomic connections, *Brain Res.*, 117 (1976) 305–312.

43 Scalia, F., The termination of retinal axons in the pretectal region of mammals, *J. comp. Neurol.*, 145 (1972) 223–257.

44 Sharpe, L. G., Pickworth, W. B. and Martin, W. R., Pupillary changes following micro-injections of opioids, sympathomimetics and cholinomimetics into the oculomotor nucleus in the dog, *Soc. Neurosci. Abstr.*, 3 (1977) 301.

45 Sillito, A. M., The pretectal light input to the pupilloconstrictor neurones, *J. Physiol.* (Lond.), 204 (1969) 36P–37P.

46 Sillito, A. M. and Zbrożyna, A. W., The localization of pupilloconstrictor function within the midbrain of the cat, *J. Physiol.* (Lond.), 211 (1970) 461–477.

47 Stone, J. and Fukuda, Y., Properties of cat retinal ganglion cells: A comparison of W-cells with X- and Y- cells, *J. Neurophysiol.*, 37 (1974) 722–748.

48 Stone, J. and Hoffmann, K. P., Very slow-conducting ganglion cells in the cat's retina: A major new functional type? *Brain Res.*, 43 (1972) 610–616.

49 Thomas, D. M., Kaufman, R. R., Sprague, J. M. and Chambers, W. W., Experimental studies of the vermal cerebellar projections in the brain stem of the cat (Fastigiobulbar tract), *J. Anat.* (Lond.), 90 (1956) 371–384.

50 Tsukahara, N., Kiyohara, T. and Ijichi, Y., The mode of cerebellar control of pupillary light reflex, *Brain Res.*, 60 (1973) 244–248.

51 Warwick, R., The ocular parasympathetic nerve supply and its mesencephalic sources, *J. Anat.* (Lond.), 88 (1954) 71–93.

52 Wilson, P. D. and Stone, J., Evidence of W-cell input to the cat's visual cortex via the C laminae of the lateral geniculate nucleus, *Brain Res.*, 92 (1975) 472–478.

53 Yoshida, K., Comparative-anatomical and experimental studies on the oculomotor nucleus and neighboring nuclei, *Acta Med. Biol.*, 1 (1953) 143–161.

SECTION II

PERIPHERAL INTERACTIONS BETWEEN EFFERENT TERMINALS AND IN PLEXUSES

In the original simpler concepts of autonomic system function the sympathetic and parasympathetic outflows were visualized as entirely separate entities interacting to maintain an intermediate state of function in visceral organs. Centers were considered to govern the action of these two antagonistically-acting outflows and it was found that in many reflexes they acted reciprocally: if one was activated, the other was inhibited. The vagi inhibited the heart and the sympathetic excited that organ; the parasympathetic initiated gastrointestinal system digestive processes and the sympathetic inhibited them; the sympathetic dilated the pupil and the parasympathetic constricted it; etc. There was no concept of peripheral interactions which might reverse these peripheral antagonistic effects.

It was soon realized, however, that sympathetic and parasympathetic actions are not always opposed. They can facilitate and supplement each other at least in certain organs such as the salivary glands. Peripheral actions may be different but not always opposed, furthermore, even when peripheral actions are antagonistic, there is often a late reversal. One of the best examples of this is "post vagus tachycardia". The claim is now made that these reversals are not entirely central in origin but may be due to peripheral interactions. There is evidence to suggest that though cholinergic transmitters certainly can block both release and action of sympathetic nerve transmitters, the catecholamines, they can also cause their release. Similarly, it is thought that in certain instances adrenergic transmitters may activate release of cholinergic materials.

Furthermore, in modern considerations of the autonomic system we no longer think in terms of only two transmitters, only four receptors, occurrence of interaction only centrally. The modern questions are: Are peripheral interactions to be thought of as purely chemical or are they in part based on anatomic interrelationships? Do branches of the sympathetic and parasympathetic fibers innervate or make synaptic contacts with each other in ganglia or in terminal arborizations? How do the two outflows interact in plexuses where they intermingle? These are questions to be discussed in the following chapters of this section.

The new advances made in study of finer structures, terminals and synapses of the autonomic system have provided structural bases for the physiological evidence of peripheral interactions. Electron microscopy has revealed much we had assumed. We now can see axonal collaterals, multiple types of synapses, and stored transmitters. The assumption that there are different types of synapses, some propagating excitation while others exert inhibitory effects, now seems not completely without support. This progress in anatomy has been accompanied by the claim that there are more than two transmitters liberated by autonomic terminals. The concept of receptors has also been enormously expanded although this has not been reviewed here.

The chapters of this section have dealt primarily with interaction at terminals. Evidence for cholinergic inhibition of adrenergic neurotransmission in the cardio-vascular system has become very convincing. It has also been found that interactions between sympathetic and parasympathetic efferents occur in organ plexuses. As a matter of fact, attention has recently reverted to a suggestion made by Langley: that plexuses of the gut comprised an "enteric nervous system". The independence of the neural complex is not accepted and we consider the plexuses of Auerbach and Meisner as parts of the autonomic system. Nevertheless, we are finding that unique functions and peripheral interactions occur therein.

CHAPTER 10

INTERACTIONS OF CHOLINERGIC, ADRENERGIC, PURINERGIC AND PEPTIDERGIC NEURONS IN THE GUT

G. Burnstock

Department of Anatomy and Embryology, University College, London, England

INTRODUCTION

The classical picture of the innervation of the gut is one of cholinergic excitatory neurons in the gut wall controlled by preganglionic cholinergic vagal and sacral parasympathetic fibers opposed by postganglionic sympathetic adrenergic inhibitory fibers (see Fig. 1A).

Two findings in the early 1960's made it necessary to revise this picture (Fig. 1B). Firstly, the application of the fluorescence histochemical method for localizing catecholamines showed that the terminal varicosities of the majority of adrenergic fibers were localized in Auerbach's and Meissner's plexuses and only supplied the smooth muscle of limited areas of the circular muscle coat[15]. The second discovery was the demonstration of powerful nonadrenergic, noncholinergic inhibitory nerves supplying the smooth muscle of the gastrointestinal tract[3,10,52]. These nerves are concerned with the propulsion of material through the alimentary canal, and are involved in reflex opening of sphincters, 'receptive relaxation' of the stomach and 'descending inhibition' during peristalsis, whereas the main role of adrenergic nerves is to modulate these activities mostly at the ganglion level (see[14]).

It seems unlikely that the nonadrenergic, noncholinergic nerves in the gut are a single population of fibers with one transmitter. Cook and Burnstock[20] showed recently that there are up to nine morphologically distinguishable neurons in the enteric plexuses, including some nerve profiles with complex mixtures of vesicles, suggesting that they may contain more than one transmitter (see[6]). Some of these neurons are responsible for the powerful nonadrenergic, noncholinergic inhibitory responses of the smooth muscle mentioned above, others may be concerned with the nonadrenergic, noncholinergic excitatory responses of the smooth muscle of certain regions of the intestine in some species[25]. Some nerves are sensory, others may represent various types of interneurons, while some may be supplying blood vessels and mucosal epithelial cells. Evidence that the nonadrenergic, noncholinergic inhibitory fibers supplying the smooth muscle of the gut are purinergic (i.e., release ATP as the principle transmitter) will be reviewed. The possibility that the various polypeptides localized by immuno-

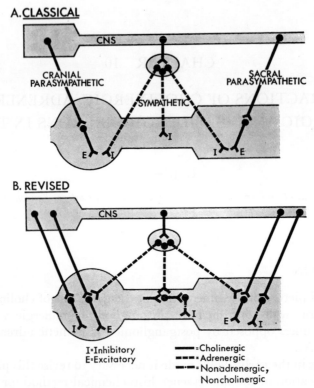

A. CLASSICAL

B. REVISED

I=Inhibitory   ━━━━━=Cholinergic
E=Excitatory   ━ ━ ━=Adrenergic
                      ━·━·=Nonadrenergic,
                           Noncholinergic

Fig. 1.   A diagrammatic representation of the innervation of the gut, showing the classical
picture and a revised picture (see text for explanation). Modified from Burnstock[4].

histochemical methods are present in sensory fibers or interneurons will then be
considered. (A discussion of the possibility that 5-hydroxytryptamine is the transmitter
in some nonadrenergic, noncholinergic excitatory nerves has been dealt with elsewhere[25,27,83].) Finally the role of presynaptic neuromodulation of transmitter release
in neuronal interaction in the gut will be discussed.

RESULTS AND DISCUSSION

*Evidence that Nonadrenergic, Noncholinergic Efferent Inhibitory Fibers to Gastro-intestinal
Muscle are Purinergic*

Five criteria are generally regarded as necessary for establishing a substance as
a neurotransmitter, namely: (1) synthesis and storage of transmitter in nerve terminals;
(2) release of transmitter during nerve stimulation; (3) postjunctional responses to
exogenous transmitter that mimic responses to nerve stimulation; (4) enzymes that
inactivate the transmitter and/or an uptake system for the transmitter or its breakdown
products; (5) drugs that produce parallel blocking or potentiating effects on the responses to both exogenous transmitter and nerve stimulation.

In experiments carried out to try to identify the transmitter in nonadrenergic,
noncholinergic inhibitory nerves supplying the gastrointestinal smooth muscle, ATP

appears to satisfy these criteria best[4,5,8]. Other substances have been explored as the possible transmitter released from nonadrenergic, noncholinergic inhibitory nerves in the gut, including 3′, 5′,-catecholamines, 5-hydroxytryptamine, cyclic adenosine monophosphate (cAMP), histamine, prostaglandins, various amino acids such as alanine, arginine, histidine, glycine, glutamic acid and γ-aminobutyric acid (GABA) and the polypeptides, enkephalin, neurotensin, vasoactive intestinal peptide (VIP), somatostatin, bradykinin and substance P. However, these substances have been rejected as contenders by most workers on the grounds that they were either inactive or did not mimic the nerve-mediated responses, that specific blocking drugs for these substances did not affect the nerve-mediated response or that their action was by stimulation of nerves and not by direct action on smooth muscle.

Storage. Both ATP and the enzyme systems that synthesize ATP occur ubiquitously in cells, so that it is not contentious that nonadrenergic inhibitory nerves are also able to produce and store ATP. Tritium-labeled adenosine is taken up by preparations of stomach and intestine and rapidly converted mostly to ^{3}H-ATP. Analysis of the radioactivity in serial frozen sections showed that when the tissue was incubated in low concentrations of ^{3}H-adenosine, most of the label was stored as ^{3}H-ATP in nerves.

Electronmicroscopic studies of axon profiles in preparations innervated by nonadrenergic, noncholinergic nerves led to the proposal that they were characterized by a predominance of 'large opaque vesicles' (LOV). These vesicles differ from the small number of 'large granular vesicles' found in both adrenergic and cholinergic nerves in that they are larger (80 to 200 nm, cf. 60 to 120 nm in diameter), have a less prominent halo between the granular core and vesicle membrane and are unaffected by 6-hydroxydopamine, which destroys adrenergic nerve terminals. Preliminary studies in our laboratory suggest that after exposure of intestine to low concentrations of ^{3}H-adenosine for short periods (45 sec) there is selective accumulation of silver grains over nerve profiles containing LOV. Indirect support for the view that ATP is contained in LOV is that the unicellular parasite *Trypanosoma cruzi*, responsible for Chaga's disease, is unable to synthesize its own adenine and the LOV in nerve profiles are damaged in the intestine of infected patients.

A fluorescence histochemical method for localizing quinacrine was introduced by Olson et al.[59]. Quinacrine is known to bind to ATP and also to regions of DNA rich in adenine and thymine. It gives positive staining of adrenal medullary cells, megakaryocytes and blood platelets, known to contain high levels of ATP. Microsomal fractions obtained by differential and sucrose-density gradient centrifugation of homogenates of purinergically-innervated preparations (taenia coli and bladder) preloaded with ^{3}H-adenosine and ^{14}C-quinacrine showed peaks of ^{14}C which corresponded to peaks of ^{3}H-ATP. Quinacrine-positive nerve cell bodies and varicose fibers have been demonstrated in gut and also in gall bladder, urinary bladder and portal vein, where pharmacological evidence for purinergic transmission has been presented, but are absent from the iris, which contains abundant adrenergic and cholinergic, but not purinergic, nerves.

Release. Early evidence for release of ATP during stimulation of purinergic nerves was as follows: (a) venous efflux of adenosine and inosine occurred from the stomach of both guinea-pigs and toads on stimulation of the vagus nerves. These compounds are likely to be the breakdown products of adenine nucleotides, because ATP introduced into the same perfusing system was quickly broken down into comparable proportions of adenosine and inosine; (b) radioactive compounds were released from guinea-pig taenia coli previously incubated in ³H-adenosine upon stimulation of the intramural nerves; and this release was blocked by tetrodotoxin.

That the release of nucleosides was due to stimulation of nonadrenergic inhibitory fibers in the vagus nerves rather than of cholinergic fibers was demonstrated by the use of the toad stomach preparation. In this preparation, all the preganglionic parasympathetic fibers in the vagus nerves make synaptic connection with nonadrenergic inhibitory, postganglionic neurons in the wall of the stomach, while the postganglionic cholinergic fibers running in the vagus nerves are of sympathetic origin. Stimulation of the vagal roots (or of the vagosympathetic trunks) resulted in increased nucleoside efflux, but stimulation of the cervical sympathetic branch of the vagus nerves did not.

The possibility that the purine nucleotides or nucleosides released from nerves are not neurotransmitter substances but are released from nerve membranes during propagation of an action potential has been considered. However, the amount of nucleosides collected during stimulation of nonadrenergic inhibitory nerves was calculated to be at least 1000-fold greater than that released as a direct result of the process of axon membrane activation during impulse propagation.

The possibility that ATP is released as a result of antidromic stimulation of enteric sensory nerves was ruled out when it was shown that the nonadrenergic inhibitory response to stimulation of the vagal nerves supplying the rabbit stomach was abolished after degeneration of the efferent, but not the afferent, component achieved by vagal section above the nodose ganglion eight days previously.

The problem of whether ATP released during stimulation of purinergic nerves comes from nerve or secondarily from muscle has been resolved recently in our laboratory[12]. It was shown that while there was a two- to six- fold increase in ATP release from the guinea-pig taenia coli or bladder during isometric responses to purinergic nerve stimulation, there was no significant release of ATP during comparable responses elicited by direct muscle stimulation. Further, the nerve-mediated release of ATP was Ca^{++} dependent; a 10-fold reduction in Ca^{++} concentration resulted in an 80–90% reduction in both the mechanical response and the ATP release[12]. This finding is consistent with that of Holman and Weinrich[37], who showed that the amplitude of the inhibitory junction potentials in the taenia coli was reduced by 80% when the external Ca^{++} was reduced 10-fold. Release from muscle was also considered unlikely, since stimulation of portions of Auerbach's plexus from turkey gizzard (heavily innervated by nonadrenergic inhibitory nerves), dissected free of the underlying muscle, still resulted in efflux of purine nucleotides, in this case mostly AMP.

Receptor activation. The form and time course of the response to exogenously-applied ATP closely mimics that in nonadrenergic inhibitory nerve stimulation. Typically, the relaxations of the gut produced by ATP and nerve stimulation rapidly reach a maximum that declines quickly; this is in contrast to the relaxations to noradrenaline and sympathetic nerve stimulation, which reach a maximum more slowly and are maintained for a longer time. The transmitter released by nonadrenergic inhibitory nerves produces inhibitory junction potentials, and ATP also causes rapid hyperpolarization of smooth muscle cells; both are due to a specific increase in K^+ conductivity. The possibility that ATP might be causing relaxation by initiating action potentials in nonadrenergic inhibitory nerves was negated by the finding that tetrodotoxin abolished the inhibitory responses of atropinized intestinal muscle to stimulation of either perivascular or intramural nerves but did not affect the relaxation produced by ATP.

In the intestine the most potent inhibitory purine compounds are ATP and ADP, which are about equipotent, with a threshold concentration for relaxation of the taenia coli of about $10^{-7}M$. AMP and adenosine have about 1/100 the potency of ATP. The following related compounds produce no effects, even with concentrations as high as $10^{-3}M$: the purine base, adenine; the deaminated nucleoside, inosine, and its mononucleotide, IMP; the pyrimidine nucleotide, uridine, and its mononucleotide UMP. The sensitivity of the gut to cAMP is also low. Of ATP and ADP, ATP is considered to be the most likely transmitter, since ^{3}H-adenosine taken up into the taenia coli is rapidly converted and stored mostly as ^{3}H-ATP, with only traces of ^{3}H-ADP detectable. Structure-activity studies of a wide variety of analogs on visceral smooth muscle have been described (see[7]).

The discovery that ATP is a potent inducer of prostaglandin synthesis[55] led Burnstock et al.[13] to suggest that ATP released from purinergic nerves may be linked with prostaglandins in peristalsis. The authors showed that the prostaglandin synthesis inhibitor, indomethacin, blocked the 'rebound contractions' that follow the inhibitory responses of the guinea-pig taenia coli to purinergic nerve stimulation and ATP.

Ultraviolet light between 340 and 380 nm produces responses in the guinea-pig taenia coli and rabbit portal vein that mimic precisely the inhibitory response to purinergic nerve stimulation and ATP[16]. UV light does not initiate impulses in purinergic nerves since its action is unaffected by tetrodotoxin, nor does it release ATP from nerve terminals. Agents which alter postjunctional responses to ATP and purinergic nerve stimulation also alter the responses to UV light. Since UV irradiation has no action on smooth muscle which is not innervated by inhibitory purinergic nerves, it may be acting on some part of the purinergic receptor complex and may provide a means of investigating the chemistry of purinergic receptors.

Burnstock[9] has recently suggested a basis for distinguishing two types of purinergic receptor according to four criteria: relative potencies of agonists, competitive antagonists, changes in levels of cAMP and induction of prostaglandin synthesis. Thus P_1 purinoceptors are most sensitive to adenosine, are competitively blocked by methylxanthines and occupation leads to changes in cAMP accumulation: while P_2 purinoceptors are most sensitive to ATP, are blocked (although not competitively) by high concentrations of quinidine, 2-substituted imidazolines, 2′ 2-pyridylisatogen and possibly by low concentrations of apamin (see below), and occupation leads to production of prostaglandin. P_2 purinoceptors on smooth muscle appear to mediate the responses of the smooth muscle of the gut to ATP released from purinergic nerves, while P_1 purinoceptors mediate the presynaptic actions of adenosine (ATP is rapidly broken down to adenosine before it is effective) on adrenergic, cholinergic and purinergic nerve terminals (see Section on neuromodulation).

Inactivation. The rapid recovery of smooth muscle after application of ATP or stimulation of nonadrenergic inhibitory nerves and the absence of long-lasting action despite continued stimulation indicates an efficient inactivation mechanism. By analogy with other neuroeffector systems, it has been argued that if the nonadrenergic inhibitory nerves act on the gut by releasing ATP, the action of ATP would be terminated by uptake into nerves or smooth muscle and/or breakdown of ATP by enzymes into compounds with greatly reduced potency.

When ATP is added to a perfusion fluid recycled through the vasculature of the stomach, very little ATP is recovered, but the perfusate contains substantially increased amounts of adenosine and inosine as well as some ADP and AMP. While there is no direct evidence for the breakdown of ATP released from nerves by enzymic activity, the gut is known to contain high levels of 5′-nucleotidase and adenosine deaminase. Mg^{++}-activated ATPase localization has been described in micropinocytotic vesicles in smooth muscle membranes closely adjacent (20 nm) to nonadrenergic, noncholinergic nerve profiles in the intestine.

An uptake mechanism for adenosine, but not nucleotides, has been demonstrated and this supports the view that ATP released from nerves is broken down to adenosine before uptake occurs, in a manner comparable to uptake of choline after breakdown of acetylcholine (ACh) released from cholinergic nerves. When the adenosine moiety of ATP is labelled with tritium and the phosphate moiety labelled with ^{32}P, the rate of uptake of ^{3}H into taenia coli is considerably greater than that of ^{32}P. Further support comes from studies of transmitter overflow at different stimulation frequencies. Stimulation at low physiological frequencies (5 Hz) shows little overflow, while stimulation at 30 Hz leads to substantial overflow. In the presence of low concentrations of the adenosine uptake-inhibitor dipyridamole, overflow at low stimulation frequencies is comparable to that at high frequencies.

Drugs. Several groups of drugs are known from early studies to block the responses to either adenine nucleotides or nucleosides in a wide variety of preparations. These include anti-malarial drugs such as mepacrine, quinine and quinidine, and methylxanthines such as caffeine, theophylline and aminophylline. Quinidine blocks nonadrenergic, noncholinergic nerve-mediated responses in the gut and bladder, but only in concentrations that give little confidence in its specificity. With the development of the P_1, P_2 purinoceptor hypothesis (see above) some of the apparently contradictory data have been clarified. It has been shown that the methylxanthines are competitive antagonists to adenosine and AMP, while several new agents which block responses of intestine to ATP have been found. These include the 2-substituted imidazoline compounds such as antazoline and phentolamine[69] and 2-2′-pyridylisatogen[38,45]. Unfortunately, these drugs are not specific for ATP. In a recent report, however, it has been claimed that very low concentrations ($10^{-8}M$) of apamin, a constituent of bee venom, selectively block both the inhibitory junction potentials in response to purinergic nerve stimulation in the intestine and the hyperpolarizations produced by ATP[78].

Immunohistochemical Localization of Polypeptides in Enteric Nerves and their Actions on Smooth Muscle

Recent immunohistochemical studies have demonstrated that some biologically active polypeptides are localized within enteric neurons of the gastrointestinal tract: these include Substance P[33,54,56,63,73], somatostatin[21,34,35], enkephalin[23,42,66] and vasoactive intestinal polypeptide[2,26,48,49]. Other vasoactive polypeptides such as neurotensin have also been found in the gut[18,50], although not localized histochemically within enteric neurons[60].

On the basis of these studies it has been claimed that the nonadrenergic, noncholinergic nerves supplying intestinal smooth muscle are 'peptidergic' rather than 'purinergic'[1,41]. However, an important criterion for the identification of a neurotransmitter is that exogenous application of the substance mimics the response to nerve stimulation, and while the responses to ATP mimic closely the rapid responses to intramural nerve stimulation in all preparations whether the tone is low, medium or high, Substance P, somatostatin, enkephalin and vasoactive intestinal polypeptide do not produce mimicking responses[19]. Substance P always causes contraction, enkephalin and somatostatin are inactive, while VIP produces very slow relaxation, taking about four mins to reach a maximum after a latency of about 60 sec (compared to a latency of about one sec at a time to maximum of about 15 secs for the responses to both ATP and nerve stimulation).

Since Substance P, enkephalin, somatostatin and VIP are clearly not the transmitters released from the nonadrenergic, noncholinergic efferent nerves supplying the intestinal musculature, other possible roles for these intraneuronal polypeptides should be considered. It is unlikely that the contractile responses to the peptides tested are produced by excitatory prostaglandins, which mask any inhibitory effects. Such a role for prostaglandins has been proposed for the contractile response of the anococcygeus to exogenous ATP[11]. However, in the present study no inhibitory responses to peptides were unmasked following inhibition of prostaglandin synthesis (see also[17]).

There is strong evidence that Substance P is a neurotransmitter in primary afferent fibers in the spinal cord and skin (see[33,51,61]) so that it is possible that it is also localized in sensory fibers in the gut (see also[33]). However, Substance P is known to have a variety of peripheral actions including contraction of intestinal longitudinal muscle[24,64,80] and dilatation of blood vessels[80].

The endogenous opiate ligands, enkephalins, have potent inhibitory actions on electrically-stimulated contractions of both the mouse vas deferens and the guinea-pig ileum[39,40]. Also, both enkephalins and morphine have been shown to inhibit neuronal firing in Auerbach's plexus[22,58] by causing membrane hyperpolarization[57]. Therefore, it seems likely that enkephalins are released from interneurons involved in modulation of nerve-mediated excitation of the intestine. Neither enkephalin nor naloxone, a potent opiate antagonist[46] had any effect on the inhibitory response to nonadrenergic intramural nerve stimulation in the guinea-pig taenia coli. It has also been suggested that neurons which display somatostatin immunoreactivity are interneurons within the enteric nervous system[21]. This is supported by the finding that somatostatin inhibits the release of acetylcholine from nerves within Auerbach's plexus of the small intestine[28] and no somatostatin-immune-reactive fibers were found in either the longitudinal or circular muscle of the ileum[21].

Intrinsic VIP-containing neurons found throughout the gut may also be interneurons, since they have been shown to innervate nerve cells in both Meissner's and Auerbach's plexuses[26]. VIP-positive nerve fibers have been observed within the circular muscle layer and muscularis mucosa of the rat stomach, duodenum and colon, but these appear to be en route to the mucosal epithelium[26]. The role of the very slow inhibitory response of the taenia coli to VIP is not clear, since it does not mimic the nerve-mediated response. Similar slow relaxations to VIP have been reported in the gall bladder, trachea and stomach[65] and canine small intestine[43].

Finally, the possibility should be considered that polypeptides are stored together with neurotransmitters in enteric nerves. Burnstock[6] has recently discussed the concept that some nerves contain more than one transmitter. Hökfelt et al.[34] have shown that some adrenergic neurons in peripheral sympathetic ganglia contain somatostatin together with noradrenaline, and earlier Von Euler[79] showed that splenic nerves contained vesicular Substance P.

Presynaptic Neuromodulation of Transmitter Release in Neuronal Interactions in the Gut

There are interactions between adrenergic, cholinergic and purinergic nerves in the gut at presynaptic as well as postsynaptic levels. Neuromodulation, defined as the regulation of release of transmitter from nerves by the action of neurohumoral agents on prejunctional receptors, is a relatively recent concept of physiological importance (see[81]). Apart from the inhibition of transmitter output by the negative feedback of noradrenaline (NA) mediated through prejunctional α-adrenoceptors, some inhibition of the activity of adrenergic nerves appears to be due to the prejunctional actions of acetylcholine (ACh), prostaglandins, ATP and adenosine. Similarly the prejunctional action of catecholamines and adenine nucleotides and nucleosides[47,72] modulates cholinergic nerve activity.

Modulation of adrenergic nerve activity by acetylcholine, ATP and adenosine. It has been known for some years that high concentrations of ACh have an inhibitory effect on the responses to sympathetic nerve stimulation; this effect is mediated through prejunctional muscarinic receptors. Low concentrations of ACh have facilitatory effects on adrenergic transmission.

Adenine nucleotides and nucleosides have also been shown to inhibit NA release from adrenergic nerves. Adenosine significantly and reversibly depresses, in a concentration-dependent manner, NA release evoked by adrenergic nerve stimulation to guinea-pig terminal ileum. Kazic and Milosavljevic[44] concluded from these and other experiments that adenosine acts by two discrete mechanisms, prejunctional inhibition and postjunctional enhancement, and that in this situation the latter mechanism dominates.

ATP-induction of prostaglandin synthesis has been described[13,55] and the possibility has been raised earlier in this article that purinergic nerves are linked with prostaglandin in physiological regulatory mechanisms. Thus it is of some interest that prostaglandins of the E series can also act as neuromodulators, reducing release of NA from adrenergic nerves[68].

Modulation of cholinergic nerve activity by catecholamines, ATP and adenosine. It has been shown that NA released from sympathetic nerve terminals reduces the release of ACh, thereby inhibiting gastrointestinal motility[62,75,76,77]. There is considerable evidence for a prejunctional site of action for adenosine on cholinergic terminals. Adenosine reduces acetylcholine release from excitatory nerves in the intestine[29,30,53,77]. Further, theophylline, which blocks adenosine action, enhances the release of ACh from intestine[70,77].

It seems likely that the modulatory actions are physiological mechanisms and not merely a pharmacological feature. The ultrastructural arrangement of nerve terminals is consistent with this hypothesis since there is frequently close apposition of adrenergic and cholinergic nerve varicosities, often enclosed within the same Schwann cell sheath (see[15]). Vizi and Knoll[77] have considered the possibility that the source of adenine nucleotides involved in prejunctional inhibition of ACh release in the intestine is either purinergic nerves or cholinergic nerves which have been claimed to release ATP together with ACh[71,82].

SUMMARY AND CONCLUSIONS

1.   Up to nine morphologically distinct neurons have been identified at the ultrastructural level in the gastrointestinal tract. About 10 substances have been claimed as established or putative neurotransmitters in the gut, including acetylcholine, noradrenaline, dopamine, 5-hydroxytryptamine, adenosine triphosphate and the polypeptides enkephalin, bradykinin, Substance P, somatostatin and vasoactive intestinal peptide. This morphological and neurochemical complexity implies that the enteric nervous system is capable of considerable integrative activity, independent of the central nervous system.

2.   Acetylcholine is contained in intramural excitatory neurons and in preganglionic parasympathetic nerves.

3.   Noradrenaline is contained in postganglionic sympathetic nerves. These terminate mostly in Auerbach's plexus, where they appear to inhibit intrinsic reflexes by presynaptic inhibition of acetylcholine release or possibly by a direct action on the cell bodies of intramural cholinergic neurons; a few directly innervate the smooth muscle of the circular coat in some regions. The presence of intramural adrenergic neurons in the gut is a rare occurrence in a limited region of the small intestine of some species.

4.   ATP appears to be the principle transmitter in nonadrenergic, noncholinergic *inhibitory* nerves that supply the smooth muscle of the esophagus, stomach, intestine and various sphincters. These intramural neurons in the stomach and distal rectum are controlled via nicotinic receptors by preganglionic parasympathetic nerves in the vagal and pelvic outflow, while throughout most of the intestine they are controlled by cholinergic interneurons and perhaps by other types of interneurons. Purinergic nerves are involved in inhibitory reflexes which facilitate passage of material through the alimentary canal by opening sphincters, increasing stomach size and expanding the intestine in front of an advancing bolus during peristalsis.

5.   5-hydroxytryptamine may be the transmitter in some of the neurons responsible for the non-adrenergic, non-cholinergic *excitatory* responses of smooth muscle.

6.   Various polypeptides have been demonstrated with immunohistochemical methods in nerves in the gut wall. Their role is still not resolved, but some (e.g., Sub-

stance P) may be contained in sensory nerves, while others (e.g., somatostatin, vaso-active intestinal peptide and enkephalin) appear to be contained in interneurons. Others may be contained in nerve fibers supplying blood vessels or mucosal epithelial cells.

7. It is possible that more than one putative neurotransmitter is stored in the same neuron, e.g., noradrenaline with somatostatin, or with acetylcholine or ATP; and Substance P with 5-hydroxytryptamine.

8. Enteric nerves interact at pre- as well as postsynaptic levels. Acetylcholine and adenosine act as presynaptic neuromodulators of noradrenaline release from adrenergic nerve terminals; and noradrenaline and adenosine act as presynaptic neuromodulators of acetylcholine release from cholinergic nerve terminals.

9. Other indirect means of modulating enteric neuron activity include the potent effects of prostaglandins, whose synthesis can be induced by ATP and peptides, neurohormones circulating in the blood and nerve-induced changes in blood flow.

REFERENCES

1 Bloom, S. R. and Polak, J. M., Peptidergic versus purinergic, *Lancet*, 1 (1978) 93.

2 Bryant, M. G., Bloom, S. R., Polak, J. M., Albuquerque, R. H., Modlin, I. and Pearse, A. G. E., Possible dual role for vasoactive intestinal peptide as gastrointestinal hormone and neurotransmitter substance, *Lancet*, 1 (1976) 991.

3 Burnstock, G., Evolution of the autonomic innervation of visceral and cardiovascular systems in vertebrates, *Pharmacol. Rev.*, 21 (1969) 247–324.

4 Burnstock, G., Purinergic nerves, *Pharmacol. Rev.*, 24 (1972) 509–581.

5 Burnstock, G., Purinergic transmission. In: L. L. Iversen, S. D. Iversen and S. H. Snyder (Eds.), *Handbook of Psychopharmacology*, Vol. 5, Plenum Press, New York, 1975, pp. 131–194.

6 Burnstock, G., Do some nerve cells release more than one transmitter? *Neuroscience*, 1 (1976) 239–248.

7 Burnstock, G., Purinergic receptors, *J. theor. Biol.*, 62 (1976) 491–503.

8 Burnstock, G., Past and current evidence for the purinergic nerve hypothesis. In: H. P. Baer and G. I. Drummond (Eds.), *Physiological and Regulatory Functions of Adenosine and Adenine Nucleotides*, Raven Press, New York, 1978, in press.

9 Burnstock, G., A basis for distinguishing two types of purinergic receptor. In: L. Bolis and R. W. Straub (Eds.), *Cell Membrane Receptors for Drugs and Hormones: A Multidisciplinary Approach*, Raven Press, New York, 1978, pp. 107–118.

10 Burnstock, G., Campbell, G., Bennett, M. and Holman, M. E., Inhibition of the smooth muscle of the taenia coli, *Nature*, 200 (1963) 581–582.

11 Burnstock, G., Cocks, T. and Crowe, R., Evidence for purinergic innervation of the anococcygeus muscle, *Brit. J. Pharmacol.*, 64 (1978) 13–20.

12 Burnstock, G., Cocks, T., Kasakov, L. and Wong, H. K., Direct evidence for release of ATP from nonadrenergic, noncholinergic ('purinergic') nerves, in the guinea-pig taenia coli and bladder, *Europ. J. Pharmacol.*, 49 (1978) 145–149.

13 Burnstock, G., Cocks, T., Paddle, B. M. and Staszewska-Barczak, J., Evidence that prostaglandin is responsible for the 'rebound contraction' following stimulation of non-adrenergic, noncholinergic ('purinergic') inhibitory nerves, *Europ. J. Pharmacol.*, 31 (1975) 360–362.

14 Burnstock, G. and Costa, M., Inhibitory innervation of the gut, *Gastroent.*, 64 (1973) 141–144.

15 Burnstock, G. and Costa, M., *Adrenergic Neurons: Their Organisation, Function and Development in the Peripheral Nervous System*, Chapman and Hall, London, 1975, 225 pp.

16 Burnstock, G. and Wong, H., Comparison of the effects of UV light and purinergic nerve stimulation on the quinea-pig taenia coli, *Brit. J. Pharmacol.*, 62 (1978) 293–302.

17 Bury, R. W. and Mashford, M. L., A pharmacological investigation of synthetic Substance P on the isolated guinea-pig ileum, *Clin. exp. Pharmac. Physiol.*, 4 (1977) 453–461.

18 Carraway, R. and Leeman, S. E., Characterization of radioimmunoassayable neurotensin in rat—Its differential distribution in central nervous system, small intestine, and stomach, *J. biol. Chem.*, 251 (1976) 7045–7052.

19 Cocks, T. and Burnstock, G., Effects of neuronal polypeptides on intestinal muscle: A comparison with non-adrenergic, non-cholinergic nerve stimulation and ATP, *Europ. J. Pharmacol.*, (in press).

20 Cook, R. D. and Burnstock, G., The ultrastructure of Auerbach's plexus in the guinea-pig. 1. Neuronal elements, *J. Neurocytol.*, 5 (1976) 171–194.

21 Costa, M., Patel, Y., Furness, J. B. and Arimura, A., Evidence that some intrinsic neurons of the intestine contain somatostatin, *Neuroscience Letters*, 6 (1977) 215–222.

22 Dingledine, R. and Goldstein, A., Effect of synaptic transmission blockade on morphine action in the guinea-pig myenteric plexus, *J. Pharm. exp. Ther.*, 196 (1976) 97–106.

23 Elde, R., Hökfelt, T., Johansson, O. and Terenius, L., Immunohistochemical studies using antibodies to leucine-enkephalin: Initial observations on the nervous system of the rat, *Neuroscience*, 1 (1976) 349–351.

24 Franco, R. and Costa, M., The effect of substance P on intestinal nerves and muscle, *Proc. Aust. Physiol. & Pharmac. Soc.*, (1978) 10 P.

25 Furness, J. B. and Costa, M., Distribution of intrinsic nerve cell bodies and axons which take up aromatic amines and their precursors in the small intestine of the guinea-pig, *Cell Tiss. Res.*, 188 (1978) 527–543.

26 Fuxe, K., Hökfelt, T., Said, I. and Mutt, V., Vasoactive intestinal polypeptide and the nervous system. Immunohistochemical evidence for localization in central and peripheral neurons, particularly intracortical neurons of the cerebral cortex, *Neuroscience Letters*, 5 (1977) 241–246.

27 Gershon, M. D., Dreyfus, C. F., Pickel, V. M., Joh, T. H. and Reis, D. J., Serotonergic neurons in peripheral nervous-system: Identification in gut by immunohistochemical localization of tryptophan hydroxylase, *Proc. nat. Acad. Sci. USA*, 74 (1977) 3086–3089.

28 Guillemin, R., Somatostatin inhibits the release of acetylcholine induced electrically in the myenteric plexus, *Endocrinology*, 99 (1976) 1653–1654.

29 Gustafsson, L., Hedqvist, P. and Fredholm, B. B., Inhibition of acetylcholine-release by adenosine, *Acta Pharm.*, 41 (1977) 49 P.

30 Hayashi, E., Mori, M., Yamada, S. and Kunitomo, M., Effects of purine compounds on cholinergic nerves—specificity of adenosine and related compounds on acetylcholine-release in electrically stimulated guinea-pig ileum, *Europ. J. Pharmacol.*, 48 (1978) 297–307.

31 Hayashi, E., Yamada, S., Mori, M. and Shinozuka, K., Effect of purine nucleotides on parasympathetic nerves. 7. Effect of some drugs on transmurally (high frequency) —induced contraction of guinea-pig isolated ileum, *Jap. J. Pharm.*, 26 (1976) 64 P.

32 Hökfelt, T., Elfvin, L. G., Elde, R. and Schultz, B. M., Occurrence of somatostatin-like immunoreactivity in some peripheral sympathetic noradrenergic neurons, *Proc. nat. Acad. Sci. USA*, 74 (1977) 3587–3591.

33 Hökfelt, T., Elfvin, L. G., Schultz, B. M., Goldstein, M. and Nilsson, G., Occurrence of substance P-containing fibers in sympathetic ganglia—Immunohistochemical evidence, *Brain Res.*, 132 (1977) 29–41.

34 Hökfelt, T., Hellerstrom, C., Effendic, S., Johansson, O., Luft, R. and Arimura, A., Immunohistochemical evidence for a widespread occurrence of somatostatin in neurosecretory cells, primary sensory neurons and endocrine-like cell systems, *Acta Endocrinol.*, 80 (1975) 134 P.

35 Hökfelt, T., Johansson, O., Effendic, S., Luft, R. and Arimura, A., Are there somatostatin-containing nerves in the rat gut? Immunohistochemical evidence for a new type of peripheral nerve, *Experientia*, 31 (1975) 852–854.

36 Hökfelt, T., Kellerth, J.-O., Nilsson, G. and Pernow, B., Experimental immunohistochemical studies on the localization and distribution of substance P in cat primary sensory neurons, *Brain Res.*, 100 (1975) 235–252.

37 Holman, M. E. and Weinrich, J. P., Effects of calcium and magnesium on inhibitory junctional transmission in smooth-muscle of guinea-pig small-intestine, *Pflügers Arch.*, 360 (1975) 109–119.

38 Hooper, M., Spedding, M., Sweetman, A. J. and Weetman, D. F., 2–2′ pyridylisatogen tosylate antagonist of inhibitory effects of ATP on smooth muscle, *Brit. J. Pharmac.*, 50 (1974) 458–459.

39 Hughes, J., Smith, T. W., Kosterlitz, H. W., Fothergill, L. A., Morgan, B. A. and Morris, H. R., Identification of two related pentapeptides from the brain with potent opiate agonist activity, *Nature*, 258 (1975) 577–579.

40 Hughes, J., Smith, T., Morgan, B. and Fothergill, L., Purification and properties of enkephalin—The possible endogenous ligand for the morphine receptor, *Life Sci.*, 16 (1975) 1753–1758.

41 Humphrey, C. S. and Fischer, J. E., Peptidergic versus purinergic nerves, *Lancet*, 1 (1978) 390.

42 Johansson, O., Hökfelt, T., Elde, R. P., Schultzberg, M. and Terenius, L., Immunohistochemical distribution of enkephalin neurons. In: E. Costa and M. Trabucchi (Eds.), *Advances in Biochemical Psychopharmacology*, Vol. 18, Raven Press, New York, 1978, pp. 51–70.

43 Kachelhoffer, J., Mendel, C., Dauchel, J., Hohmatter, D. and Grenier, J. F., The effects of VIP on intestinal motility. Study on *ex vivo* perfused isolated canine jejunal loops, *Amer. J. Digest. Diseases*, 21 (1976) 957–962.

44 Kazic, T. and Milosavljevic, D., Influence of adenosine, cAMP and db-cAMP on responses of the isolated terminal guinea-pig ileum to electrical stimulation, *Archs int. Pharmacodyn.*, 223 (1976) 187–195.

45 Kazic, T. and Milosavljevic, D., Influence of pyridylisatogen tosylate on contractions produced by ATP and by purinergic stimulation in terminal ileum of guinea-pig, *J. Pharm. Pharmac.*, 29 (1977) 542–545.

46 Klee, W. A., Endogenous opiate peptides. In: H. Gainer (Ed.), *Peptides in Neurobiology*, Plenum Press, New York, 1977, pp. 357–396.

47 Langer, S. Z., Presynaptic receptors and their role in the regulation of transmitter release, *Brit. J. Pharmac.*, 60 (1977) 481–498.

48 Larsson, L.-I., Ultrastructural localization of a new neuronal peptide (VIP), *Histochem.*, 54 (1977) 173–176.

49 Larsson, L.-I., Fahrenkrug, J., Schaffalitzy de Muckadell, O., Sundler, F., Hakanson, R. and Rehfeld, J. F., Localization of vasoactive intestinal polypeptide (VIP) to central and peripheral neurons, *Proc. nat. Acad. Sci. USA*, 73 (1976) 3197–3200.

50 Leeman, S. E., Mroz, E. A. and Carraway, R. E., Substance P and Neurotensin. In H. Gainer (Ed.), *Peptides in Neurobiology*, Plenum Press, New York, 1977, pp. 99–144.

51 Lembeck, F., Zur Frage der zentralen Übertragung afferenter Impulse. III. Mitteilung. Das Vorkommen und die Bedeutung der Substanz P in den dorsalen Wurzeln des Ruckenmarks, *Naunyn-Schmiederbergs Arch. Pharmakol.*, 219 (1953) 197–213.

52 Martinson, J. and Muren, A., Excitatory and inhibitory effects of vagus stimulation on gastric motility in the cat, *Acta physiol. scand.*, 57 (1963) 309–316.

53 Mori, M., Yamada, S., Takamura, S. and Hayashi, E., Effect of purine nucleotides on acetylcholine output from cholinergic nerves in guinea-pig ileum, *J. Jap. Pharmacol.*, 23 (1973) 137 P.

54 Mroz, E. A. and Leeman, S. E., Substance P, *Vitamins and Hormones*, 35 (1977) 209–281.

55 Needleman, P., Minkes, M. S. and Douglas, J. R., Stimulation of prostaglandin biosynthesis by adenine nucleotides. Profile of prostaglandin release by perfused organs, *Circulation Res.*, 34 (1974) 455–460.

56 Nilsson, G., Larsson, L. I., Hakansson, R., Brodin, E., Sundler, F. and Pernow, B., Localization of substance P-like immunoreactivity on mouse gut, *Histochemistry*, 43 (1975) 97–99.

57 North, R. A. and Tonini, M., Hyperpolarization by morphine of myenteric neurones. In: H. W. Kosterlitz (Ed.), *Opiates and Endogenous Opioid peptides*, North Holland, Amsterdam, 1976, pp. 205–212.

58 North, R. A. and Williams, J. T., Enkephalin inhibits firing of myenteric neurones, *Nature*, 264 (1976) 460–461.

59 Olson, L., Alund, M. and Norberg, K., Fluorescence—Microscopical demonstration of a population of gastrointestinal nerve fibers with a selective affinity for quinacrine, *Cell Tiss. Res.*, 171 (1976) 407–423.

60 Orci, L., Baetens, D., Rufener, C., Brown, M., Vale, W. and Guillemin, R., Evidence for immunoreactive neurotensin in dog intestinal mucosa, *Life Sci.*, 19 (1976) 559–561.

61 Otsuka, M. and Konishi, S., Release of substance P-like immunoreactivity from isolated spinal cord of newborn rat, *Nature*, 264 (1976) 83–84.

62 Paton, W. D. M. and Vizi, E. S., The inhibitory action of noradrenaline and adrenaline on acetylcholine output by guinea-pig ileum longitudinal muscle strip, *Brit. J. Chemother.*, 35 (1969) 10–18.

63 Pearse, A. G. E. and Polak, J. M., Immunocytochemical localization of substance P in mammalian intestine, *Histochemistry*, 41 (1975) 373–375.

64 Pernow, B., Effect of substance P on smooth muscle. In: M. Schachter (Ed.), *Polypeptides which Affect Smooth Muscle and Blood Vessels*, Pergamon Press, Elmsford, New York, 1960, pp. 163–170.

65 Piper, P. J., Said, S. E. and Vane, J. R., Effects on smooth muscle preparations of unidentified vasoactive peptides from intestine and lung, *Nature*, 225 (1970) 1144–1146.

66 Polak, J. M., Sullivan, S. N., Bloom, S. R., Facer, P. and Pearse, A. G. E., Enkephalinlike immunoreactivity in the human gastrointestinal tract, *Lancet*, 1 (1977) 972–974.

67 Rutherford, A. and Burnstock, G., Neuronal and non-neuronal components in the overflow of labelled adenine compounds from guinea-pig taenia coli, *Europ. J. Pharmacol.*, 48 (1978) 195–202.

68 Sakato, M. and Shimo, Y., Possible role of prostaglandin El on adrenergic neurotransmission in guinea-pig taenia coli, *Europ. J. Pharmacol.*, 40 (1976) 209–214.

69 Satchell, D., Burnstock, G. and Dann, P. Antagonism of the effects of purinergic nerve stimulation and exogenously applied ATP on the guinea-pig taenia coli by 2-substituted imidazolines and related compounds, *Europ. J. Pharmacol.*, 23 (1973) 264–269.

158   G. Burnstock

70   Sawynok, J. and Jhamandas, K. H., Inhibition of acetylcholine release from cholinergic nerves by adenosine, adenine nucleotides and morphine—Antagonism by theophylline, *J. Pharmac. exp. Ther.*, 197 (1976) 379–390.

71   Silinsky, E. M. and Hubbard, J. I., Release of ATP from rat motor nerve terminals, *Nature*, 243 (1973) 404–405.

72   Story, D. F., Allen, G. S., Glover, A. B., Hope, W., McCulloch, M. W., Rand, M. J. and Sarantos, C., Modulation of adrenergic transmission by acetylcholine, *Clin. & exp. Pharmacology & Physiology*, 2 (1975) 27–33.

73   Sundler, F., Hakansson, R., Larsson, L.-I., Brodin, E. and Nilsson, G., In: U.S. Von Euler and B. Pernow (Eds.), *Substance P: Nobel symposium 37*, Raven Press, New York, 1977, pp. 59–65.

74   Vizi, E. S., Acetylcholine release from guinea-pig ileum by parasympathetic ganglion stimulants and gastrin-like-polypeptides, *Brit. J. Pharmac. Chemother.*, 47 (1973) 765–777.

75   Vizi, E. S., The role of α-adrenoceptors situated in Auerbach's plexus in the inhibition of gastrointestinal motility, In: E. Bülbring and M. F. Shuba (Eds.), *Physiology of Smooth Muscle*, Raven Press, New York, 1976, pp. 357–367.

76   Vizi, E. S. and Knoll, J., The effect of sympathetic nerve stimulation and guanethidine on parasympathetic neuroeffector transmission; The inhibition of acetylcholine release, *J. Pharm. Pharmac.*, 23 (1971) 918–925.

77   Vizi, E. S. and Knoll, J., The inhibitory effect of adenosine and related nucleotides on the release of acetylcholine, *Neuroscience*, 1 (1976) 391–398.

78   Vladimirova, A. I. and Shuba, M. F., Strychnine, hydrastine and apamin effect on synaptic transmission in smooth muscle cells, *Neurophysiology* (U.S.S.R.), 10 (1978) 295–299.

79   Von Euler, U. S., Substance P in subcellular particles in peripheral nerves, *Ann. N. Y. Acad. Sci.*, 104 (1963) 449–463.

80   Von Euler, U. S. and Gaddum, J. H., An unidentified depressor substance in certain tissue extracts, *J. Physiol.* (Lond.), 72 (1931) 74 P.

81   Westfall, T. C., Local regulation of adrenergic neurotransmission, *Physiol. Rev.*, 57 (1977) 659–728.

82   Whittaker, V. P., Dowdall, M. J. and Boyne, A. F., The storage and release of acetylcholine by cholinergic nerve terminals: Recent results with non-mammalian preparations, *Biochem. Soc. Sym.*, 36 (1972) 49–68.

83   Wood, J. D., Neurophysiology of the enteric nervous system. This volume, pp. 177–193.

CHAPTER 11

CHOLINERGIC INHIBITION OF ADRENERGIC NEUROTRANSMISSION IN THE CARDIOVASCULAR SYSTEM

Paul M. Vanhoutte* and Matthew N. Levy**

*Department of Medicine, University of Antwerp, Belgium, and
**Department of Investigative Medicine, The Mount Sinai Hospital of
Cleveland, Cleveland, Ohio, USA

INTRODUCTION

The heart and certain blood vessels are innervated by both adrenergic and cholinergic neurons[4,14]. Ordinarily the direct effects of the sympathetic and parasympathetic neurotransmitters on the peripheral effector cells oppose each other. Thus, the sympathetic transmitter, norepinephrine, excites, while the cholinergic messenger, acetylcholine, depresses both cardiac function and blood vessel tone in the intact organism. The general belief is that neurogenic alteration of the activity of the cardiovascular effector cells depends on the summation of the opposing effects of the liberated amounts of adrenergic and cholinergic transmitters. There is little doubt that in the heart and certain blood vessels, acetylcholine can indeed oppose the direct excitatory effect of norepinephrine, although the action of acetylcholine on both cardiac and vascular smooth muscle cells can be extremely complex[14,36,38]. The present discussion is concerned mainly with the role played by the cholinergic transmitter in modulating the function of the adrenergic nerve endings in the heart and in the blood vessel wall[5,14,23,29,30,35-38,45].

RESULTS AND DISCUSSION

The Heart

In 1934, Rosenblueth and Simeone[26] reported that, in the cat, the absolute decrease in heart rate evoked by a given vagal stimulus was more pronounced the greater the level of heart rate produced by tonic cardiac sympathetic stimulation. Just a year later, Samaan[27] demonstrated that, in both cats and dogs, the chronotropic response to vagal stimulation was considerably greater when the background level of sympathetic activity was increased. These two early observations are explained most logically by an inhibitory effect of the vagal neurotransmitter on the release of norepinephrine in the heart; such an inhibitory effect has been demonstrated beyond doubt in more recent work.

P. M. Vanhoutte and M. N. Levy

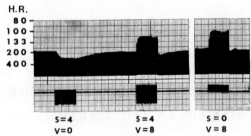

Fig. 1.   Demonstration of the preponderance of the vagus over the sympathetic nerves in controlling heart rate. Original recording of an experiment performed on a canine isovolumetric left ventricle preparation. At the event marks (lower tracings), the frequencies (in herz) of sympathetic (S) and vagal (V) stimulation are shown. Note that the absolute values of the increase in rate during sympathetic stimulation alone (S=4; V=0) and of the decrease during vagal stimulation alone (S=0; V=8) are comparable. Combined stimulation of sympathetic and vagal nerves (S=4; V=8) results in a decrease in heart rate similar to that produced by vagal stimulation alone. (From reference 17; by permission.)

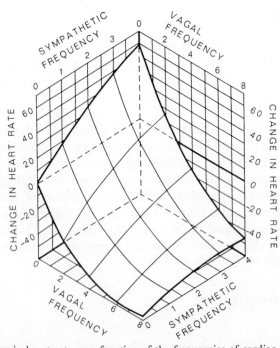

Fig. 2.   Changes in heart rate as a function of the frequencies of cardiac sympathetic and vagal stimulation. The response surface represents the mean data for 10 animals. The accentuated antagonism between the two parts of the autonomic nervous system may be appreciated by contrasting the slopes of the opposing edges of the surface. Considering the edges parallel to the sympathetic frequency axis, it is apparent that a change in sympathetic activity has a much greater effect on heart rate in the absence of vagal activity than when the vagi are stimulated at 8 Hz. On the other hand, contrasting the edges parallel to the vagal frequency axis reveals that the vagi have a much greater negative chronotropic effect when the sympathetic nerves are stimulated at 4 Hz than in the absence of sympathetic stimulation. (From reference 17; by permission.)

Parasympathetic-sympathetic antagonism and the control of heart rate and myocardial contractility. Vagal influences on heart rate greatly preponderate over sympathetic effects. In the dog, for example, the frequencies of sympathetic and vagal stimulation can be adjusted so that they each produce changes in the heart rate of equal magnitude, but of opposite direction (Fig. 1). When such vagal and sympathetic stimuli are applied simultaneously the heart rate decreases almost as if there were no sympathetic stimulation at all (Fig. 1[17]). This accentuated antagonism between vagal and

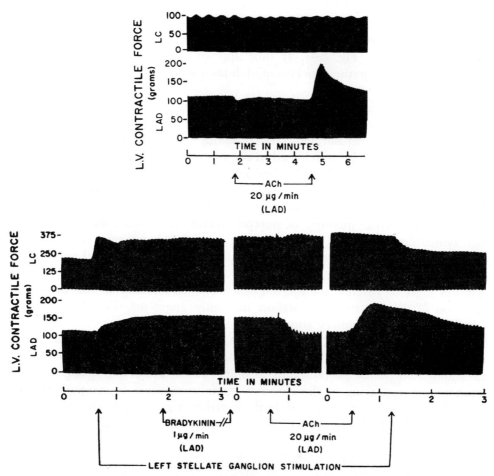

Fig. 3.   The effects of acetylcholine (ACh) infused into the left anterior descending coronary artery (LAD) of a dog, on the contractile force of segments of the left ventricular myocardium in regions supplied by that artery and by the left circumflex coronary artery (LC). Panel A: Infusion of ACh, in the absence of sympathetic stimulation, causes only a slight decrease in contractile force in the region of the LAD during the infusion; after cessation of infusion, there is a transient increase of contractile force. Panel B: Infusion of ACh, during left stellate ganglion stimulation, causes a more pronounced depression of contractile force. Another coronary vasodilator (bradykinin) does not influence contractile force appreciably. (Modified from reference 10; by permission of the American Heart Association.)

sympathetic effects on heart rate can be demonstrated for a wide range of stimulation frequencies (Fig. 2[17]).

In the dog, intracoronary infusions of acetylcholine have minimal depressant effects on ventricular contractility in the absence of a background of sympathetic activity. By contrast, during tonic sympathetic stimulation, the same infusions of acetylcholine have substantial negative inotropic effects (Fig. 3[10]). In the same species, vagal stimulation usually evokes slight to moderate reductions in peak left ventricular pressure (Fig. 4[15]). When ventricular contractility is first enhanced by cardiac sympathetic stimulation, vagal stimulation elicits a much greater reduction in peak left ventricular pressure (Fig. 4). The antagonism between the two divisions of the autonomic nervous system is variable, and it depends on the degree of activation of the autonomic nerves (Fig. 5[21]). It thus appears that the peripheral interaction between vagal and sympathetic nerves modulates both the chronotropic and inotropic behavior of the heart[14].

Parasympathetic inhibition of peripheral adrenergic neurotransmission. In the isolated perfused rabbit heart, stimulation of the sympathetic nerves augments the appearance of norepinephrine in the perfusate. Infusions of acetylcholine markedly reduce the amount of norepinephrine released in response to standard stimuli applied to the sympathetic nerves (Fig. 6[2,18]). This inhibition of the evoked release of adrenergic transmitter is obtained not only with exogenous acetylcholine, but also with endogenously-released cholinergic transmitter. Indeed, in the isolated rabbit atrium, vagal stimulation reduces the quantity of norepinephrine overflowing during stimulation of the sympathetic nerves[19]. These observations strongly suggest, at least for the isolated rabbit heart, that the acetylcholine liberated from the vagal nerve endings exerts an inhibitory effect on the peripheral adrenergic nerve terminals[23]. A similar conclusion must be reached for the dog's heart studied *in situ*. In this preparation, stimulation of the left stellate ganglion markedly augments the overflow of norepinephrine into the coronary sinus blood. When the vagus nerves are stimulated simultaneously with the sympathetic nerves, the rate of norepinephrine overflow is markedly reduced (Fig. 7[16]). The curtailment of norepinephrine overflow by vagal stimulation can be prevented by atropine. In the intact dog heart, most of the norepinephrine appearing in the coronary sinus in response to sympathetic stimulation is derived from nerve terminals in the ventricular walls, and hence the reduction in norepinephrine overflow produced by vagal stimulation probably reflects an inter-

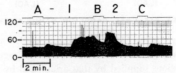

Fig. 4. Demonstration that vagal nerve stimulation (A, B and C: cervical vagi stimulated at 20 Hz, with supramaximal voltage, for the time shown by the event marker) causes a much larger decrease in myocardial contractility during sympathetic nerve stimulation (left stellate ganglion stimulated at 2 Hz, with supramaximal voltage, between marks 1 and 2) than in absence of sympathetic stimulation. Original recording of the changes in left ventricular pressure in a canine isovolumetric left ventricle preparation. (From reference 15; by permission of MIT Press.)

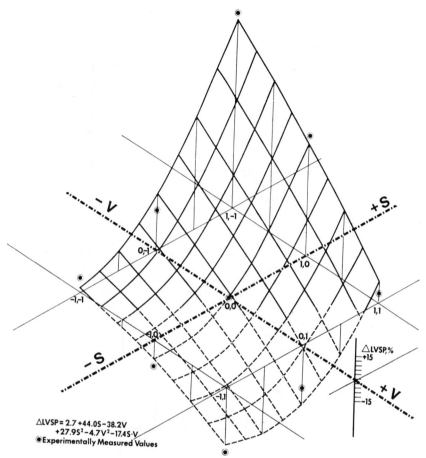

Fig. 5. Changes in myocardial contractility, measured as changes in left ventricular systolic pressure (△LVSP), as a function of the intensity of cardiac sympathetic (S) and vagal (V) stimulation in a canine isovolumetric left ventricle. The lower left edge of the surface indicates the change in left ventricular systolic pressure (LVSP) at a low constant level of sympathetic activity (denoted by −S) as vagal activity is changed from low (−V) to high (+V) levels. It is evident that LVSP does not change appreciably over the prevailing range of vagal stimulation intensities. The upper right edge of the surface represents the change in LVSP over the same range of vagal activities, but at a constant high level of sympathetic activity (+S). It is clear from the figure that with a high background of sympathetic activity, a progressive increase in the intensity of vagal stimulation evokes a pronounced reduction in LVSP. (From reference 21; by permission.)

action occurring largely in the ventricles. It thus appears that the pronounced antagonism between the vagal and sympathetic systems in the control of both heart rate and myocardial contractility can be attributed in part to prejunctional inhibition of peripheral adrenergic neurotransmission.

Blood Vessels

In 1965, de la Lande and Rand[6] reported that acetylcholine markedly depressed

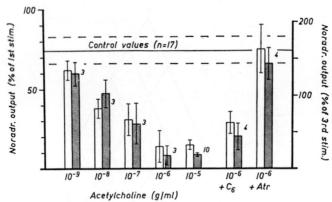

Fig. 6.   The effect of different concentrations of acetylcholine (ACh) on the output of norepinephrine (NE) evoked by sympathetic nerve stimulation in the perfused rabbit
heart. The cardiac sympathetic nerves were stimulated for three successive 10-min
periods. The various concentrations of ACh were present only during the second
period. The heights of the bars represent the mean output of NE during the second
period, expressed as percentages of the first (open bars) and third (closed bars)
stimulation periods. It is evident that the output of NE decreases as the concentration
of ACh is increased. The effect of ACh is not appreciably influenced by hexamethonium (C_6), but it is abolished by atropine (Atr). (From reference 18; by permission.)

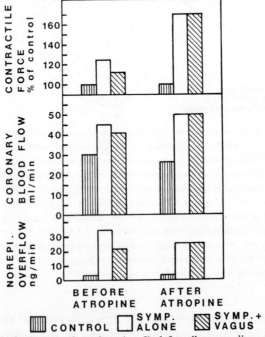

Fig. 7.   In anesthetized, open chest dogs (n=6), left stellate ganglion stimulation (2 Hz)
produces an increase in ventricular contractile force, coronary blood flow and
norepinephrine (NE) overflow into the coronary sinus blood. Concomitant vagal
stimulation (15 Hz) significantly curtails these sympathetically-mediated changes
in contractile force, coronary blood flow and NE overflow. The effects of vagal
stimulation are abolished by atropine (1 mg/kg). (From reference 16; by permission
of the American Heart Association.)

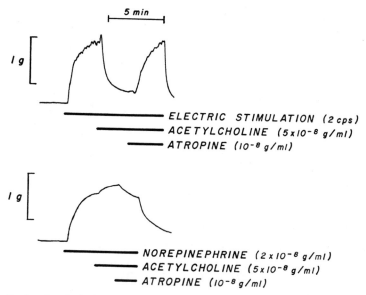

Fig. 8. During electrical stimulation (top) of an isolated saphenous vein of the dog, acetylcholine causes a marked relaxation, whereas during contraction caused by norepinephrine (bottom), it causes a further increase in tension. Since the response to electrical
stimulation is due to the release of endogenous norepinephrine, this paradoxical
effect of acetylcholine suggest that it inhibits adrenergic neurotransmission. Both
effects of acetylcholine are inhibited by atropine. (From reference 40; by permission
of the American Heart Association.)

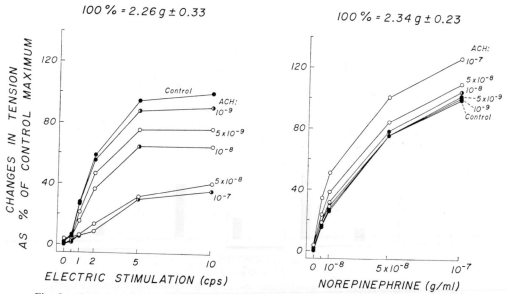

Fig. 9. Opposite effect of increasing doses of acetylcholine on the reactions of six dog saphenous vein strips to electrical stimulation at five different frequencies (left) and to
norepinephrine at four different concentrations (right) (means, n=6). (From
reference 40; by permission of the American Heart Association.)

the constrictor responses to periarterial nerve stimulation in the isolated rabbit ear artery; these observations were confirmed in the same preparation with a variety of muscarinic agonists by different authors[2,11,24,25,31]. Likewise, in the isolated rat mesenteric arteries, the cholinergic transmitter inhibits selectively the vasoconstriction caused by sympathetic nerve stimulation[20]. In the isolated saphenous vein of the dog concentrations of acetylcholine that do not affect basal tension cause a dose-dependent relaxation during sympathetic nerve stimulation. By contrast, similar doses of acetylcholine cause a further increase in tension when added to strips contracted by exogenous norepinephrine (Figs. 8 and 9). These findings suggested that, in the saphenous vein of the dog, acetylcholine has a dual action. At the prejunctional level it inhibits the release of norepinephrine from the adrenergic nerve endings, thus leading to relaxation of the venous wall during sympathetic nerve stimulation. At the smooth muscle level, on the other hand, the direct effect of acetylcholine is to cause contraction[40]. These initial observations prompted a series of experiments to confirm, analyze and assess the importance of the prejunctional effect of acetylcholine on adrenergic neurotransmission in the blood vessel wall.

Inhibitory effect on release of ³H-norepinephrine. To confirm the inhibitory effect of

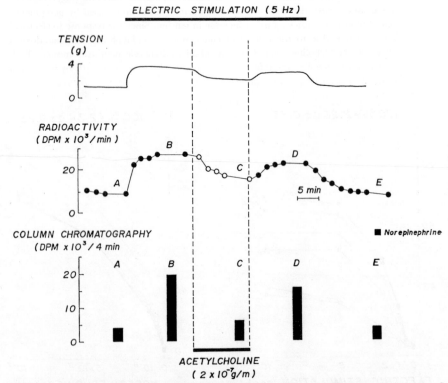

Fig. 10. Demonstration that acetylcholine decreases the contractile response (upper) of dog's saphenous vein strip to nerve stimulation by inhibiting the release of nor-epinephrine (lower). Experiment performed on a vein previously incubated with ³H-norepinephrine. The middle trace shows the total radioactivity of the superfusate (³H-norepinephrine plus its metabolites). (From reference 39; by permission.)

acetylcholine on the release of adrenergic transmitter during sympathetic nerve stimulation, saphenous veins of the dog were incubated with ^{3}H-norepinephrine and mounted for superfusion and isometric tension recording. The superfusate was analyzed to determine the amounts of labeled transmitter present[39]. Electrical stimulation augmented the overflow of ^{3}H-norepinephrine; acetylcholine caused a reversible depression of the evoked release of labeled transmitter (Fig. 10). This is direct evidence in support of the conclusion that during sympathetic nerve stimulation acetylcholine has a prejunctional inhibitory effect[35,36,39,40].

Ubiquity of the phenomenon. Studies performed on isolated strips of different arteries and veins of the dog confirm that the inhibitory effect of acetylcholine on adrenergic neurotransmission can be demonstrated in isolated blood vessels from a variety of vascular beds[32,34,44]. In those blood vessels where the cholinergic transmitter causes relaxation of the smooth muscle cells by its direct depressing effect, the prejunctional inhibitory action occurs at lower concentrations and is more potent. Thus, the response to sympathetic nerve stimulation is depressed to a greater extent than that to exogenous norepinephrine (Fig. 11[32,34]). As mentioned before, the same holds for blood vessels such as those in the rabbit ear and the rat mesentery[11,20,24,31]. Measurement of the effects of acetylcholine on the overflow of ^{3}H-norepinephrine in rabbit ear arteries and dog pulmonary arteries[1, 31, 34] confirms that in these vessels the dilator effect of acetylcholine rests for an important part upon the inhibition of the release of adrenergic neurotransmission by nerve impulses (Fig. 12). In the pulmonary and mesenteric veins of the dog, acetylcholine, even in small amounts, augments the contractile response to sympathetic nerve stimulation. This is because

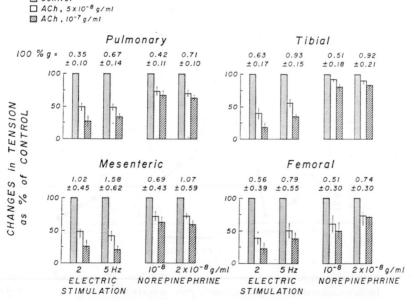

Fig. 11.   Demonstration in four different arteries of the dog that acetylcholine (ACh) depresses the response to nerve stimulation more than that to exogenous norepinephrine. (From reference 34; by permission of the American Heart Association.)

168 P. M. Vanhoutte and M. N. Levy

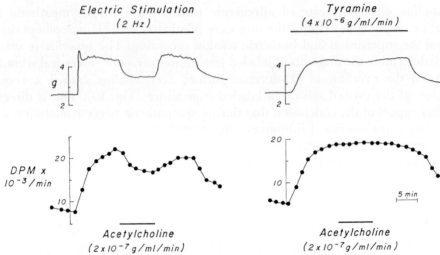

Fig. 12. Comparison of the effects of the same concentration of acetylcholine on tension and total ³H-efflux induced by electrical stimulation (left) or by tyramine (right) in the same pulmonary artery strip. During superfusion with tyramine, the ³H-efflux is unaltered by acetylcholine; the slight relaxation is due to the direct inhibitory effect of acetylcholine on the smooth muscle cells. During nerve stimulation, this direct effect is greatly reinforced by the inhibition of adrenergic neurotransmission. (From reference 34; by permission of the American Heart Association.)

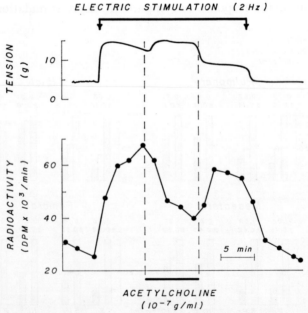

Fig. 13. Demonstration in the dog's mesenteric vein that although acetylcholine causes a further contraction during sympathetic nerve stimulation (upper) this must be due to the direct effect of the drug on the smooth muscle cells, since at the same time the amount of ³H-norepinephrine released is greatly reduced (lower). (From reference 34; by permission of the American Heart Association.)

in those vessels the vascular smooth muscle cells are exquisitely sensitive to the direct stimulatory effect of acetylcholine (see refs. 29, 36, 38), which then obscures the prejunctional inhibitory effect. Hence it is easy to show in mesenteric veins that during electrical stimulation acetylcholine depresses the evoked release of ^{3}H-norepinephrine at a time where the tension augments (Fig. 13[34]). From these different observations on isolated vessels it is tempting to conclude that acetylcholine can inhibit adrenergic neurotransmission throughout the vascular tree[35, 36].

Occurence in the intact organism. The prejunctional inhibitory effect of acetylcholine on adrenergic neurotransmission can easily be demonstrated in the intact animal. Thus, in the anesthetized dog, acetylcholine depresses the constrictor responses of the lateral saphenous vein (perfused at constant flow with autologous blood) to lumbar sympathetic chain stimulation, but not that to exogenous norepinephrine (Fig. 14[40]). In the blood-perfused hind leg of the same species, acetylcholine markedly reduces the vasoconstriction induced by sympathetic nerve stimulation, but affects that caused by the infusion of norepinephrine to a lesser extent. Vasodilators such as isoproterenol have the opposite effect (Fig. 15[33]). When combined with studies on isolated blood vessels, the experiments in the intact animal imply that the prejunctional effect of acetylcholine should be accounted for every time the drug is given to a vascular bed under sympathetic control[35, 36].

Physiological importance. In the heart, it is relatively easy to conclude that vagal inhibition of adrenergic neurotransmission is part of the normal regulatory mechanisms. Likewise, in the blood vessel wall the question of importance is whether the

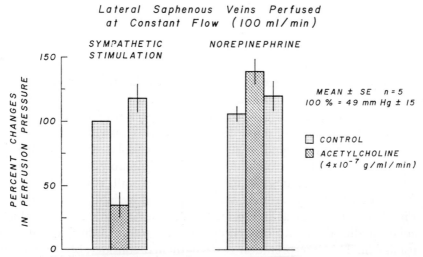

Fig. 14. Effect of acetylcholine on venoconstrictions of similar magnitude obtained either by lumbar sympathetic stimulation or by norepinephrine. Acetylcholine decreases the venoconstriction caused by sympathetic nerve stimulation (left) but augments that caused by norepinephrine infusions (right) in lateral saphenous vein perfused at constant flow (100 ml/min) in intact dogs. The stimulation frequency and the norepinephrine concentration were selected in each experiment to cause comparable venoconstrictions. (From reference 29; by permission.)

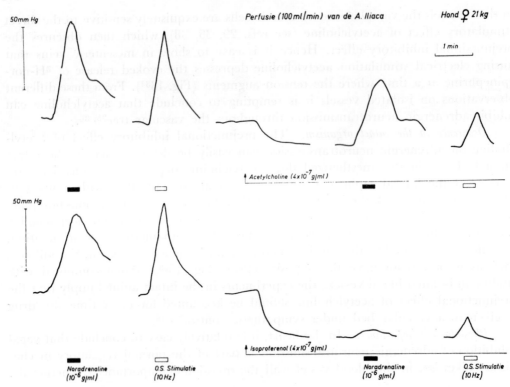

50mm Hg

Perfusie (100 ml/min) van de A. Iliaca

Hond ♀ 21 kg

1 min

↑ Acetylcholine (4x10⁻⁷ g/ml)

50mm Hg

↑ Isoproterenol (4x10⁻⁷ g/ml)

Noradrenaline (10⁻⁶ g/ml)   O.S. Stimulatie (10 Hz)   Noradrenaline (10⁻⁶ g/ml)   O.S. Stimulatie (10 Hz)

Fig. 15.   Demonstration, in a dog hind leg perfused at constant flow (100 ml/min) with autologous blood, that acetylcholine (upper), unlike isoproterenol (lower), depresses
the response to sympathetic nerve stimulation (O. S. stimulatie) more than that to
exogenous norepinephrine (noradrenaline). (From reference 33; by permission.)

prejunctional inhibitory effect of the cholinergic transmitter is only of pharmacological
interest, or plays a role in neurogenic cholinergic vasodilatation. Arteries, and in particular arterioles, of many vascular beds are innervated both by adrenergic and cholinergic fibers (see refs. 3, 4, 12, 28, 36, 38). In these vessels the cholinergic and adrenergic nerve terminals are in close apposition[8,13] and this provides the morphological
basis for neurogenic prejunctional regulation. In the isolated gastric artery of the
dog transmural electrical field stimulation, which presumably activates both adrenergic and cholinergic nerve endings in the blood vessel wall, causes contraction. This
contraction is augmented by atropine but is depressed by inhibitors of acetylcholinesterase (Fig. 16[32]). The logical interpretation for those observations is that during
field stimulation the liberated acetylcholine causes partial inhibition of adrenergic
neurotransmission. This interpretation is strengthened considerably by data obtained
in the intact animal. Indeed, in the blood-perfused stomach studied *in situ* in the dog,
vagal stimulation reduces the constrictor response to sympathetic nerve stimulation
significantly more than that to exogenous norepinephrine (Fig. 17[32]). Such a difference
is explained most logically if the acetylcholine released by the vagal nerve endings is
able to depress peripheral adrenergic neurotransmission in the gastric blood vessel
wall. These morphological, pharmacological and physiological findings thus support

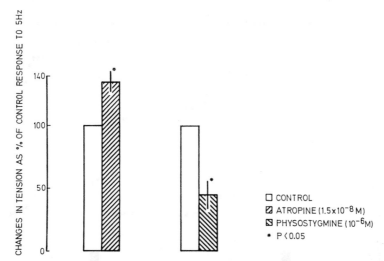

Fig. 16.   Since atropine (left) augments and physostigmine (right) depresses the response of canine gastric arteries to electrical field stimulation, the latter must activate both cholinergic and adrenergic nerve endings; the endogenously released acetylcholine causes partial inhibition of adrenergic neurotransmission. This inhibition is blocked by the muscarinic antagonist, and enhanced by the inhibitor of acetylcholinesterase. (From reference 32; by permission.)

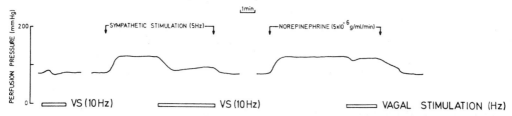

Fig. 17.   Demonstration that in the blood-perfused stomach of the intact dog, vagal stimulation (VS; 10 Hz) depresses the response to sympathetic (coeliac ganglion) stimulation much more than that to exogenous norepinephrine. (From reference 32; by permission.)

the hypothesis that cholinergic neurogenic vasodilatation can be due in part to a decreased release of norepinephrine in those vascular beds where the sympathetic nerve endings are activated.

Mechanism of Action

Acetylcholine still inhibits adrenergic neurotransmission in the presence of α-adrenolytic or β-adrenolytic agents, and does not require prostaglandin-mediated mechanisms to alter the function of the adrenergic nerve terminals[7,42]. Other muscarinic agonists also depress the evoked release of norepinephrine[2,24,25,31]. The inhibitory effects of acetylcholine and vagal stimulation on adrenergic neurotransmission are abolished by atropine, but not by nicotinic antagonists (Fig. 8; see refs. 11, 20, 24, 31, 32, 34, 40). Thus, both in the heart and in the peripheral blood vessels it appears that acetylcholine binds to muscarinic receptors on the adrenergic nerve

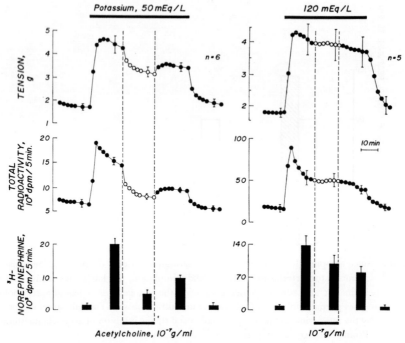

Fig. 18.   Acetylcholine causes relaxation (upper) of dog's saphenous vein superfused with 50 mEq/1K$^+$ (left) due to a decrease in the release of norepinephrine (middle and bottom); it does not do so during the exposure to 120 mEq/1K$^+$ (right). Note that with 120 mEq/1K$^+$ the release of ^{3}H-norepinephrine is much greater than with 50 mEq/l. (From reference 41; redrawn for reference 30; reprinted from *Federation Proceedings*, 37, 1978, 191–194.)

endings. The activation of these receptors causes inhibition of the release of adrenergic transmitter evoked by nerve impulses. Acetylcholine inhibits the release of ^{3}H-norepinephrine evoked by electrical stimulation or moderate increases in K$^+$-concentration, but does not inhibit its pharmacological displacement obtained with tyramine[34,39,40,41,44]. This suggests that acetylcholine interferes specifically with the exocytotic process[37]. Since the inhibitory effect is seen in various Ca^{++} concentrations, and is not blocked by tetrodotoxin[41,43] it cannot be explained in terms of specific interferences with Ca^{++} or Na$^+$ exchanges or with spike electrogenesis[22,36]. Because acetylcholine inhibits the release of ^{3}H-norepinephrine evoked by 50 mEq/1K$^+$ (which causes only partial depolarization of the adrenergic nerve endings), but not that seen with 120 mEq/l of the ion (Fig. 18[41]), the most likely explanation for the prejunctional inhibitory effect of the cholinergic transmitter is that it causes hyperpolarization of the adrenergic nerve terminals[9,41].

CONCLUSION

In the heart and in the blood vessel wall acetylcholine markedly and reversibly inhibits the release of norepinephrine evoked by sympathetic nerve activity. It does

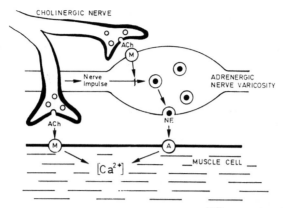

NE : norepinephrine
ACh : acetylcholine
A : adrenergic receptor
M : muscarinic receptor

Fig. 19.   Summary of the prejunctional effects of acetylcholine on adrenergic nerve terminals
in the heart and the blood vessel wall. Acetylcholine, whether liberated from cholinergic nerve endings or exogenously added, inhibits the release of norepinephrine,
presumably by causing hyperpolarization of the terminal. This inhibitory effect
combines with the direct action on the effector cells (cardiac or vascular smooth
muscle). ACh: acetylcholine; NE: norepinephrine; A: adrenergic receptor; M:
muscarinic receptor.

so by activation of muscarinic receptors, which presumably results in hyperpolarization
of the adrenergic nerve terminals and subsequent depression of the exocytotic process.
If acetylcholine is given to the heart or to a vascular bed when they are submitted to
an increased sympathetic activity, the prejunctional inhibitory effect of acetylcholine
greatly reinforces the direct depressant effect it has on cardiac and vascular effector
cells. Hence, the action of acetylcholine on the adrenergic nerve terminals explains
part of the depressor effect of the drug in the intact organism. Evidence has accumulated suggesting that the prejunctional effect of acetylcholine is important not only
when it is exogenously added, but also when it is endogenously liberated from cholinergic nerve terminals. It is likely that, both in the heart and in the blood vessel
wall, acetylcholine released in the vicinity of the adrenergic nerve endings switches
off the existing release of norepinephrine. Such a mechanism undoubtedly greatly
increases the efficacy of the inhibitory cholinergic messenger to counteract the excitatory effects of the adrenergic transmitter (Fig. 19).

REFERENCES

1   Allen, G. S., Glover, A. B., McCulloch, M. W., Rand, M. J. and Story, D. F., Modulation by acetylcholine of adrenergic transmission in the rabbit ear artery, *Brit. J.
Pharmacol.*, 54 (1975) 49.
2   Allen, G. S., Rand, M. J. and Story, D. F., Effect of the muscarinic agonist McN-A-343
on the release by sympathetic nerve stimulation of (^{3}H)—noradrenaline from rabbit
isolated ear arteries and guinea-pig atria, *Brit. J. Pharmacol.*, 51 (1974) 29–34.

3 Bell, C., Autonomic nervous control of reproduction: Circulatory and other factors, *Pharmacol. Rev.*, 24 (1972) 657–736.

4 Brody, M. J., Histaminergic and cholinergic vasodilator systems. In: P. M. Vanhoutte and I. Leusen (Eds.), *Mechanisms of Vasodilatation*, S. Karger, Basel, 1978, pp. 266–277.

5 Burnstock, G. and Costa, M., *Adrenergic Neurons*, Chapman and Hall, Ltd., London, 1975, 225 pp.

6 de la Lande, I. S., and Rand, M. J., A simple isolated nerve—blood vessel preparation, *Aust. J. exp. Biol. med. Sci.*, 43 (1965) 639–656.

7 Fuder, H. and Muscholl, E., The effect of methacholine on noradrenaline release from the rabbit heart perfused with indomethacin, *Naunyn-Schmiedeberg's Arch. Pharmacol.*, 285 (1974) 127–132.

8 Graham, J. D. P., Lever, J. D. and Spriggs, T. L. B., An examination of adrenergic axons around pancreatic arterioles of the cat for the presence of acetylcholinesterase by high resolution autoradiographic and histochemical methods, *Brit. J. Pharmacol.*, 33 (1968) 15.

9 Haeusler, G., Thoenen, H., Haefely, W. and Huerlimann, A., Electrical events in cardiac adrenergic nerves and noradrenaline release from the heart induced by acetylcholine and KCl, *Naunyn-Schmiedeberg's Arch. Pharmacol.*, 261 (1968) 389–411.

10 Hollenberg, M., Carriere, S. and Barger, A. C., Biphasic action of acetylcholine on ventricular myocardium, *Circulation Res.*, 16 (1965) 527–536.

11 Hume, W. R., de la Lande, I. S. and Waterson, J. G., Effect of acetylcholine on the response of the isolated rabbit ear artery to stimulation of the perivascular sympathetic nerves, *Eur. J. Pharmacol.*, 17 (1972) 227–233.

12 Iwayama, T., Furness, J. B. and Burnstock, G., Dual adrenergic and cholinergic innervation of the cerebral arteries of the rat, *Circulation Res.*, 26 (1970) 635–646.

13 Kadowitz, P. J., Knight, D. S., Hibbs, R. G., Ellison, J. P., Joiner, P. D., Brody, M. J. and Hyman, A. L., Influence of 5- and 6-hydroxydopamine on adrenergic transmission and nerve terminal morphology in the canine pulmonary vascular bed, *Circulation Res.*, 39 (1976) 191–199.

14 Levy, M. N., Sympathetic-parasympathetic interactions in the heart, *Circulation Res.*, 29 (1971) 437–445.

15 Levy, M. N., Neural control of the heart: Sympathetic-vagal interactions. In: J. Baan, A. Noordergraaf and J. Raines (Eds.), *Cardiovascular System Dynamics*, M. I. T. Press, Cambridge, 1978, pp. 365–370.

16 Levy, M. N. and Blattberg, B., Effect of vagal stimulation on the overflow of norepinephrine into the coronary sinus during cardiac sympathetic nerve stimulation in the dog, *Circulation Res.*, 38 (1976) 81–85.

17 Levy, M. N. and Zieske, H., Autonomic control of cardiac pacemaker activity and atrioventricular transmission, *J. appl. Physiol.*, 27 (1969) 465–470.

18 Löffelholz, K. and Muscholl, E., A muscarinic inhibition of the noradrenaline release evoked by postganglionic sympathetic nerve stimulation, *Naunyn-Schmiedeberg's Arch. Pharmacol.*, 265 (1969) 1–15.

19 Löffelholz K., and Muscholl, E., Inhibition by parasympathetic nerve stimulation of the release of the adrenergic transmitter, *Naunyn-Schmiedeberg's Arch. Pharmacol.*, 267 (1970) 181–184.

20 Malik, K. U. and Ling, G. M., Modification by acetylcholine of the response of rat mesenteric arteries to sympathetic stimulation, *Circulation Res.*, 25 (1969) 1–9.

21 Martin, P. J., Levy, M. N. and Zieske, H., Analysis and simulation of the left ventricular response to autonomic nervous activity, *Cardiovascular Res.*, 3 (1969) 396–410.

22 McGrath, M. A. and Vanhoutte, P. M., Vasodilation caused by peripheral inhibition

of adrenergic neurotransmission. In: P. M. Vanhoutte and I. Leusen (Eds.), *Mechanism of Vasodilatation*, S. Karger, Basel, 1978, pp. 248–257.

23 Muscholl, E., Muscarinic inhibition of the norepinephrine release from peripheral sympathetic fibres. In: *Pharmacology and the Future of Man, Proc. 5th Int. Congr. Pharmacol.*, San Francisco, S. Karger, Basel, Vol. 4, 1973, p. 440.

24 Rand, M. J. and Varma, B., The effects of cholinomimetic drugs on responses to sympathetic nerve stimulation and noradrenaline in the rabbit ear artery, *Brit. J. Pharmacol.*, 38 (1970) 758–770.

25 Rand, M. J. and Varma, B., Effects of the muscarinic aganist McN-A-343 on responses to sympathetic nerve stimulation in the rabbit ear artery. *Brit. J. Pharmacol.*, 43 (1971) 536–542.

26 Rosenblueth, A. and Simeone, F. A., The interrelations of vagal and accelerator effects on the cardiac rate, *Amer. J. Physiol.*, 110 (1934) 42–55.

27 Samaan, A., The antagonistic cardiac nerves and heart rate, *J. Physiol. (Lond.)*, 83 (1935) 332–340.

28 Schenk, E. A. and Elbadawi, A., Dual innervation of arteries and arterioles. A histochemical study, *Z. Zellforsch. Mikrosk. Anat.*, 91 (1968) 170–177.

29 Shepherd, J. T. and Vanhoutte, P. M., *Veins and their Control*, W. B. Saunders Co., London, 1975, 269 pp.

30 Shepherd, J. T., Lorenz, R. R., Tyce, G. M. and Vanhoutte, P. M., Acetylcholine-inhibition of transmitter release from adrenergic nerve terminals mediated by muscarinic receptors, *Fed. Proc.*, 37 (1978) 191–194.

31 Steinsland, O. S., Furchgott, R. F. and Kirpekar, S. M., Inhibition of adrenergic neurotransmission by parasympathomimetics in the rabbit ear artery, *J. Pharmacol. exp. Ther.*, 184 (1973) 346–356.

32 Van Hee, R. and Vanhoutte, P. M., Cholinergic inhibition of adrenergic neurotransmission in the canine gastric artery, *Gastroenterology*, 74 (1978) 1266–1270.

33 Vanhoutte, P. M., *Cholinergische Mechanismen in Vasculair glad Spierweefsel*, University of Antwerp, 1973, 181 pp.

34 Vanhoutte, P. M., Inhibition by acetylcholine of adrenergic neurotransmission in vascular smooth muscle, *Circulation Res.*, 34 (1974) 317–326.

35 Vanhoutte, P. M., Inhibition by acetylcholine of adrenergic neurotransmission in vascular smooth muscle. In: E. Bülbring and M. F. Schuba (Eds.), *Physiology of Smooth Muscle*, Raven Press, New York, 1976, pp. 369–377.

36 Vanhoutte, P. M., Cholinergic inhibition of adrenergic transmission, *Fed. Proc.*, 36 (1977) 2444–2449.

37 Vanhoutte, P. M., Adrenergic neuroeffector interaction in the blood vessel wall, *Fed. Proc.*, 37 (1978) 181–186.

38 Vanhoutte, P. M., Heterogeneity in vascular smooth muscle. In: G. Kaley and B. M. Altura (Eds.), *Microcirculation*, Vol. II, University Park Press, Baltimore, 1978, pp. 181–309.

39 Vanhoutte, P. M., Lorenz, R. R. and Tyce, G. M., Inhibition of norepinephrine-^{3}H release from sympathetic nerve endings in veins by acetylcholine, *J. Pharmacol. exp. Ther.*, 185 (1973) 386–394.

40 Vanhoutte, P. M. and Shepherd, J. T., Venous relaxation caused by acetylcholine acting on the sympathetic nerves, *Circulation Res.*, 32 (1973) 259–267.

41 Vanhoutte, P. M. and Verbeuren, T. J., Inhibition by acetylcholine of the norepinephrine release evoked by potassium in canine saphenous veins, *Circulation Res.*, 39 (1976) 263–269.

42   Vanhoutte, P. M. and Verbeuren, T. J., Inhibition by acetylcholine of ³H-Norepineph-
     rine release in cut aneous veins after alpha-adrenergic blockade, *Arch. int. Pharmacodyn.*,
     221 (1976) 344–346.
43   Vanhoutte, P. M., Verbeuren, T. J. and Collis, M. G., Muscarinic inhibition of ad-
     renergic neurotransmission is not due to a decrease of Ca⁺⁺ entry in the adrenergic nerve
     endings, *J. de Pharmacol.* (Paris), 8 (1977) 556–557.
44   Verbeuren, T. J. and Vanhoutte, P. M., Acetylcholine inhibits potassium evoked release
     of ³H-norepinephrine in different blood vessels of the dog, *Arch. int. Pharmacodyn.*, 221
     (1976) 347–350.
45   Westfall, T. C., Local regulation of adrenergic neurotransmission, *Physiol. Rev.*, 57 (1977)
     659–728.

CHAPTER 12

NEUROPHYSIOLOGY OF THE ENTERIC NERVOUS SYSTEM

J. D. Wood

Department of Physiology, University of Kansas Medical Center,
Kansas City, Kansas, USA

INTRODUCTION

The term "enteric nervous system" was introduced by J. N. Langley to describe the neural elements of the gastrointestinal tract[41]. Langley distinguished enteric ganglia from other autonomic ganglia on the basis of histological differences between the ganglion cells and on indications that enteric ganglia contained interneurons that did not receive direct synaptic input from parasympathetic preganglionic fibers. This concept of the unique nature of the enteric nervous system has been supported strongly by results of subsequent histoanatomical and neurophysiological investigations. These studies indicate that both the structural and neurophysiological characteristics of the enteric ganglia resemble more closely the neural tissue of the central nervous system than other autonomic ganglia[12,21,77,79].

The present review will support further the view that the enteric nervous system is an independent integrative network which programs and coordinates gastrointestinal functions. It will become apparent that the functional properties are analogous to those of the central nervous system and that the earlier concept of the enteric ganglia functioning only as simple relay-distribution centers for information transmitted in cranio-sacral efferent fibers is no longer tenable. The ganglia do indeed receive command signals transmitted from the central nervous system along parasympathetic and sympathetic pathways; however, this constitutes only one kind of input to a nervous system that also contains pattern-generating circuitry and integrative circuitry for processing sensory information derived from receptors along the gut.

The neurophysiology of the enteric nervous system is best known in the small intestine; therefore, the present discussion will concentrate on nervous control of motor function in the small bowel. The various aspects of the neuroeffector system will be considered in the following order: 1) properties of the effector system; 2) sensory reception; 3) final common pathways; 4) integrative circuitry; 5) extrinsic nervous input.

RESULTS AND DISCUSSION

Effector System

The effectors for intestinal motility are essentially the longitudinal and circular muscle layers of the bowel. The two muscle coats differ in both ultrastructural characteristics and in mechanisms of nervous control. The principal ultrastructural difference is scarcity of nexuses in the longitudinal muscle coat and abundance of nexuses in the circular muscle coat[23]. Transmission at the myoneural appositions in the longitudinal muscle is mediated by the excitatory action of acetylcholine and this layer does not appear to receive inhibitory innervation[14,25,57]. Acetylcholine is only weakly excitatory on the circular muscle layer[14,22] and the principal control is exerted by nonadrenergic-noncholinergic (purinergic) inhibitory neurons[8,77,79].

Mixing and propulsion of the luminal contents of the intestine are accomplished primarily by mechanical forces generated by the circular muscle layer. Any theory which attempts to explain the mechanism of neural control of this layer must take into account two well-established and fundamental physiological properties of the circular muscle. Firstly, the muscle behaves as an electrical syncytium (i.e., a three-dimensional core conductor). Regions of fusion (nexuses) between plasma membranes of contiguous muscle fibers function as intercellular pathways of low electrical resistance which provide for propagation of excitation between adjacent cells[1,6,46,67]. In the presence of tetrodotoxin and in the absence of all neuronal influence, the electrical connections between muscle cells account for the three-dimensional spread of excitation throughout the intestinal segment, which occurs when a localized stimulus is applied to any point on the tissue[71]. Secondly, organized excitation of the network of electrically-coupled muscle cells is initiated by myogenic pacemaker mechanisms (electrical slow waves) which are omnipresent and appear to be generated in the longitudinal muscle layer[2,59]. These inherent properties of the muscle preclude a mechanism of neural control that utilizes only direct neuronal excitation of the muscle. The basis for control of the circular muscle layer appears to be neuronal inhibition of the inherently excitable myogenic system. An inhibitory control mechanism answers the fundamental questions of why each and every cycle of the electrical slow wave does not trigger action potentials and associated contraction in the circular muscle coat (only one-third of the slow waves trigger spikes in the circular muscle of the dog in vivo[59]) and why excitation usually does not spread over great extents of the conductile syncytium when spikes are triggered in local regions, as is the case when segmentation patterns of motility predominate in the intestine.

Final Common Pathways

Motor neurons of the central nervous system receive input from afferents arising in different parts of the body and from many different interneurons. Discharge of motor neurons represents the final decision of the integrative circuitry and the final pathway from the nervous system. The same concept can be applied to the enteric nervous system from which there are two well-established final common pathways; namely, a cholinergic excitatory pathway to longitudinal muscle and a purinergic inhibitory pathway to the circular muscle.

The endings of the cholinergic neurons are at the surfaces of the enteric ganglia and the interganglionic fiber tracts[21,57]; and after release, acetylcholine traverses relatively long diffusion pathways to the longitudinal muscle. Cholinergic junction potentials can also be recorded in some of the circular muscle cells[30], but these are rare and species dependent[14]. This cholinergic component of the circular muscle may be associated with tonic contractile activity as opposed to phasic contraction of segmentation and peristaltic movements[69].

The presence of the intrinsic nonadrenergic inhibitory ganglion cells in the intestine has now been confirmed by several different laboratories[8,55,71,73]. These cells appear to be ubiquitous at all levels of the gut in all vertebrate species[9] and they are no doubt of important functional significance in control of the motor activity of the musculature. The evidence presented below suggests that the intrinsic inhibitory neurons are continuously active in nonsphincteric regions of the bowel and that their general function in the intestine is continuous suppression of the autogenous activity of the circular muscle.

The first line of evidence for continuous neuronal inhibition of the muscle is that some of the ganglion cells of Auerbach's plexus of dog, cat, guinea-pig and rabbit small intestine show continuous-patterned discharge of action potentials[53,54,70,76]. One function of this neuronal activity appears to be continuous inhibition of the spontaneous myogenic activity of the circular musculature because in segments of intestine *in vitro*, in which neuronal discharge in the myenteric plexus is prevalent, muscle action potentials and associated contractile activity are absent. Myogenic pacemaker potentials (electrical slow waves) are always present and when the neuronal discharge is blocked experimentally with tetrodotoxin, every cycle of the electrical slow waves triggers intense discharge of muscle action potentials and large-amplitude contractions[4,5,55,68,70,71,72,73].

Many different situations, such as application of local anesthetic drugs, long periods of cold storage and congenital absence of enteric ganglion cells, all of which involve functional ablation of enteric neurons, are associated with conversion from a hypoirritable condition of the circular muscle to a hyperirritable state[71,74]. When ongoing activity of the enteric neurons can be demonstrated, neither mechanical stimulation[71] nor electrical stimulation[37,69] effectively elicit contractile responses of the circular muscle. Following neuronal blockade, both electrical and mechanical stimulation readily trigger muscle action potentials and waves of contractile activity which may be propagated for distances of several centimeters in either direction along the longitudinal axis of an isolated segment of intestine[69,71]. These observations together suggest that blockade of the enteric ganglion cells releases the circular muscle from an inhibitory influence and this permits excitation and conduction that are mediated by myogenic mechanisms.

The evidence suggests that tonically active inhibitory neurons continuously suppress myogenic activation of the circular muscle. If this is the case, then it is implicit that the various patterns of intestinal motor activity are dependent upon integrated disinhibition of the muscle. In normal motor function, it is probable that integration of the activity of the intrinsic neurogenic inhibitory system determines: 1) whether a particular cycle of the electrical slow waves triggers a response in the circular muscle; 2) the number of muscle fibers activated in parallel and consequently the force of the contractile response triggered by a particular slow wave; 3) the distance over which excitation spreads within the electrical syncytium; 4) the direction of spread of excitation within the syncytium[77,79].

Sensory Receptors

The term "peristaltic reflex" suggests the existence of classical reflex arcs within the enteric nervous system. Representations of such connections have been searched for in the intestine, but have never been identified morphologically. Apparent reflex pathways have been demonstrated many times by pharmacological experiments on the isolated intestine[38], and a clear demonstration was recently made with electrophysiological recording from enteric neurons[25,30]. A corollary to "peristaltic reflex" is "sensory receptor" and both chemo- and mechano-receptors have been demonstrated in the gastrointestinal tract. Discharge patterns characteristic of both fast-

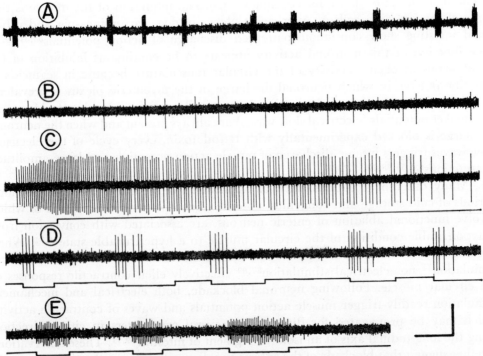

Fig. 1.   Examples of the types of enteric neurons that are detected by extra-cellular recording electrodes. A: Erratic burst-type unit. B: Single spike unit. C: Tonic-type mechano-sensitive neuron. This unit was activated to discharge by transient mechanical deformation of the ganglionic surface (downward deflection of bottom trace) and continued to discharge for prolonged time after removal of stimulus. Compare with Fig. 2C. D: Fast-adapting mechanoreceptor. This unit discharged only at the onset of mechanical distortion of the ganglion indicated by downward deflection of bottom trace. E: Slowly-adapting mechanoreceptor. This unit discharged throughout mechanical stimulation. Vertical calibration: 75 μV. Horizontal calibration: A, 1.6 sec; B–E, 3.3 sec.

and slowly-adapting mechanoreceptors have been recorded in gastrointestinal afferent fibers within the vagal [15,33,45,56] and splanchnic nerves[60,65].

Direct electrical recording from single units within Auerbach's plexus reveals three different kinds of neurons which respond with an increase in rate of discharge to mechanical distortion of the ganglion[43,70]. One kind of mechano-sensitive unit behaves like a typical slowly-adapting mechanoreceptor (Fig. 1E) and another like a fast-adapting mechanoreceptor (Fig. 1D). The third kind of mechanosensitive cell is activated by mechanical stimulation to discharge long trains of spikes of 30 to 40 sec duration (Fig. 1C). The latter have been termed "tonic-type enteric neurons" and are believed to be interneurons that are activated by input derived from mechano-receptors[43,75,79]. The generator region of the mechanoreceptors in Auerbach's plexus appears to be located within the periganglionic connective tissue[43,54]. The mechano-receptors in Auerbach's plexus are neither excited nor desensitized by serotonin[78]; however, serotonin mimics the action of electrical stimulation of presynaptic fibers to the tonic-type mechanosensitive neurons and high concentrations of serotonin (1 μm) desensitizes the cells to the endogenous transmitter substance[44,86].

Iggo discovered vagal afferents that connected with acid and alkaline receptors in the mucosa of the stomach[32] and indirect evidence suggests the presence of osmo-receptors, tryptophan receptors and glucose receptors within the small intestine[13].

The enteric sensory receptors no doubt provide both the enteric nervous system and the central nervous system with a steady flow of information on conditions within the lumen and the wall of the bowel.

Integrative Circuitry

Peristaltic propulsion of an intraluminal bolus occurs within isolated segments of intestine without extrinsic innervation *in vitro*[7,20]. Contractile activity persists, but peristaltic propulsion does not occur after blockade of nervous function with tetrodo-toxin *in vitro*[20]. This indicates that the contractile activity of the intestinal musculature during peristalsis is dependent upon intact integrative circuitry within the enteric nervous system and occurs independent of input from the central nervous system. During peristalsis, it can be assumed that intramural sensory receptors furnish the integrative circuitry with information on parameters such as bolus size, rate and direction of bolus movement. The integrative circuitry processes the sensory informa-tion and generates organized excitatory and inhibitory outflow to the musculature in much the same manner as internuncial circuitry within the spinal cord organizes motor outflow during reflex responses. Knowledge of the neural circuits and inte-grative functions within the enteric nervous system is fundamental to understanding gastrointestinal function; however, neurophysiological studies on this system are still in their infancy and the following discussion can provide only preliminary insight into how the system functions.

The gastrointestinal tract is characterized by rhythmic, stereotyped motor movements. This is mentioned here to point out the similarities to neural generation of rhythmic motor behavior in other systems; especially in the invertebrate phyla where one or a few ganglia generate nervous outflow which drives rhythmic, stereo-typed motor patterns of behavior[3,35]. Three properties are common to these "simple" motor systems. Firstly, the motor outflow patterns consist of rhythmically-timed bursts of spikes that arise either from specific connectivity within an ensemble of neurons and cannot be traced to any individual neuron or that are derived from endogenous activity of a single neuron. Secondly, the preprogrammed sequence of rhythmic motor behavior is elicited by activation of single "command neurons". Thirdly, the motor behavior may be initiated and modulated by sensory input, but the stereotyped sequence of motor events continues in the absence of sensory input. The notion of a motor program, as apposed to a reflex arc, offers an heuristic concept for the rhythmic motor activity of the intestine. Motor activity in the intestine occurs in two distinct patterns, with the particular pattern dictated by the intraluminal digestive state. The predominant postprandial motor pattern is rhythmic segmentation[10], and the interdigestive pattern is represented by the so-called migrating myoelectric complex[64]. Each of these two motor patterns can be thought of as representing the outflow from a "prewired" motor program within the neural circuitry of the enteric nervous system. Sensory input, circulating hormones and commands from the central nervous system represent mechanisms by which one or the other of the motility programs may be selected.

Auerbach's plexus (myenteric plexus) and Meissner's plexus (submucous plexus) comprise the integrative circuitry of the enteric system. The electrical activity of ganglion cells within the two plexuses is qualitatively similar[54]. The two plexuses are interconnected by neural fibers[63]; and although the two are separated spatially, they probably function together as a unit.

Both spontaneous and stimulus-evoked patterns of spike discharge can be recorded extracellularly and intracellularly from single neuronal units within myenteric and submucous ganglia[83]. Figure 1 illustrates the units that have been classified into the following categories on the basis of characteristic patterns of spike discharge[79]:

  A. Mechanosensitive neurons   1. Mechanoreceptors   a. Slowly-adapting
                                                           b. Fast-adapting

                                  2. Tonic-type enteric neurons

  B. Single-spike neurons
  C. Burst-type neurons   1. Steady bursters
                                  2. Erratic bursters

Tonic-type enteric neurons. These ganglion cells (Fig. 1C) appear to be interneurons that are activated by synaptic input derived either directly or indirectly from mechanoreceptors[43,75,79]. Figure 2 shows that stimulation of the synaptic input to these cells in the guinea-pig myenteric plexus produces a slow EPSP that is associated with a decreased ionic conductance of the somal membrane and prolonged spike discharge lasting for 10 to 40 sec[83,84]. Microiontophoresis of serotonin (5-HT) onto these neurons mimics the slow EPSP and several kinds of evidence suggest that 5-HT is the chemical transmitter[44,86]. These neurons are multipolar as indicated by focal mapping with a stimulating electrode, and the somal membranes behave differently from the membranes of the cell's processes. In the absence of the excitatory transmitter substance (5-HT), the somal membranes either cannot be activated to spike discharge by intrasomatic depolarizing current injection or the spike threshold is high and the cells do not discharge repetitively to depolarizing current. Higher excitability of the

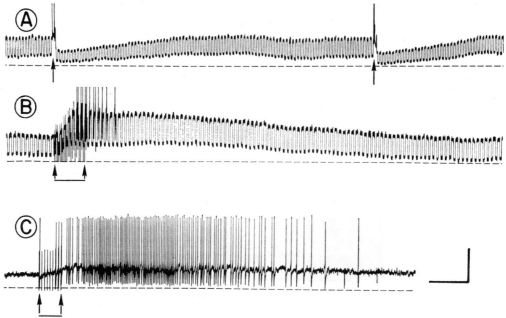

Fig. 2. Slow EPSP in myenteric neuron of guinea-pig small intestine. A: Action potentials followed by prolonged hyperpolarizing after-potentials associated with decreased input resistance during low excitability state of the cell. Action potentials (arrows) were elicited by a depolarizing current pulse applied during repetitive intrasomatic injection of rectangular hyperpolarizing current pulses. B: Repetitive stimulation of interganglionic fiber tract (arrows) elicited depolarization and increase in input resistance that outlasted the period of stimulation by several seconds. Membrane was hyperpolarized 10 mV beyond resting potential by steady current injection to reduce spike discharge. Some spikes still occurred at the offset of the hyperpolarizing pulses during and immediately after fiber tract stimulation. C: Slow EPSP and tonic spike discharge elicited by fiber tract stimulation (arrows). Vertical calibration: A and B, 20 mV; C, 40 mV. Horizontal calibration: A and B, 1.1 sec; C, 3.3 sec.

processes relative to the soma can be demonstrated by electrotonic spread of anti-dromic spikes into the soma during electrical stimulation of the cell's processes[85,87]. The action potentials in the processes of the tonic-type neurons are blocked by tetro-dotoxin[85]; whereas the somal spikes are tetrodotoxin-resistant, calcium-dependent spikes[24,50,85]. In the absence of 5-HT, action potentials in the soma are followed by prolonged hyperpolarizing after-potentials of 10 to 20 sec duration[27,47,85]. The slow after-hyperpolarization (Fig. 2A) appears to reflect an increased potassium con-ductance triggered by influx of calcium[47].

The characteristics of the somal membranes of the tonic-type enteric neurons when they are in the low excitability state can be summarized as follows: 1) action potentials followed by prolonged hyperpolarizing after-potentials; 2) relatively low input resistance; 3) no spontaneous discharge; 4) either no spikes in response to injection of a depolarizing current pulse or one to three spikes only at the onset of a depolarizing current pulse[82,84,87]. Both microiontophoretic application of 5-HT and electrical stimulation of interganglionic fiber tracts convert the somal membranes to a state of augmented excitability (slow EPSP). The characteristics of the augmented excitability state are: 1) increased input resistance; 2) membrane depolarized by 10 to 20 millivolts relative to resting potential; 3) disappearance of hyperpolarizing after-potentials; 4) spontaneous spike discharge; 5) spike discharge throughout a depolarizing current pulse with spike frequency a direct function of current intensity[44,86,87]. Earlier workers referred to this population of myenteric ganglion cells as either AH-cells[25,27] or Type II cells[47] and suggested that they were sensory neurons because no synaptic input could be demonstrated. This postulation is no longer tenable.

Intracellular recording from the soma shows that extracellular electrical stimulation of the ganglion cell's processes elicits spikes which electrotonically invade the

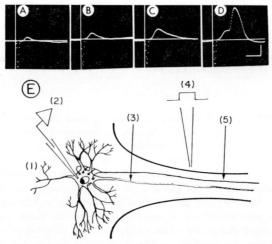

Fig. 3.   Functional significance of the slow EPSP in myenteric neurons. A through D: Intracellular recordings of progressive changes in electrotonic potentials within the soma during repetitive stimulation of the fiber tract. Stimuli were applied to the fiber tract at a frequency of 1 Hz and A through D represent the first, fifth, eighth and tenth respective stimuli. Note that the amplitude of the electrotonic potentials increased and the rate of decay decreased as the slow EPSP developed with consecutive stimulus pulses. In D, spike threshold was reached and the some fired a spike. E: Diagram of the experiment. An electrode (2) recorded electrical changes in the cell soma (1). Fiber tract stimulation (4) activated both the cell's axon (3) and presynaptic fibers to the cell (5). The somal membrane had high resting conductance and antidromic spikes from the axon (3) produced only small electrotonic potentials in the soma (A). During repetitive stimulation of the presynaptic fiber (5) the slow EPSP and associated increase in input resistance and time constant of the somal membrane were reflected by increased amplitude and decreased rate of decay of the electrotonic potentials. These observations suggest that the soma may function as a rate which permits transmission of information from its dendrites (1) to axons (3) only during the slow EPSP which can be elicited by input from an adjacent ganglion. The axon of the tonic-type neuron projects to the adjacent ganglion, thus establishing bidirectional flow of information between the two ganglia. The electrical records were plotted from computer memory. The initial downward deflection is the stimulus artifact. Vertical calibration: 20 mV. Horizontal calibration: 2 msec.

soma (Fig. 3). Spontaneously-occurring spikes in the processes also are observed to spread electrotonically into the soma[84]. The probability that the passive current flow from these axonal or dendritic spikes will trigger a somal action potential is greatly increased during the augmented excitability of the slow EPSP[87]. The myenteric ganglia contain a dense synaptic neuropil[13,21] in which neural integrative function takes place, and one aspect of the functional significance of the slow EPSP is that it provides a mechanism by which the soma of the multipolar neuron can gate or switch the transmission of information between the dendritic processes and axon at opposite poles of the soma (refer to Fig. 3). Spike activity from the neuropil is restricted to the dendritic tree in the absence of the slow EPSP; whereas during the slow EPSP, the soma relays dendritic spikes to the axon at the opposite pole of the soma.

A second aspect of the functional significance of the tonic-type neurons is that neural models of peristalsis require sustained discharge by a particular type of enteric neuron in order to account for the observed delays of several seconds between stimulus and coordinated responses, and to account for sustained neural influence at the effector[29]. The behavior of the tonic-type neurons fits the requirements for a neuronal unit whose functional significance would be production of either prolonged excitation or inhibition at neuronal and neuro-effector junctions within the gut wall[79].

Single-spike units. These neurons continuously discharge single action potentials at relatively low frequencies and with no consistent pattern to the activity on extra-cellular records (Fig. 1B). The large variation in interspike intervals of single-spike neurons produces broad, platykurtic interspike-interval histograms with relatively large values for the coefficient of variation[75,78]. The rate of discharge of single-spike units is increased by acetylcholine and other nicotinic agonists in the myenteric plexus of both the cat[70] and guinea-pig[18,61] and the discharge rate of some of these cells is reduced by norepinephrine acting at α-receptors[61]. The feline single-spike units do not require synaptic input for spontaneous discharge, because they continue to generate spikes in the presence of elevated concentrations of magnesium[80]. However, the discharge pattern appears to be influenced by synaptic input because spike-interval statistics are altered in the presence of elevated magnesium[80]. The cholinergic receptors on single-spike neurons are activated by nicotine in the presence of elevated magnesium[80]. Morphine depresses the ongoing discharge of some single-spike units in guinea-pig small bowel, and the firing rate of some of these units is increased by serotonin[16,52] and caerulein[66]. The excitatory effects of 5-HT, caerulein and nicotine are prevented by pretreatment with morphine both in preparations in normal physio-logical solutions[16,66] and in preparations with synaptic transmission depressed by elevated magnesium and lowered calcium in the bathing solution[17,52]. Intracellular recording suggests that the mechanism of action of morphine is hyperpolarization of the somal membranes[51]. Morphine does not produce a depressive effect burst-type on myenteric neurons of the cat[19].

Intracellular recordings from single-spike neurons in guinea-pig myenteric plexus also show continuous discharge of spikes[83,84]. There is large variation in duration of interspike interval and this produces broad, platykurtic interspike-interval histo-grams that closely resemble interspike-interval histograms for extracellularly-recorded activity. Spontaneous single spikes that are detected by intracellular electrodes sometimes are superimposed upon a fluctuating baseline that appears to reflect continuous synaptic bombardment of the cell membrane[84].

Tonic-type neurons sometimes show periods of spontaneous discharge of single spikes. This probably reflects a tonic release of the putative transmitter (5-HT) because continuous electrical stimulation of the interganglionic fiber tracts at low frequency (0.5 to 1 Hz) elicits maintained discharge of single spikes in these cells[84] and application of methysergide or norepinephrine prevents this. The single-spike activity probably does not represent a homogeneous population of enteric neurons.

Burst-type neurons. Burst-type units in extracellular studies refer to neurons which periodically discharge bursts of spikes with silent interburst intervals (Fig. 1A). This discharge occurs in the absence of any overt stimulation and it continues steadily for several hours in segments of intestine *in vitro*. Burst-type units are distinguished as either steady bursters or erratic bursters on the basis of regularity of interburst intervals[79].

Steady bursters discharge with relatively low variance of interburst interval[78]. Frequency-distribution histograms of interburst intervals for these cells are sometimes multimodal, and the additional peaks on the histograms are distinct multiples of the time interval represented by the first peak[76,80]. This implies that the timing of the bursts is determined by an endogenous oscillatory pacemaker mechanism and that generation of spikes fails during some cycles of the continuously-running oscillator[77].

Contrary to the steady bursters, the discharge patterns of erratic bursters are dominated by irregular interburst intervals and by periodic conversion to continuous discharge of either single spikes or doublets of spikes. Variations in the duration of interburst intervals of some erratic bursters are repeated systematically in cyclical patterns. In these cases, each cycle of activity consists of the following sequential changes in spike discharge: 1) a silent period of relatively long duration; 2) a series of bursts at regular intervals; 3) progressive decrease in intervals separating successive bursts; 4) continuous discharge of spikes[75].

Many different pharmacological agents have been tested on burst-type neurons[55,61,70]. In general, only agents that are active at cholinergic synapses seem to alter the ongoing discharge of these units. Acetylcholine stimulates some, but not all, of the tested burst units[55,70], and both muscarinic and nicotinic receptor-blocking drugs stop the discharge of some, but not all, of the burst units[55,70].

Unlike the erratic bursters, the firing patterns of the steady bursters are unaltered by a number of pharmacological compounds, including acetylcholine, that are either putative neurotransmitter substances or antagonists of transmission at specific chemical synapses in the central and autonomic nervous systems[70]. The steady-burster neurons continue to discharge in the presence of elevated magnesium; whereas, the erratic bursters are reversibly blocked by elevated magnesium[80]. This is consistent with the view that the steady-burster neurons may be endogenous oscillators that do not receive synaptic input from other neurons and that the second population of erratic-burst-type neurons, which are activated by acetylcholine and blocked by cholinergic antagonists, may be driven by input from the endogenous oscillators.

Neither serotonin nor the serotonin antagonist, methysergide, alters the discharge of the burst-type units[55,70] (and unpublished observations).

Intracellular studies have not detected a counterpart of the steady-burster neurons. This may be because ganglion cells of the myenteric plexus are highly variable in size and shape[12,21], and it is unlikely that all neurons, especially the smaller ones, are sampled in intracellular studies.

A counterpart of the erratic burster has been detected in intracellular studies[83,84]. Ongoing patterns of spike activity characteristic of the erratic bursters occur in the processes distal to the cell soma and these spikes electrotonically invade the soma where they are recorded by the intracellular microelectrode[83,84].

The functional significance of the continuous discharge of the burst-type units might be tonic release of inhibitory transmitter substance and production of ongoing inhibition at the circular muscle layer[79]. It has been proposed that the steady bursters are endogenous oscillators which drive nonspontaneously-active inhibitory neurons (erratic bursters) to release their transmitter at the circular muscle[77,79]. In this model, disinhibition of the circular muscle occurs either when the excitatory drive on the purinergic inhibitory neurons is removed by presynaptic inhibition of acetylcholine release from the steady-burst type neurons or by presynaptic inhibition of release of the inhibitory transmitter substance from the erratic burster[71,73,77,79].

Interneuronal interactions. Multi-unit extracellular records from both cat and guinea-pig often contain indications of inhibitory and excitatory interactions between two myenteric neurons[81]. One kind of excitatory interaction is sequential temporal coupling (driver-follower interaction) between the discharge of pairs of different burst-type neurons[54,70]. A second excitatory interaction is synchronous discharge of two different burst-type units in which the two cells appear to share a common presynaptic fiber[77,78]. Excitatory interaction between slowly-adapting mechano-receptors and tonic-type neurons was mentioned in an earlier section. Inhibitory interactions are observed as inhibition of burst-type discharge by activity of a second neuron[54,78]. The discharge of the inhibitory units in these cases is not tightly coupled to a particular phase of the burst and may occur at various times during a burst. The inhibitory discharge sometimes precedes the burst discharge, in which case the frequency of spikes in the burst is reduced.

Intracellular recording from guinea-pig enteric neurons has provided a synaptic basis for the inhibitory interactions observed on extracellular recordings. These synaptic events consist of both stimulus-evoked and spontaneous inhibitory post-synaptic potentials (IPSPs) in myenteric neurons[83,84] and stimulus-evoked IPSPs in ganglion cells of Meissner's plexus[28]. The stimulus-evoked IPSPs in both plexuses have exceptionally long latencies (>200 msec). Reversal potential for the IPSPs is 20 to 40 mV more negative than the resting potential, and the IPSPs appear to be mediated by an increased potassium conductance. In both plexuses, cholinergic EPSPs can be recorded in the same neurons that show IPSPs. Microiontophoresis of dopamine and norepinephrine mimics the IPSP in submucous neurons[28].

Extrinsic Input

Vagal input. The vagi at the level of the diaphragm contain an average of 56,138 afferent fibers and only 1,736 efferent fibers[31]. The enteric nervous system in the small intestine contains a minimum of 2×10^7 ganglion cells[62]. This great disparity in numbers between preganglionic fibers and enteric ganglion cells brings to question the functional relationship between vagal input and gastrointestinal motor function. The early theory was the concept of divergence and "mother cells"[42]; however, it is difficult to conceptualize how a divergence ratio of $1:1 \times 10^4$ could accomplish the coordinated control that is observed along the bowel. A later and more tenable view was that enteric reflex arcs functioned independent of preganglionic para-sympathetic fibers[40]. I would propose further that the enteric nervous system contains subsets of neurons that are preprogrammed for control of the basic rhythmic motility patterns and that these preexisting programs receive command inputs that are trans-mitted from the central nervous system along vagal fibers. This provides an expla-nation for the potent influence of a very small number of vagal efferent fibers on motility; and is analogous to other well-studied neural control systems in which activa-tion of single "command neurons" releases extensive coordinated motor responses[3,35].

Sympathetic input.   Sympathetic pathways carry command signals from the central nervous system which function to shut down gastrointestinal blood flow and motility. This is a well known component of the blanket-like response of the sympathetic nervous system to stressful environmental circumstances[11]. It is now clear that part of the mechanism of sympathetic shutdown of the bowel is mediated by input that acts on presynaptic terminals to prevent release of excitatory transmitter substances within the enteric nervous system.

Neurohistochemical observations[34,48,49] suggest that a vast majority of the post-ganglionic sympathetic fibers to the gut synapse directly with enteric ganglion cells. Stimulation of sympathetic nerves inhibits vagal transmission to the cat small intes-tine[36], and catecholamines are known to be inhibitors of the release of acetylcholine from cholinergic enteric neurons[39,58]. Intracellular recording shows that norepinephrine blocks the fast cholinergic synaptic potentials induced by electrical stimulation in Auerbach's plexus of guinea-pig small bowel, but does not block potential changes produced by exogenous acetylcholine[26,47]. This is a strong indication that norepineph-rine acts presynaptically to prevent acetylcholine release. Likewise, norepinephrine blocks the slow EPSP and augmented excitability in tonic-type enteric neurons of guinea-pig small bowel and this action is blocked by the α-adrenergic blocker, phen-tolamine[44,88]. Three kinds of evidence indicate that the blocking action of norepine-phrine on the slow EPSP is inhibition of release of 5-HT from serotonergic nerve terminals. Firstly, norepinephrine does not affect the depolarizing potential and augmented excitability produced by microiontophoretic application of 5-HT. Second-ly, norepinephrine does not block the excitatory effects of adding 5-HT to the per-fusion solution and addition of 5-HT to a perfusion solution containing norepineph-rine reverses suppression of excitability produced by norepinephrine. Thirdly, addition of norepinephrine at the onset of the EPSP and the augmented excitability do not alter the time course of the response[88].

CONCLUSIONS

The experimental findings reviewed in this paper suggest that the ganglia of the enteric division of the autonomic nervous system are simple integrative systems ("scattered little brains along the alimentary canal", according to the terminology of Dr. C. McC. Brooks) analogous to ganglia of the nervous systems of invertebrate animals in terms of functional properties, ease of study and relative simplicity. Thus, continued investigation of the neurophysiology of this system offers returns for two disciplines. For the neurophysiologist, the system provides a useful model for analysis of information processing and pattern generation by small ensembles of mammalian neurons. For the gastroenterologist, neurophysiological study of the mechanisms by which the enteric nervous system integrates and programs the various patterns of gastrointestinal motility and other gut functions offers a better understanding of normal and pathologic gastrointestinal function.

Some of the work described here was supported by National Science Foundation Grant GB-31292, National Institutes of Health Grant AM 16813, National Institutes of Health Career Development Award AM 70726 and the Alexander von Humboldt Foundation.

REFERENCES

1 Barr, L., Berger, W. and Dewey, M. M., Electrical transmission at the nexus between smooth muscle cells, *J. gen. Physiol.*, 51 (1968) 347–368.

2 Bass, P., *In vivo* electrical activity of the small bowel. In: C. F. Code (Ed.), *Handbook of Physiology, Section 6, Alimentary Canal, Vol. IV*, American Physiological Society, Washington, D. C., 1968, pp. 2051–2074.

3 Bentley, D., Control of cricket song patterns by descending interneurons, *J. comp. Physiol.*, 116 (1977) 19–38.

4 Biber, B. and Fara, J., Intestinal motility increased by tetrodotoxin lidocaine and procaine, *Experientia*, 29 (1973) 551–552.

5 Bortoff, A. and Miller, R., Stimulation of intestinal muscle by atropine, procaine and tetrodotoxin, *Amer. J. Physiol.*, 229 (1975) 1609–1613.

6 Bozler, E., Conduction, automaticity and tonus of visceral muscle, *Experientia*, 4 (1948) 312–318.

7 Brann, L. and Wood, J. D., Motility of the large intestine of piebald lethal mice, *Amer. J. digest. Dis.*, 21 (1976) 633–640.

8 Burnstock, G., Purinergic neurons, *Pharmacol. Rev.*, 34 (1972) 509–581.

9 Campbell, G. and Burnstock, G., Comparative physiology of gastrointestinal motility. In: C. F. Code (Ed.), *Handbook of Physiology, Section 6, Alimentary Canal, Vol. IV*, American Physiological Society, Washington, D. C., 1968, pp. 2213–2266.

10 Cannon, W. B., Peristalsis, segmentation and the myenteric reflex, *Amer. J. Physiol.*, 30 (1912) 114–128.

11 Cannon, W. B., *Bodily Changes in Pain, Hunger, Fear, and Rage*, D. Appleton Co., Ed. 2, 1929.

12 Cook, R. D. and Burnstock, G., The ultrastructure of Auerbach's plexus in the guinea-pig. I. Neuronal elements, *J. Neurocytol.*, 5 (1976) 171–194.

13 Cooke, A. R., Localization of receptors inhibiting gastric emptying in the gut, *Gastroenterol.*, 72 (1977) 875–880.

14 Daniel, E. E., Taylor, G. S., Daniel, V. P. and Holman, M. E., Can nonadrenergic inhibitory varicosities be identified structurally? *Can. J. Physiol. Pharmacol.*, 55 (1977) 243–250.

15 Davison, J. S., Response of single vagal afferent fibers to mechanical and chemical

stimulation of the gastric and duodenal mucosa in cats, *Q. J. exp. Physiol.*, 57 (1972) 405–416.

16   Dingledine, R. A., Goldstein, A. and Kendig, J., Effects of narcotic opiates and serotonin on the electrical behavior of neurons in the guinea pig's Auerbach's plexus, *Life Sci.*, 14 (1974) 2299–2309.

17   Dingledine, R. and Goldstein, A., Effect of synaptic transmission blockade on morphine action in the guinea pig myenteric plexus, *J. Pharmacol. exp. Ther.*, 196 (1976) 97–106.

18   Ehrenpreis, S., Sato, T., Takayanagi, I., Comaty, J. E. and Takagi, K., Mechanism of morphine block of electrical activity in ganglia of Auerbach's plexus, *European J. Pharmacol.*, 40 (1976) 303–309.

19   Erwin, D. N., Ninchoji, T. and Wood, J. D., Effects of morphine on electrical activity of single myenteric neurons in cat small bowel, *European J. Pharmacol.*, 47 (1978) 401–405.

20   Frigo, G. M. and Lecchini, S., An improved method for studying the peristaltic reflex in the isolated colon, *Br. J. Pharmacol.*, 39 (1970) 346–356.

21   Gabella, G., Fine structure of the myenteric plexus in the guinea-pig ileum, *J. Anat.*, 111 (1972) 69–97.

22   Harry, J., The action of drugs on the circular muscle strip from the guinea-pig isolated ileum, *Brit. J. Pharmacol.*, 20 (1963) 399–417.

23   Henderson, R. M., Duchon, G. and Daniel, E. E., Cell contacts in duodenal smooth muscle layers, *Amer. J. Physiol.*, 221 (1971) 564–574.

24   Hirst, G. D. S. and Spence, I., Calcium action potentials in mammalian peripheral neurones, *Nature* (Lond.), 243 (1973) 54–56.

25   Hirst, G. D. S. and McKirdy, H. C., A nervous mechanism for descending inhibition in guinea pig small intestine, *J. Physiol.* (Lond.), 238 (1974) 129–144.

26   Hirst, G. D. S. and McKirdy, H. C., Presynaptic inhibition at mammalian peripheral synapse, *Nature* (Lond.), 250 (1974) 430–431.

27   Hirst, G. D. S., Holman, M. E. and Spence, I., Two types of neurons in the myenteric plexus of duodenum in the guinea pig, *J. Physiol.* (Lond.), 236 (1974) 303–326.

28   Hirst, G. D. S. and Silinsky, E. M., Some effects of 5-hydroxytryptamine, dopamine and noradrenaline on neurones in the submucous plexus of guinea-pig small intestine, *J. Physiol.* (Lond.), 251 (1975) 817–832.

29   Hirst, G. D. S. and McKirdy, H. C., Synaptic potentials recorded from neurons of the submucous plexus of guinea-pig small intestine, *J. Physiol.* (Lond.), 249 (1975) 369–385.

30   Hirst, G. D. S., Holman, M. E. and McKirdy, H. C., Two descending nerve pathways activated by distension of guinea-pig small intestine, *J. Physiol.* (Lond.), 244 (1975) 113–127.

31   Hoffman, H. H. and Schnitzlein, H. N , The number of vagus nerves in man, *Anat Rec.*, 139 (1969) 429–435.

32   Iggo, A., Gastric mucosal chemoreceptors with vagal afferent fibers in the cat, *Q. J. exp. Physiol.*, 42 (1957) 398–409.

33   Iggo, A., Gastrointestinal tension receptors with unmyelinated afferent fibers in the vagus of the cat, *Q. J. exp. Physiol.*, 42 (1957) 130–143.

34   Jacobowitz, D., Histochemical studies of the autonomic innervation of the gut, *J. Pharmacol. exp. Ther.*, 149 (1965) 356–364.

35   Kennedy, D., Evoy, W. H. and Hanawalt, J. T., Release of coordinated behavior in crayfish by single central neurons, *Science*, 154 (1966) 917–919.

36   Kewenter, J., The vagal control of the jejunal and ileal motility and blood flow, *Acta. physiol. scand. Suppl.*, 251 (1965) 3–68.

37 Kobayashi, M., Prosser, C. L. and Nagai, T., Electrical interaction between muscle layers of cat intestine, *Amer. J. Physiol.*, 211 (1966) 1281–1291.

38 Kosterlitz, H. W. and Lees, G. M., Pharmacological analysis of intrinsic intestinal reflexes, *Pharmacol. Rev.*, 16 (1964) 301–339.

39 Kosterlitz, H. W., Lydon, R. J. and Watt, A. J., The effects of adrenaline, noradrenaline and isoprenaline on inhibitory alpha- and beta-adrenoreceptors in the longitudinal muscle of the guinea-ileum, *Br. J. Pharmacol.*, 391 (1970) 398–413.

40 Kuntz, A., On the occurrence of reflex arcs in the myenteric and submucous plexuses, *Anat. Rec.*, 13 (1922) 193–210.

41 Langley, J. N., *The Autonomic Nervous System*, W. Heffer & Sons, 1921, Part 1.

42 Langley, J. N., Connexions of the enteric nerve cells, *J. Physiol.* (Lond.), 56 P (1922) 39.

43 Mayer, C. J. and Wood, J. D., Properties of mechanosensitive neurons within Auerbach's pleux of the small intestine of the cat, *Pflügers Arch.*, 357 (1975) 35–49.

44 Mayer, C. J. and Wood, J. D., Excitatory action of serotonin on somal membranes of myenteric neurons of guinea pig small bowel, *Fed. Proc.*, 37 (1978) 227.

45 Mei, N., Mechanorecepteurs Vageaux Digestive chez le chat, *Exp. Brain Res.*, 11 (1970) 502–514.

46 Nagai, T. and Prosser, C. L., Electrical parameters of smooth muscle cells, *Amer. J. Physiol.*, 204 (1963) 915–924.

47 Nishi, S. and North, R. A., Intracellular recording from the myenteric plexus of the guinea-pig ileum, *J. Physiol.* (Lond.), 231 (1973) 471–491.

48 Norberg, R. A., Adrenergic innervation of the intestinal wall studied by fluorescence microscopy, *Int. J. Neuropharmacol.*, 3 (1964) 379–382.

49 Norberg, K. A. and Sjoqvist, R., New possibilities for adrenergic modulation of synaptic transmission, *Pharmacol. Rev.*, 18 (1966) 743–751.

50 North, R. A., Calcium-dependent slow after-hyperpolarization in myenteric plexus neurones with tetrodotoxin-resistant action potentials, *Br. J. Pharmacol.*, 49 (1973) 709–711.

51 North, R. A., Effects of morphine on myenteric plexus neurones, *Neuropharmacology*, 15 (1976) 719–721.

52 North, A. R. and Williams, J. T., Extracellular recording from the guinea-pig myenteric plexus and the action of morphine, *European J. Pharmacol.*, 45 (1977) 23–33.

53 Nozdrachev, A. D., Katchalov, U. P. and Bnetov, A. V., Spontaneous discharge of neurons in myenteric plexus of the intestine of rabbits, *Fisiol. Zh. USSR*, 61 (1975) 725–730.

54 Ohkawa, H. and Prosser, C. L., Electrical activity in myenteric and submucous plexuses of cat intestine, *Amer. J. Physiol.*, 222 (1972) 1412–1419.

55 Ohkawa, H. and Prosser, C. L., Functions of neurons in enteric plexuses of cat intestine, *Amer. J. Physiol.*, 222 (1972) 1420–1426.

56 Paintal, A. S., Responses from mucosal mechanoreceptors in the small intestine of the cat, *J. Physiol.* (Lond.), 139 (1957) 353–368.

57 Paton, W. D. M. and Zar, M. A., The origin of acetylcholine released from guinea-pig intestine and longitudinal muscle strips, *J. Physiol.* (Lond.), 194 (1968) 13–33.

58 Paton, W. D. M. and Vizi, E. S., The inhibitory action of noradrenaline on acetylcholine output by guinea-pig ileum longitudinal muscle strip, *Br. J. Pharmacol.*, 35 (1969) 10–28.

59 Prosser, C. L. and Bortoff, A., Electrical activity of intestinal muscle under *in vitro* conditions. In: C. F. Code (Ed.), *Handbook of Physiology, Section 6, Alimentary Canal, Vol. IV*, American Physiological Society, Washington, D. C., 1968, pp. 2025–2050.

60 Ranieri, F., Mei, N. and Crousillat, J., Les afferences splanchniques provenant des mechanorecepteurs gastrointestinaux et peritoneaux, *Exp. Brain Res.*, 16 (1973) 276–290.

61 Sato, T., Takayanagi, I. and Takagi, K., Pharmacological properties of electrical activities obtained from neurons in Auerbach's plexus, *Jap. J. Pharmacol.*, 23 (1973) 665–671.

62 Sauer, M. E. and Rumble, C. T., The number of nerve cells in the myenteric and the submucous plexuses of the small intestine of the cat, *Anat. Rec.*, 96 (1946) 373–381.

63 Schofield, G. C., Anatomy of muscular and neural tissues in the alimentary canal. In: C. F. Code (Ed.), *Handbook of Physiology, Section 6, Alimentary Canal, Vol. IV*, American Physiological Society, Washington, D. C., 1968, pp. 1579–1677.

64 Szurszewski, J. H., A migrating electric complex of the canine small intestine, *Amer. J. Physiol.*, 217 (1969) 1757–1763.

65 Szurszewski, J. H. and Weems, W. A., A study of peripheral input to and its control by postganglionic neurones of the inferior mesenteric ganglion, *J. Physiol.* (Lond.), 256 (1976) 541–556.

66 Takayanagi, I., Sato, T. and Takagi, K., Action of 5-hydroxytryptamine on electrical activity of Auerbach's plexus in the ileum of the morphinedependent guinea pig, *European J. Pharmacol.*, 27 (1974) 252–254.

67 Tomita, T., Electrical properties of mammalian smooth muscle. In: E. Bülbring, A. F. Brading, A. W. Jones and T. Tomita (Eds.), *Smooth Muscle*, Williams and Wilkins Co., 1970, pp. 197–243.

68 Tonini, M., Lecchini, S., Frigo, G. and Crema, A., Action of tetrodotoxin on spontaneous electrical activity of some smooth muscle preparations, *European J. Pharmacol.*, 29 (1974) 236–240.

69 Wood, J. D. and Perkins, W. E., Mechanical interaction between longitudinal and circular axes of the small intestine, *Amer. J. Physiol.*, 218 (1970) 762–768.

70 Wood, J. D., Electrical activity from single neurons in Auerbach's plexus, *Amer. J. Physiol.*, 219 (1970) 159–169.

71 Wood, J. D., Excitation of intestinal muscle by atropine, tetrodotoxin and xylocaine, *Amer. J. Physiol.*, 222 (1972) 118–125.

72 Wood, J. D. and Harris, B. R., Phase relationships of the intestinal muscularis: effects of atropine and xylocaine, *J. appl. Physiol.*, 32 (1972) 734–736.

73 Wood, J. D. and Marsh, D. R., Effects of atropine, tetrodotoxin and lidocaine on rebound excitation of guinea-pig small intestine, *J. Pharmacol. exp. Ther.*, 184 (1973) 590–602.

74 Wood, J. D., Electrical activity of the intestine of mice with hereditary megacolon and absence of enteric ganglion cells, *Amer. J. Dig. Dis.*, 18 (1973) 447–488.

75 Wood, J. D., Electrical discharge of single enteric neurons of guinea-pig small intestine, *Amer. J. Physiol.*, 225 (1973) 1107–1113.

76 Wood, J. D. and Mayer, C. J., Patterned discharge of six different neurons in a single enteric ganglion, *Pflügers Arch.*, 338 (1973) 247–256.

77 Wood, J. D., Neurophysiology of ganglia of Auerbach's plexus, *Am. Zool.*, 14 (1974) 973–989.

78 Wood, J. D. and Mayer, C. J., Discharge patterns of single enteric neurons of the small intestine of the cat, dog and guinea-pig. In: E. E. Daniel (Ed.), *Fourth International Symposium on Gastrointestinal Motility*, Mitchell Press, 1974, pp. 387–408.

79 Wood, J. D., Neurophysiology of Auerbach's plexus and control of intestinal motility, *Physiol. Rev.*, 55 (1975) 307–324.

80   Wood, J. D., Effects of elevated magnesium on discharge of myenteric neurons of cat small bowel, *Amer. J. Physiol.*, 229 (1975) 657–662.

81   Wood, J. D., Neuronal interactions within ganglia of Auerbach's plexus of the small intestine. In: Bülbring and M. F. Shuba (Eds.), *Physiology of Smooth Muscle*, Raven Press, 1976, pp. 321–330.

82   Wood, J. D. and Mayer, C. J., Intracellular study of electrical behavior in tonic type myenteric neurons of guinea pig small bowel, *Fed. Proc.*, 37 (1978) 227.

83   Wood, J. D. and Mayer, C. J., Electrical activity of myenteric neurons: Comparison of results obtained with intracellular and extracellular methods of recording. In: H. Duthie (Ed.), *Gastrointestinal Motility in Health and Disease*, MTP Press Ltd., 1978, pp. 311–320.

84   Wood, J. D. and Mayer, C. J., Intracellular study of electrical activity of Auerbach's plexus in guinea-pig small intestine, *Pflügers Arch.*, 374 (1978) 265–275.

85   Wood, J. D., Mayer, C. J., Ninchoji, T. and Erwin, D. N., Effects of depleted calcium on electrical activity of neurons in Auerbach's plexus, *Amer. J. Physiol.*, 236 (1979) C 78–86.

86   Wood, J. D. and Mayer, C. J., Serotonergic activation of tonic-type enteric neurons in guinea-pig small bowel, *J. Neurophysiol.*, 42 (1979) 582–593.

87   Wood, J. D. and Mayer, C. J., Intracellular study of tonic-type enteric neurons in guinea-pig small intestine, *J. Neurophysiol.*, 42 (1979) 569–581.

88   Wood, J. D. and Mayer, C. J., Adrenergic inhibition of serotonin release from neurons in guinea-pig Auerbach's plexus, *J. Neurophysiol.*, 42 (1979) 594–603.

SECTION III

INTERACTIONS IN AUTONOMIC SYSTEM GANGLIA

In the previous section there was discussion of peripheral interactions within the autonomic system in the modulation of tissue activities. What occurs in the ganglia of the myenteric plexuses has been mentioned. The chapters of the present section deal chiefly with the ganglia which lie between the central nervous system and peripheral plexuses. There probably are similarities and dissimilarities in ganglia of all categories. The important question is: What does occur within the ganglia which is of significance to the function of the autonomic system; what interactions and integrations can occur within these peripheral aggregates of neurons?

New anatomical and electrophysiological studies have revived the ancient concept that ganglia are integrative centers. Certainly, interactions occur there. There are fast and slow processes, at least two transmitters act there and both excitatory and inhibitory actions occur within the ganglia.

Evidence for catecholamine-mediated inhibition in ganglionic transmission is reviewed and new facts are presented. Both pre- and postsynaptic inhibition occur. Comparisons are made with what occurs at other synapses and it is felt that inhibitory hyperpolarization is generated here as elsewhere by a selective increase in potassium conductance.

Another chapter emphasizes the unique interactions between sacral parasympathetic and lumbar sympathetic inputs to pelvic ganglia. This reinforces the story of integrative action and interactions within ganglia.

Our excursion into the analyses of interaction in ganglia concludes with a discussion of acetylcholine and serotonin receptors in mammalian sympathetic ganglionic neurons; nicotinic receptors and 5-HT-receptors, but no muscarinic receptors are present. It is also of interest that the density of ACh receptors is not homogeneous in different portions of the ganglionic soma membrane.

CHAPTER 13

SLOW POSTSYNAPTIC ACTIONS IN GANGLIONIC FUNCTIONS

Benjamin Libet

Department of Physiology, University of California, School of Medicine,
San Francisco, California, USA

INTRODUCTION

Synaptic transmission in autonomic ganglia has been traditionally viewed in terms of a basic similarity with that at the neuromuscular junction, with the addition of certain limited integrative functions. The synaptic actions were thought to be based only on a unitary type of postsynaptic response, the EPSP elicited by a nicotinic action of preganglionically-released acetylcholine (ACh), and the integrative interactions among separate EPSP's were made possible by both a divergence and a convergence of the preganglionic nerve fibers onto the principal neurons or ganglion cells (see Fig. 1). (These aspects have been reviewed by others[6,67,76,83].) However, during the 1960's and early 1970's the existence of several additional types of postsynaptic responses to preganglionic ACh-inputs was definitively established[48,56,58]. These include a slow (s-) IPSP and a slow (s-) EPSP[22,45,48,51], as well as a novel type of synaptic action in which one transmitter (dopamine, DA) can induce a long-lasting modulatory enhancement of the responses to another transmitter ACh[58]. These slow PSP's and the DA-modulatory action (which is independent of any PSP) have introduced new kinds of potentialities into the modes of synaptic interactions and integrations in autonomic ganglia. Reviews of the slow PSP's have appeared[34,48,67,76]. In the present paper the unique characteristics and mechanisms of these slow synaptic actions will be reviewed briefly; recent developments on these actions, as

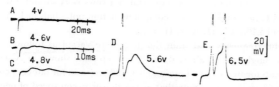

Fig. 1. (Fast) EPSP's and action potentials, elicited by different strengths of preganglionic stimulus, recorded intracellularly in rabbit SCG. The longer latency EPSP components, added by the slower preganglionic fibers excited by stronger stimuli, could induce multiple firing in this cell (see also Wallis and North[83]). Time calibration in B applies to B–E. (From Libet and Tosaka, 1969[57].)

well as the issue of their significance for ganglion functions, will be emphasized and elaborated on. An even slower "late s-EPSP" response has also been described for frog ganglion[69] and subsequently for dog superior cervical ganglion (SCG)[13]. This component appears best during both nicotinic and muscarinic blockade, and its mechanisms, transmitter and significance under physiological conditions are still obscure; it will not be considered further in this paper.

RESULTS AND DISCUSSION

Components of the Ganglionic Potentials

The ganglionic potentials elicited by orthodromic (preganglionic nerve) inputs, in a preparation not treated with blocking agents, represent a complex variety of components which partially overlap and algebraically summate with each other in time. Recordings are remarkably similar in form whether made with surface electrodes (one on ganglion and one on postganglionic nerve, at least two to three mm away) or with an intracellular microelectrode, except for a degree of asynchrony in the compound action potentials of the surface population response—(compare Figs. 1, 2 and and 3). It is possible to dissociate the various components by taking advantage of their individual sensitivities to different blocking agents, etc.

Curarized ganglia. The "fast" (f)EPSP's and the action potentials with their after-potentials that the EPSP's can generate can be suppressed by a nicotinic blocker like d-tubocurarine (d-TC).

The curarized rabbit SCG thus exhibits a depressed EPSP, followed by a hy-

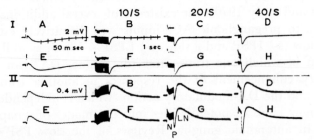

Fig. 2. Orthodromic responses to trains of repetitive stimuli; surface recordings of untreated rabbit SCG in section I, and after curarization (dihydro-β-erythroidine, 7.5 μg/ml) in section II. For horizontal rows A–D. stimulus strength was slightly submaximal for the preganglionic B fiber group, while for rows E–H stimuli it was supramaximal for B and C preganglionics (see compound action potentials in I, A vs. I, E, and the compound EPSP's in II, A vs. II, E).

Stimulus frequency and train duration were varied as follows: Vertical column under A, single volley, all at the faster sweep scale shown in A; column under B, 10/sec train for two sec; column under C, 20/sec train for one sec; column under D, 40/sec train for 0.5 sec. (Note that at the slower sweep speed of one sec per div., in columns under B–D, only the peak and bottom outlines of action potentials or fast EPSP's during the stimulus train are visible, not the separate individual responses actually making up the train.)

Voltage scale in I, A applied to all of section I; that in II, A to all of section II. (From R. M. Eccles and Libet, 1961[22].)

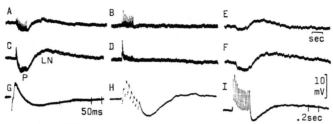

Fig. 3. Fast and slow PSP's recorded intracellularly, within same ganglion cells (of rabbit SCG). A–D, one cell curarized moderately: Supramaximal stimulus train for one sec, at 10/sec in A–B and at 40/sec in C–D; atropine sulfate (0.3 μg/ml) in B and D selectively eliminates both the s-IPSP and s-EPSP, leaving the depressed fast (f) EPSP's unchanged.

E–F, another cell more strongly curarized, stimuli at 10/s and 40/s, respectively, s-IPSP and s-EPSP appear even though (f) EPSP's are completely depressed.

G–H, another cell curarized more weakly and a similar cell in I, recorded at faster sweep speeds (50 msec/div. in G, 0.2 sec/div. in H and I); see (f) EPSP, s-IPSP with single preganglionic volley in G, and repetitive (f) EPSP's, plus s-IPSP and s-EPSP in H and I (stimulated with a 20/sec and 40/sec train respectively). (From Libet and Tosaka, 1969[57].)

perpolarizing s-IPSP and then by a depolarizing s-EPSP, as shown in Figs. 2-II and 3[22,48]. With a single maximal preganglionic volley the slow PSP's are relatively small or even absent (Fig. 3G). With brief repetition of preganglionic volleys, the partially curarized EPSP's are summated during the train of stimuli and, in surface recordings, this constitutes a negative or "N" wave (Figs. 2-II and 3). The s-IPSP overlaps with the summated EPSP's, pulling the net potential down in the hyperpolarizing direction during the train and leading into a net hyperpolarization, the surface-recorded "P" wave, following the train (Fig. 2-II, B–D and E–H; Fig. 3A, C, H and I). The s-EPSP has the longest synaptic delay of all these three (about 200–300 msec)[47]; after a short train of stimuli (0.25–1 sec) it therefore appears predominantly following the peak of the s-IPSP as a later (surface)-negative or "LN" wave (see Fig. 2-II, B–D and E–H; Fig. 3A, C and E–I). Preganglionic B fibers can elicit most or all of both slow PSP's in rabbit SCG (see Fig. 2-II, B–D vs. F–H), though it is reported that only the preganglionic C group elicits s-IPSP in rat SCG[20] (see also for frog ganglion, below). The s-IPSP requires a higher frequency (40/sec) for its optimal production in rabbit SCG at 37°C (see Fig. 2-II, D and H). Consequently, with a low frequency of preganglionic volleys the LN wave (s-EPSP) may begin to appear as a depolarizing hump (or "shift in the base-line"), superimposed on the summated EPSP's during a sufficiently long train of stimuli (for example, Fig. 2-II, B). Although stimulation of the mixed preganglionic fibers elicits all three PSP's in this temporally overlapping fashion, there is evidence that a given preganglionic fiber may elicit purely an s-IPSP or s-EPSP in a given ganglion cell[57]. (A note of caution about conditions that may make slow PSP's appear to be abnormally small or nonexistent will be discussed in the later section on "physiological significance".)

In the frog's curarized paravertebral ganglia, the picture is qualitatively similar but with some interesting differences[60,79,80]. Unlike mammalian ganglia, each frog ganglion cell is innervated by only one preganglionic fiber, with some rare excep-tions[7,80]; and the single EPSP is usually more than adequate to fire the cell, as it is in the case of neuromuscular junctions. Furthermore, the postganglionic axon from each cell is itself either a myelinated B or an unmyelinated C fiber in accordance with whether its preganglionic input is a B or C fiber, respectively[80]! For the IXth and Xth ganglia of the paravertebral chain at least, there is an anatomical separation of the B- and C-fiber inputs; purely B-fiber inputs originate in spinal nerves anterior (ceph-alad) to VIII, while purely C fiber inputs originate in VIII and probably IX[60,75,27a]. It is thus possible to investigate conveniently the physiological and morphological relationships of the "B" group of ganglion cells separately from the "C" group. It turned out that the s-IPSP is elicited predominantly by preganglionic C fibers[60] (see Fig. 4), and that the s-IPSP response is exhibited essentially exclusively in the "C" group of ganglion cells[79,80]. (B cells are perhaps capable of a relatively small equivalent response when their resting membrane potentials are at least at −60 mV or more[42,67].) It should also be noted that the s-EPSP response in frog ganglia is very small and inconsistent when recorded as a population response of intact ganglion cells by a surface electrode on the ganglion[60]; the s-EPSP is larger in the B cells with intracellular recordings[41,69,76,80], but the impaled cells are almost invariably damaged

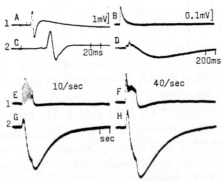

Fig. 4.　Responses of frog ganglion to stimulation of anatomically separate preganglionic B and C groups of fibers. Surface-recordings of paravertebral ganglion IX; A and C before, and all the rest after partial curarization (dihydro-β-erythroidine, four μg/ml). For horizontal rows #1, stimulus electrodes on the paravertebral chain anterior to ganglion VII could excite only the B fiber input; for rows #2, electrodes on the preganglionic ramus from VIII spinal nerve could excite only C fiber input. This is seen in the latencies for the compound action potential in tracings A and C, which give conduction velocities of about 2.5 m/sec and about 0.5 m/sec respectively[3a]; these are appropriate to B fibers and the faster C fibers, respectively, at 20°C.

After curarization, responses to a single preganglionic B volley (in tracing B) shows only (f) EPSP, while a single preganglionic C volley (in tracing D) elicits EPSP and s-IPSP. With one-sec trains of stimuli at 10/sec (E, G) and 40/sec (F, H), note the large s-IPSP's in G and H during and after the trains of preganglionic C volleys (stimulating ramus VIII). With B fiber inputs (E and F) only a small s-IPSP is elicited by the 40/sec train; there is typically little or no evidence of any s-EPSP in these intact frog ganglia, as seen here, although a small s-EPSP did appear in some ganglia. (From Libet et al., 1968[60].)

and somewhat depolarized. Since depolarization introduces the possibility of an entirely different slow depolarizing response to ACh (see below), it seems likely that the "physiological" s-EPSP in frog ganglia is rudimentary compared to that in the higher vertebrates. The weak physiological s-EPSP mechanism could account for the reported inability to obtain consistent depolarizing responses to cyclic GMP in frog ganglia[12]; see further discussion below.

Untreated ganglia. In ganglia not treated with any blocking agents, EPSP's can induce firing of ganglion cells. This in turn leads to both an early after-potential, best seen after a single action potential (Fig. 1E and Fig. 2-I, A), and later, more prolonged after-hyperpolarization that is substantial only after a train of spikes and is referred to as posttetanic-hyperpolarization (see Fig. 2-I, B–D, F–H; Fig. 5). Descriptions in the literature have in some cases tended to confuse the analysis and views about these after-hyperpolarizations, in referring to them simply by their polarity (P component, for surface positivity) without distinguishing them sharply from, for example, the P (s-IPSP) component of the curarized ganglion. It can in

GANGLIONIC POTENTIALS

(40/SEC., 1 SEC. TRAINS
SUP. CERV. GANG., RABBIT, IN VIVO.

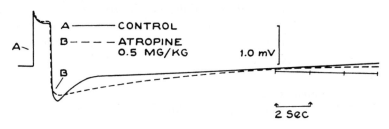

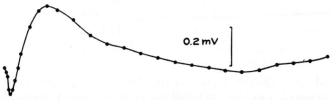

PLOT OF A MINUS B
(AT 5-FOLD AMPLITUDE)

Fig. 5.   Effect of atropine on the posttetanic after-potential, of uncurarized rabbit SCG *in vivo*. Surface-recording of ganglionic response to 40/sec, one sec train of supramaximal preganglionic stimuli; A, before and B, after injecting atropine i. v., 0.5 mg/kg. Tracings are redrawn from originals and show the peaks of the action potentials during the stimulation, outlined as a continuous line. Note that amplitude of the s-EPSP component, eliminated by atropine, is approximately 25% that of the compound action potentials. Relative amplitude of the s-IPSP (initial hyperpolarizing component eliminated) is smaller, but this may be misleading since it is generated in parallel with the true after-potential (that remains after atropine); the latter could mask part of the s-IPSP contribution. (Modified from Libet, 1964[45].)

fact be shown that the after-potentials of untreated ganglia can contain a number of electrically overlapping components in them[34,45].

Atropinized ganglia. If atropine is added, it should eliminate any s-IPSP and s-EPSP components that include a muscarinic-cholinergic step in their synaptic pathway (as in Fig. 3B and D). The changes produced by atropine added to the uncurarized ganglion, in the amplitude and form of the posttetanic after-potentials, are in accord with the presence and contribution of s-IPSP and s-EPSP components to the original response[20,34a,45], see Fig. 5. The remaining after-potential may contain an additional s-IPSP component, mediated via a nonmuscarinic cholinergic step that releases norepinephrine, NE (rather than DA), as the direct transmitter[51]. When this second s-IPSP component is also eliminated by additional selective blockade[51], the unchanged ganglionic action potentials are now followed by "pure" after-potentials; the latter are direct sequelae of the firing, similar to those in other neurones, and are not due to separate synaptic processes. Even the after-potentials consist of two components: The "early" after-potential is a hyperpolarization due to a temporarily-sustained rise in K^+-conductance after each spike[7,34,67]. A later, much longer after-potential appears in substantial form after a brief repetitive train of spikes. This posttetanic after-hyperpolarization is due to activation of the electrogenic Na-K pump as a result of the net increase in intracellular Na^+ concentration that occurs during a period of repetitive action potentials, as initially shown for other neurons[62,72]; in sympathetic ganglia this component, or its equivalent, that follows a large depolarization by ACh (acting nicotinically) can be selectively eliminated by ouabain or by Li^+-replacement of Na^+[62].

Special Features of the Slow Postsynaptic Potentials

The slow PSP's have characteristics strikingly different from all the well-known (f)PSP's, including the (f)EPSP in autonomic ganglion cells. They have durations of many seconds, rather than of msec. Synaptic delays are extraordinarily long; for s-IPSP's these are about 25 msec in rabbit SCG[47] and 100 msec in frog paravertebral ganglion[60], while for s-EPSP they are 200–300 msec in rabbit SCG[47]. Slow PSP's are relatively weak after a single preganglionic volley, but build up to maximal values upon brief periods of repetition at moderate frequencies of input[22] (see Fig. 2). The electrogenic mechanisms that develop these PSP's are not based on increases in membrane conductances for various ions[40,48], as is the case for all (f)PSP's[21]; this issue will be considered further below.

In spite of these unique characteristics, the slow hyperpolarizing and depolarizing responses to preganglionic inputs fulfill the crucial criteria demanded for establishing chemically-mediated PSP's. (Incidentally, the often-employed criterion of an increase in membrane conductance is obviously erroneous if applied generally and rigidly when judging whether an unknown potential change may qualify as a PSP. One should not confuse the particular electrogenic mechanism for a response with the question of whether its physiological production and role are those of a PSP.) The s-IPSP and s-EPSP are both recordable in most of the same ganglion cells of the rabbit SCG that exhibit the (f)EPSP's[57] (Fig. 3), and they appear in the appropriate types of neurons in frog ganglia[69,79,80]. They can affect cell excitability in the expected manner[20,45]. The slow PSP's are demonstrable in the complete absence of (f)EPSP's or of action potentials in the ganglion cells (see Fig. 3)[22,45,47,57,60,79]; they cannot therefore be regarded as some kinds of direct or indirect after effects of processes initiated by EPSP's or action potentials. The slow PSP's are mediated by specific chemical transmitters, upon whose presynaptic functional content and release they are dependent (see low Ca effects[47]; ACh release for all[22]; DA required for s-IPSP[56]); and they are mediated by specific postsynaptic receptors which differ from those for the (f)EPSP's, as evidenced in part by the differential sensitivities to nicotinic, muscarinic and adrenergic blocking agents[22,48], and in their special electrogenic mechanisms and their sensitivities to loss of oxidative metabolism[40,42,48]. A diagram schematizing many of these points in relation to the intraganglionic pathways for the various responses is given in Fig. 6.

Ganglionic Interneurons and Catecholamine Transmitters

The preganglionic fibers that elicit the (f)EPSP, s-IPSP and s-EPSP. These fibers appear to release only ACh at their terminals. This is supported not only by ultrastructural studies[23] but also by the finding that botulinum toxin eliminates all these postsynaptic responses[22]. Evidence from studies on release of NE by orthodromic input[71] led to one proposal that a substantial number of preganglionic fibers in the rabbit SCG may be noradrenergic, rather than cholinergic; however, morphological evidence now appears to exclude this possibility[16], and another explanation for the origin of NE release must be sought. Recent findings that substance P is present in some nerve fibers that form a plexus around ganglion cells[37] suggest that all the possi-

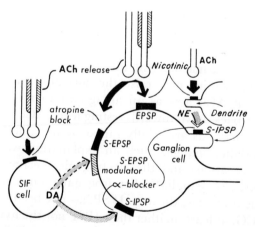

Fig. 6. Schema of intraganglionic synaptic connections, for mediation of fast and slow PSP's and of synaptic modulation of the s-EPSP by DA. All preganglionic fibers release ACh. Direct transmitter for one s-IPSP component is DA, released from SIF cell-interneurons excited by a muscarinic action of ACh. Transmitter for another s-IPSP component is NE, released by a nonmuscarinic, presumably nicotinic, action of ACh—see text; a possible pathway via a dendro-dendritic junction is shown in upper right portion of diagram. (Modified from Libet, 1977[50] and from Libet, 1970[48].)

ble types of synaptic actions in sympathetic ganglia may not yet have been discovered. To this should be added the evidence that some sensory fibers may also be making efferent synaptic contacts with some elements in ganglia[33].

Second transmitter required for s-IPSP. The s-IPSP of the curarized sympathetic ganglion is blocked by atropine[22,59]; and an equivalent hyperpolarization can be elicited by ACh or by the muscarinic agonists MCh (acetyl-β-methylcholine) or BCh (bethanechol)[41,48,57]. Nevertheless, additional evidence overwhelmingly supports the view that this muscarinic cholinergic action is actually an indirect one, exciting an intraganglionic interneuron to release the direct inhibitory transmitter[22,48,55,80]. Such an arrangement is analogous in principle to the "conversion" of an excitatory transmitter into an inhibitory transmitter via an interneuron, a principle that was proposed and developed for the mammalian central nervous system by Eccles[21]; this principle appears to be operative in peripheral sympathetic ganglia also, with an excitatory action of ACh on an interneuronal structure (see below) "converted" into an inhibitory action by synaptic release of DA[49].

In the presence of a low Ca/Mg medium that abolishes presynaptic release of transmitters in ganglia[47], the initial hyperpolarizing response to ACh (with dTC present), or to MCh or BCh, is eliminated—leaving only an enlarged slow depolarizing response[48,55]. These effects were demonstrated for both rabbit SCG[48] and frog paravertebral ganglia[55]. They show that the release of a second transmitter by the muscarinic agent is necessary for producing the s-IPSP, but not for the s-EPSP, types of response. These effects of low Ca/Mg have recently been confirmed for rabbit SCG at the single cell level, with local iontophoretic applications of ACh[18,68].

Cautions on use of nicotine. In the case of frog ganglia treated with nicotine instead of a curarizing agent, it was shown that ACh could elicit a direct hyperpolarizing response that was not abolished by low Ca/Mg[85], a finding that we confirmed[55]. It became clear that two different types of hyperpolarizing responses can be elicited by ACh, and that the direct response of nicotinized frog ganglion cells to ACh should be regarded as one of pharmacological interest, not related to the physiological s-IPSP[55]. For example, nicotine may raise the normally low resting g_{Na} membrane conductance for Na$^+$; if ACh acts as an antagonist to nicotine in this respect, it would tend to bring g_{Na} back down towards resting level. ACh would then be reducing ("inactivating") a g_{Na} that was artificially raised by nicotine[55], and this could lead to a direct hyperpolarizing change. Such an explanation would be in accordance with the reported observations and the electrogenic mechanism proposed for this response in nicotine-treated ganglia[85]. For frog ganglion C cells not treated with nicotine, direct investigation of g_m during s-IPSP has not been carried out. In neurons of untreated rabbit SCG, at least, neither the s-IPSP nor the hyperpolarizing response to DA or NE show any change in membrane conductance[19,40,41]; see further below. The induction by nicotine of cellular capacities for nonphysiological types of responses to ACh, both hyperpolarizing[55] and depolarizing[42], has led to considerable confusion in considering the natures of the physiological s-IPSP and s-EPSP responses in autonomic ganglia. Unfortunately, nicotine was used extensively by some investigators to block the nicotinic actions of ACh in frog ganglia at a time before it was clearly realized that these interesting capacities for interactions between pharmacological actions by nicotine and ACh exist. (This issue is discussed again below, in "electrogenic mechanisms".) Readers and investigators are advised to maintain an alert distinction between those reported findings in which nicotine was not employed and those in which nicotine was employed as a blocking agent in the medium.

"Interneuronal" monoaminergic structures. The hypothesis for an adrenergic type of interneuron in the pathway leading to the s-IPSP was originally proposed as the best way of explaining the existing combination of physiological and pharmacological evidence[22]. Subsequently, small monoaminergic neurons, "small-intensely-fluorescent" (SIF) cells, uniquely distinct from the principal neurons (ganglion cells), were histologically demonstrated in many autonomic ganglia (reviewed in refs. 26 and 27, see Fig. 7). It was definitively established that SIF cells can qualify morphologically as interneurons; at least some of them were found to make efferent-type synaptic contacts with principal neurons in rat SCG, in addition to their receiving afferent-type contacts made by preganglionic cholinergic fiber terminals (reviewed in ref. 88).

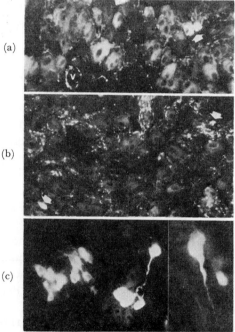

(a)

(b)

(c)

Fig. 7. Fluorescence photomicrographs of superior cervical ganglion of rabbit (formaldehyde reaction). The ganglion cells exhibit a varying degree of green catecholamine fluorescence (a); some of the cells are entirely nonfluorescent. A few more intensely fluorescent fibers are seen between the ganglion cells. Sympathetic nerves enclose small blood vessel (v). Arrow indicates small group of small, intensely fluorescent (SIF) cells with an intense yellow-green fluorescence. × 170. (b) demonstrates the abundancy of intensely greenfluorescent beaded fibers running close to the ganglion cells everywhere in the ganglion. Arrows indicate SIF cells. × 100. (c) various aspects of these SIF cells occur in small groups (left; × 160) and issue processes (middle; × 160) that sometimes can be seen to have a beaded appearance (right; × 520). (From Libet and Owman, 1974[56].)

SIF cells may be grouped according to the specific catecholamines they contain: Thus far DA has been identified as the monoamine in SIF cells of rat[2,4] and rabbit SCG's[56] and, by indirect evidence, in SCG's of monkey[14], cow[5] and possibly cat[5]; but NE is the monoamine in SIF cells of guinea pig SCG and NE plus epinephrine (E) in those of its inferior mesenteric ganglion[15,25]. SIF cells may also be grouped by their structural characteristics[87]: "Type I" cells are relatively isolated and few in number but give rise to long processes that ramify extensively among the principal ganglion cells[56] (see Fig. 7); they are regarded as the interneurons[87]. "Type II" cells occur in larger clusters, near fenestrated blood vessels and lack conspicuous processes; they have been termed "paraneurons", since they do not make efferent synaptic contacts with other neurons[14].

"*Loose synapses*".   It has often been assumed that the specialized efferent synaptic contact (200 Å cleft, etc.) characteristic of classical chemical synapses is essential for producing all transmitter-mediated synaptic actions in ganglia; such efferent synapses from SIF cells have actually been demonstrated in SCG's of rat (see above), of rabbit (Dail, personal communication), and probably of monkey[14]. However, the long synaptic delays for the slow PSP's (see above) make it feasible to consider the possibility that such close contacts may not necessarily be required for all modes of chemical transmission[46,49]. This would be true even if the bulk of each such delay were due to postsynaptic processes for the slow PSP's (see below). Release of transmitter might occur "*en passage*", in a manner already proposed by Burnstock[11] for smooth muscle innervation, from the beaded varicosities of the fine fiber networks found to be closely apposed to and surrounding the ganglion cells. In rabbit SCG these fine networks (see Fig. 7) have been shown to contain DA, and therefore they presumably originate in the SIF cells[56]. Perhaps this alternative of more remote release "*en passage*" can explain the apparent absence in frog ganglia of efferent adrenergic synaptic specializations of the classical (200 Å cleft) type[84]; it was noted above that, except in the case of ganglia treated with nicotine, the evidence appears to require that intraganglionic release of a catecholamine mediates the s-IPSP in frog ganglia as well[55].

The much greater delay for the onset of the DA modulatory action (on the s-EPSP response to ACh) has not yet been definitively quantified, but it would appear to be no less than 30 sec and could be as long as two to four min[61]. Such a delay could even accommodate a neurosecretory type of delivery at even greater distances, for example by release from the axonless type II SIF cells[49,87], especially if an intraganglionic portal circulation were to be involved[14,88]. Indeed, three kinds of actual sites of release of catecholamine by SIF cells, made apparent by either preganglionic or muscarinic stimulation, have recently been demonstrated histologically in the rat SCG by Grillo[33]: Extruded material related to dense core vesicles appeared (1) at classical-type chemical synapses, (2) at nonjunctional membrane specializations called "synaptoids" and (3) at "sheathless portions of an SIF cell surface bordering on the interstitial space and, in some cases, a fenestrated blood vessel".

A potential additional interneuronal type of arrangement resides in the dendrodendritic contacts, which have been described in rat SCG[81] and cat inferior mesenteric ganglion[24]. Small dendritic protrusions (termed "accessory dendrites")[24], which contain a raised concentration of dense-core vesicles, make contact with dendrites of other ganglion cells. Elfvin[24] has even observed preganglionic fiber terminations onto the "presynaptic" side of such dendro-dendritic contacts, and has suggested that this may provide a pathway by which ACh activates the synaptic release of NE intraganglionically.

DA and NE as intraganglionic transmitters. The selective blockade of s-IPSP by α-adrenergic antagonists[22,48,55,60], the augmentation of its amplitude and duration by inhibitors of COMT[55,59] (in a manner analogous to the action of anticholinesterases on ACh responses), the presence of catecholamine-containing "chromaffin" cells[10] and the ability of exogenous catecholamine to elicit some postsynaptic hyperpolarization[63], had all suggested that a catecholamine transmitter was involved[22,48]. The criteria for establishing the identity of the actual transmitter have been fulfilled by DA, in the case of the s-IPSP produced via a muscarinic-ACh pathway in rabbit SCG[48,52,56]. (i) The appropriate interneurons (SIF cells) and the monoamine-containing fibers surrounding ganglion cells contain DA (see above), and release DA upon suitable preganglionic or direct cholinergic stimulation[56]. (ii) Depletion of DA from SIF cells and its replenishment by uptake from exogenous DA are accompanied by a loss and restoration, respectively, of the s-IPSP response[56,58]. Exogenous NE or E are incapable of restoring the s-IPSP. (iii) The postsynaptic actions of DA are identical in nature with those in the s-IPSP, i.e., hyperpolarization with no change in membrane conductance, etc.[19,41,58].

NE or E can also elicit a postsynaptic hyperpolarization similar to the s-IPSP[41,48], but they are clearly not the actual transmitters for the s-IPSP that is mediated via a muscarinic-ACh pathway in the rabbit SCG. However, we have more recently developed strong evidence for the existence of another s-IPSP component in the SCG of the rabbit (and probably guinea pig), one that is mediated by a nonmuscarinic ACh pathway; this s-IPSP component appears definitely to utilize NE, not DA, as the inhibitory transmitter [51](Libet et al. unpublished). The intraganglionic pathway for this NE-mediated s-IPSP is still not established; one obvious possibility is that offered by the dendro-dendritic junctions[24], with preganglionic ACh activation of a nicotinic type of receptor on the presynaptic, NE-containing dendritic element (see Fig. 6).

DA-Modulatory Action on the s-EPSP

DA was found to exert another postsynaptic action in the rabbit SCG, in addition to its role as inhibitory transmitter. After a brief single exposure to DA, the slow depolarizing responses to ACh or MCh (or BCh) can be enhanced by 50–100% for at least some hours, see Fig. 8[58]. The effect can be induced by an amount of DA too small to produce any hyperpolarization, and it appears to be mediated via a different type of postsynaptic receptor than the one for the s-IPSP[52]. NE and E were virtually ineffective for this modulatory change (e.g., Fig. 8), in contrast to their hyperpolarizing capacities.

A prolonged modulatory effect can also be demonstrated for the s-EPSP response itself and it can be induced via physiological routes. Prevention of the inactivation by COMT of endogenous DA, released intraganglionically, was by itself able to pro-

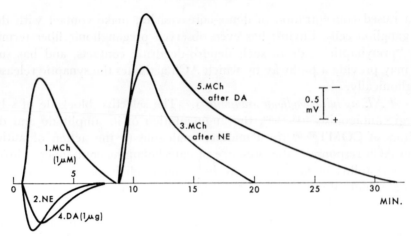

Fig. 8. Modulation of slow muscarinic depolarizations by DA. Surface-recorded responses
of rabbit SCG (22°C) in a sucrose-gap superfusion chamber; ganglion pretreated
with BCh, to deplete intraganglionic DA and eliminate the initial hyperpolarizing
component normally seen in the responses to methacholine (MCh) (Libet and
Owman, 1974[56]). First test shown (#1) is response to a single-bolus injection of one μM
of MCh into ganglionic superfusate. Test #2, response to NE, one μg dose. Test #3,
repeat MCh, as in test 1, shortly after hyperpolarizing response to NE has finished.
Test #4, one μg dose of DA, injected after conclusion of response #3. Test #5, repeat
MCh, as in test 1, shortly after hyperpolarizing response to DA has finished. The
substantial increase in amplitude and duration of the MCh-response seen in test #5
after DA, but not in test #3 after NE, can be exhibited by succeeding tests with MCh
for some hours even though no further DA is applied. (From experiments reported
by Libet and Tosaka, 1970[58].)

duce a considerable enhancement of s-EPSP (as well as of s-IPSP) responses[59]. In
more recent experiments a long conditioning train of preganglionic volleys was shown
to produce selective enhancement of s-EPSP's, one that depended on availability
of functionally releasable DA in SIF cells[43]. Similar evidence of a more indirect
nature had already been obtained; in this, tests of atropine-sensitive "after discharges"
recorded in the postganglionic nerve (presumably generated by the s-EPSP in the
ganglion cells) showed a prolonged enhancement after preganglionic conditioning[66,82].

We have then a novel type of synaptic action, in which one transmitter (DA)
can selectively induce a long-lasting change in the postsynaptic responses to another
transmitter (ACh, acting muscarinically here). The molecular nature of the enduring
neuronal change whose development is induced initially by a brief exposure to DA,
and the cellular site at which it controls the amplitude and duration of s-EPSP
responses, are yet to be discovered. However, some clues to the possible kinds of
neuronal changes are available, since cAMP appears to mediate this DA action and
cGMP can antagonize it in a time-dependent way (see below). In any case, the
DA-modulatory action and the time-dependent "disruptability" of its retention
by cGMP show striking formal similarities to long-lasting functional changes in
reactivities of the brain. The action has been proposed as at least the partial basis of
a possible model for synaptic coupling into the production of a neuronal memory
trace[61].

Intracellular Mediation of Slow Synaptic Actions

Electrogenesis of slow PSP's.   Both the s-IPSP and s-EPSP responses appear with
no increases in membrane conductances (g_m), in contrast to most other PSP's[40].
Some decreases in g_m (i.e., increases in resistance) can be observed under special
conditions (see below), but "normal" ganglion cells, with resting potentials in the
range of -60 to -70 mV and not treated with nicotine, have exhibited no detectable
change in g_m, as studied in s-IPSP of rabbit cells[40,41] and in s-EPSP's of rabbit[35]
and frog[70] cells. Consequently, electrogenesis of both the s-IPSP and s-EPSP appear
to involve mechanisms other than those mediated by changes in ionic conductances.
The only obvious present alternatives would seem to lie in the activation of electrogenic pumps for some appropriate ions. Thus far, identification of any such electrogenic pump has not been achieved[40,42,48,55].

a) *Some alternatives for s-IPSP.*   Activation of the Na-K pump, acting electro-
genically, has been proposed as the mechanism of the s-IPSP[69]. The evidence for that
proposal was largely based on tests of sensitivity of s-IPSP's to ouabain, in frog ganglia
blocked by nicotine. But nicotine treatment makes possible a direct hyperpolarizing
response to ACh that is unrelated to the physiological s-IPSP[55] (see above). Partially
curarized ganglia of either frog or rabbit showed no difference between the ouabain
sensitivities of EPSP and s-IPSP[40,48] that could not be explained on the basis of depolarized presynaptic terminals[62]. Indeed, when the factor of early depression of
presynaptic function by ouabain was excluded, by testing for direct postsynaptic
hyperpolarizing responses to DA or NE applied exogenously, these postsynaptic
equivalents of the s-IPSP responses were clearly insensitive to either ouabain[54,62] or
to replacement of extracellular Na$^+$ by Li$^+$[62].

More recently, the possibility of electrogenesis of the s-IPSP by an increase in
g_K has been introduced by Nishi[68]. This is based on membrane changes during a
large hyperpolarization when ACh is applied iontophoretically in the vicinity of a
ganglion cell in rabbit SCG; this response required release of an intraganglionic
transmitter, as already shown for the hyperpolarizing response to ACh or BCh added
to the external medium in bulk[48]. It is difficult to assess the relationship of these
findings on the large ACh-induced response to relationships with the s-IPSP itself.
No change in g_m has been found either during an s-IPSP[40,41], or during direct hyperpolarization by the direct inhibitory transmitter, DA[19]. Even with hyperpolarizations
elicited by the iontophoretic ACh, no changes in g_m appeared when these responses
were in a "submaximal" range[18,68]. Also, shifts in membrane potential produce
changes in the s-IPSP (or in the direct hyperpolarizations elicited by NE or DA)
that would not appear to conform to those expected for a response due to an increase
in g_K, either in rabbit[40,41], or in frog ganglia[40,69]. Perhaps the conditions under
which a large hyperpolarization is induced by iontophoretic ACh permit the development of another hyperpolarizing component that is additional to or in parallel with
the one that is equivalent to the recorded s-IPSP. Such an additional type of component might also be mediated via a release of DA; indeed, another apparently
DA-mediated type of s-IPSP in neurons of myenteric plexuses seems to be based
completely on electrogenesis via an increase in g_K[36].

b) *Some alternatives for s-EPSP.* Analysis of these alternatives has been subject to some confusion, stemming largely from the fact that s-EPSP's can exhibit a decrease in g_m under certain special though not physiological conditions. The s-EPSP's even in curarized ganglia can be accompanied by a small (approximately 10–20%) decrease in g_m[40], but only when the membrane potentials are in a depolarized range of less than -60 mV[35,41]. In frog ganglia treated with nicotine, the decrease in g_m during the s-EPSP (as well as the amplitudes of the s-EPSP responses) can be greatly enlarged[41]; but, in this case also, the decrease in g_m is only evident when membrane voltages are allowed to depolarize in a range less than -60 mV[70]. Therefore, the proposal by Weight and Padjen[85] that the s-EPSP is produced by a decrease ("inactivation") of g_K could apply only to a component of the response which develops in depolarized cells, especially when nicotinized[42]; this component or type of s-EPSP is best regarded as due to an interesting antagonism by ACh against the increase of (resting) g_K that accompanies delayed rectification of depolarized and nicotinized cells[35,42]. The "physiological" s-EPSP, elicited in cells with resting potentials of about -70 mV, would show little or nothing of a component based on a change in g_K[35,42]; its electrogenesis must involve a mechanism other than one based on increases or decreases in ionic conductances.

Roles of cyclic nucleotides. The present version of these roles is schematized in Fig. 9; this is based on the following considerations[12]:

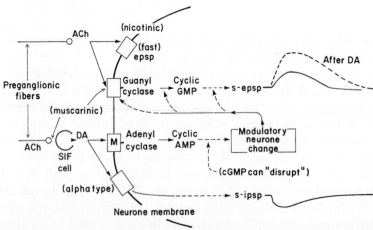

Fig. 9. Schema for postsynaptic intracellular mediation of responses to ACh and DA inputs. ACh action on muscarinic-type receptors leads to s-EPSP response via mediation by cGMP. DA may act on two types of receptors: on an α-adrenergic type that elicits the s-IPSP response, and on a "modulator" (M) receptor (Libet, 1979[53]). The M receptor activates adenyl cyclase to produce more cAMP, which induces, via a series of unknown reactions, an enduring change in the neuron. This latter altered molecular state or product modifies (enhances) the s-EPSP responses to the ACh inputs (see dashed s-EPSP response "after DA"). The general possible sites for this action are indicated by dashed lines leading from the "modulatory neuronal change". The process for developing the modulatory molecular change, but not the latter's final nature or effectiveness on the s-EPSP, can be antagonized or "disrupted" by cyclic GMP. (Modified from Libet et al., 1975[61].)

a) Adenosine 3', 5'-cyclic monophosphate (cAMP) concentrations were found to rise in certain mammalian sympathetic ganglia when they were exposed either to exogenous DA or to conditions that could synaptically release endogenous DA (reviewed in refs. 31, 32 and 53). This suggests that cAMP could be an intracellular mediator for either one or both of the synaptic actions of DA. It was initially proposed by Greengard and his colleagues (reviewed in ref. 32) that cAMP mediates the hyperpolarizing response to DA, i.e., the s-IPSP response. Subsequent evidence led Libet et al.[61] to propose that cAMP mediates the DA-modulatory action on the s-EPSP, i.e., the induction by DA of the long-lasting enhancement of slow muscarinic depolarizing responses to ACh (see above). An analysis of the full evidence presently available indicates that cAMP does not mediate the s-IPSP response to DA, but it strongly supports the role for cAMP in the DA-modulatory action (on the s-EPSP)[52,53]. The basis for this conclusion may be briefly and partially summarized here:

(i) A postsynaptic action appropriate to the DA action in question should be demonstrable for exogenous cAMP. There is presently no suitable evidence that cAMP can elicit any postsynaptic hyperpolarization, as expected for the role in an s-IPSP (reviewed in ref. 53). Trials in which an intracellular technique was employed have yielded uniformly negative results. It has been reported that cAMP did elicit a hyperpolarizing response, when recorded extracellularly in a sucrose-gap superfusion chamber[65]; however, it now appears that these apparently positive responses are actually variable and easily misleading artifacts, producible when switching from one superfusion channel to another in this technique[53]. On the other hand, cAMP can completely mimic the DA-modulatory action, even at the low concentration of 0.1 mM[53,61]. This ability has recently been demonstrated even with an intracellular iontophoretic injection of cAMP[43]; the long-lasting enhancement of s-EPSP responses, produced by the cAMP, appeared with no accompanying changes in membrane potential or resistance.

(ii) Inhibition of phosphodiesterase should tend to augment those actions of DA that may be mediated by cAMP. In apparent support of the proposed role for cAMP in the s-IPSP response, McAfee and Greengard[65] found that theophylline could augment both the s-IPSP and the hyperpolarizing response to exogenous DA. It now turns out, however, that this action of theophylline cannot be attributed to the inhibition of phosphodiesterase by this drug and is instead due to another additional cellular effect by theophylline[53]. Indeed, the inability of more specific and potent inhibitors of phosphodiesterase to augment the s-IPSP[53] argues against the proposed s-IPSP role for cAMP.

The effects of phosphodiesterase inhibition in relation to the DA-modulatory role for cAMP are more difficult to assess, since they are potentially multiple and even mutually opposite in direction[53]. Nevertheless, the phosphodiesterase inhibitors have been found to have effects that were at least compatible with a cAMP role as mediator of the DA-induction of the modulatory change in the muscarinic responses to ACh, i.e., in the s-EPSP[53].

(iii) The relative timing of the physiological vs. the cAMP-chemical processes appears to argue against the role in the s-IPSP, but in favor of that in the DA-modulatory action (on the s-EPSP)[53]. Synaptic delays for s-IPSP's are in the range of about

25 msec (rabbit SCG at 37°C) to 100 msec (frog ganglion at 22°C)[47,60]; and peak amplitudes of s-IPSP's are achieved by about 150 msec or 500–600 msec, at 37°C and 22°C, respectively. These time characteristics are very long when compared to the analogous values for fast PSP's, but they appear to be far too short to accommodate the times required for cAMP changes and actions. The rise in ganglionic cAMP, following a 20-sec period of preganglionic nerve stimulation, was found to require minutes to be detectable and to require about five to 10 minutes to achieve the peak rise[1]. Furthermore, the putative sequence of enzymatic activities set into motion by cAMP[31] appears to operate with time constants of at least hundreds of msec for each step, and would add substantial time before the final physiological change could appear[53]. On the other hand, development of the neuronal changes that mediate the DA-modulation of the s-EPSP does indeed appear to require minutes[61], even when cAMP is injected intracellularly[43].

    b)   Guanosine 3′, 5′-cyclic monophosphate (cGMP) was suggested as the intracellular mediator of the s-EPSP response to ACh, on the basis of the slow depolarizing response elicited by cGMP at $50 \mu M$[65]. The two further crucial conditions that must be established for such a role appear now to have been fulfilled: (i) *Muscarinic cholinergic action* can induce a substantial rise in cGMP concentration within ganglion cells of bovine SCG[31,39]; and preganglionic nerve stimulation was reported to raise cGMP in frog ganglia[86]. (ii) *In the lower concentration range* of 25 to 100 μM, cGMP has now been consistently shown to be able to elicit a depolarization of ganglion cells (rabbit SCG), with no change in membrane conductance attributable to cGMP action[35]. This unique type of depolarization is in accord with that expected for the s-EPSP itself (see above). (When cGMP was in a higher concentration range of 250 to 1000 μM, it elicited an even larger depolarization which was accompanied by a large increase in membrane conductance that was independent of the level of membrane potential[35]. This second type of depolarization may be a nonspecific one and can lead to confusion in evaluating the physiological role of cGMP. It may be related to the increases in conductance which can be elicited by either cGMP or cAMP when injected intracellularly in sufficient amounts[28,74], and it may explain the cGMP depolarization of a nonsynaptic structures like peripheral nerves[65]. (The extraordinary synaptic delay of the s-EPSP, 200–300 msec[47], its electrogenesis by a mechanism other than that of changes in ionic conductance[35,40,41] and its special sensitivity to loss of oxidative metabolism[40,48], all indicate that a series of energy-consuming reactions lie between the ACh-receptor combination and the final appearance of the slow depolarization[48]; this situation lends itself to mediation by a nucleotide such as cGMP.

    Another kind of postsynaptic effect of cGMP in this system has been discovered[61]; in this system, cGMP can fully antagonize the development of the long-lasting modulatory change in the s-EPSP by cAMP. This effect is remarkably time-dependent; cGMP can antagonize or "disrupt" the modulatory process only if it is applied during the initial period of five to 15 min after exposure to DA or cAMP[61]. Some preliminary evidence indicates that cGMP produced endogenously by a strong muscarinic action on ganglion cells may also be capable of producing such a disruptive effect on the DA-modulatory change in the s-EPSP.

It should be noted, if cAMP mediates the DA-modulatory action on s-EPSP and if cGMP mediates the s-EPSP response itself, the physiological role of cAMP would be to synergize rather than to oppose the role of cGMP. The two nucleotides would, in sympathetic ganglia, not follow the proposed rule "that cAMP and cGMP act in a dualistic opposing fashion"[30,39,78]. However, it is possible that the additional capability of cGMP to antagonize the cAMP modulatory action[61] may become physiologically significant when cGMP levels in the cell achieve sufficiently high values; the cGMP could then prevent any enhancement by cAMP of the cGMP-mediated s-EPSP, in a kind of negative-feedback manner. If so, there could, depending on the conditions, be both synergistic and opposing interactions between the two nucleotides, in relation to actions on the long-lasting modulation of the post-synaptic responses elicited by the synaptic transmitter ACh.

Physiological Significance of Slow Synaptic Actions

An adequate answer to this question, in relation to the normal operations of the autonomic nervous system in the intact animal, still awaits further investigation by those working in that area. One available approach to studying this question consists in employing selective pharmacological blockade of both slow PSP's by atropinic agents, in concentrations that have no effect on the nicotinically-mediated (fast) EPSP's or on the postganglionic firing produced by the EPSP's[8,20,22,45]. In addition, the s-IPSP is selectively sensitive to α-adrenergic antagonists[22,58], although it is difficult to achieve as full a blockade of the orthodromically-elicited s-IPSP with a "cleaner" competitive antagonist like dihydroergotamine than it is with agents like phenoxybenzamine or dibenamine which have weak atropinic side effects[48,55]. Of course, atropine and α-adrenergic antagonists can affect autonomic responses by their effects at the more peripheral effector sites; their use in studying slow PSP roles at the ganglionic level therefore requires analysis of discharge responses in postganglionic nerves.

Some studies employing such an approach have already shown that at least the potentialities for significant physiological participation by an *s-EPSP* do exist (see Brown[9], deGroat[17], Janig[38], and related findings for myenteric plexus, Wood[89]).

A role for the *s-IPSP* in regulating ganglionic excitability has always been more difficult to establish[20,34a,45], because any s-IPSP contribution to depressed excitability appears in parallel with after-hyperpolarizing potentials due to firing of ganglion cells. The ability of individual preganglionic nerve fibers to elicit a pure s-IPSP in a given ganglion cell does exist[57]. Therefore, the potentiality appears to exist for the selective inhibition of one functional class of ganglion cells coupled with excitation of another class, in a manner reminiscent of reciprocal inhibition in the spinal cord[48]. Any such differential effects would presumably have to be limited to relatively crude and large groupings of ganglion cells; the inhibitory interneurons, the SIF cells, are few in number[88], and each must therefore innervate hundreds or even thousands of ganglion cells[49,50,56]. The present possibility for selective activation of such fibers (for s-IPSP) in substantial numbers, among the total in a "mixed" preganglionic nerve, lies in studying responses or actions organized by the central nervous system portions of the intact autonomic nervous system—in the case of responses that appear to involve inhibition at ganglionic levels[3,17,29]. The alternative possibility of eliciting ganglionic inhibition via an anatomically selective group of "inhibitory" fibers apparently can occur[17].

Are the slow PSP's large enough to be significant?   It has been argued by some[67,76] that the amplitudes of s-IPSP and s-EPSP responses recorded intracellularly are generally too small to be physiologically significant. Even the direct application of exogenous DA or of ACh often gives rise, respectively, to postsynaptic hyperpolarizing or muscarinic-depolarizing responses that are relatively small[19] or absent[77]. However, one must be reminded that both of the slow PSP's are much more labile than is the (f)EPSP or the action potential. The slow PSP's are easily depressed by a number of now specifiable conditions, which will be discussed below as possible explanations of the observed smaller amplitudes.

a)   Resting membrane potentials.   Both the s-IPSP and s-EPSP are much more sensitive than the (f)EPSP to changes in resting potential in the range close to the presumed normal one of about -60 to -70 mV; they are both depressed markedly by either depolarization or hyperpolarization and appear to be near their maxima at a resting potential of about -70 mV[40,41]. The different responses in nicotinized frog ganglia may have somewhat different characteristics, as noted above (see refs. 40, 41 and 70). Most intracellular recordings in sympathetic ganglion cells, especially in mammalian ganglia, are made on partially damaged cells with resting potentials already depolarized below the -60 to -70 mV range, because of the special difficulties with impalement by the microelectrode in these structures. Consequently one would expect these slow PSP's to be small compared to what they would be in intact cells. In fact, recordings of the population responses of intact ganglion cells, by means of surface electrodes, often exhibit amplitudes of s-IPSP's and s-EPSP's that are quite substantial[22,45,48]. If the amplitude of similarly recorded, relatively synchronous compound action potentials of the same population of neurons are taken to reflect actual transmembrane changes of 100 mV or more, the cellular amplitudes of the slow PSP's (as estimated from the ratios of PSP/action potential in surface recordings) could reach levels of 25 mV and more. Indeed, there is evidence that the s-EPSP's in intact ganglion cells can be large enough to fire the cells directly; this is based on the selective elimination by atropine of prolonged postganglionic after-discharges that follow brief preganglionic trains (e.g., Brown[9]; McIsaac[66]).

b)   Loss of s-IPSP with depletion of DA *in vitro*.   After excision of the rabbit SCG from the animal there is a progressive, though not linear, loss of the s-IPSP response with time[56], which can progress to complete abolition of the s-IPSP. This loss is speeded up by repeated stimulations of the preganglionic nerve, but it is quite substantial even with no stimulation. The state of s-IPSP response is correlated with the DA content of the SIF cells[56]. The s-IPSP response is virtually completely abolished when total DA concentration in SIF cells has been cut by about 50%; and the "lost" s-IPSP can be restored, at least in part, by temporary exposure to DA[58], which results in a re-uptake of DA by depleted SIF cells[56]. Obviously, any inferences about s-IPSP amplitudes in relation to the physiological significance of this PSP could be strongly colored by the state of functional DA in the interneurons during a given experiment. This variable factor could be responsible for differences between reports of incidence and amplitudes of s-IPSP's in samplings of ganglion cells within a given ganglion.

c) Sensitivity of s-EPSP to loss of oxidative metabolism. The s-EPSP was found to be selectively depressed by various conditions that reduce oxidative metabolism: anoxia, azide, cyanide and dinitrophenol[40,48]. Such a factor could account, for example, for the inability of Larrabee and Bronk[44] to detect heterosynaptic post-tetanic potentiation (PTP) in the stellate ganglion of cat; in their classic investigation of PTP they found that potentiation of test responses was restricted to those elicited homosynaptically, by the same orthodromic line that had been tetanically stimulated, and concluded that PTP was purely a presynaptic function. However, it was later shown by Libet[45] that a large component of heterosynaptic PTP could also be exhibited by this ganglion; this had a time course not so different from the homosynaptic component, but it was clearly due to a postsynaptic change, the s-EPSP. The failure to detect such a heterosynaptic PTP in the earlier study[44] might easily have been due to a reduction in blood flow to the ganglion, brought about by compression of blood vessels by the chamber applied to the ganglion *in vivo*. In addition, we have found that excessive stretch or tension on the rabbit SCG in a chamber tends to depress the s-EPSP or the slow muscarinic depolarizing responses to ACh[57] (Hsu and Libet, unpublished).

There is good reason to believe, therefore, that both the s-IPSP and s-EPSP can be sufficiently large, under normal physiological conditions, to affect neuronal excitability levels and firing in significant ways. (See also, for parasympathetic ganglia[17,89].) The inhibiting effect of the hyperpolarizing s-IPSP would be limited to the change it could produce in the amount of superimposed depolarization needed to achieve the firing threshold; as was pointed out by Nishi[67], there would not be the additional depressant effect on size of the (f)EPSP's that can result from the drop in g_m during the fast IPSP's.

Is presynaptic depression by DA (or NE) more significant than s-IPSP responses to DA (or NE)? When applied exogenously, the catecholamines have been shown to depress the amount of ACh released by presynaptic terminals (reviewed[67,68]). This presynaptic action of exogenous catecholamines appears to be more effective than the postsynaptic action. It was therefore proposed[19,67] that the presynaptic depressant, rather than the postsynaptic hyperpolarizing action, can account for most of the observed depression of "ganglionic transmission" by exogenous catecholamines, a depression first described by Marrazzi[64]. However, one must distinguish an action based solely on the effect of an exogenously applied agent (that may be purely pharmacological, albeit potent, in nature) from an action that can be developed by the endogenous dopamine, released via morphologically-existent routes and in conditions that are physiological. In contrast to the case for the s-IPSP (postsynaptic inhibition), there is as yet no firm evidence that presynaptic inhibition by catecholamines is actually producible by preganglionic nerve impulses. Also, there is no morphological evidence for adrenergic terminations onto cholinergic presynaptic terminals; i.e., no axo-axonal synapses have been found in which the presynaptic terminals contain dense core vesicles (Elfvin; Grillo, personal communications), whereas those containing clear vesicles have been described[24,33]. (A finding that haloperidol enhanced the s-IPSP response of cat SCG[28a] has been interpreted as being due to an action on DA-releasing presynaptic terminals, in which haloperidol would antagonize a presumed inhibitory effect of DA on these terminals. However, there are alternative possibilities for interpreting this finding; for example, haloperidol may block the postsynaptic DA-modulatory receptor[52] and thereby make more DA available for binding to the postsynaptic s-IPSP receptor.)

Significance of the special features of slow PSP's.

a)   Durations.   The relatively long durations of the slow PSP's are obviously compatible with and appropriate to the tonic operations and slow types of reactions that characterize the autonomic nervous system.

b)   Absence of increases in conductance.   Since there are no increases in g_m, the slow PSP's can provide long-lasting changes in membrane potential without significant intracellular losses or gains of certain species of ions, and there is therefore no need to expend energy to restore ionic balances. The s-IPSP and s-EPSP can thus provide relatively sustained changes in neuronal excitability much more efficiently than could the (fast)EPSP.

c)   Decreases in conductance?   It has been proposed that a decrease in g_m during an s-EPSP could serve to reduce the shunting effects of the resting g_m on (fast)EPSP's; in this view, the chief function of the s-EPSP would thus lie in enlarging any (f)EPSP's elicited during the course of the s-EPSP, rather than in direct effects of s-EPSP depolarization on membrane excitability[73]. However, this proposed role for the s-EPSP could not ordinarily be a physiologically significant one; it could only come into play in cells that are considerably depolarized (e.g., by impalement for intracellular recordings). An s-EPSP elicited when resting potentials are about −70 mV would show no appreciable change in g_m[35] (see above) and would not produce any enlargement of EPSP responses.

SUMMARY

Slow s-IPSP's and s-EPSP's are exhibited by various autonomic ganglia of vertebrates, the s-EPSP being particularly prominent and ubiquitous in mammalian sympathetic ganglia. The direct transmitter for s-IPSP's is apparently in all cases a catecholamine, released intraganglionically by the action of preganglionic ACh inputs on interneuronal-type structures. Dopamine (DA) is found to be the specific transmitter for one s-IPSP in rabbit sympathetic cervical ganglion (SCG); more recent evidence indicates that norepinephrine is the transmitter for another s-IPSP component that is mediated via a nonmuscarinic pathway in the ganglion.

Electrogenesis of either s-IPSP's or s-EPSP's elicited under physiologically normal conditions is not accompanied by or dependent on any increases or decreases in ionic conductances of the membrane. (In depolarized cells, the raised resting conductance for K^+, the so-called delayed rectification, can apparently be reversed by ACh, leading to another slow depolarizing component accompanied by a decrease in conductance. Treatment of frog ganglia with nicotine can greatly accentuate the latter type of response of the B cells to ACh; it can also make possible a direct hyperpolarizing response of the C cells to ACh. These abnormal and different slow depolarizing or hyperpolarizing responses should not be confused with the "physiological" s-EPSP and s-IPSP, respectively.)

Cyclic AMP (cAMP) appears to mediate the intracellular induction of a second postsynaptic action of DA; in this a brief action by DA leads to a modulatory enhancement of the s-EPSP responses to ACh that lasts for hours. cAMP appears not to mediate the hyperpolarizing s-IPSP response to DA. Cyclic GMP (cGMP) does appear to be the intracellular mediator for slow muscarinic depolarizing response to ACh, the s-EPSP. (In sufficient amounts, cGMP can also antagonize induction of the enduring modulatory change, in the s-EPSP responses, that is otherwise elicited by exposure to DA, or to cAMP.)

The unique features of the s-IPSP's and s-EPSP's constitute potentially important modes of postsynaptic responses in sympathetic ganglia. They provide for relatively long-lasting interactions of heterosynaptic inputs, both excitatory and inhibitory, and can thereby greatly increase the available kinds of ganglionic integrations. Evidence indicates that the slow PSP's of intact ganglionic neurons can be sufficiently large to be physiologically significant; conditions that can lead to the recording of relatively small or even absent PSP's are analyzed.

The full participation and impact of the s-IPSP's and s-EPSP's in physiological operations of the autonomic nervous system are yet to be established. The possible physiological role of the enduring modulatory action by synaptically-released DA, on the s-EPSP responses to ACh, is presently even more obscure. In any case, however, the existence of such types of synaptic processes provides models for possible analogous postsynaptic actions which could be of fundamental importance in mediating slow and enduring functional events in the brain.

This research was supported by U.S. Public Health Service Research Grant NS-00884 from the National Institute of Neurological and Communicative Disorders and Stroke.

REFERENCES

1   Aleman, V., Bayon, A. and Molina, J., Functional changes of synapses, *Adv. behav. Biol.*, 10 (1974) 115–124.

2   Baker, N. A., Redick, J. A., Schnute, W. J. and Van Orden, L. L. III, Neurotransmitter identification in small, fluorescent cells of rat paracervical ganglia by microspectrofluorometry and immunohistochemistry, *(Soc.) Neurosci. Abstr.*, 4th Ann. Meeting (1974) 126.

3   Beck, L., DuCharme, D. W., Gebber, G. L., Levin, J. A. and Pollard, A. A., Inhibition of adrenergic activity at a locus peripheral to the brain and spinal cord, *Circulation Res.* Suppl. I, Vols. 28 and 29 (1966) I-55–I-69.

3a   Bishop, G. H. and O'Leary, J., Pathways through the sympathetic nervous system in the bullfrog, *J. Neurophysiol.*, 1 (1938) 442–454.

4   Björklund, A., Cegrell, L., Falck, B., Ritzén, M. and Rosengren, E., Dopamine-containing cells in sympathetic ganglia, *Acta physiol. scand.*, 78 (1970) 334–338.

5   Black, A. C., Jr., Chiba, T., Wamsley, J. K., Bhalla, R. C. and Williams, T. H., Interneurons of sympathetic ganglia: Divergent cyclic AMP responses and morphology in cat and cow, *Brain Res.*, 148 (1978) 389–398.

6 Blackman, J. G. and Purves, R. D., Ganglionic transmission in the autonomic nervous system, *N. Z. med. J.*, 67 (1968) 376–384.

7 Blackman, J. G., Ginsborg, B. L. and Ray, C., Synaptic transmission in the sympathetic ganglion of the frog, *J. Physiol.* (Lond.), 167 (1963) 355–373.

8 Brimble, M. J., Wallis, D. I. and Woodward, B., Facilitation and inhibition of cell groups within the superior cervical ganglion of the rabbit, *J. Physiol.* (Lond.), 226 (1972) 629–652.

9 Brown, A. M., Cardiac sympathetic adrenergic pathways in which synaptic transmission is blocked by atropine sulphate, *J. Physiol.* (Lond.), 191 (1967) 271–288.

10 Bülbring, E., The action of adrenaline on transmission in the superior cervical ganglion, *J. Physiol.* (Lond.), 103 (1944) 55–67.

11 Burnstock, G., Interactions of cholinergic, adrenergic, purinergic and peptidergic neurons in the gut. This volume, pp. 145–158.

12 Busis, N. A., Weight, F. F. and Smith, P. A., Synaptic potentials in sympathetic ganglia: Are they mediated by cyclic nucleotides? *Science*, 200 (1978) 1079–1081.

13 Chen, S. S., Effects of divalent cations and of catecholamines on the late response of the superior cervical ganglion, *J. Physiol.* (Lond.), 253 (1975) 443–457.

14 Chiba, T., Black, A. C., Jr. and Williams, T. H., Evidence for dopamine-storing interneurons and paraneurons in rhesus monkey sympathetic ganglia, *J. Neurocytol.*, 6 (1977) 441–453.

15 Dall, W. G., Jr., Histochemical and fine structural studies of SIF cells in the major pelvic ganglion of the rat. In: O. Eränkö (Ed.), *SIF Cells: Structure and Function of the Small, Intensely Fluorescent Sympathetic Cells*, U.S. Government Printing Office, Washington, D. C., 1976, pp. 8–18.

16 Dail, W. G., Jr. and Wood, J., Studies on the possibility of an extraganglionic source of adrenergic terminals to the superior cervical ganglion, *(Soc.) Neurosci. Abstr.*, III (1977) 248.

17 De Groat, W. C., Booth, A. M. and Krier, J., Interaction between sacral parasympathetic and lumbar sympathetic inputs to pelvic ganglia. This volume, pp. 234–247.

18 Dun, N. J. and Karczmar, A. G., Involvement of the interneuron in the generation of the slow inhibitory postsynaptic potential in mammalian sympathetic ganglia, *Proc. nat. Acad. Sci. USA*, 75 (1978) 4029–4032.

19 Dun, N. and Nishi, S., Effects of dopamine on the superior cervical ganglion of the rabbit, *J. Physiol.* (Lond.), 239 (1974) 155–164.

20 Dunant, Y. and Dolivo, M., Relations entre les potentials synaptiques lents et l'excitabilite du ganglion sympathique chez le Rat, *J. Physiol.* (Paris), 59 (1967) 281–294.

21 Eccles, J. C., *The Physiology of Synapses*, Springer, Berlin, 1964, 316 pp.

22 Eccles, R. M. and Libet, B., Origin and blockade of the synaptic responses of curarized sympathetic ganglia, *J. Physiol.* (Lond.), 157 (1961) 484–503.

23 Elfvin, L.-G., The ultrastructure of the superior cervical sympathetic ganglion of the cat. II. The structure of the preganglionic end fibers and the synapses as studied by serial sections, *J. Ultrastruct. Res.*, 8 (1963) 441–476.

24 Elfvin, L.-G., Ultrastructural studies on the synaptology of the inferior mesenteric ganglion of the cat, *J. Ultrastruct. Res.*, 37 (1971) 411–425.

25 Elfvin, L.-G., Hökfelt, T. and Goldstein, M., Fluorescence microscopical, immunohistochemical and ultrastructural studies on sympathetic ganglia of the guinea pig, with special reference to the SIF cells and their catecholamine content, *J. Ultrastruct. Res.*, 51 (1975) 377–396.

26 Eränkö, O., *SIF Cells: Structure and Function of the Small, Intensely Fluorescent Sympathetic Cells*, U.S. Government Printing Office, Washington, D. C., 1976, 260 pp.

27 Eränkö, O. and Eränkö, L., Small intensely fluorescent, granule-containing cells in the sympathetic ganglion of the rat, *Progr. Brain Res.*, 34 (1971) 39–52.

27a Francini, F. and Urbani, F., Pathways and synapses location in the lumbar sympathetic trunk of the frog (*Rana esculenta*), *Arch. Fisiol.*, 68 (1970–71) 182–197.

28 Gallagher, J. P. and Shinnick-Gallagher, P., Cyclic nucleotides injected intracellularly into rat superior cervical ganglion cells, *Science*, 198 (1977) 851–852.

28a Gardier, R. W., Tsevdos, E. J. and Jackson, D. B., The effect of pancuronium and gallamine on muscarinic transmission in the superior cervical ganglion, *J. Pharmac. exp. Ther.*, 204 (1978) 46–53.

29 Gebber, G. L. and Beck, L., Reflex inhibition of sympathetic vasoconstrictor activity at a peripheral locus, *Circulation Res.*, 18 (1966) 714–728.

30 Goldberg, N. D., O'Dea, R. F. and Haddox, M. K., Cyclic GMP. In: P. Greengard and G. A. Robinson (Eds.), *Advances in Cyclic Nucleotide Research*, Vol. 3, Raven Press, New York, 1973, pp. 155–223.

31 Greengard, P., Possible role for cyclic nucleotides and phosphorylated membrane proteins in postsynaptic actions of neurotransmitters, *Nature*, 260 (1976) 101–108.

32 Greengard, P. and Kebabian, J. W., Role of cyclic AMP in synaptic transmission in the mammalian peripheral nervous system, *Fed. Proc.*, 33 (1974) 1059–1067.

33 Grillo, M. A., Ultrastructural studies on catecholamine release from SIF cells, *J. cell Biol.*, 75 (1977) 118a.

34 Haefely, W., Electrophysiology of the adrenergic neuron. In: H. Blaschko and E. Muscholl (Eds.), *Handbook of Experimental Pharmacology*, Vol. 33, Springer-Verlag, Berlin, 1972, pp. 661–725.

34a Haefely, W., Muscarinic postsynaptic events in the cat superior cervical ganglion *in situ*, *Naunyn-Schmiedeberg's Arch. Pharmacol.*, 281 (1974) 119–143.

35 Hashiguchi, T., Ushiyama, N., Kobayashi, H. and Libet, B., Does cyclic GMP mediate the slow excitatory postsynaptic potential: Comparison of changes in membrane potential and conductance, *Nature*, 271 (1978) 267–268.

36 Hirst, G. D. S. and Silinsky, E. M., Some effects of 5-hydroxytryptamine, dopamine and noradrenaline on neurones in the submucous plexus of guinea-pig small intestine, *J. Physiol.* (Lond.), 251 (1975) 817–832.

37 Hökfelt, T., Elfvin, L.-G., Schultzberg, M., Fuxe, K., Said, S. I., Mutt, V. and Goldstein, M., Immunohistochemical evidence of vasoactive intestinal polypeptide-containing neurons and nerve fibers in sympathetic ganglia, *Neuroscience*, 2 (1977) 885–896.

38 Jänig, W., Reciprocal reaction patterns of sympathetic subsystems with respect to various afferent inputs. This volume, pp. 263–274.

39 Kebabian, J. W., Steiner, A. L. and Greengard, P., Muscarinic cholinergic regulation of cyclic guanosine 3′, 5′-monophosphate in autonomic ganglia: Possible role in synaptic transmission, *J. Pharmac. exp. Ther.*, 193 (1975) 474–488.

40 Kobayashi, H. and Libet, B., Generation of slow postsynaptic potentials without increase in ionic conductance, *Proc. nat. Acad. Sci. USA*, 60 (1968) 1304–1311.

41 Kobayashi, H. and Libet, B., Actions of noradrenaline and acetylcholine on sympathetic ganglion cells, *J. Physiol.* (Lond.), 208 (1970) 353–372.

42 Kobayashi, H. and Libet, B., Is inactivation of potassium conductance involved in slow postsynaptic excitation of sympathetic ganglion cells? Effects of nicotine, *Life Sci.*, 14 (1974) 1871–1883.

43 Kobayashi, H., Hashiguchi, T. and Ushiyama, N., Postsynaptic modulation by cyclic

AMP, intra- or extra-cellularly applied, or by stimulation of preganglionic nerve, in mammalian sympathetic ganglion cells, *Nature*, 271 (1978) 268–270.

44 Larrabee, M. G. and Bronk, D. W., Prolonged facilitation of synaptic excitation in sympathetic ganglia, *J. Neurophysiol.*, 10 (1947) 139–154.

45 Libet, B., Slow synaptic responses and excitatory changes in sympathetic ganglia, *J. Physiol.* (Lond.), 174 (1964) 1–25.

46 Libet, B., Slow synaptic responses in autonomic ganglia. In: D. R. Curtis and A. K. McIntyre (Eds.), *Studies in Physiology*, Springer-Verlag, Berlin, 1965, pp. 160–165.

47 Libet, B., Long latent periods and further analysis of slow synaptic responses in sympathetic ganglia, *J. Neurophysiol.*, 30 (1967) 494–514.

48 Libet, B., Generation of slow inhibitory and excitatory postsynaptic potentials, *Fed. Proc.*, 29 (1970) 1945–1956.

49 Libet, B., The SIF cell as a functional dopamine-releasing interneuron in the rabbit superior cervical ganglion. In: O. Eränkö (Ed.), *SIF Cells: Structure and Function of the Small, Intensely Fluorescent Sympathetic Cells*, U.S. Government Printing Office, Washington, D. C., 1976, pp. 163–177.

50 Libet, B., The role SIF cells play in ganglionic transmission. In: E. Costa and G. L. Gessa (Eds.), *Nonstriatal Dopaminergic Neurons, Adv. in Biochem. Psychopharmacol.*, Vol. 16, Raven Press, New York, 1977, pp. 541–546.

51 Libet, B., Roles of intraganglionic catecholamines in slow synaptic actions, *Proc. int. Union physiol. Sci.*, 12 (1977) 558.

52 Libet, B., Dopaminergic synaptic processes in the superior cervical ganglion: models for synaptic actions. In: A. Horn, J. Korf and B. H. C. Westerink (Eds.), *The Neurobiology of Dopamine*, Academic Press, Inc., London, (1979) in press.

53 Libet, B., Which postsynaptic action of dopamine is mediated by cyclic AMP? *Life Sci.*, 24 (1979) 1043–1058.

54 Libet, B. and Kobayashi, H., Generation of adrenergic and cholinergic potentials in sympathetic ganglion cells, *Science*, 164 (1969) 1530–1532.

55 Libet, B. and Kobayashi, H., Adrenergic mediation of the slow inhibitory postsynaptic potential in sympathetic ganglia of the frog, *J. Neurophysiol.*, 37 (1974) 805–814.

56 Libet, B. and Owman, CH., Concomitant changes in formaldehyde-induced fluorescence of dopamine interneurones and in slow inhibitory postsynaptic potentials of rabbit superior cervical ganglion, induced by stimulation of preganglionic nerve or by a muscarinic agent, *J. Physiol.* (Lond.), 237 (1974) 635–662.

57 Libet, B. and Tosaka, T., Slow inhibitory and excitatory postsynaptic responses, in single cells of mammalian sympathetic ganglia, *J. Neurophysiol.*, 32 (1969) 43–50.

58 Libet, B. and Tosaka, T., Dopamine as a synaptic transmitter and modulator in sympathetic ganglia; a different mode of synaptic action, *Proc. nat. Acad. Sci. USA*, 67 (1970) 667–673.

59 Libet, B. and Tosaka, T., Dopaminergic synaptic actions in sympathetic ganglia, *Fed. Proc.*, 30 (1971) 323.

60 Libet, B., Chichibu, S. and Tosaka, T., Slow synaptic responses and excitability in sympathetic ganglia of the bullfrog, *J. Neurophysiol.*, 31 (1968) 383–395.

61 Libet, B., Kobayashi, H. and Tanaka, T., Synaptic coupling into the production and storage of a neuronal memory trace, *Nature*, 258 (1975) 155–157.

62 Libet, B., Tanaka, T. and Tosaka, T., Different sensitivities of acetylcholine-induced "after-HP" compared to dopamine-induced hyperpolarization, to ouabain or to lithium-replacement of sodium, in rabbit sympathetic ganglia, *Life Sci.*, 20 (1977) 1863–1870.

63 Lundberg, A., Adrenaline and transmission in the sympathetic ganglion of the cat, *Acta physiol. scand.*, 26 (1952) 251–263.

64 Marrazzi, A. S., Adrenergic inhibition at sympathetic synapses, *Amer. J. Physiol.*, 127 (1939) 738–744.

65 McAfee, D. A. and Greengard, P., Adenosine 3', 5'-monophosphate: electrophysiological evidence for a role in synaptic transmission, *Science*, 178 (1972) 310–312.

66 McIsaac, R. J., Afterdischarge on postganglionic sympathetic nerves following repetitive stimulation of the preganglionic nerve to the rat superior cervical ganglion *in vitro*, *J. Pharmac. exp. Ther.*, 200 (1977) 107–116.

67 Nishi, S., Ganglionic transmission. In: J. H. Hubbard (Ed.) *The Peripheral Nervous System*, Plenum, New York, 1974, pp. 225–255.

68 Nishi, S., The catecholamine-mediated inhibition in ganglionic transmission. This volume, pp. 223–233.

69 Nishi, S. and Koketsu, K., Early and late after-discharges of amphibian sympathetic ganglion cells, *J. Neurophysiol.*, 31 (1968) 109–121.

70 Nishi, S., Soeda, H. and Koketsu, K., Unusual nature of ganglionic slow EPSP studied by a voltage-clamp method, *Life Sci.*, 8 (1969) 33–42.

71 Noon, J. P., McAfee, D. A. and Roth, R. H., Norepinephrine release from nerve terminals within the rabbit superior cervical ganglion, *Naunyn-Schmiedeberg's Arch. Pharmacol.*, 291 (1975) 139–162.

72 Ritchie, J. M. and Straub, R. W., The hyperpolarization which follows activity in mammalian non-medullated fibres, *J. Physiol.* (Lond.), 136, (1957) 80–97.

73 Schulman, J. A. and Weight, F. F., Synaptic transmission: Long-lasting potentiation by a postsynaptic mechanism, *Science*, 194 (1976) 1437–1439.

74 Shinnick-Gallagher, P., Williams, B. J. and Gallagher, J. P., Biochemical and electrophysiological studies of cyclic nucleotides and their effects in the rat superior cervical ganglion, (*Soc.*) *Neurosci. Abstr.*, II (2) (1976) 800.

75 Skok, V. I., Conduction in tenth ganglion of the frog sympathetic trunk, *Fed. Proc.*, 24: Transl. Suppl. (1965) T363–T367.

76 Skok, V. I., *Physiology of Autonomic Ganglia*, Igaku Shoin, Ltd., Tokyo, 1973, 197 pp.

77 Skok, V. I. and Selyanko, A. A., Acetylcholine and serotonin receptors in mammalian sympathetic ganglion neurons. This volume, pp. 248–253.

78 Stone, T. W., Taylor, D. A. and Bloom, F. E., Cyclic AMP and cyclic GMP may mediate opposite neuronal responses in the rat cerebral cortex, *Science*, 187 (1975) 845–847.

79 Tosaka, T. and Libet, B., Slow postsynaptic potentials recorded intracellularly in sympathetic ganglia of frog, *Intern. Congr. Physiol. Sci.*, *23rd*, Tokyo, 1965, p. 386.

80 Tosaka, T., Chichibu, S. and Libet, B., Intracellular analysis of slow inhibitory and excitatory postsynaptic potentials in sympathetic ganglia of the frog, *J. Neurophysiol.*, 31 (1968) 396–409.

81 Van Orden, L. S. III, Burke, J. P., Geyer, M. and Lodoen, F. V., Localization of depletion-sensitive and depletion-resistant norepinephrine storage sites in autonomic ganglia, *J. Pharmac. exp. Ther.*, 174 (1970) 56–71.

82 Volle, R. L., Enhancement of postganglionic responses to stimulating agents following repetitive preganglionic stimulation, *J. Pharmac. exp. Ther.*, 136 (1962) 68–74.

83 Wallis, D. I. and North, R. A., Synaptic input to cells of the rabbit superior cervical ganglion, *Pflügers Arch.*, 374 (1978) 145–152.

84 Watanabe, H. and Burnstock, G., Postsynaptic specializations at excitatory and inhibitory cholinergic synapses, *J. Neurocytol.*, 7 (1978) 119–133.

85 Weight, F. F. and Padjen, A., Acetylcholine and slow synaptic inhibition in frog sympathetic ganglion cells, *Brain Res.*, 55 (1973) 225–228.

86 Weight, F. F., Petzold, G. and Greengard, P., Guanosine 3′, 5′-monophosphate in sympathetic ganglia: Increase associated with synaptic transmission, *Science*, 186 (1974) 942–944.

87 Williams, T. H., Black, A. C., Jr., Chiba, T. and Bhalla, R. C., Morphology and biochemistry of small intensely fluorescent cells of sympathetic ganglia, *Nature*, 256 (1975) 315–317.

88 Williams, T. H., Chiba, T., Black, A. C., Jr., Bhalla, R. C. and Jew, J., Species variation in SIF cells of superior cervical ganglia: are there two functional types? In: O. Eränkö (Ed.), *SIF Cells: Structure and Function of the Small, Intensely Fluorescent Sympathetic Cells*, U.S. Government Printing Office, Washington, D. C., 1976, pp. 143–162.

89 Wood, J. D., Neurophysiology of the enteric nervous system. This volume, pp. 177–193.

CHAPTER 14

THE CATECHOLAMINE-MEDIATED INHIBITION IN GANGLIONIC TRANSMISSION

Syogoro Nishi

Department of Physiology, Kurume University School of Medicine, Kurume, Japan

INTRODUCTION

The sympathetic ganglion has long been regarded as a prototype of a mono-synaptic system in which impulse transmission is mediated by the nicotinic action of acetylcholine (ACh). Studies in the last two decades have disclosed that the ganglion possesses not only the nicotinic system but also a muscarinic system[15,49,50] and in some vertebrates an additional noncholinergic[4-7,38] transmission system. Moreover, presynaptic[8,9,13,37] and postsynaptic[15] inhibitory systems, both of which are mediated by a catecholamine, have also been found. This paper will describe first the nature of the presynaptic adrenoceptor which can be activated either by epinephrine, norepinephrine or dopamine and subserves as the site to initiate presynaptic inhibition. Secondly, the slow inhibitory postsynaptic potential (slow IPSP), i.e., the hyper-polarizing response associated with the activation of the postsynaptic dopaminoceptor[28,30] will be considered with particular reference to its electrogenesis.

RESULTS AND DISCUSSION

Presynaptic Inhibition

The depressant action of epinephrine on ganglionic transmission, originally reported by Marrazzi[35], has been shown by many investigators[2,15,36,42]. Yet the mechanism of this depression has not been elucidated completely. Lundberg[33] suggested that epinephrine hyperpolarizes the postsynaptic membrane, but this change in membrane potential is not always present when transmission is depressed by epinephrine. Paton and Thompson[43] proposed that epinephrine has a dual action on the ganglion cells; it may not only reduce the ACh output from presynaptic terminals but also depress postsynaptic sensitivity to the transmitter. Contrary to their common blocking action, an enhancement of transmission has also been found when lower doses of catecholamines were administered[2,3,34,47]. Furthermore, blocking doses of catecholamines have been observed to potentiate the ganglionic response to ACh[20,25]. Costa et al.[10] showed that ganglionic transmission is enhanced following administration of dibenamine or after depletion of ganglionic catecholamines with reserpine.

In 1966, De Groat and Volle[11] disclosed that sympathetic ganglia contain two pharmacologically distinctive sites; one, which is blocked by α-adrenergic blocking agents, mediates catecholamine-induced inhibition and ganglionic hyperpolarization, and the other, which is blocked by β-adrenergic blocking agents, mediates catecholamine-induced facilitation and ganglionic depolarization. Thus, they demonstrated the existence of postsynaptic α- and β-adrenoceptors which are, respectively, responsible for the inhibitory and facilitatory actions of catecholamines on the ganglion.

Several years later, Christ and Nishi[8] found that epinephrine or norepinephrine inhibits the orthodromic impulse transmission in rabbit superior cervical ganglion (SCG) cells by reducing the amplitude of EPSP generated at the nicotinic subsynaptic membrane. They reached the conclusion that the depression of EPSP induced by pressor amines is primarily caused by the decrease in transmitter output and that this action is exerted through an α-adrenoceptive site at the presynaptic nerve terminals.

This section will describe a) how the concept of adrenergic presynaptic inhibition has been formulated, b) what the mechanism underlying the catecholaminergic presynaptic inhibition is, and c) whether dopamine, which has been identified as being liberated from the intraganglionic chromaffin-like cells[28], can depress transmission presynaptically.

Catecholamine-induced depression of EPSP. Superfusion of rabbit SCG with a solution containing 10 μM epinephrine causes in many cells a rapid blockade of the orthodromic action potential, which leaves an EPSP with a markedly attenuated amplitude and rate of rise[8]. The minimum effective concentration of epinephrine ranges between one μM and five μM among different cells and 10 μM of epinephrine reduces EPSP amplitude by 30–70%. Norepinephrine and isoproterenol at concentrations of 10 μM also depress the EPSP amplitude, but their blocking actions are much weaker and slower than that of epinephrine. The order of depressant potency is epinephrine, norepinephrine and isoproterenol. An α-adrenergic blocking agent, such as phenoxybenzamine or dihydroergotamine, which does not in itself affect the EPSP at a concentration of 10 μM, quite effectively antagonizes the blocking action of epinephrine. The α-blocking action of phenoxybenzamine and dihydroergotamine develops very slowly; thus they have to be given for at least 10 min before epinephrine. Furthermore, they are relatively irreversible, as epinephrine is ineffective for several hours after withdrawal of the α-blocker from the perfusing medium. In contrast, the β-adrenergic blocking agents, such as propranolol and dichlorisoproterenol, show no antagonistic influence on epinephrine action. This experimental evidence indicates that the depressant action of epinephrine or norepinephrine is exerted via an α-adrenoceptive site.

Depression of impulse transmission with 10 μM epinephrine, which is completed in a few min, is not associated with any change in the resting membrane potential. Prolonged perfusion with 10 μM epinephrine for more than five min generally produces a small depolarization not exceeding five mV. The same concentration of epinephrine does not alter electrotonic potentials induced by small current pulses. Moreover, the threshold level, amplitude or time course of cell-body action potential is also unaffected by 10 μM epinephrine. Only when the epinephrine concentration is raised to one mM is there a consistent slow depolarization of five to 15 mV which is occasionally preceded by a short-lasting hyperpolarization less than five mV in amplitude. It can be surmised therefore that a lowering of membrane excitability is an unlikely mechanism of epinephrine blockade since the threshold depolarization is not altered. Also, epinephrine does not appear to reduce EPSP amplitude by increasing cell membrane conductance, since there is no change in electrotonic potentials. Moreover, the inability of epinephrine to hyperpolarize the cell membrane at a concentration at which blockade of transmission occurs, or even at much higher concentrations, indicates that hyperpolarization is not the primary mechanism of epinephrine blockade.

One of the crucial observations in regard to the site of catecholamine-induced blockade is that epinephrine does not alter the amplitude and time course of the postsynaptic depolarization induced by ACh applied either by superfusion or iontophoresis[8,37]. A typical example of the effect of epinephrine on the EPSP and the iontophoretically-elicited ACh potential of a single SCG cell of the rabbit is shown in Fig. 1. It can be seen that epinephrine depresses the EPSP but has no effect on the ACh potential. This characteristic action of epinephrine is most easily explained by hypothesizing a presynaptic site for the blocking action of epinephrine.

Presynaptic mechanism of catecholamine action. It can be assumed then that activation of the presynaptic adrenoceptive site brings about a reduction of ACh output from the terminals. Indeed, the study of spontaneous and evoked EPSP's in the presence and absence of epinephrine substantiated this assumption[8,37]. Table 1 summarizes the frequency and amplitude of miniature EPSP's in five SCG cells (rabbit) superfused with a Krebs solution containing 20 mM KCl, before and after addition of epinephrine (10 μM). It is seen in the Table that epinephrine markedly decreases the frequency of miniature EPSP's but only slightly influences their amplitude. The

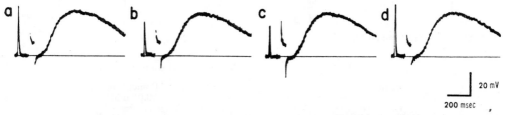

20 mV

200 msec

Fig. 1. Effect of epinephrine on the fast EPSP and ACh-potential recorded from a rabbit SCG cell. Records a and b were obtained, respectively, before and two min after control solution was switched to an epinephrine (0.01 mM) solution. Note the selective depression of the EPSP by epinephrine. Immediately after record b was taken, control solution was introduced again. Records c and d were taken one and three min after completion of epinephrine perfusion. The resting membrane potential was maintained at approximately −80 mV by applying a continuous anodal current to prevent spike generation by the EPSP and ACh-potential. The ACh was iontophoretically applied to the cell membrane from an ACh-filled microelectrode by current pulses of 0.5 μA with 50-msec duration (from Nishi, 1970[37]).

data shows clearly that epinephrine impairs the spontaneous release of transmitter with almost no effect on the quantal size of the transmitter. In Table 2 are shown the quantal contents of evoked EPSP of six SCG cells (rabbit) superfused with low Ca-high Mg solutions before and after addition of epinephrine (10 μM). The data yields that 10 μM of epinephrine reduces the quantal content by nearly 60%. This reduction in quantal content occurs without significant alteration in quantal size. Thus, in keeping with its effect on the spontaneous release of transmitter, epinephrine decreases the quantal release by nerve impulse but manifests no noticeable postsynaptic effects.

What then is the mechanism by which catecholamines decrease the release of transmitter? The most obvious possibility involves a change in the resting membrane potential of the nerve terminals. Christ and Nishi[9], however, found that epinephrine does not alter the threshold of the presynaptic nerve terminal nor the terminal membrane potential measured by the sucrose-gap technique[24]. This finding is consistent with the forementioned evidence that epinephrine decreases miniature EPSP frequency and decreases EPSP amplitude, since changes in the presynaptic membrane potential should affect miniature EPSP frequency and EPSP amplitude in a reciprocal manner[12,17,18,31,48]. The inability of epinephrine to change the threshold of the nerve terminal also eliminates the possibility that epinephrine produces its effect by a local anesthetic action. Such an action should cause a significant increase in threshold.

Table 1.   Effect of epinephrine on miniature EPSP's.

Frequency			Amplitude		
Control (n/sec)	Epinephrine (n/sec)	(% decrease)	Control (mV)	Epinephrine (mV)	(% decrease)
0.97	0.88	9	0.76	0.73	4
0.89	0.73	18	0.63	0.63	0
1.68	0.72	57	0.65	0.62	5
6.20	2.01	68	1.27	1.01	3
1.61	0.61	62	1.04	1.11	13
		43±11*			5±1.9*

* Mean ±1 SE (from Nishi, 1970[37]).

Table 2.   Effect of epinephrine on quantal content.

	Control				Epinephrine (0.01 mM)		
Failures	[Ca] (mM)	[Mg] (mM)	m	Failures	m	% decrease	q'/q
89	0.5	5.5	0.81	161	0.22	73	1.07
94	0.5	3.5	0.76	113	0.57	25	1.02
60	0.5	5.5	1.21	182	0.10	92	0.95
132	0.5	2.5	0.42	150	0.29	31	0.92
119	0.5	2.5	0.52	133	0.41	21	1.06
83	0.5	2.5	0.88	188	0.06	93	0.85
						56±12*	0.98±0.03*

* Mean ±1 SE (from Nishi, 1970[37]).

The decrease of quantal release, without potential changes in the nerve terminal membrane, indicate that epinephrine acts directly on the release mechanism. Although the steps involved in excitation-release coupling have not been completely elucidated, the best known step in the release mechanism is the influx of calcium ions during the action potential[19]. Epinephrine could produce blockade by decreasing the entry of calcium ions. In fact it was found that epinephrine is much less effective in a high-Ca medium; a five-fold increase in external Ca from two mM to 10 mM decreases the depressant effect of epinephrine to approximately one fourth[9]. This is in favor of the idea that the release site may be completely activated in 10 mM of Ca medium; thus a decrease in Ca entry by epinephrine cannot appreciably alter the quantal release.

Quantal content (m) of the EPSP is dependent on the number of quanta readily available for release (n) and the probability of release for each quantum (p), according to the relationship $m = np$. The EPSP's of rabbit SCG neurons decline in amplitude when the presynaptic nerve is stimulated at frequencies of 30–50 Hz. After the initial decline, the EPSP amplitude levels off to a constant value. This is probably the point at which mobilization equals release. The initial decline is due to depletion of n[32,45,46]. When m of each EPSP in the head of the train is plotted against depletion, namely the sum of previous m in a train, the slope of the line is equal to p and the intercept of the X axis is equal to n[16]. As mentioned earlier, epinephrine decreases m, and it is interesting to examine by this method whether the epinephrine action is due to a decrease in n, or p or both. p is well known to be dependent upon the amount of Ca influx at the nerve terminal. Christ and Nishi's analysis of rabbit SCG neurons[8] indicated that the decrease in m by epinephrine is primarily due to a decrease in n; p is not significantly decreased. The EPSP's in guinea-pig myenteric neurons are also presynaptically depressed by catecholamines[41]. Analysis of the myenteric neuron EPSP with the aid of a computer program by North and Nishi[41] and Katayama and Nishi showed clearly that the decrease in m by catecholamines is due to a reduction in p. It is difficult to understand why epinephrine decreases n in SCG neurons, while the result obtained from myenteric neurons is consistent with the concept that the activation of the presynaptic α-adrenoceptor causes a reduction of Ca entry which in turn results in the decrease of transmitter liberation.

Dopamine and presynaptic inhibition. Since dopamine-containing neurons have been identified in the sympathetic ganglion[1,26,44] and since preganglionic stimulation actually induces liberation of dopamine from the intraganglionic chromaffin-like cells[28], it is worthwhile to investigate whether dopamine can depress ganglionic transmission presynaptically like other catecholamines[13]. Dun and Nishi[13] have shown that dopamine decreases miniature EPSP frequency without affecting their amplitude, and that dopamine decreases quantal content of evoked EPSP's without changing quantal size and without altering the amplitude of ACh-induced depolarization. Thus the dopamine action is characteristically similar to that of pressor amines; it decreases liberation of ACh from the presynaptic terminals. In addition to the presynaptic action, dopamine often causes a hyperpolarization of the postsynaptic membrane. This hyperpolarization, however, is small, only a few mV in amplitude, and not associated with any appreciable change in membrane conductance. It is conceivable therefore that the primary role of endogenous dopamine would be to mediate pre-synaptic inhibition rather than postsynaptic inhibition.

Postsynaptic Inhibition

A train of tetanic preganglionic stimuli produces in deeply curarized sympathetic ganglia a slow surface-positive potential (P potential) followed by a long-lasting surface-negative potential[14,15]. Eccles and Libet[15] postulated that an adrenergic substance, which is liberated from the intraganglionic chromaffin-like cells in response to the muscarinic action of endogenous ACh, encounters an α-adrenoceptive site on ganglion cells, and that this interaction results in the P potential. Intracellular recordings from curarized sympathetic ganglia proved that the P potential is truly an extracellular counterpart of a hyperpolarizing postsynaptic potential, which can be generated in the absence of any cellular discharge[29]. The P potential has since been referred to as the slow IPSP. Although the depressant action of the slow IPSP on the excitability of mammalian ganglion neurons has not been clearly demonstrated, it has been shown in amphibian sympathetic ganglia that a marked inhibition of afterdischarge occurs at the same time as the generation of P potential[23].

Inhibitory transmitter. Libet[28] and Libet and Tosaka[30] have shown recently that dopamine is the only catecholamine able to restore the slow IPSP of the ganglion in which catecholamines of chromaffin-like cells were believed to be depleted by bethanechol. They found, moreover, that incubation of ganglia with diethyldithio-carbamate, which inhibits the enzymatic conversion of dopamine to norepinephrine, specifically enhances the slow IPSP. Based on these findings Libet and Tosaka[30] proposed that dopamine is the transmitter that physiologically mediates the slow IPSP. More recently, Libet and Owman were able to identify dopamine, by means of formaldehyde histochemistry and cytospectrofluorometry, localized to the intra-ganglionic small intensely fluorescent (SIF) cells (chromaffin-like cells) in the rabbit SCG, and also to the characteristically beaded fibers forming a network in close contact with virtually all ganglion cell bodies. They measured the changes in the dopamine content of SIF cells in conjunction with changes in the slow IPSP of the ganglion under various conditions. The results well supported the hypothesis[27,30] that a dopamine interneuron is activated muscarinically by preganglionic nerve impulses and mediates the production of slow IPSP in sympathetic ganglion cells.

Electrogenesis of the slow IPSP. Several different hypotheses have been proposed for the ionic mechanism of slow IPSP based on the extraordinary behavior of the slow IPSP in various experimental conditions. For example, the slow IPSP recorded from the surface of nicotinized bullfrog ganglia[23,38,39] is diminished and eventually abolished by depolarization, whereas it is markedly enhanced by moderate hyper-polarization. When the applied hyperpolarization is strong enough to nullify or reverse the afterhyperpolarization of a ganglionic action potential, the slow IPSP tends to decrease. A much stronger hyperpolarization eventually abolished the slow IPSP but cannot reverse the polarity of the response. In curarized rabbit ganglion cells, the slow IPSP is decreased in amplitude by progressive reduction of membrane potential and is nullified by a 20-mV depolarization. On the other hand, the amplitude of the slow IPSP is increased by moderate hyperpolarization of 10–30 mV, although further hyperpolarization consistently produces a decrease in amplitude and the IPSP can usually be nullified by hyperpolarization somewhat greater than 30 mV. It should be pointed out that no alteration in membrane conductance is detected during the slow IPSP in either frog or rabbit ganglion cells[21,40].

Koketsu and Nishi[23] and Nishi and Koketsu[38,39] found in nicotinized frog sympathetic ganglia that alteration of the external Cl has little effect on the slow IPSP but also reported that the slow IPSP is depressed or abolished by ouabain, low temperature or the removal of the external K ions and is enhanced markedly after loading the ganglia with Na. On the basis of these results, they suggested that the slow IPSP is caused by synaptic activation of an electrogenic Na pump. Kobayashi and Libet[21], on the other hand, reported that removal of the extracellular K does not depress the slow IPSP; and further the depressant action of ouabain on the slow IPSP is not specific because there is also depression of the fast EPSP. They suggested that the electrogenetic mechanism of the slow IPSP may involve active transport, but that a ouabain-sensitive Na-K pump or a Cl pump are excluded as the generator. Weight and Padjen[51] proposed the alternative hypothesis that the slow IPSP is generated by a fall in Na conductance induced by transmitter action.

It should be mentioned that although the slow IPSP can be readily recorded from the surface of a curarized ganglion, intracellular recording of this response is difficult owing to its occurrence in a limited number of cells and its small amplitude. In addition, the slow IPSP generally occurs concomitantly with the slow EPSP which is produced by the muscarinic action of ACh on the ganglion cells. These properties have hampered the study of the slow IPSP and also contributed to the diversity of suggestions on its electrogenesis.

One of the most anomalous features reported is that the slow IPSP is not associated with any significant change in membrane conductance. However, the slow IPSP recorded intracellularly is, in general, only a few mV in amplitude. With such a small amplitude, it is difficult to asertain there is no conductance change.

With the expectation that a denervation supersensitivity would occur in the muscarinic site on the chromaffin-like cells and also in the dopamine receptor on the principal ganglion cells, Lees and Nishi chronically decentralized the rabbit SCG, usually for over 14 days, and applied acetylcholine iontophoretically to various points in the vicinity of a ganglion cell from which membrane potentials were recorded intracellularly.

When the acetylcholine electrode was successfully placed at an ideal position by the trial-and-error method, there occurred a slow hyperpolarizing response which was very similar in time course to the slow IPSP. The induced hyperpolarization increased its amplitude up to 20 to 25 mV in proportion to the strength of current pulses ejecting ACh from the ACh electrode. A relatively fast depolarizing response preceding the hyperpolarizing response was nicotinic in nature, and it was reversibly blocked by hexamethonium, leaving the hyperpolarizing response alone. When the control Krebs solution was switched to a low Ca–high Mg Krebs solution, the hyperpolarizing response slowly and gradually decreased in amplitude. Upon returning to the control solution, the hyperpolarizing response regained its amplitude in only a matter of some ten seconds, indicating that this response is not the product of a direct action of acetylcholine on the ganglion cell, but it is mediated by an element which liberates a hyperpolarizing substance when the element is activated by ACh. Atropine abolished this hyperpolarizing response, and phentolamine, a typical α-adrenergic blocking agent, depressed the hyperpolarizing response selectively. All these characteristics of the hyperpolarizing response are in keeping with the disynaptic mechanism of the slow IPSP suggested originally by Eccles and Libet[15]. The most crucial nature of this hyperpolarizing response was that it was associated with a small but definite reduction in membrane resistance (Fig. 2A). Furthermore, in contrast to the initial depolarizing response, the hyperpolarizing response was increased in amplitude by reducing the membrane potential level, while it was decreased and reversed by hyperpolarizing the membrane. The reversal level which could be clearly seen after eliminating the preceding depolarization by hexamethonium (Fig. 2B), was found to be approximately −95 mV on the average.

Based on the close pharmacological similarity of ACh-induced hyperpolarization to the slow IPSP and also on the disynaptic characteristic of ACh-induced hyperpolarization, Lees and Nishi have been inclined to assume that the hyperpolarizing response is the slow IPSP elicited by stimulation of chromaffin-like cells by the muscarinic action of ACh applied by iontophoresis. If this is the case, the slow IPSP in the rabbit SCG would be produced by an increased conductance to potassium ions. It can be surmised further that the slow IPSP induced by tetanic stimulation of the preganglionic trunk would be contaminated by various factors, which mask the essential nature of the slow IPSP. Such factors could possibly be the activation of an electrogenic Na-pump by a rise in external potassium after tetanic activation of presynaptic nerve terminals and a concomitant production of slow EPSP which is known to be associated with a reduction in membrane conductance[22,52].

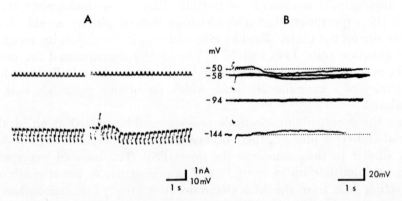

Fig. 2.   A: Reduction of membrane resistance during ACh-induced hyperpolarization of a rabbit SCG neuron. Left and right records show electrotonic potentials elicited repetitively before (left) and during (right) the hyperpolarizing response evoked by ACh iontophoretically applied by a pulse of 0.2 μA with a duration of 100 msec. Upper trace: current pulses delivered through the cell membrane. B: reversal of ACh-induced hyperpolarizing response of a rabbit SCG neuron. The levels of membrane potential at which the responses were evoked are indicated in mV.

CONCLUSIONS

The sympathetic ganglion is endowed with pre- and postsynaptic inhibitory systems both of which are mediated normally by dopaminergic neurons in the ganglion. Should a situation in which excessive impulses invade the ganglion arise, a large amount of dopamine would be liberated into the intraganglionic fluid and minimize ACh liberation from the presynaptic nerve terminals and at the same time safeguard the postganglionic outflow of discharges by antagonizing the excitatory postsynaptic currents with a dopamine-produced hyperpolarizing current. Our most recent experiment indicates that the ACh-induced slow hyperpolarization is disynaptic in nature and its pharmacological characteristic is essentially similar to that of the slow IPSP. Moreover the hyperpolarization is generated by a selective increase in potassium conductance.

This study was supported in part by the Ministry of Education, Science and Culture of Japan.

REFERENCES

1 Björklund, A., Cegrell, L., Falck, B., Ritzén, M. and Rosengren, E., Dopamine-containing cells in sympathetic ganglia, *Acta physiol. scand.*, 78 (1970) 334–338.
2 Bülbring, E., The action of adrenaline on transmission in the superior cervical ganglion, *J. Physiol.* (Lond.), 103 (1944) 55–67.
3 Bülbring, E. and Burn, J. H., An action of adrenaline on transmission in sympathetic ganglia which may play a part in shock, *J. Physiol.* (Lond.), 101 (1942) 289–303.
4 Chen, S. S., Late contraction of nictitating membrane of the dog, *Amer. J. Physiol.*, 217 (1969) 1205–1210.
5 Chen, S. S., Transmission in superior cervical ganglion of the dog after cholinergic suppression, *Amer. J. Physiol.*, 221 (1971) 209–213.
6 Chen, S. S., Late discharges in dog's sympathetic ganglia, *Can. J. Physiol.*, 50 (1972) 263–269.
7 Chen, S. S., Effects of divalent cations and of catecholamines on the late response of the superior cervical ganglion, *J. Physiol.* (Lond.), 253 (1975) 443–457.
8 Christ, D. D. and Nishi, S., Site of adrenaline blockade in the superior cervical ganglion of the rabbit, *J. Physiol.* (Lond.), 213 (1971) 107–117.
9 Christ, D. D. and Nishi, S., Effects of adrenaline on nerve terminals in the superior cervical ganglion of the rabbit, *Br. J. Pharmac.*, 41 (1971) 331–338.
10 Costa, E., Revzin, A. M., Kuntzman, R., Spector, S. and Brodie, B. R., Role for ganglionic norepinephrine in sympathetic synaptic transmission, *Science*, 133 (1961) 1822–1823.
11 De Groat, W. C. and Volle, R. L., The actions of the catecholamines on transmission in the superior cervical ganglion of the cat, *J. Pharmac. exp. Ther.*, 154 (1966) 1–13.
12 del Castillo, J. and Katz, B., Changes in end-plate activity produced by presynaptic polarization, *J. Physiol.* (Lond.), 124 (1954) 586–604.
13 Dun, N. and Nishi, S., Effects of dopamine on the superior cervical ganglion of the rabbit, *J. Physiol.* (Lond.), 239 (1974) 155–164.

14 Eccles, R. M., Responses of isolated curarized sympathetic ganglia, *J. Physiol.* (Lond.), 117 (1952) 196–217.

15 Eccles, R. M. and Libet, B., Origin and blockade of the synaptic responses of curarized sympathetic ganglia, *J. Physiol.* (Lond.), 157 (1961) 484–503.

16 Elmqvist, D. and Quastel, D. M., A quantitative study of end-plate potentials in isolated human muscle, *J. Physiol.* (Lond.), 178 (1965) 505–529.

17 Hubbard, J. I. and Willis, W. D., Hyperpolarization of mammalian motor nerve terminals, *J. Physiol.* (Lond.), 163 (1962) 115–137.

18 Hubbard, J. I. and Willis, W. D., The effects of depolarization of motor nerve terminals upon the release of transmitter by nerve impulses, *J. Physiol.* (Lond.), 194 (1968) 381–405.

19 Katz, B. and Miledi, R., The role of calcium in neuromuscular facilitation, *J. Physiol.* (Lond.), 195 (1968) 481–492.

20 Kewitz, H. and Reinert, H., Prüfung Pharmakologischer Wirkungen oberen sympathischen Halsganglion bei verschiedenen Erregungzuständen, *Arch. exp. Pathol. Pharmakol.*, 215 (1952) 547–555.

21 Kobayashi, H. and Libet, B., Generation of slow postsynaptic potentials without increases in ionic conductance, *Proc. nat. Acad. Sci. USA*, 60 (1968) 1304–1311.

22 Kobayashi, H. and Libet, B., Actions of norepinephrine and acetylcholine on sympathetic ganglion cells, *J. Physiol.* (Lond.), 208 (1970) 353–372.

23 Koketsu, K. and Nishi, S., Characteristics of the slow inhibitory postsynaptic potential of bullfrog sympathetic ganglion cells, *Life Sci.*, 6 (1967) 1827–1836.

24 Koketsu, K. and Nishi, S., Cholinergic receptors at sympathetic preganglionic nerve terminals, *J. Physiol.* (Lond.), 196 (1968) 293–310.

25 Konzett, H., Sympathomimetica und Sympathicolytica am isoliert durchströmten Ganglion Cervicale superius der Katze, *Helv. physiol. pharmac. Acta*, 8 (1950) 245–258.

26 Lavery, R. and Sharman, D. F., The estimation of small quantities of 3, 4-dihydroxyphenylethylamine in tissues, *Br. J. pharmac. Chemother.*, 24 (1965) 538–548.

27 Libet, B., Generation of slow inhibitory and excitatory postsynaptic potentials, *Fed. Proc.*, 29 (1970) 1945–1056.

28 Libet, B. and Owman Ch., Concomitant changes in formaldehyde-induced fluorescence of dopamine interneurones and in slow inhibitory postsynaptic potentials of the rabbit superior cervical ganglion, induced by stimulation of the preganglionic nerve or by a muscarinic agent, *J. Physiol.* (Lond.), 237 (1974) 635–662.

29 Libet, B. and Tosaka, T., Slow postsynaptic potentials recorded intracellularly in sympathetic ganglia, *Fed. Proc.*, 25 (1966) 270.

30 Libet, B. and Tosaka, T., Dopamine as a synaptic transmitter and modulator in sympathetic ganglia: A different mode of synaptic action, *Proc. nat. Acad. Sci. USA*, 67 (1970) 667–673.

31 Liley, A. W., The effects of presynaptic polarization on the spontaneous activity at the mammalian neuromuscular junction, *J. Physiol.* (Lond.), 134 (1956) 427–443.

32 Liley, A. W. and North, K. A. K., An electrical investigation of effects of repetitive stimulation on mammalian neuromuscular junction, *J. Neurophysiol.*, 16 (1953) 509–527.

33 Lundberg, A., Adrenaline and transmission in the sympathetic ganglion of the cat, *Acta physiol. scand.*, 26 (1952) 251–263.

34 Malméjac, J., Action of adrenaline on synaptic transmission and on adrenal medullary secretion, *J. Physiol.* (Lond.), 130 (1955) 497–512.

35 Marrazzi, A. S., Adrenergic inhibitoin at sympathetic synapses, *Amer. J. Physiol.*, 127 (1939) 738–744.

36 Matthews, R. J., The effect of epinephrine, levarterenol and DL-isoproterenol on transmission in the superior cervical ganglion of the cat, *J. Pharmac. exp. Ther.*, 116 (1956) 433–443.

37 Nishi, S., Cholinergic and adrenergic receptors at sympathetic preganglionic nerve terminals, *Fed. Proc.*, 29 (1970) 1957–1965.

38 Nishi, S. and Koketsu, K., Early and late after-discharges of amphibian sympathetic ganglion cells, *J. Neurophysiol.*, 31 (1968) 109–121.

39 Nishi, S. and Koketsu, K., Analysis of slow inhibitory postsynaptic potential of bullfrog sympathetic ganglion, *J. Neurophysiol.*, 31 (1968) 717–728.

40 Nishi, S. and Koketsu, K., Underlying mechanisms of ganglionic slow IPSP and post-tetanic hyperpolarization of pre- and postganglionic elements, *Proc. Int. Union Physiol. Sci.*, VII (1968) 321.

41 North, R. A. and Nishi, S., Properties of the ganglion cells of the myenteric plexus of the guinea-pig ileum determined by intracellular recording. *Proceedings of the Fourth International Symposium on Gastrointestinal Motility*, Banff, Canada, (1973) 667–676.

42 Pardo, E. G., Cato, J., Gijon, E. and Alonso de Florida, F., Influence of several adrenergic drugs on synaptic transmission through the superior cervical and the ciliary ganglia of the cat, *J. Pharmac. exp. Ther.*, 139 (1963) 296–303.

43 Paton, W. D. M. and Thompson, J. W., The mechanism of action of adrenaline on the superior cervical ganglion of the cat, *Int. Physiol. Congr.*, 19 (1953) 664.

44 Schumann, H. J., Nachweis von Oxytryamin (Dopamin) in sympathischen Nerven und Ganglion, *Arch. exp. Path. Pharmak.*, 227 (1956) 566–573.

45 Takeuchi, A., The long-lasting depression in neuromuscular transmission of frog, *Jap. J. Physiol.*, 8 (1958) 102–113.

46 Thies, R. E., Neuromuscular depression and apparent depletion of transmitter in mammalian muscles, *J. Neurophysiol.*, 28 (1965) 427–442.

47 Trendelenburg, U., Modification of transmission through the superior cervical ganglion of the cat, *J. Physiol.* (Lond.), 132 (1956) 529–541.

48 Vladimirova, I. A., Effect of electrical polarization of motor nerve endings on transmission of single impulses, *Fed. Proc.*, 23 (1964) T1127–T1128.

49 Volle, R. L., The actions of several ganglion blocking agents on the postganglionic discharge induced by diisopropyl phosphorofluoridate (DFP) in sympathetic ganglia, *J. Pharmac. exp. Ther.*, 135 (1962) 45–53.

50 Volle, R. L. and Koelle, G. B., The physiological role of acetylcholinesterase (AChE) in sympathetic ganglia, *J. Pharmac. exp. Ther.*, 133 (1961) 223–240.

51 Weight, F. F. and Padjen, A., Slow synaptic inhibition: Evidence for synaptic activation of sodium conductance in sympathetic ganglion cells, *Brain Res.*, 55 (1973) 219–224.

52 Weight, F. F. and Votava, J., Slow synaptic excitation in sympathetic ganglion cells: Evidence for synaptic inactivation of potassium conductance, *Science*, 170 (1970) 755–758.

CHAPTER 15

INTERACTION BETWEEN SACRAL PARASYMPATHETIC AND LUMBAR SYMPATHETIC INPUTS TO PELVIC GANGLIA

W. C. de Groat, A. M. Booth and J. Krier

Department of Pharmacology, School of Medicine, University of Pittsburgh, Pittsburgh, Pennsylvania, USA

INTRODUCTION

The pelvic plexus of the cat is a complicated network of ganglia and nerve fibers through which important autonomic reflexes are transmitted to the urinary bladder and large intestine[12,34,35,36]. The plexus is formed by afferent and efferent fibers branching from: (1) the pelvic nerve, (2) the hypogastric nerve and (3) the caudal sympathetic chain[29,34,35,36]. The pelvic nerve contains sacral parasympathetic preganglionic axons which provide the major excitatory input to the urinary bladder and large intestine, whereas the hypogastric nerve provides an inhibitory input to these organs and an excitatory input to the anal and urethral sphincters. Pathways from the sympathetic chain are primarily vasomotor[33,34,35].

Ganglia in the pelvic plexus and on the surface of the urinary bladder are more complex than prevertebral and paravertebral ganglia since they contain various types of principal ganglion cells (adrenergic, cholinergic and purinergic)[9,28,29,32,33], as well as adrenergic small intensely fluorescent cells (SIF cells) which seem to mediate synaptic interactions between sympathetic and parasympathetic pathways in the pelvic plexus. An anatomical substrate for ganglionic interactions between the sympathetic and parasympathetic systems was first indicated by histofluorescence studies[28,32,33], which showed that adrenergic terminals occur in close apposition to nonadrenergic, presumably parasympathetic, neurons in vesical ganglia of the cat. The terminals remained after decentralization of the ganglia indicating that they were of intraganglionic origin, possibly arising from SIF cells[32,33]. More recent studies[9] of the rat pelvic ganglia using electron microscopy have identified afferent cholinergic inputs to SIF cells, and efferent contacts from SIF cells to nonadrenergic ganglion cells. Various histochemical and morphological evidence indicated that the majority of SIF cells in the rat pelvic ganglion contain norepinephrine.

A possible synaptic modulatory function of SIF cells in vesical and pelvic ganglia

was suggested[28,32,33] based on known effects of exogenous and endogenous catecholamines in other autonomic ganglia. For example, the work of Marrazzi[41] and
Bulbring[3] established that exogenous catecholamines have both inhibitory and
facilitatory effects on ganglionic transmission. De Groat and Volle[23,24] showed in the
superior cervical ganglion of the cat that the inhibitory responses were mediated by
α-receptors and associated with ganglionic hyperpolarization, whereas the facilitatory responses were mediated by β-receptors and associated with ganglionic depolarization. Evidence for a physiological role of adrenergic inhibition in the superior
cervical ganglia of the rabbit was provided by Eccles and Libet[27] and later by Libet
and co-workers[38,39] who showed that endogenously-released catecholamines produced
a hyperpolarization (slow IPSP) of the ganglion cells. Various evidence, which will
be reviewed in detail by other contributors to this volume[39,43], indicated that the
hyperpolarizing potential was mediated by dopamine released from SIF cells and
that these cells were in turn activated by preganglionic cholinergic axons. Various
mechanisms for the production of slow IPSP's have been suggested including activation of adenylate cyclase and increased synthesis of cyclic AMP[31], although this
mechanism now seems unlikely on the basis of recent findings[25,30,39,43]. It should
be mentioned also that adrenergic inhibition elicited in ganglia by exogenous
catecholamines has a presynaptic component, i.e., a depression of acetylcholine
release[7,26,43], but this has yet to be demonstrated for catecholamines released endogenously.

Thus the potential exists for both inhibitory and facilitatory interactions between
sympathetic and parasympathetic inputs to pelvic ganglion cells. The present studies
were undertaken to examine these interactions in pelvic ganglia of the urinary bladder
and large intestine of the cat. In the course of this work we used multiunit recording
techniques *in situ* and to a limited extent intracellular recording *in vitro*. The results
indicate that transmission in bladder and intestinal ganglia differ considerably with
regard to the integration of sympathetic and parasympathetic inputs and also in
regard to sensitivity to exogenous catecholamines.

METHODS

Experiments were performed on cats anesthetized with dial-urethane or chloralose. Ganglia on the serosal surface of the urinary bladder or distal colon[14,35,36]
were exposed through a midline abdominal incision and postganglionic fibers were
prepared for monophasic recording. Branches of the pelvic nerve (preganglionic)
to each ganglion were sectioned and the peripheral stump was mounted on stimulating electrodes. Sympathetic postganglionic nerves including the hypogastric and
lumbar colonic nerves were also isolated and placed on stimulating electrodes. Postganglionic action potentials were recorded by standard techniques and averaged with
a digital computer. Activity of the bladder and intestine was monitored by measuring
intraluminal pressures with water-filled open-ended cannulae or balloons. Drugs
were administered through a cannula inserted into the aorta via the renal artery or
inferior mesenteric artery.

Experiments were also conducted on pelvic ganglia, *in vitro*. Ganglia from the

surface of the bladder or from the pelvic plexus along with the pelvic and hypogastric nerves were rapidly isolated and transferred to a recording chamber, where
they were superfused with Kreb's solution maintained at 34–36°C. Preganglionic
and postganglionic nerves were drawn into suction electrodes for either stimulation
or recording. Intracellular recording from ganglion cells was obtained with micropipettes filled with 3M KCl or 2M K citrate.

RESULTS

Facilitation in Parasympathetic Pathways to Pelvic Ganglia

Investigations of the micturition and defecation reflex pathways revealed that
continuous stimulation of afferent fibers in the pelvic nerve at relatively low frequencies (0.5–2 Hz) produced a gradual recruitment or facilitation of the evoked
discharges in parasympathetic postganglionic pathways to the bladder[17] and colon[15].
It was not determined, however, whether the facilitation was related to increased
transmission in central pathways or in peripheral ganglia. Experiments on decentralized ganglia have examined this question with multiunit and intracellular recording.

As shown in Fig. 1A continuous stimulation of preganglionic axons in the pelvic
nerves or sacral ventral roots elicited responses in vesical postganglionic nerves which
gradually increased in amplitude. Depending on the frequency of stimulation (one
to four Hz) the discharge increased two to 13 times over control levels obtained at
low frequencies (0.25 Hz) of stimulation (Fig. 1D). The number of shocks necessary
to produce maximal facilitation ranged from 17 to 45 (mean 27) in different experiments and seemed to be unrelated to the frequency of stimulation[20]. The facilitation
of transmission persisted for several minutes after termination of the stimulus. Facilitation was considerably smaller in colonic ganglia. As shown in Fig. 1B, D the evoked
responses in colonic postganglionic nerves increased one to two times over control
values at frequencies of preganglionic stimulation between two to four Hz[13,14]. A
similar divergence in facilitation in the two ganglion preparations was observed with
regard to the duration and magnitude of the facilitatory response to a single stimulus.
In bladder ganglia a conditioning stimulus to the preganglionic nerve markedly
(two to seven times) increased the response to a second stimulus for intervals up to
1000 msec, whereas in colonic ganglia the facilitation was much smaller and of very
short duration (100 msec) (Fig. 1C).

Slow EPSP's which are mediated via muscarinic receptors and blocked by
atropine have been implicated in recruitment in sympathetic ganglia[37]. However,
facilitation in pelvic ganglia was not affected by atropine. This and other indirect
data obtained with homo- and heterosynaptic conditioning procedures indicated that
facilitation was mediated by a presynaptic mechanism which enhanced the release
of acetylcholine from the preganglionic nerve terminals[20].

Facilitation in pelvic ganglia was also demonstrated with intracellular recordings
in vitro[1]. Two populations of ganglion cells were studied: (1) cells on the surface of the
urinary bladder and (2) cells in the pelvic plexus. The function and the effector
organs innervated by the latter cells are unknown.

Recordings were obtained from 80 bladder ganglion cells which had resting

GANGLIONIC FACILITATION

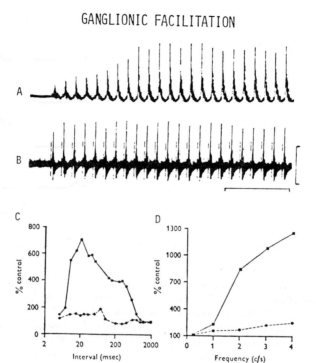

Fig. 1. Facilitation of transmission in vesical (A) and colonic (B) parasympathetic ganglia by repetitive stimulation (six Hz) of preganglionic axons in the sacral ventral roots. Horizontal calibration is equivalent to one second. Vertical calibration represents 250 μV in A and 100 μV in B. C: homosynaptic testing in colonic (●⋯●) and bladder (■—■) ganglia. The test response was elicited by supramaximal stimulation of the preganglionic nerves in the S2 ventral root at frequencies of 0.4 Hz. Single conditioning stimuli were also applied to the same preganglionic nerves at supramaximal intensities at frequencies of 0.4 Hz. The ordinate is the area of the colonic and vesical response expressed as the % control response while the abscissa is the interval in milliseconds between the conditioning and test stimuli. D: maximum facilitation obtained in parasympathetic ganglia of the colon (●⋯●) and bladder (■—■) during different frequencies of stimulation of preganglionic of fibers in the S2 ventral root. The ordinate is the area of the postganglionic discharge expressed as the % control response. The abscissa is the frequency of stimulation. Each point represents the computer average of ten responses. Parts C and D reproduced with permission from *Journal of Physiology*.

membrane potentials between 40–65 mV (mean 50 mV), action potentials ranging between 60–120 mV (mean 74 mV) and membrane resistances between five–84 Mohm (mean 26 Mohm). Forty cells in the pelvic plexus had similar properties. The cells could be fired at high frequencies (50–100 Hz) by intracellular depolarizing current but only fired synaptically at frequencies up to 10–15 Hz.

EPSP's elicited by submaximal preganglionic stimulation below the threshold for firing the cells were markedly facilitated at frequencies of stimulation above one Hz. Maximal facilitation occurred during the first 10–15 stimuli (Fig. 2A) and

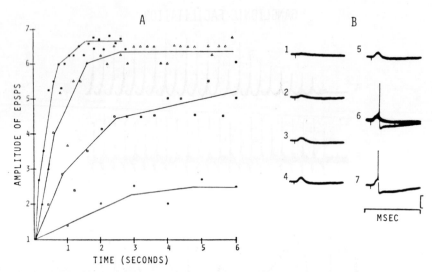

Fig. 2.   Facilitation of EPSP's in bladder parasympathetic ganglion cells by repetitive stimulation of the preganglionic fibers in the pelvic nerve. A: time course of facilitation.
The abscissa is time in seconds after the initiation of a stimulus train and the ordinate
is the amplitude of EPSP's in arbitrary units. Records are included for frequencies of
stimulation at 1 Hz (O), 2.5 Hz (□), 5 Hz (△) and 7.2 Hz (■). B: records from another
cell showing a series of EPSP's evoked at a frequency of one Hz. Records 1–7 represent
the responses evoked by first, second, fourth, tenth, twelfth, sixteenth and twenty-
fifth stimuli in the train. Horizontal calibration is 100 msec, vertical calibration
20 mV. The spike is truncated.

was maintained at low frequencies but not at higher frequencies. The amplitude
of the EPSP's increased five to six times during the first one to two sec after the onset
of five to seven Hz stimulation. Some cells did not fire to supramaximal preganglionic
stimulation at low frequencies but did discharge at higher frequencies of stimulation
(Fig. 2B) as expected from results of the *in situ* experiments described above. The
firing threshold for most cells ranged from six–18 mV. When cell firing was blocked
by hyperpolarizing the membrane, EPSP amplitudes at the maximum of the facilitation ranged from 20–40 mV. The enhancement of EPSP's persisted for one to two
min following termination of stimulation. Similar results were obtained with cells in
bladder ganglia and in the pelvic plexus.

The period of facilitation following single shocks was also explored using homo-
and heterosynaptic conditioning procedures. Stimulation of one preganglionic input
to a cell facilitated the EPSP's elicited by a subsequent stimulus to that same input for
200–500 msec, but did not alter the responses elicited by stimulation of another
preganglionic pathway. This indicates that the facilitation occurred via a presynaptic
mechanism.

A considerable number of cells in the pelvic plexus and a smaller number in
bladder ganglia exhibited spontaneous firing and low amplitude potentials having
the appearance of EPSP's. The firing but not the synaptic potentials could be blocked
by hyperpolarizing the cells or by repetitive stimulation (10–30 Hz, for 10 sec) of the

preganglionic input to the cells. The synaptically-evoked depression lasted for two–10 sec.

Sympathetic Input to Pelvic Ganglia

The influence of the sympathetic nerves on transmission in pelvic ganglia has been studied primarily with multiunit recording from postganglionic nerves *in situ*. It was shown that electrical stimulation of the hypogastric nerves at frequencies (five–30 Hz) which depressed the activity of the urinary bladder and colon produced inhibition and facilitation in bladder ganglia[18,19,21,44] but did not alter transmission in colonic ganglia (Fig. 3A)[14]. Inhibition was the primary effect but was followed by facilitation in 50% of the experiments[19]. Stimulation of the lumbar colonic nerves which contain the principal inhibitory pathways to the colon also had no effect on colonic ganglionic transmission[14]. Consistent with those observations, intra-arterial injection of norepinephrine (one–100 μg) or dopamine (10–100 μg) did not depress transmission in colonic ganglia but markedly depressed transmission in bladder ganglia (Fig. 3B). Transmission in both ganglia was depressed by other synaptic depressants, e.g., gamma aminobutyric acid (0.1–one mg) and tetraethylammonium (one–four mg). Thus, unlike most other autonomic ganglia[10,43] colonic ganglia appear to be resistant to exogenous catecholamines.

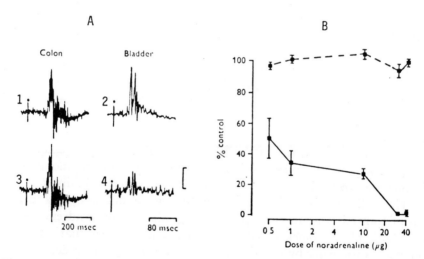

Fig. 3. Adrenergic inhibition in colonic and bladder parasympathetic ganglia. A: effects of stimulation of the ipsilateral hypogastric nerve (HGN 20 Hz, 20 V) on transmission in colonic and bladder ganglia. Discharges were recorded in postganglionic fibers to the colon and bladder and were elicited by electrical stimulation of preganglionic fibers in the S2 ventral root. Records 1 and 2 are control responses while records 3 and 4 were obtained during electrical stimulation of the hypogastric nerve. B: the effects of graded doses of norepinephrine on transmission in colonic and bladder ganglia. The ordinate represents the amplitude of the postganglionic discharge expressed as the % control response while the abscissa is the dose of norepinephrine on a log scale. Each point on the colonic (■···■) and bladder curve (■—■) represents the mean of four experiments. Reproduced with permission from *Journal of Physiology*.

Adrenergic inhibition and facilitation in bladder ganglia could be differentiated pharmacologically. Inhibition was elicited by agonists with α-receptor-stimulating actions (e.g., epinephrine, norepinephrine and dopamine) but was not mimicked by a selective β-receptor stimulant, isoproterenol, which produced only facilitation[19]. The inhibitory effects of endogenous and exogenous catecholamines were blocked by the administration of α-adrenergic blocking agents[19,45]. Treatment with α-blocking agents enhanced or unmasked facilitatory responses to norepinephrine and epinephrine, but not to dopamine[19]. The administration of propranolol, a β-blocking agent blocked the facilitation produced by isoproterenol but did not consistently affect the facilitation produced by injected norepinephrine or hypogastric nerve stimulation.

Adrenergic inhibition in bladder ganglia could also be elicited by activation of reflex pathways in the spinal cord[21]. As described in another paper[12] in this volume, the urinary bladder is subject to a feedback inhibition via the hypogastric nerve. Tension receptor afferents from the bladder travelling in the pelvic nerve to the sacral spinal cord elicit reflex firing in sympathetic efferents in the hypogastric nerve[16]. Electrical stimulation of this afferent pathway leads to reflex inhibition of transmission in bladder ganglia as well as inhibition of the detrusor smooth muscle via activation of β-receptors and contraction of the trigonal or internal sphincter region of the bladder[21]. These three reflex responses seem to be organized as a unit to promote the maintenance of urinary continence.

Electrophysiological evidence indicates that the peripheral pathway for the inhibitory reflex to bladder ganglia is composed in part of preganglionic axons that pass directly through the inferior mesenteric ganglion to make synaptic connections with inhibitory neurons in the pelvic plexus[19,44]. For example, it was shown that electrical stimulation of preganglionic fibers to the inferior mesenteric ganglia produced inhibition in the bladder ganglia even after transmission in the inferior mesenteric ganglia was blocked by the topical application of nicotine. Furthermore, after transection of the hypogastric nerve pharmacological activation of adrenergic inhibitory pathways in the plexus by the administration of cholinomimetic agents (acetylcholine and acetyl-B-methylcholine) elicited adrenergic inhibition in bladder ganglia[44]. This is illustrated in Fig. 4A. Acetyl-B-methylcholine produced a biphasic depression of transmission; the late phase being blocked by α-adrenergic blocking agents and both phases blocked with atropine. This suggests that cholinomimetic agents depress transmission by two different mechanisms: (1) a direct depression via muscarinic receptors and (2) activation of adrenergic inhibitory neurons via muscarinic receptors (Fig. 4B). Atropine did not block inhibition elicited by hypogastric stimulation, indicating that the adrenergic inhibitory neurons must be activated synaptically also by non-muscarinic receptors (Fig. 4B). By analogy with excitatory receptors on other peripheral adrenergic neurons, it seems likely that these receptors on inhibitory neurons are of the nicotinic type.

The mechanism underlying adrenergic inhibition in bladder ganglia has not been resolved. It is known that the inhibition occurs at a long latency (100–600 msec) after a train of pulses to the hypogastric nerve, suggesting that it might be mediated by a slow inhibitory process, such as the slow IPSP which has been identified in the

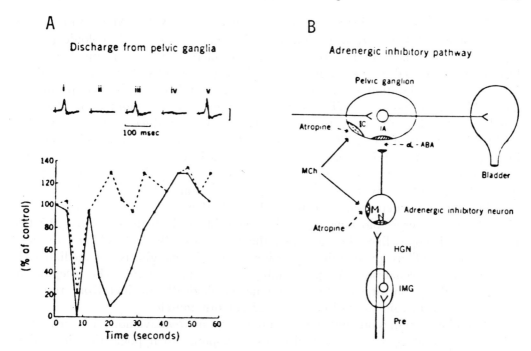

A

Discharge from pelvic ganglia

100 msec

B

Adrenergic inhibitory pathway

Fig. 4. Adrenergic inhibition in bladder parasympathetic ganglia. A: time course of ganglionic inhibitory effects to injection of acetyl-B-methylcholine (MCh five µg, i.a.).
Record i is the control discharge, and records ii, iii, iv, and v were taken 8, 12,
20, and 44 seconds, respectively, after an injection of MCh (five µg). Vertical calibration is 200 µv. Below is a graph of the depression by MCh (five µg) of the discharge,
before (solid line) and after (dashed line) the administration of dihydroergotamine
(200 µg). B: diagram of the proposed adrenergic inhibitory pathway, which is
activated by electrical stimulation of the hypogastric nerves (HGN); or by an
administered cholinomimetic agent (MCh). Muscarinic (M) and non-muscarinic
(N) receptors are depicted on adrenergic inhibitory neurons, and inhibitory cho-
linoceptive (IC) and inhibitory adrenoceptive (IA) sites are shown in the pelvic
ganglion. The latter receptors are not shown on any particular neural element since
their specific location has not been determined. The α-adrenergic blocking agent is
shown as α-ABA, and the inferior mesenteric ganglion is shown as IMG. The preganglionic nerve to the IMG is shown passing directly through the ganglion to synapse
with the adrenergic inhibitory neuron. Reproduced with permission from *Science*.

superior cervical ganglion (SCG) of the rabbit[38]. Recently it was proposed that slow
IPSP's are generated by activation of adenylate cyclase and increased synthesis of
cAMP[31]. To test this possibility experiments were conducted to examine the effects
of exogenous cAMP and theophylline, a phosphodiesterase inhibitor, on transmission
in bladder ganglia[22]. The intra-arterial injection of massive doses of cAMP and
dibutyryl cAMP (10–20 µmol) had virtually no effect on ganglionic transmission.
Furthermore, theophylline, which reportedly enhances slow IPSP's in the SCG did
not enhance adrenergic inhibition in bladder ganglia as expected if the inhibition
were mediated by the cAMP system.

In the course of these experiments, it was noted that although cAMP was ineffective as a ganglionic depressant, related nucleotides, AMP, ADP, ATP as well as adenosine, did depress transmission in bladder ganglia but not in colonic ganglia. Adenine, inosine and cGMP were inactive. A purinergic mechanism involving ATP has been implicated in postganglionic excitatory transmission in the bladder[4,6] but purinergic inhibition in bladder ganglia has not been considered previously. The inhibitory response to ATP in ganglia occurred at threshold doses (0.05–0.1 μmol, i.a.) which were one-tenth the dose necessary to produce an excitatory effect on bladder smooth muscle. The depressant effects of ATP were probably mediated in part via a postsynaptic depression since ATP blocked the direct excitation of the ganglion cells by tetramethylammonium. Evidence at other cholinergic synapses indicates that ATP may have a presynaptic depressant action as well[5].

The ganglionic depressant effects of ATP and other nucleotides were not antagonized by α-adrenergic blocking agents but were blocked by theophylline (0.5–two mg, i.a.)[22]. Theophylline did not block the excitatory effect of ATP on detrusor smooth muscle. Thus, purinergic depression in bladder ganglia is not mediated via an adrenergic mechanism and presumably occurs via receptors (P_1 receptors as characterized by Burnstock[5]) that are pharmacologically distinct from receptors involved in purinergic excitation in vesical smooth muscle.

Preliminary studies on vesical ganglia of the cat *in vitro* have not yet been successful in demonstrating adrenergic inhibition in response to hypogastric stimulation. We have shown, however, that sympathetic pathways in the hypogastric nerve provide an excitatory input to some neurons in the pelvic plexus. As illustrated in Fig. 5, this input from hypogastric nerve was weak, commonly producing only small EPSP's in response to single volleys. However, when transmission was facilitated by trains of stimuli (15–30 Hz, 100–200 msec train duration) EPSP's reached sufficient amplitude to fire the cells. The same cells also received an excitatory input from the pelvic nerve (Fig. 5A) which elicited large EPSP's and firing. The identify of the transmitter in the sympathetic excitatory pathway has not been established.

A similar excitatory input from the hypogastric nerve to ganglion cells in the pelvic plexus has been demonstrated in the guinea-pig[2]. This excitatory response was depressed by d-tubocurarine, indicating that it occurred via a cholinergic mechanism.

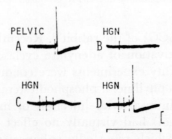

Fig. 5. Response of a ganglion cell in the pelvic plexus to stimulation of the pelvic nerve (A) and the hypogastric nerve (HGN) with single shocks (B) and trains of stimuli (C, 15 Hz and D, 20 Hz). Vertical calibration is 20 mV, horizontal calibration is 500 msec.

SUMMARY

A comparison of synaptic transmission in extramural ganglia of the urinary bladder and colon revealed numerous differences that were unexpected based on the apparently similar functions of these two ganglionic systems. Indeed, vesical and colonic ganglia seem to lie at two extremes in terms of their potential for modulating central autonomic outflow and as possible sites for sympathetic-parasympathetic interactions.

Bladder ganglia are subject to adrenergic inhibitory and possibly facilitatory controls which can be demonstrated following the injection of exogenous catecholamines or during either electrical stimulation or reflex activation of the sympathetic innervation to the bladder. On the other hand, transmission in extramural colonic ganglia was completely resistant to injected catecholamines or stimulation of the sympathetic inhibitory pathways to the colon. The site of sympathetic inhibition in the colon, therefore, must be in the myenteric plexus or in the colonic smooth muscle.

Temporal facilitation was observed in both vesical and colonic ganglia but was considerably more prominent in the former. Potentials evoked in vesical postganglionic nerves in response to stimulation of preganglionic fibers gradually increased in amplitude reaching seven–20 times control levels during continuous stimulation at frequencies greater than three to four Hz whereas facilitation in colonic ganglia under similar conditions ranged from a one-and-a half to two-fold increase. These data suggest that the subliminal fringe in colonic ganglia is small. Transmission must occur with a high safety factor so that a large percentage of the ganglion cells are activated with single preganglionic volleys. The ganglia seem to serve as simple relay stations, with very little capability of modifying the neuronal activity arising in the central nervous system. It is possible, however, that they provide an input into the myenteric plexus which has more complicated functions[8] and where centrally- and peripherally-generated activities are integrated to provide a final input to the colonic smooth muscle.

In bladder ganglia, transmission was relatively inefficient at low frequencies of stimulation. The subliminal fringe was large and the majority of the ganglion cells only discharged when trains of stimuli were applied to the preganglionic nerves. These characteristics matched the properties of the central reflex pathway, in which reflexes were minimal at low frequencies of stimulation but exhibited marked recruitment during repetitive stimulation at frequencies of one to five Hz. The reflex pathway seems to function as a gating circuit being activated only periodically and responding in an all-or-none fashion. It maintains the excitatory input to the bladder at or near zero during urine accumulation, when intravesical pressure and afferent firing are low, but responds maximally once a critical level of intravesical pressure is reached. Vesical ganglia must play an important role in this gating mechanism since they can "filter out" low frequency preganglionic activity but seem to amplify the intense firing which occurs during micturition[11]. The existence of the latter recruiting mechanism as well as adrenergic inhibitory and facilitatory mechanisms in vesical ganglia provides the basis for a potentially complex ganglionic modulation of the parasympathetic outflow to the bladder.

Facilitation in the parasympathetic ganglionic pathway to the bladder seems to be mediated by a presynaptic mechanism, which enhances the release of acetylcholine from the preganglionic nerve terminals. The amplitude of EPSP's increased markedly during facilitation induced by trains of stimuli without any evidence for a change in postsynaptic excitability or for the generation of slow EPSP's which have been implicated in facilitation in sympathetic ganglia[37]. It has been suggested by analogy with presynaptic facilitatory mechanisms at the neuromuscular junction[40] that facilitation in bladder ganglia is related to the accumulation of calcium in the presynaptic terminals with each stimulus, thereby leading to the gradual increase in the quantal release of transmitter during repetitive stimulation[20].

Less information is available about the mechanisms underlying adrenergic inhibition and facilitation in bladder ganglia. It is known that the responses occur via the activation of different receptors and it is tempting to speculate that these responses may be generated, respectively, by hyperpolarization and depolarization of the ganglion cells as noted in sympathetic ganglia[23,24]. However, this has not yet been confirmed with intracellular recording. A presynaptic adrenergic inhibitory mechanism may also be important in bladder ganglia since it has been demonstrated in guinea-pig pelvic[42] and myenteric plexus[29]. A role for adenylate cyclase and cAMP in adrenergic inhibition in bladder ganglia seems unlikely. The administration of exogenous cAMP did not mimic adrenergic inhibition. Furthermore theophylline, a phosphodiesterase inhibitor, which reportedly enhances slow IPSP's in the superior ganglion of the rabbit did not alter adrenergic inhibitory responses in bladder ganglia.

Transmission in the bladder and pelvic ganglia may be subject to other synaptic modulatory mechanisms. ATP and related nucleotides elicited prominent inhibitory responses in the bladder ganglia. This raises the possibility of purinergic inhibitory mechanisms. In addition the hypogastric nerve provided weak excitatory inputs to ganglia in the pelvic plexus. This was also noted in the pelvic ganglia of the guinea pig, where the responses have been identified as cholinergic[2]. Finally spontaneous firing and/or spontaneous EPSP's were observed in decentralized colonic ganglia in situ[15] and in isolated pelvic ganglia in vitro, suggesting that parasympathetic ganglion cells may receive excitatory inputs from peripherally located neurons (i.e., afferents or interneurons) as well as from preganglionic neurons in the central nervous system. The transmitters involved in these peripheral pathways have not been identified.

This research was supported in part by Grant NB 07923 from the National Institute of Neurological Diseases and Stroke and in part by fellowships from the Benevolent Foundation of Scottish Rite Freemasonry and the NIH. W. C. de Groat was a recipient of a Research Center Development Award from NINDS.

REFERENCES

1 Booth, A. M. and de Groat, W. C., A study of recruitment in vesical parasympathetic ganglia (VPG) of the cat using intracellular recording techniques, *Fed. Proc.*, 37 (1978) 526.

2 Blackman, J. G., Crowcroft, P. J., Devine, C. E., Holman, M. E. and Yonemura, K., Transmission from preganglionic fibres in the hypogastric nerve to peripheral ganglia of male guinea-pigs, *J. Physiol.* (Lond.), 201 (1968) 723–743.

3 Bülbring, E., The action of adrenaline on transmission in the superior cervical ganglion, *J. Physiol.* (Lond.), 103 (1944) 55–67.

4 Burnstock, G., Purinergic transmission. In: L. Iversen, S. Iversen and S. Synder (Eds.), *Handbook of Psychopharmacology*, New York, Plenum Publishing 5, 1975, pp. 131–194.

5 Burnstock, G. A., Basis for distinguishing two types of purinergic receptor, In: L. Bolis and R. W. Straub (Eds.), *Cell Membrane Receptors for Drugs and Hormones: A Multidisplinary Approach*, Raven Press, New York, 1978, pp. 107–118.

6 Burnstock, G., Cocks, T., Crowe, R. and Kasakub, L., Purinergic innervation of the guinea-pig urinary bladder, *Br. J. Pharmac.*, 61 (1978) 125–138.

7 Christ, D. D. and Nishi, S., Site of adrenaline blockade in the superior cervical ganglion of the rabbit, *J. Physiol.* (Lond.), 213 (1971) 107–117.

8 Costa, M. and Furness, J. B., The peristalic reflex: An analysis of the nerve pathways and their pharmacology, *Arch. Pharmacol.*, 294 (1976) 47–60.

9 Dail, W. C., Histochemical and fine structural studies of SIF cells in the major pelvic ganglion of the rat. In: O. Fränkö (Ed.), *SIF Cells, Structure and Function of the Small Intensely Fluorescent Sympathetic Cells*, Fogarty International Center Proceedings No. 30 U.S. Government Printing Office, Washington, D. C., 1976, pp. 8–18.

10 de Groat, W. C., Actions of the catecholamines in sympathetic ganglia, *Circulation Res.*, 20–21, Suppl. 3 (1967) 135–145.

11 de Groat, W. C., Nervous control of the urinary bladder of the cat, *Brain Res.*, 87 (1975) 201–211.

12 de Groat, W. C., Booth, A. M., Krier, J., Milne, R. J., Morgan, C. and Nadelhaft, I., Neural control of the urinary bladder and large intestine. This volume, pp. 50–67.

13 de Groat, W. C. and Krier, J., Preganglionic C-fibers: A major component of the sacral autonomic outflow to the colon of the cat, *Pflügers Arch.*, 359 (1975) 171–176.

14 de Groat, W. C. and Krier, J., An electrophysiological study of the sacral parasympathetic pathway to the colon of the cat, *J. Physiol.* (Lond.), 260 (1976) 425–445.

15 de Groat, W. C. and Krier, J., The sacral parasympathetic reflex pathway regulating colonic motility and defecation in the cat, *J. Physiol.* (Lond.), 276 (1978) 481–500.

16 de Groat, W. C. and Lalley, P. M., Reflex firing in the lumbar sympathetic outflow to activation of vesical afferent fibres, *J. Physiol.* (Lond.), 226 (1972) 289–309.

17 de Groat, W. C. and Ryall, R. W., Reflexes to sacral parasympathetic neurones concerned with micturition in the cat, *J. Physiol.* (Lond.), 200 (1969) 87–108.

18 de Groat, W. C. and Saum, W. R., Adrenergic inhibition in mammalian parasympathetic ganglia, *Nature New Biol.*, 231 (1971) 188–189.

19 de Groat, W. C. and Saum, W. R., Sympathetic inhibition of the urinary bladder and of pelvic ganglionic transmission in the cat, *J. Physiol.* (Lond.), 214 (1972) 297–314.

20 de Groat, W. C. and Saum, W. R., Synaptic transmission in parasympathetic ganglia in the urinary bladder of the cat, *J. Physiol.* (Lond.), 256 (1976) 137–158.

21 de Groat, W. C. and Theobald, R. J., Sympathetic inhibitory reflexes to the urinary

bladder and bladder ganglia evoked by electrical stimulation of vesical afferents, *J. Physiol.* (Lond.), 259 (1976) 223–237.

22   de Groat, W. C. and Theobald, R. J., Effects of ATP, cyclic AMP and related nucleotides on transmission in parasympathetic ganglia, *Pharmacologist*, 18 (1976) 185.

23   de Groat, W. C. and Volle, R. L., The actions of the catecholamines on transmission in the superior cervical ganglion of the cat, *J. Pharmac. exp. Ther.*, 154 (1966) 1–13.

24   de Groat, W. C. and Volle, R. L., Interactions between the catecholamines and ganglionic stimulating agents in sympathetic ganglia, *J. Pharmac. exp. Ther.*, 154 (1966) 200–215.

25   Dun, N. and Karczmar, G., A comparison of the effect of theophylline and cyclic adenosine 3′: 5′-monophosphate on the superior cervical ganglion of the rabbit by means of the sucrose-gap method, *J. Pharmac. exp. Ther.*, 202 (1977) 89–96.

26   Dun, N. and Nishi, S., Effects of dopamine on the superior cervical ganglion of the rabbit, *J. Physiol.* (Lond.), 239 (1974) 155–164.

27   Eccles, R. M. and Libet, B., Origin and blockade of the synaptic responses of curarized sympathetic ganglia, *J. Physiol.* (Lond.), 157 (1961) 484–503.

28   El-Badawi, A. and Schenk, E. A., A new theory of the innervation of bladder musculature. Part 3. Post-ganglionic synapses in uretero-vesico-urethral autonomic pathways, *J. Urol.* (Baltimore), 105 (1971) 372–374.

29   Gabella, G., *Structure of the Autonomic Nervous System*, John Wiley and Sons, Inc., New York, 1976.

30   Gallagher, J. P. and Shinnick-Gallagher, P., Cyclic nucleotides injected intracellularly into rat superior ganglion cells, *Science*, 198 (1977) 851–852.

31   Greengard, P. and Kebabian, J. W., Role of cyclic AMP in synaptic transmission in the mammalian peripheral nervous system, *Fed. Proc.*, 33 (1974) 1059–1067.

32   Hamberger, B. and Norberg, K. A., Adrenergic synaptic terminals and nerve cells in bladder ganglia of the cat, *Int. J. Neuropharmacol.*, 4 (1965) 41–45.

33   Hamberger, B. and Norberg, K. A., Studies on some systems of adrenergic synaptic terminals in the abdominal ganglia of the cat, *Acta. physiol scand.*, 65 (1965) 235–242.

34   Langley, J. N. and Anderson, H. K., On the innervation of the pelvic and adjoining viscera. Part I. The lower portion of intestine, *J. Physiol.* (Lond.), 18 (1895) 67–105.

35   Langley, J. N. and Anderson, H. K., The innervation of the pelvic and adjoining viscera. Part II. The bladder, *J. Physiol.* (Lond.), 19 (1895) 71–84.

36   Langley, J. N. and Anderson, H. K., The innervation of the pelvic and adjoining viscera. V. Position of the nerve cells on the course of the efferent nerve fibres, *J. Physiol.* (Lond.), 19 (1896) 131–139.

37   Libet, B., Slow synaptic responses and excitatory changes in sympathetic ganglia, *J. Physiol.* (Lond.), 174 (1964) 1–25.

38   Libet, B., Generation of slow inhibitory and excitatory postsynaptic potentials, *Fed. Proc.*, 29 (1970) 1945–1956.

39   Libet, B., Slow postsynaptic actions in ganglionic functions. This volume, pp. 197–222.

40   Magelby, K. L. and Zengel, J. E., A quantitative description of tetanic and post-tetanic potentiation of transmitter release at the frog neuromuscular junction, *J. Physiol.* (Lond.), 245 (1975) 183–208.

41   Marrazzi, A. S., Electrical studies on the pharmacology of autonomic synapses. II. The action of a sympathomimetic drug (epinephrine) on sympathetic ganglia, *J. Pharmac. exp. Ther.*, 65 (1939) 395–404.

42   McLachlan, E. M., Interaction between sympathetic and parasympathetic pathways

in the pelvic plexus of the guinea pig, *Proceedings of the Australian Physiological and Pharmacological Society*, 8 (1977) 15.

43 Nishi, S., The catecholamine-mediated inhibition in ganglionic transmission. This volume, pp. 223–233.

44 Saum, W. R. and de Groat, W. C., Parasympathetic ganglia: Activation of an adrenergic inhibitory mechanism by cholinomimetic agents, *Science*, 175 (1972) 659–661.

45 Saum, W. R. and de Groat, W. C., Antagonism by bulbocapnine of adrenergic inhibitoin in parasympathetic ganglia in the urinary bladder, *Brain Res.*, 37 (1972) 340–344.

CHAPTER 16

ACETYLCHOLINE AND SEROTONIN RECEPTORS IN MAMMALIAN SYMPATHETIC GANGLION NEURONS

V. I. Skok and A. A. Selyanko

Bogomoletz Institute of Physiology, Kiev, U.S.S.R.

INTRODUCTION

It has long been known that transmission through the mammalian sympathetic ganglion occurs by means of activation of nicotinic receptors (see review[13]). In amphibian sympathetic ganglia activation of nicotinic receptors is followed by an increase in sodium and potassium permeabilities of the neuronal membrane[7,8,9]. In mammalian sympathetic ganglion the ionic mechanisms underlying activation of nicotinic receptors has not yet been studied in detail.

There are also muscarinic[4,10,14], adrenergic[4] and serotonin or 5-hydroxytryptamine (5-HT)[2,5,16] receptors in the neurons of mammalian sympathetic ganglia. Muscarinic and adrenergic receptors are thought to modulate transmission through the ganglion. The role of 5-HT receptors remains unknown.

The aim of the present work was to study the properties of acetylcholine (ACh) and 5-HT receptors in the mammalian sympathetic ganglion, particularly their distribution in the ganglion and the ionic mechanisms involved in their activation.

METHODS

The experiments were performed on the isolated superior cervical ganglion (SCG) of the rabbit. The ganglion was kept in saline solution (see ref. 3) at 37°C, equilibrated with O_2 (95%) and CO_2 (5%).

Intracellular electrodes were filled with 2.5 M KCl and had a resistance of from 90 MΩ to 200 MΩ. The drugs given were applied iontophoretically through double-barrel micropipettes with one barrel filled with ACh (2.5 M) and another barrel filled with 5-HT (0.13 M). The intensity and duration of iontophoretic current were $1 \times 10^{-8} - 3 \times 10^{-7}$ A and two–20 msec, respectively. To shift the membrane potential level, a current was passed through the membrane using either the same intracellular electrode used for recording of membrane potential (and bridge circuit) or another intracellular electrode.

The impalement of the cell with intracellular electrodes[3] and the approach to the cell for iontophoretic micropipette placement were made under visual control using Nomarski differential interference optics. For orthodromic stimulation of the cell a single shock 0.5 msec in duration was applied to preganglionic fibers through a suction electrode. For more details relative to methods used, see ref. 12.

RESULTS

The effect of iontophoretic application of ACh was studied in 61 neurons. In all cases ACh was applied to the soma membrane, for it was difficult to visualize the dendrites through a differential interference microscope. ACh evoked depolarizations (ACh potential) with rising times ranging approximately from 10 to 50 msec.

It has been shown that when ACh is applied iontophoretically through a micropipette with a tip diameter of about 0.1 μm, the diameter of the activated receptor area is found to be approximately 8 μm (see ref. 11). The diameter of soma in the neurons studied was not less than 35 μm. It thus was possible to activate locally different portions of the soma membrane.

By accepting the concept that the amount of applied ACh is linearly proportional to the electrical charge transferred through the iontophoretic micropipette, the ACh sensitivities of different portions of the soma membrane could be compared in terms of the electric charges necessary to evoke ACh potentials of similar amplitudes. ACh potentials could be evoked from any portion of the soma membrane but the maximal

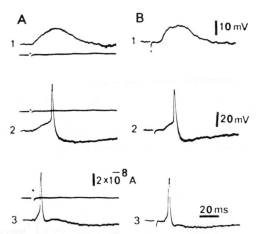

Fig. 1. Responses evoked by iontophoretic application of ACh compared with the responses to single orthodromic stimuli. A: the responses to iontophoretic application of ACh with the current monitored in the lower trace (1) or in the upper trace (2, 3). B: the responses to a single orthodromic stimulus recorded from the same cell that gave the responses in A. The iontophoretic current (A) and the orthodromic stimulus (B) are subthreshold in record 1 and increase in their intensities from record 2 to record 3. Note the same time scale which applies in A and B is shown in B 3. Voltage scale for record A 1 is shown in record B 1 and that for the other records is given in record B 2 (see [12]).

difference in ACh sensitivities between neighboring portions of the membrane differed by a factor of four; in order to excite some areas four times more ACh was required than needed to excite others. It thus follows that each portion of the soma membrane possesses ACh receptors but their densities differ markedly. ACh potential evoked from the most sensitive portion of the membrane approached in its time course that of the EPSP (Fig. 1).

We did not observe slow ACh potentials with rising times of several hundreds mseconds such as characterize potentials evoked by activation of muscarinic receptors in amphibian sympathetic[8] and parasympathetic[6] ganglia. It can be concluded that the soma membrane of mammalian sympathetic ganglion neurons does not possess muscarinic receptors such as are presumably located in the dendrites.

The effect of membrane potential levels on the amplitude of ACh potentials and EPSP's was studied by using the extrapolation method except in the case of a few neurons where two intracellular electrodes were used. In the latter case the depolarizing current passed through the membrane was strong enough to decrease the amplitude of ACh potential to zero and even to cause an actual reversal (Fig. 4).

The mean value ($\pm$S.E.) of the reversal potential for ACh potential (E_{ACh}) and for EPSP(E_{EPSP}) was -16.5 ± 1.2 mV (n=21) and -14.4 ± 1.6 mV (n=23), respectively; the difference between these values was statistically nonsignificant.

In one group of neurons both E_{ACh} and E_{EPSP} were much more negative than mentioned above. This was apparently due to the increase in cell input resistance when strong hyperpolarizing currents were applied, i.e., to nonaccuracy of the extrapolation method (for details see ref. 12). This fact can explain unusually low values of E_{EPSP} observed in our earlier experiments[13].

In order to know what ionic channels are opened by ACh and by transmitters, the effects of changes in external concentrations of sodium and potassium ions upon E_{ACh} and E_{EPSP} were studied. In sodium-deficient solutions sucrose was substituted for 76 mM of NaCl. In potassium-rich solutions KCl was substituted for eight mM of NaCl. In potassium-deficient solutions sucrose was substituted for four mM of KCl. In chloride-deficient solutions sodium glutamate was substituted for 137.9 mM of NaCl.

A decrease in external concentrations of sodium or potassium shifted E_{ACh} and E_{EPSP} towards more negative values, while an increase in external concentration

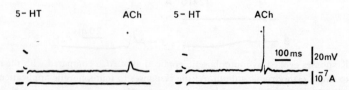

Fig. 2. Responses evoked by iontophoretic application of ACh in a neuron which did not respond to iontophoretic application of 5-HT. The iontophoretic charge transferred through the micropipette during the application of 5-HT was approximately 10 times higher than during the application of ACh (pulse duration 30 ms and two ms, respectively). In the left recording the dose of ACh is subthreshold and in the right recording is suprathreshold for spike generation.

of potassium shifted them to the opposite side. Changes in external concentration of chloride did not change E_{ACh} or E_{EPSP}. These results confirm the well-known postulate that ACh is an excitatory transmitter in mammalian sympathetic ganglion, and indicate that ACh increases the postsynaptic membrane permeabilities to sodium and potassium ions in a fashion similar to what is known to occur at nicotinic synapses in amphibian neuro-muscular junctions[15] and in amphibian sympathetic ganglia[8,9].

The effect of 5-HT was studied in 13 neurons. In seven neurons 5-HT did not evoke any change in membrane potential although ACh applied to the same neuron from another barrel of the iontophoretic micropipette evoked depolarization and firing. An example of such response is shown in Fig. 2. This neuron did not respond even to a dose of 5-HT 10 times higher than the dose of ACh which evoked a depolarization and spike.

It has been found that when small-diameter iontophoretic micropipettes are used the transfer number for 5-HT does not differ much from that for ACh: The values are 0.18 and 0.24, respectively[1]. On the other hand the threshold dose of 5-HT for depolarizing the whole ganglion is even lower than that of ACh[16]. These observations rule out the possibility that the dose of 5-HT applied in our experiments was subthreshold. It thus can be concluded that no 5-HT receptors were found in about half the neurons studied.

In the remaining six neurons of the 13 studied 5-HT evoked depolarization (5-HT potential) and firing. An example of such a response is shown in Fig. 3. In its time course the 5-HT-potential differs markedly from the ACh potential: The former is much slower and has a much longer rising time. This makes the participation of 5-HT receptor activation in conduction through the ganglion of single orthodromic volleys unlikely, but leaves the possibility open that such receptor activation may modulate transmission through the ganglion.

An alternative possibility is that 5-HT receptors play no special role in the ganglion with respect to synaptic input as, for example, is the case with respect to 5-HT receptors found in the soma membrane of afferent neurons (see ref. 7).

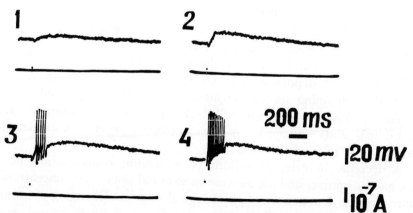

Fig. 3.   Responses evoked by iontophoretic application of 5-HT. The dose of 5-HT increases from record 1 to record 4.

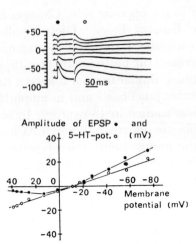

Fig. 4. Reversal potential for EPSP and 5-HT potential recorded on the same sweep. Current was passed through the membrane and membrane potential was recorded using two different intracellular electrodes. Both EPSP and 5-HT potential reversed at −14 mV. The graph presents data, some of which are illustrated in the top. Each dark circle and light circle represents, respectively, single EPSP and single 5-HT potentials.

The reversal potential for 5-HT potential estimated in three neurons was similar to the reversal potential for EPSP and the ACh potential. The results obtained from one of the neurons are shown in Fig. 4. These data indicate that the ionic mechanisms underlying the effects of ACh and 5-HT on the postsynaptic membrane are similar.

SUMMARY

1. The effects of an excitatory transmitter, exogenous acetylcholine (ACh) and 5-hydroxytryptamine (5-HT) on the postsynaptic membrane of the neurons of rabbit isolated SCG were studied using orthodromic stimulation and local iontophoretic application of ACh and 5-HT.

2. ACh applied locally to the soma membrane evoked nicotinic depolarization (ACh potential) and did not evoke muscarinic depolarization. The ACh sensitivity of the soma membrane differed markedly in its different parts.

3. 5-HT evoked depolarization and spikes in six neurons from 13 neurons studied; in the remaining seven neurons no response was observed.

4. The reversal potential for EPSP (E_{EPSP}) and ACh potential (E_{ACh}) was −14.4±1.6 mV and −16.5±1.2 mV, respectively; reversal potential for 5-HT potential was close to these values.

5. A decrease in external sodium or potassium concentration made E_{EPSP} and E_{ACh} more negative, and an increase in external potassium concentration made them more positive than in normal physiological solution. Changing of external chloride concentration did not influence E_{EPSP} or E_{ACh}.

6. It has been concluded that: i) The soma membrane possesses nicotinic recep-

tors and (in some neurons) 5-HT receptors but does not possess muscarinic receptors; ii) excitatory transmitters and exogenous ACh (as well as probably 5-HT) increase membrane permeabilities to sodium and potassium ions; iii) the density of ACh receptor distribution is not homogeneous in different portions of the soma membrane.

REFERENCES

1 Bradley, P. B. and Candy, J. M., Iontophoretic release of acetylcholine, noradrenaline, 5-hydroxytryptamine and D-lysergic acid from micropipettes, *Brit. J. Pharmacol.*, 40 (1970) 194–201.

2 De Groat, W.C. and Lalley, P.M., Interaction between picrotoxine and 5-hydroxytryptamine in the superior cervical ganglion of the cat, *Brit. J. Pharmacol.*, 48 (1973) 233–244.

3 Eccles, R.M., Intracellular potentials recorded from a mammalian sympathetic ganglion, *J. Physiol.* (Lond.), 130 (1955) 572–584.

4 Eccles, R.M. and Libet, B., Origin and blockade of the synaptic responses of curarized sympathetic ganglia, *J. Physiol.* (Lond.), 157 (1961) 484–503.

5 Haefely, W., The effects of 5-hydroxytryptamine and some related compounds on the cat superior cervical ganglion *in situ.*, *Naunyn-Schmiedeberg's Arch. Pharmacol.*, 281 (1974) 145–165.

6 Hartzell, H.C., Kuffler, S.W., Stickgold, R. and Yoshikami, D., Synaptic excitation and inhibition resulting from direct action of acetylcholine on two types of chemoreceptors on individual amphibian parasympathetic neurones, *J. Physiol.* (Lond.), 271 (1977) 817–846.

7 Higashi, H., 5-hydroxytryptamine receptors on visceral primary afferent neurons in the nodose ganglion of the rabbit, *Nature*, 267 (1977) 448–450.

8 Koketsu, K., Cholinergic synaptic potentials and the underlying ionic mechanisms, *Fed. Proc.*, 28 (1969) 101–112.

9 Nishi, S. and Koketsu, K., Electrical properties and activities of single sympathetic neurons in frogs, *J. cell. comp. Physiol.*, 55 (1960) 15–30.

10 Nishi, S. and Koketsu, K., Early and late after-discharges of amphibian sympathetic ganglion cells, *J. Neurophysiol.*, 31 (1968) 109–121.

11 Roper, S., The acetylcholine sensitivity of the surface membrane of multiply-innervated parasympathetic ganglion cells in the mudpuppy before and after partial denervation, *J. Physiol.* (Lond.), 254 (1976) 455–473.

12 Selyanko, A. A. and Skok, V. I., Activation of nicotinic acetylcholine receptors in mammalian sympathetic ganglion neurons, *Progr. Brain Res.*, 49 (1979) 241–252

13 Skok, V. I., *Physiology of Autonomic Ganglia*, Igaku Shoin, Tokyo, 1973.

14 Takeshige, Ch. and Volle, R. L., Bimodal response of sympathetic ganglia to acetylcholine following eserine or repetitive preganglionic stimulation, *J. Pharmac. exp. Ther.*, 138 (1962) 66–73.

15 Takeuchi, A. and Takeuchi, N., On the permeability of endplate membrane during the action of transmitter, *J. Physiol.* (Lond.), 154 (1960) 52–67.

16 Wallis, D. and Woodward, B., Membrane potential changes induced by 5-hydroxytryptamine in the rabbit superior cervical ganglion, *Brit. J. Pharmacol.*, 55 (1975) 199–212.

SECTION IV

REFLEX ACTIONS AND INTERACTIONS

In order to analyze the components of autonomic system response, reflex actions evoked by various stimuli must be studied. There are at least two major categories of autonomic reflex, if one thinks of them in terms of efferent nerve action. There are those dependent on autonomic nerves such as salivary and cardiac reflexes. There are other reflexes such as vomiting and somatomotor responses for which autonomic nerves are not essential but to which the autonomic system contributes.

A more common practice is to identify reflexes by the sensors which trigger them. This is quite satisfactory if one does not forget that these same stimuli which evoke sympathetic and parasympathetic responses likewise activate respiratory and somatomotor effectors.

As pointed out by certain contributors to this section, neither reflexes nor centers should be considered purely autonomic. Even in the simplest reflexes somatic and autonomic responses occur together and secondary reactions often result. To be sure, the balance of involvement differs; there are viscerovisceral reflexes involving principally the autonomic, but recent work has shown that even reflexes evoked by stimulating visceral afferents, such as intracardiac receptors, have a widespread effect. The following chapters will deal with several types of reflexes.

The fact that cardiovascular reactions are evoked by excitation of muscle afferents seems physiologically appropriate. Just as the autonomic system is not essential to vomiting, it is involved in and responsible for some components of the general reaction. Active muscles require an enhanced blood supply and this requires a shift of blood volume as well as an augmented cardiac output.

It is equally important that vasomotor reactions should be evoked by other types of stimuli. Recent analyses of responses in vasoconstrictor neurons supplying skeletal muscle and skin and in the sudomotor system initiated by various afferent inputs from the skin surface and from the interior of the body have shown very definite reciprocal patterns. Muscle vasoconstrictors and skin vasoconstrictors respond in a reciprocal fashion to cutaneous nociceptors and arterial chemoreceptors. Apparently, muscle vasoconstrictors and sudomotor systems are regulated in an "excitatory mode" while skin vasoconstrictors are "regulated in an inhibitory mode". The major point is that very definite patterns of response are evoked by peripheral afferents.

CHAPTER 17

VOMITING AND RELATED REFLEXES

H. L. Borison

Department of Pharmacology and Toxicology, Dartmouth Medical School,
Hanover, New Hampshire, USA

INTRODUCTION

The autonomic nervous system is not essential to the act of vomiting but, as in many other reflexes and behavioral reactions, it is involved. The autonomic efferents which supply the glands, blood vessels and muscles of the gastrointestinal system are responsible for some components of the general reactions evoked by stimuli which produce vomiting.

DISCUSSION AND CONCLUSIONS

Cannon's View of Vomiting

Walter B. Cannon[5] was the first to use X-rays for observation of stomach movements associated with vomiting. Injection of apomorphine in the cat caused the stomach to become divided into two parts by a contraction at the incisura angularis. This was followed by a flattening of the diaphragm and a quick jerk of the abdominal muscles which forced the contents of the upper part of the stomach out through the esophagus. Cannon concluded: "In the process of ridding the gastric mucosa of irritants, therefore, the stomach plays a relatively passive role".

The Nonessential Role of the Autonomic Nervous System

A half-century later, Kuntz[9] devoted less than a page of his book on the autonomic nervous system to the mechanism of vomiting. He briefly stated how the vagus, splanchnic, phrenic and lower thoracic nerves participate in the process. Wang and Borison[14] at about the same time demonstrated by surgical means that the autonomic innervation of the stomach and small intestine is not essential for vomiting. Indeed, chronic vagotomy promotes the occurrence of vomiting. A simple pharmacologic experiment that proves the nonessential role of the autonomic nervous system in vomiting is the administration of a ganglionic blocking drug which interrupts all autonomic pre- to post-ganglionic transmission yet spares the performance of vomiting[10].

The Respiratory Mechanics of Vomiting

It was already clear to Cannon[5] that the striated muscles of the diaphragm and abdominal wall generate the force needed to evacuate the stomach through the mouth. However, the precise interplay of the thoracic and abdominal components that operate in the retching (pre-expulsion) and the expulsion phases of the vomiting act were not elucidated until the pressure changes occurring in the chest and abdomen were recorded simultaneously with cineradiographic and electromyographic observations[11,12]. These studies revealed that during the retching phase, a series of large negative pressure pulses are produced in the thorax synchronously with postive pressure pulses in the abdomen. The trans-diaphragm synergistic pressure pulses in retching cause the gastric contents repeatedly to move forth and back between stomach and esophagus without escaping into the oropharynx. Sudden conversion of the intrathoracic pressure pulse from negative to postive then marks the phase of expulsion whence the vomitus is forcibly ejected through the open mouth. Thus, the raising of the gastric contents is a complex motor event executed by the voluntary respiratory muscles in a highly stereotyped pattern of expression. Moreover, it is evident that the autonomic nervous system is not indispensable for the act of vomiting. Nevertheless, autonomic involvement is by no means excluded.

The Problem of Definition

The triad of nausea, retching and expulsion describes the entire emetic process. The three components, however, are separate functional entities which can occur independently of each other and in any combination. While vomiting *per se* is a neatly delineated mechanical form of behavior, the prodromes of vomiting are so varied as to defy general description. Indeed, vomiting can even occur without subjective warning which is said to happen in cerebrospinal fluid hypertension. Rapid intravenous injection of apomorphine in the dog can induce vomiting in the time taken for the first pass of blood-borne drug through the brain, that is, in less than a minute. By contrast, the vomiting of motion sickness may develop after hours of perturbation of the non-acoustic vestibular apparatus. Other vomiting reactions—as after exposure to high-energy radiation, in uremia or in certain forms of chemical intoxication—occur in two distinct time frames resulting from different early and late pathophysiological disturbances.

The mechanical part of divers vomiting syndromes is undoubtedly consistent in its somatic motor organization, due allowance being made for more or less retching activity preceding each expulsion of vomitus. On the other hand, it is fair to state that the extent of autonomic expression over the gamut of vomiting reactions is directly related to the time required for development of the emetic syndrome. Accordingly, given sufficient anticipation, vomiting may be preceded by salivation, sweating, facial pallor, tachycardia, weak pulse, feeling of faintness, headache, diarrhea, etc., attributable to parasympathetic and sympathetic neural discharges.

The autonomic effects related to vomiting are thus mostly associated with the premechanical development of "nausea". Curiously, all the autonomic signs of motion sickness occurring prodromal to vomiting have been observed in a "decorticate" man subjected to a rough airplane journey[7]. Motion-induced salivation and vomiting are

elicitable in the mid-brain transected dog[1]; however, the general autonomic con-
comitants of motion sickness have not been assessed in the decerebrate animal.

The Vomiting Center—Somatic or Autonomic?

In 1949, Borison and Wang[3] localized an electrically reactive region for vomiting
in the lateral reticular formation of the medulla oblongata in decerebrate cats.
Electrical stimulation yielded stimulus-bound expulsion of vomitus, that is, with
no measurable delay and with no afterdischarge. Another region, dorsolateral to the
vomiting locus, yielded coughing and retching responses to electrical stimulation
but no expulsion of the gastric contents. These results provided the basis for assigning
separate control loci for the functions of retching and expulsion in the vomiting
syndrome.

There is a growing tendency among medical scientists to include all automatic
and subconscious forms of behavior in the autonomic sphere of influence. By such
reasoning it could be argued speciously that subcortical control of body posture is an
autonomic function. This undiscriminating point of view must also be considered
inappropriate for respiratory regulation, which is a somatomotor reflex process.
On the other hand, there is no denying that the visceral effector system interacts with
the somatic effector system in every homeostatic function. It seems most prudent to
this writer, therefore, that reflex control centers in the brain remain undesignated—
neither "somatic" nor "autonomic"—since their *modus operandi* is the integration of
all available effector machinery encompassing somatic, autonomic and endocrine
outputs of the central nervous system.

A Specialized Chemoreceptor for Vomiting in the Brain

Early pharmacologists believed that "centrally-acting" emetic drugs stimulated
the vomiting center directly. In fact, this belief provided the rationale for the original
localization of the vomiting center in the dorsal vagal nuclei where topical application
of various substances evoked vomiting[8]. This kind of reasoning required that the
neural circuitry responsible for coordinating the complex behavior of emesis should
itself be sensitive to chemical activation in such a way that the sequence and pattern
of motor events would follow a preset schedule of functional expression. However,
it was discovered by Wang and Borison[15] that the medullary chemoresponsive region
was in fact situated superficial to the vagal nuclei (soon found to be the area
postrema[2]). Its ablation in surviving animals did not at all interfere with the performance of vomiting; only the emetic sensitivity to certain chemicals was irrevocably
abolished. This chemoresponsive locus has come to be known as the medullary emetic
chemoreceptor trigger zone or CTZ. Thus, the vomiting "center" in the reticular
formation, where the act of vomiting is programmed and controlled, is not chemically
reactive but it translates codified signals delivered to it from specialized sensors for
chemical or physical stimuli into appropriate action.

There is no place for special sensors such as the area postrema or the non-acoustic
vestibular apparatus in the classic definitions of the sympathetic and parasympathetic
divisions of the autonomic nervous system. Moreover, no afferent nerve has an exclusive reflex influence upon a visceral or somatic motor pathway. Hence, it seems

irrational to place any sensory input for vomiting under the umbrella of "autonomic innervation" regardless of its source.

"Autonomic Drugs" and Vomiting

In the formative years of elucidating the chemical nature of junctional transmission in visceral effectors, it became fashionable to tie together the autonomic mediators and their modifiers by the label of "autonomic drugs". With the continously expanding list of substances involved in synaptic transmission everywhere in the nervous system, use of the "autonomic" qualifier for neuroactive drugs is now meaningless and confusing. Hence, while many agents that affect autonomic neural transmission also cause vomiting, the two types of effects undoubtedly reflect independent actions of those agents.

Rumination and Appetite

Unlike vomiting, regurgitation for the purpose of rechewing the gastric contents is a normal cyclic alimentary function in ruminants. Sheep spend approximately 30 percent of their daily existence ruminating, day and night. It occurred to us that the area postrema might serve the physiologic role of a feedback sensor for rumination. We were wrong since ablation of the area postrema performed on sheep in our laboratory did not affect the daily pattern of rumination[4]. However, we found that a selective drug effect on rumination was abolished. In our hands, digitalis did not cause vomiting in the normal sheep; rather, it produced a protracted inhibition of rumination. Following extirpation of the area postrema, digitalis no longer inhibited rumination. In nonruminant species, digitalis causes a loss of appetite that long outlasts the occurrence of vomiting. Ablation of the area postrema done by us in cats not only rendered the animals immune to the emetic action of digitalis, they no longer showed signs of anorexia. Oddly enough, the hindbrain is practically always disregarded by investigators studying the control of appetite.

Is an "Endogenous Opiate" Involved in the Control of Vomiting?

It has long been known that morphine both initiates and suppresses vomiting. Most other narcotics, however, rarely cause vomiting although they do act as emetic suppressants. We found that prior treatment of cats with a small dose of the narcotic antagonist naloxone converted all narcotic drugs into active emetic substances[6]. This was interpreted to mean that the narcotics normally suppress their own emetic influence and that naloxone unmasked the emetic effect by antagonizing the suppressant action. We demonstrated in addition that the narcotic emetic stimulation is exercised at the CTZ whereas the inhibitory action occurs downstream in the reflex path, probably at the vomiting center itself. The recent postulated existence of specific opiate receptors and endogenous opiate ligands in the brain[13] raises the question whether an individual's susceptibility to nausea and vomiting might be adjusted from moment to moment by the balance of stimulant and inhibitory actions of endogenous morphine-like substances.

Therapeutic Implications

Vomiting is said to be second to pain as the presenting complaint for medical help. It is the most common sign of poisoning; it is a frequent side effect of drug therapy; it is the first sign of acute overexposure to high-energy radiation; and it is the greatest deterrent of modern cancer chemotherapy. Vomiting has caused untold misery and economic loss, yet anti-emetic therapy is still dispensed by trial and error. At the present time, the only sure way chemically to block vomiting is by antagonizing the offending agent at its receptor site when such a fortunate pharmacological matching condition happens to exist. Unfortunately most causes of vomiting are not chemically identifiable nor is a drug available that can selectively interrupt the emetic reflex arc at a common point of convergence of inputs. The possibility that an endogenous opiate substance may serve as a dedicated neurotransmitter in the central control of vomiting provides the first rational approach in the search for an effective general anti-emetic drug.

REFERENCES

1   Bard, P., Woolsey, C. N., Snider, R. S., Mountcastle, V. B. and Bromiley, R. B., Determination of central nervous mechanisms involved in motion sickness, *Fed. Proc.*, 6 (1947) 72.

2   Borison, H. L. and Brizzee, K. R., Morphology of emetic chemoreceptor trigger zone in cat medulla oblongata, *Proc. Soc. exp. Biol. Med.*, 77 (1951) 38–42.

3   Borison, H. L. and Wang, S. C., Functional localization of central coordinating mechanism for emesis in cat, *J. Neurophysiol.*, 12 (1949) 305–313.

4   Bost, J., McCarthy, L. E., Colby, E. D. and Borison, H. L., Rumination in sheep: Effects of morphine, deslanoside, and ablation of area postrema, *Physiol. Behavior*, 3 (1968) 877–881.

5   Cannon, W. B., The movements of the stomach studied by means of the Röntgen rays, *Amer. J. Physiol.*, 1 (1898) 359–382.

6   Costello, D. J. and Borison, H. L., Naloxone antagonizes narcotic self-blockade of emesis in the cat, *J. Pharmac. exp. Ther.*, 203 (1977) 222–230.

7   Doig, R. K., Wolf, S. and Wolff, H. G., Study of gastric function in a "decorticate" man with gastric fistula, *Gastroenterol.*, 23 (1953) 40–44.

8   Hatcher, R. A., Mechanism of vomiting, *Physiol. Rev.*, 4 (1924) 479–504.

9   Kuntz, A., *The Autonomic Nervous System*, Philadelphia, Lea and Febiger (1953).

10 Laffan, R. J. and Borison, H. L., Emetic action of nicotine and lobeline, *J. Pharmac. exp. Ther.*, 121 (1957) 468–476.

11 McCarthy, L. E. and Borison, H. L., Respiratory mechanics of vomiting in decerebrate cats, *Amer. J. Physiol.*, 226 (1974) 738–743.

12 McCarthy, L. E., Borison, H. L., Spiegel, P. K. and Friedlander, R. M., Vomiting: Radiographic and oscillographic correlates in the decerebrate cat, *Gastroenterol.*, 67 (1974) 1126–1130.

13 Snyder, S. H., Opiate receptors and internal opiates, *Sci. Am.*, 236 (1977) 44–56.

14 Wang, S. C. and Borison, H. L., Copper sulfate emesis: A study of afferent pathways from the gastrointestinal tract, *Amer. J. Physiol.*, 164 (1951) 520–526.

15 Wang, S. C. and Borison, H. L., A new concept of organization of the central emetic

mechanism: Recent studies on the sites of action of apomorphine, copper sulfate and cardiac glycosides, *Gastroenterol.*, 22 (1952) 1–12.

CHAPTER 18

RECIPROCAL REACTION PATTERNS OF SYMPATHETIC SUBSYSTEMS WITH RESPECT TO VARIOUS AFFERENT INPUTS

Wilfrid Jänig

Physiologisches Institut, Universität Kiel, Kiel, Federal Republic of Germany

INTRODUCTION

The somatomotor system has been analyzed rigorously using the Sherringtonian approach. By looking at the monosynaptic stretch reflex circuit and its integration into various spinal and supraspinal neuronal circuits at the single neuron level it can be seen that our knowledge of the neural circuitry regulating the activity of the final common motor path during various functional states is developing fairly well. Recently some ideas have evolved concerning the hierarchical organization of spinal and supraspinal neuronal circuits, based on the analytical cellular approach to the neuronal motor system and on the understanding of these analytical data in the behavioral context[5,23-26,28].

The sympathetic nervous system has been looked at more as a unitary system from the functional point of view. This approach has given valuable insight relative to the overall capacity of the system to regulate various functions in the body for maintenance of homeostasis, to adaptation of the inner milieu and to the integration of the sympathetic actions during motor performances of organisms[3,4]. However, this approach has given only minor insight into the central neuronal machinery involving homeostasis-maintaining reactions of the sympathetic subsystems. Furthermore, it may have hindered an analytical approach and studies of single neurons which were so successful in the somatosensory and in the somatomotor systems. This analytical approach using neurophysiological, neuroanatomical, neuropharmacological and biochemical methods is the only one which will tell us how the machinery of the sympathetic subsystems works and finally how the fine differentiated adaptations made by these subsystems are brought about. Some ten years ago use of this analytical approach, in which recordings were made from single neurons and axons with fine electrodes, began in studies of the sympathetic nervous system but the standards of use and the knowledge acquired are far below the level of attainment in studies of the somatomotor and sensory systems.

In the following pages of this chapter some organizational aspects of the sympathetic subsystems' projection to the hindlimb and tail of the cat—the vasoconstrictor systems supplying skin and skeletal muscle and the sudomotor system to the sweat glands in the hind paw of the cat—will be discussed. It will be stressed that the post- and preganglionic neurons reveal typical reaction patterns with respect to various afferent inputs and that these reaction patterns are largely reciprocally organized in the three sympathetic subsystems under study.

METHODS

Most experiments were performed on cats anesthetized by α-chloralose (50 to 60 mg/kg, i.p. or i.v.), but some of the spinal cats were anesthetized by Ketamine hydrochloride (20 mg/kg per hour). The animals were immobilized by sodium triethiodide (Flaxedil) and artificially ventilated (end-expiratory CO_2 4%). Blood pressure measured by an intracarotid or an intrafemoral catheter was always above 110 mm Hg. Body core temperature measured intraesophageally was kept at 38 to 38.5°C by a heating pad.

The following types of preparations were used, the specific methods applied have been described in the respective papers quoted and as far as necessary in the text and figure legends: 1) Brain-intact cats in which postganglionic fibers were dissected from the deep peroneal nerve (muscle nerve) and/or from the superficial peroneal nerve (skin nerve) or from the skin nerves to the tail; the lumbar sympathetic trunk (LST) also was exposed for stimulation in these experiments[6-9,14]. 2) Brain-intact cats in which postganglionic fibers were dissected from the deep peroneal and from the superficial peroneal nerves without exposing the LST; in this type of preparation the baroreceptor afferents were excited by pressure steps in a carotid "blind sack"; only the carotid sinus nerve to the "blind sack" being left intact, all other buffer nerves as well as the vagal nerves being cut. The chemoreceptor afferents were excited by quick injections of small amounts (0.1–0.2 ml) of CO_2-Ringer solution into the external carotid artery (Jänig, Rieckman and Szulczyk, unpublished observations). 3) Brain-intact and chronic spinal cats (71–129 days after low thoracic section) in which the activities of postganglionic fibers dissected from the medial plantar nerve and innervating the hairless skin of the hind foot were recorded with respect to the skin potentials. The LST was not exposed or stimulated in these experiments[16,19]. 4) Brain-intact cats in which activity of preganglionic neurons from lumbar segments L_2 and L_3 was investigated by recordings from single preganglionic axons dissected from the LST between lumbar ganglia L_4 and L_5[20].

RESULTS

In recent years postganglionic neurons supplying skeletal muscle (lateral gastrocnemius muscle, peroneal muscles), hairy skin (of tail and hind leg) and hairless skin of the hind foot have been investigated in brain-intact and spinal cats with regard to various peripheral afferent inputs. The results of these investigations led to criteria for discriminating between vasoconstrictor neurons supplying muscle (MVC), vasoconstrictor neurons supplying skin (CVC) and sudomotor neurons (SM) on the basis of their typical reaction patterns. The same reaction patterns were found in preganglionic lumbar neurons without knowing the target organs of the respective preganglionic neurons[20]. The above-mentioned sympathetic subsystems had a resting activity under the experimental conditions maintained. Other sympathetic subsystems to the hind limb and tail, such as the vasodilatator neurons to skin[7] and muscle[14] and the pilomotor neurons to the tail[9], have no resting activity and generally cannot be activated by the afferent inputs mentioned in this paper and their activity will not be described in detail.

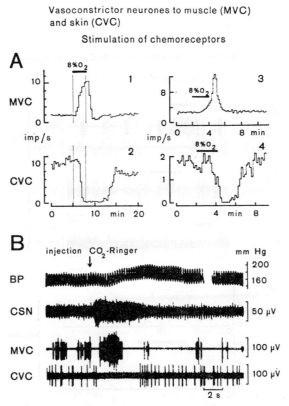

Fig. 1.   Effects of systemic hypoxia and direct chemoreceptor stimulation on MVC and CVC neurons. A: Respiration of the preparations with a mixture of 8% O_2 in N_2. A_1, A_2: Activity in a single postganglionic neuron to the skeletal muscle (MVC) and in a bundle of postganglionic neurons to the hairy skin (CVC) recorded simultaneously. A_3, A_4: Single preganglionic neurons with properties similar to those of MVC-(A_3) and CVC-neurons (A_4). B: Reaction of blood pressure (BP), afferent fibers in left carotid sinus nerve (CSN), muscle vasoconstrictor neurons (MVC) supplying peroneal skeletal muscle and a single cutaneous vasoconstrictor neuron (CVC) supplying hairy skin of the superficial peroneal nerve on a bolus-injection of 0.2 ml CO_2-Ringer into the external carotid artery through the laryngeal artery. A_1, A_2 from[6]; A_3, A_4 from[20]; B from Jänig, Rieckmann and Szulczyk, unpublished observations.

Muscle (MVC) and Cutaneous (CVC) Vasoconstrictor Neurons

MVC neurons are under the strong control and CVC neurons are under the
weak control of the barorecepter afferents. This has been tested by recording the
cardiac rhythmicity from post-R-wave histograms[8,16] or by recording the inhibition
of vasoconstrictor neurons resulting from pressure steps applied in an isolated carotid
"blind sack" with one intact sinus nerve (Jänig, Rieckmann and Szulczyk, unpublished observations). Comparative investigations of the same population of MVC
and CVC neurons with both techniques led to the conclusion that both methods of
determining the influence of the baroreceptor afferents on the vasoconstrictor neurons
delivered the same results: Vasoconstrictor neurons with cardiac rhythmicity are
inhibited upon stimulation of baroreceptor afferents by pressure steps; vasoconstrictor neurons without cardiac rhythmicity are not. The cardiac rhythmicity

Vasoconstrictor neurones to muscle (MVC) and skin(CVC)

Noxious cutaneous stimulation

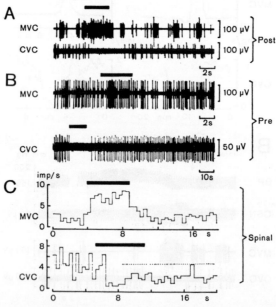

Fig. 2. Effects of noxious cutaneous stimulation on MVC and CVC neurons. A: Postganglionic neurons supplying skeletal muscle and postganglionic neurons supplying hairy
skin, simultaneous recording. Same preparation as in Fig. 1B. B: Preganglionic
lumbar neurons with functional properties similar to those of MVC and CVC
postganglionic neurons. C: Postganglionic bundles supplying lateral gastrocnemius
muscle (MVC) and hairy skin of the superficial peroneal nerve (CVC) in low thoracic
chronic spinal cats. The upper histogram was obtained from eight successive trials
in a cat 48 days after spinalization. The lower histogram was obtained from five
successive trials in a spinal cat 96 days after spinalization. In all records the toes of
the ipsilateral hind foot were stimulated manually with toothed forceps during the
time periods indicated by the black bars. A from Jänig, Rieckmann and Szulczyk,
unpublished observations; B from[20]; C from[13].

determined from post-R-wave histograms is the more sensitive indicator of baroreceptor influence on the vasoconstrictor neurons (Jänig, Rieckmann and Szulczyk,
unpublished observations).

Stimulation of chemoreceptor afferents either by respiring the animal with a
gas mixture of 8% O_2 in N_2 (Fig. 1A$_{1,2}$) or by quick injections of small amounts of
Ringer solution saturated with CO_2 into a common carotid artery (Fig. 1B) induced
excitation of the MVC and inhibition in the majority of the CVC. The reflex action
elicited in the MVC and CVC by injection of CO_2-Ringer solution into a common
carotid artery was preceded by an excitation of afferents in the carotid sinus nerve
(CSN in Fig. 1B). The short excitation of the MVC is followed by an increase in
blood pressure, leading to an inhibition of the activity in MVC but none in the CVC
(Fig. 1B; see increased pulsatile discharges in CSN; the CVC had only weak cardiac
rhythmicity; note that the excitation of the MVC is preceded by a short-lasting inhibition probably produced by the distension of the carotid artery).

The same type of reciprocal pattern (excitation of MVC and inhibition of CVC)
could be produced by stimulation of cutaneous nociceptors induced by mechanical
(Fig. 2A) or by radiant heat stimuli. These reflexes can also be seen in chronic spinal
animals and are therefore probably based on spinal neuronal mechanisms (Fig. 2C;
see also[19]).

Most lumber preganglionic neurons with resting activity which project to
sympathetic chain ganglia caudal to L_4 have the same properties as postganglionic
CVC and MVC neurons[20]. These preganglionic neurons are either excited by stimulation of chemoreceptor and/or cutaneous nociceptor afferents and have cardiac
rhythmicity or are inhibited by stimulation of chemoreceptor and/or cutaneous
nociceptor afferents and have weak or no cardiac rhythmicity (Fig. 1A$_{3,4}$; Fig. 2B).

Sudomotor (SM) and Cutaneous Vasoconstrictor (CVC) Neurons

Postganglionic SM neurons were identified with respect to atropine-sensitive skin
potentials recorded from the hairless skin of the central, large pad of the left hind foot
(see [16,19]; lower records in Fig. 3A–C). These neurons are activated by vibrational
stimuli applied to the experimental frame or to one of the footholders in which the
hind feet were embedded. The discharges in the single SM neuron in Fig. 3A were
fairly well correlated with the fast transient skin potentials evoked by the vibrational
stimulation (see dotted parallel lines connecting discharges and peaks of skin potentials). This observation argues that many SM neurons discharged synchronously
during vibrational stimulation in this experiment.

There are several arguments that this solitary selective activation of the SM
neurons is brought about by the activation of Pacinian corpuscles in the hind paws:
1. The vibrational stimuli used in our laboratory leads to selective activation of afferent
fibers from Pacinian corpuscles[18,27]; other sensitive types of cutaneous receptors such
as those connected with guard or down hairs[1] are not activated by this type of stimulus
(Jänig and Younkin, unpublished observations). 2. Afferent group II fiber stimulation
of the medial plantar nerve (which contains the majority of large diameter afferents
from the Pacinian corpuscles in the hind foot) excites the SM neurons (Jänig and
Kümmel, unpublished observations). 3. Air jet stimulation applied to the toes of one

hind foot activates the SM neurons whereas airjet stimulation applied tangentially to the skin of the lower and/or upper hind leg, thus providing a maximal afferent input from hair follicle receptor afferents, does not activate the SM neurons (see [17,19]).

Cutaneous vasoconstrictor (CVC) neurons innervating the hind paw were either not affected by vibrational stimuli or—more rarely—inhibited (Fig. 3B). Noxious cutaneous stimuli inhibited CVC neurons and excited the SM neurons (Fig. 3C). Excitation of the SM neurons by noxious stimuli in brain-intact chloralose anesthetized animals was normally weak[16]. In lightly anesthetized (with Ketamine or Methohexital) brain-intact cats the effects of noxious cutaneous stimulation on the SM system were mostly stronger[17].

Cutaneous vasoconstrictor (CVC) and sudomotor (SM) neurones

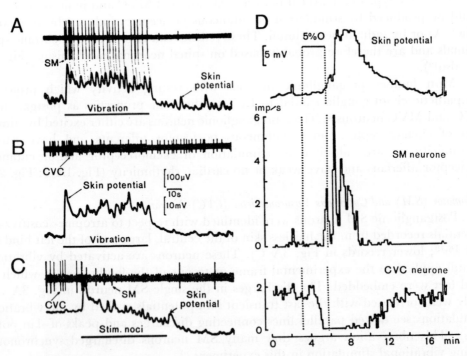

Fig. 3.   Effects of vibrational stimuli (A, B), noxious cutaneous stimuli (C) and chemoreceptor stimulation (D) on CVC and SM neurons. Neuronal activity recorded from filaments dissected from the medial plantar nerve. Skin potential recorded from the central (large) pad of the ipsilateral hind foot. A, B: Single fiber preparations. Note that the discharges of the neuron in A are followed, with one exception, by small transient skin potentials during the vibrational stimulation. C: Multifiber preparation; two postganglionic axons (SM, CVC) could be discriminated. The small signals were recorded from other, most likely CVC, axons. D: Simultaneous recording of skin potential and activity of an SM and a CVC neuron before, during and after respiration of the animal with 5% O_2 in N_2. The skin potential was recorded in an analog mode. Bin width 10s. From[16].

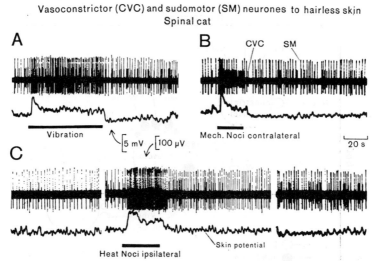

Fig. 4. Reaction of a postganglionic SM neuron and a CVC neuron to vibrational and noxious cutaneous stimuli in a chronic spinal cat. Activity recorded from postganglionic axons in a filament dissected from the medial plantar nerve. Skin potential recorded from the central (large) pad of the ipsilateral hind foot. Vibrational stimulus produced by tapping on the experimental frame (see[17]). Mechanical noxious stimulus applied to one of the toes of the contralateral hind foot. Noxious heat stimulus produced by radiant heat of 55°C applied to the toes of the ipsilateral hind foot (Jänig and Spilok, unpublished observations).

This reaction pattern of SM and CVC neurons to cutaneous stimuli has also been observed in chronic spinal cats (Fig. 4). Vibrational stimulation activates SM neurons and does not affect or—more rarely—inhibits CVC neurons (Fig. 4A). Noxious stimulation of the contralateral hind paw mostly activates both SM and CVC neurons (Fig. 4B); noxious stimulation of the toes of the ipsilateral hind paw mostly activates the SM neurons and inhibits the CVC neurons (Fig. 4C).

Stimulation of peripheral chemoreceptor afferents by systemic hypoxia or systemic hypercapnia leads to excitation of the SM neurons and to inhibition of the CVC neurons supplying the hairless skin of the hind paw (Fig. 3D). Essentially the same pattern has been observed upon stimulation of warm receptors in the spinal cord[30] in brain-intact and in chronic spinal animals[7]; (Jänig and Kümmel, unpublished observations). These warm stimuli activate SM neurons only transiently.

COMMENTS

The effects of the most potent afferent inputs so far investigated in our laboratory on the vasoconstrictor systems supplying skeletal muscle and hairy and hairless skin and on the SM system are schematized in Fig. 5. Details about the functional and static properties of these sympathetic subsystems and of other sympathetic subsystems to hind limb and tail being investigated in our laboratory are not described in this paper but in the respective publications referred to herein[6-9,13-17,19,20]. Figure 5 shows

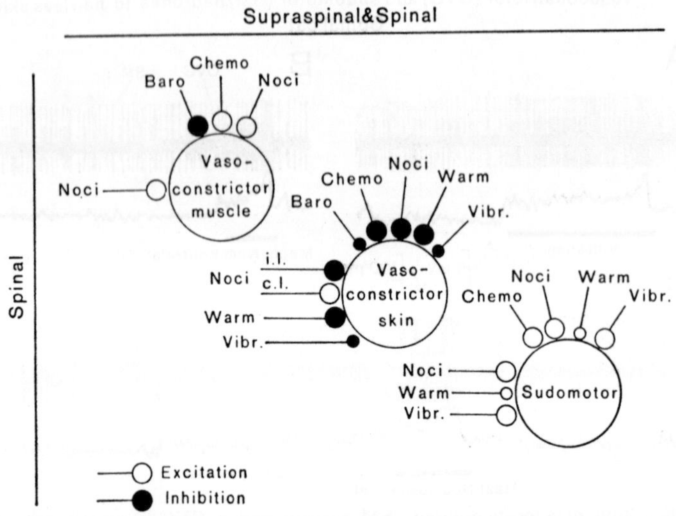

Fig. 5. Organization of vasoconstrictor systems (MVC, CVC) and sudomotor system (SM) in brain-intact animals (supraspinal and spinal) and in spinal animals (spinal) with respect to various afferent inputs. The open and closed small cycles represent the overall excitatory and inhibitory effects on the respective system. Baro: Effect of baroreceptor stimulation by pressure steps in the carotid blindsack or by pulsatile blood pressure. Chemo: Effect of chemoreceptor stimulation by systemic hypoxia or by quick injections of CO_2-Ringer into the external carotid artery. Noci: Effect of cutaneous nociceptor stimulation by mechanical or radiant heat stimuli (i. l., ipsilateral; c. l., contralateral). Vibr.: Effect of Pacinian corpuscle stimulation in the hind paws by vibrational stimuli produced by tapping on the experimental frame. Warm: Effect of warm receptor stimulation in the spinal cord by spinal cord warming.

that, first, MVC and CVC systems and, second, CVC and SM systems, are largely reciprocally organized with respect to specific afferent inputs. The important exception to this reciprocal organization is the effect of the baroreceptor afferents on the vasoconstrictor systems. These afferents have no effect on the SM system.

The reciprocal organization can be shown to exist in brain-intact preparations (inputs from top in Fig. 5) as well as to some extent in chronic spinal preparations (inputs from the left side in Fig. 5). It is most obvious from Fig. 5 that the CVC system is largely controlled in an inhibitory mode by the different afferent inputs whereas the MVC and the SM systems are regulated in an excitatory mode. These reciprocal reaction patterns reflect the functional synergy between different sympathetic subsystems. It must be assumed that these rather uniform patterns are based on simple neuronal interconnections in the spinal cord and brain stem. Neuronal network with excitatory and inhibitory interneurons should be able to produce these reciprocal reaction patterns.

Occasional chance observations on totally deafferented animals (buffer nerves and vagal nerves cut) in which the activity in postganglionic neurons supplying skeletal muscle and hairy skin have been recorded simultaneously and in which the arterial blood pressure was about 100 mm Hg, support this assumption (Jänig,

Mense and Torigata, unpublished observations). In six of eleven cats it was observed that when the activity in the MVC increased spontaneously (without any stimulus applied to the animal), this increase of activity in the MVC was accompanied by a decrease in the activity in CVC neurons and was followed by an increase in blood pressure (Fig. 6A, B). Simultaneous increase and decrease in activity in MVC and CVC neurons, respectively, were nearly mirror images of one another in some experiments (Fig. 6A), indicating a close reciprocal neuronal linkage between both systems in the neuraxis.

On the basis of these reciprocal reaction patterns preganglionic sympathetic neurons can be classified and, in this way, indirectly identified with respect to the target organs they regulate. In the future it perhaps will be more important for the reciprocal reaction patterns to serve as conceptual frame for the analysis of the neuronal circuits in the neuraxis which enable regulation of the sympathetic subsystems to occur.

A functional interpretation of these reciprocal reaction patterns can, for the time being, only be conjectured. It must be emphasized that Fig. 5 is neither a model nor a wiring diagram; it expresses and summarizes for the three sympathetic subsystems the effects caused by activation of various afferent channels. These effects can be looked upon as reflexes in the Sherringtonian sense (which may be especially justified

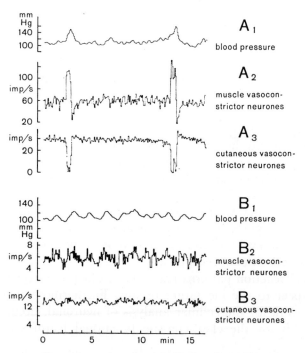

Fig. 6. Spontaneous fluctuations of resting activity in MVC and CVC neurons in two preparations (A, B) with buffer and vagal nerves cut. Multifiber preparations dissected from the deep peroneal nerve (muscle vasoconstrictor neurons) and from the superficial peroneal nerve (nerve supplying hairy skin). Simultaneous recordings. Bin width five sec. From Jänig, Mense and Torigata (unpublished observations).

for the spinal preparation; but see[19]); however they can also be thought of as disturbances of ongoing regulations. The reactions are artificially produced under controlled experimental conditions. They do not tell us how the sympathetic subsystem works under various functional conditions such as heat load, arousal, stress, work, etc.

The afferent input systems belong to feedback systems (e.g., from baro-, chemo-, warm-receptors, Fig. 5) or to open-loop systems (e.g., from nociceptors, Fig. 5). It must be assumed that the same afferent channel feeds at various levels into yet unknown neuronal machineries. This is especially obvious for the neuronal substrates which bring about temperature regulation[30], but has also been established for the inputs from baro- and chemoreceptors[10,22] and for the input from various cutaneous afferents (spinal and supraspinal reflexes, see [21,29]). These neuronal interactions must be conceived of as having some sort of closely intertwined organizations which are represented on diverse levels in complex functions[2,22]. Pre- and postganglionic neurons are the final common motoneurons of these neuronal mechanisms. Eventually an analysis such as summarized in Fig. 5 may lead in future to the elaboration of spinal and supraspinal neuronal wiring diagrams. The understanding of the functions of these wiring diagrams can only be accomplished in the context of various autonomic regulations.

SUMMARY

Reciprocal reaction patterns with respect to various afferent inputs from the skin surface and from the interior of the body have been described for the following three sympathetic subsystems: the vasoconstrictor system supplying skeletal muscle (MVC), the vasoconstrictor system supplying skin (CVC), and the sudomotor system (SM). The MVC and SM systems are largely regulated in an excitatory mode, whereas the CVC system is predominantly regulated in an inhibitory mode.

The MVC system and the CVC system are reciprocally organized with respect to the afferent inputs from cutaneous nociceptors and from arterial chemoreceptors. The CVC system supplying hairless skin and the sudomotor system are reciprocally organized with respect to afferent inputs from cutaneous nociceptors, from arterial chemoreceptors, from spinal warm receptors and from vibrational receptors (Pacinian corpuscles) in the foot pads. These reciprocal organizations can also be shown to exist at the spinal cord level for inputs from cutaneous nociceptors, from spinal warm receptors and from vibrational receptors.

The reciprocal reaction patterns may serve to help one recognize preganglionic neurons with respect to specific target organs. Furthermore they may serve as a conceptual framework for the cellular analysis of neuronal circuits in the neuraxis which are the basis for the characteristic functional features of the sympathetic subsystems.

Supported by the Deutsche Forschungsgemeinschaft.

REFERENCES

1 Burgess, P. R. and Perl, E. R., Cutaneous mechanoreceptors and nociceptors. In: A. Iggo (Ed.), *Handbook of Sensory Physiology*, Vol. *II*, *"Somato-sensory System"*, Springer-Verlag, Berlin—Heidelberg—New York, 1973, pp. 29–78.

2 Calaresu, R. F., Faiers, A. A. and Mogenson, G. J., Central neural regulation of heart and blood vessels in mammals, *Progress in Neurobiology*, 5 (1975) 1–35.

3 Cannon, W. B., *Bodily Changes in Pain, Hunger, Fear and Rage*, D. Appleton & Co., New York, 2nd ed. 1929.

4 Cannon, W. B., *The Wisdom of the Body*, W. W. Norton & Co., New York, 1932, revised 1939.

5 Granit, R., The functional role of the muscle spindles—facts and hypotheses, *Brain*, 98 (1975) 531–556.

6 Gregor, M. and Jänig, W., Effects of systemic hypoxia and hypercapnia on cutaneous and muscle vasoconstrictor neurones to the cat's hindlimb, *Pflügers Arch.*, 368 (1977) 71–81.

7 Gregor, M., Jänig, W. and Riedel, W., Response patterns of cutaneous postganglionic neurones to the hind limb on spinal cord heating and cooling in the cat, *Pflügers Arch.*, 363 (1976) 135–140.

8 Gregor, M., Jänig, W. and Wiprich, L., Cardiac and respiratory rhythmicities in cutaneous and muscle vasoconstrictor neurones to the cat's hind limb, *Pflügers Arch.*, 370, (1977) 299–302.

9 Grosse, M. and Jänig, W., Vasoconstrictor and pilomotor fibers in skin nerves to the cat's tail, *Pflügers Arch.*, 361 (1976) 221–229.

10 Hilton, S. M., Ways of viewing the central nervous control of the circulation—Old and new, *Brain Res.*, 87 (1975) 213–219.

11 Horeyseck, G. and Jänig, W., Reflexes in postganglionic fibers within skin and muscle nerves after mechanical non-noxious stimulation of skin, *Exp. Brain Res.*, 20 (1974) 115–123.

12 Horeyseck, G. and Jänig, W., Reflexes in postganglionic fibers within skin and muscle nerves after noxious stimulation of skin, *Exp. Brain Res.*, 20 (1974) 125–134.

13 Horeyseck, G. and Jänig, W., Reflex activity in postganglionic fibers within skin and muscle nerves elicited by somatic stimuli in chronic spinal cats, *Exp. Brain Res.*, 21 (1974) 155–168.

14 Horeyseck, G., Jänig, W., Kirchner, F. and Thämer, V., Activation and inhibition of muscle and cutaneous postganglionic neurones to hind limb during hypothalamically induced vasoconstriction and atropine-sensitive vasodilation, *Pflügers Arch.*, 361 (1976) 231–240.

15 Jänig, W., Central organization of somatosympathetic reflexes in vasoconstrictor neurones, *Brain Res.*, 87 (1975) 305–312.

16 Jänig, W. and Kümmel, H., Functional discrimination of postganglionic neurones to the cat's hind paw with respect to the skin potentials recorded from the hairless skin, *Pflügers Arch.*, 371 (1977) 217–225.

17 Jänig, W. and Räth, B., Electrodermal reflexes in the cat's paws elicited by natural stimulation of skin, *Pflügers Arch.*, 369 (1977) 27–32.

18 Jänig, W., Schmidt, R. F. and Zimmermann, M., Single unit responses and the total afferent outflow from the cat's foot pad upon mechanical stimulation, *Exp. Brain Res.*, 6 (1968) 100–115.

19   Jänig, W. and Spilok, N., Functional organization of the sympathetic innervation supplying the hairless skin of the hind paws in chronic spinal cats, *Pflügers Arch.*, 377 (1978) 25–31.

20   Jänig, W. and Szulczyk, P., Functional properties of lumbar preganglionic neurons, *Brain Res.*, (1979) submitted.

21   Koizumi, K. and Brooks, C. McC., The integration of autonomic system reactions: A discussion of autonomic reflexes, their control and their association with somatic reactions, *Ergebn. Physiol.*, 67 (1972) 1–68.

22   Korner, P. I., Integrative neural cardiovascular control, *Physiol. Rev.*, 51 (1971) 312–367.

23   Lundberg, A., Ascending spinal hind limb pathways in the cat, *Progress in Brain Res.*, 12 (1964) 135–163.

24   Lundberg, A., Excitatory control of the Ia inhibitory pathway. In: P. Anderson and J. K. S. Jansen (Eds.), *Excitatory Synaptic Mechanisms*, Universitetsforlaget, Oslo-Bergen-Tromsö, 1970, pp. 333–340.

25   Lundberg, A., The significance of segmental spinal mechanisms in motor control, *4th Internat. Biophysics Congress, Moscow: International Union for Pure and Applied Physics*, 1972, pp. 1–13.

26   Lundberg, A., Control of spinal mechanisms from the brain. In: D. B. Tower (Ed.), *The Nervous System, Vol. 1, The Basic Neurosciences*, Raven Press, New York, 1975, pp. 253–265.

27   Lynn, B., The form and distribution of receptive fields of Pacinian corpuscles found in and around the cat's large foot pad, *J. Physiol.* (Lond.), 217 (1971) 755–771.

28   Phillips, C. G. and Porter, R., *Corticospinal neurones. Their role in movement*, Academic Press, London—New York—San Francisco, 1977.

29   Sato, A. and Schmidt, R. F., Somatosympathetic reflexes: Afferent fibers, central pathways, discharge characteristics, *Physiol. Rev.*, 53 (1973) 916–947.

30   Simon, E., Temperature regulation: The spinal cord as a site of extra-hypothalamic thermoregulatory functions, *Rev. Physiol. Biochem. Pharmacol.*, 71 (1974) 1–76.

CHAPTER 19

THE EFFECTS OF SOMATIC AFFERENT ACTIVITY ON THE HEART RATE

A. Sato*, Y. Sato* and R. F. Schmidt**

*2nd Department of Physiology, The Tokyo Metropolitan Institute of Gerontology,
Tokyo, Japan, and
**The Physiologisches Institut der Universität Kiel,
Kiel, Fed. Rep. Germany

INTRODUCTION

Despite extensive experimental tests, Hunt's (1895)[8] ingenious postulate of specific "pressor" and "depressor" somatosensory afferent fibers has never been satisfactorily confirmed. To the contrary, it has been shown by many workers that the occurrence of such pressor or depressor responses depended not only, or at least not completely, on the diameter of the activated fiber population, but on other parameters, such as the frequency and duration of the tetanic stimulation, the location of the afferent input and, particularly, the condition of the animal (*cf.* McDowall[16] for the early literature and others[10,14,15] for later contributions).

On the efferent side a further important aspect has been introduced by Johansson[10] when showing that the same somatic afferent volley by no means has to have the same effect on the sympathetic outflows to functionally different vascular beds. These findings are but one aspect of the long-neglected individuality of sympathetic subsystems which is now much more generally recognized (see for instance in this volume the contributions of Jänig[9] and Sato et al.[23]).

In regard to the afferent side it is also more and more appreciated that graded electrical stimulation of afferent nerves is only an extremely crude substitute for the naturally-occurring modes of activating the various sensory modalities. In particular there are very few if any situations indeed where electrical stimulation unequivocally activates but one type of cutaneous or muscle receptor. The only rather clear-cut example in this respect is the activation of the Group Ia afferents from primary muscle spindles by low strength stimuli (although a contamination by Ib fibers is always difficult to exclude). But, alas, these sense organs do not seem to appreciably influence any sympathetic outflow[26]. Those which do, like the nociceptive afferents, cannot be stimulated in isolation, not even under a complete conduction block of the thick afferent fibers, since the cutaneous as well as the muscle nerves also contain plenty of non-nociceptive fine afferents.

In the studies concerned with the pressor and depressor effects of somatic afferent activity, little notice has been taken of the changes in heart rate induced by these inputs[10]; and there are only sporadic and short reports from other laboratories addressing themselves directly to this subject[13,20,21]. Nevertheless, these reports definitely indicate that somatic afferent activity does induce reflex changes in the sympathetic outflow to the heart which can clearly be separated from effects induced either by alterations of the vagal outflow, or by humoral effects or by more indirect reflex actions via the baro- or chemo-receptor afferents.

The present contribution is part of a systematic effort by this laboratory to characterize in detail the direct reflex effects of somatosensory input on the heart rate. Preceding studies on cats and rats have dealt with the heart rate changes induced by noxious and non-noxious thermal and mechanical skin stimulation[1,27]. In the endeavor briefly summarized here, the effects of electrical stimulation of cutaneous and muscle nerves as well as those of a chemical activation of muscular nociceptors have been analyzed.

METHODS

The experiments were performed on 15 adult cats anesthetized with chloralose and urethane (initially 50–60 mg/kg and 100–120 mg/kg, i.p., respectively, additional doses as required). The general experimental procedures, such as immobilization with gallamine thriethiodide, adjustment of artificial respiration, the recording of systemic blood pressure from the right common carotid artery, control and regulation of body temperature, cutting of both vagus nerves early in the experiment and the recording of heart rate by a pulse rate tachometer have recently been described[11].

In the experiments using electric nerve stimulation the major cutaneous and muscle nerves of the left hind limb were cut and prepared for bipolar stimulation (cf. Sato et al.[24], for details). The thresholds for various fiber groups and stimulus strengths for their maximum activation were determined by recording the centripetal volleys several centimeters proximal to the stimulating electrodes. The stimulus strength for the most excitable fibers was called 1.0T. The threshold for Group IV or C fibers was always near 100T, and the Group IV volley usually reached its maximum before 400T. Since 1.0T was usually around 50 mV, a stimulus strength of 20 V has been considered to excite all Group IV fibers.

Chemical stimulation of muscle afferent units was performed by injection of algesic substances such as bradykinin triacetate (Brad.), 5-hydroxytryptamine creatine sulphate (5-HT), and potassium chloride (K^+) via a catheter into the left saphenous artery. In these experiments the left hind limb was denervated except for the nerve branches to the triceps surae, flexor digitorum longus, flexor hallucis longus and plantaris muscles. A complete transection of the left hind limb except for the femoral artery and vein, and the occlusion of these vessels during the chemical stimulation were necessary because otherwise the effects on heart rate and blood pressure induced by bradykinin and 5-HT after their influx into the general circulation interfered appreciably with the changes evoked by the excitation of muscle afferent units.

For the injection of chemicals the following technique was adopted: The test solution (0.3–0.5 ml) was injected into the catheter, the femoral artery and vein were occluded and 30 sec later the test substances were injected with one ml Tyrode. Sixty to 90 seconds later, sometimes 120 sec later, circulation was restored. The amount of test solution necessary for maximal heart rate changes (usually 0.4 or 0.5 ml) was determined at the beginning of each experiment. The occlusion itself and placebo injections of Tyrode solution had no effects. Cutting the sciatic nerves made all effects disappear, but there was no change in the response patterns following removal of the suprarenal glands. (For a more detailed description of the method of chemically exciting muscle afferent units and for its application in the present experiments see Mense and Schmidt[19] and others[3,4,12,18,25].)

RESULTS AND DISCUSSION

Heart Rate Changes Induced by Afferent Volleys in Cutaneous Nerves

In anesthetized cats with the central nervous system intact, a reflex increase in heart rate was found by Kaufman et al.[11] after natural stimuli such as pinching (noxious mechanical stimulation), rubbing (non-noxious mechanical stimulation), warming and cooling (thermal stimuli) were applied to the skin of the neck, chest, abdomen or perineum. It was shown by these authors that this cutaneo-cardiac acceleration reflex was produced mainly by a reflex increase in the discharges of the cardiac sympathetic efferent nerves, and only to a small extent by a reflex decrease in the discharges of the cardiac vagal efferent nerves. In rats, corresponding cardiac acceleration reflexes were produced purely as a result of a reflex increase in cardiac sympathetic activity[27]. In view of these findings, both vagus nerves were cut in the present experiments.

Repetitive electrical stimulation of all Group II fibers in a cutaneous nerve did not change the heart rate (or blood pressure) irrespective of the duration or the frequency of the tetanus. However, volleys in cutaneous Group III fibers usually produced small to intermediate increases in heart rate. In a few cases no effects on the heart rate were seen, and in two series cutaneous Group III volleys induced slight bradycardic effects.

A comparison of these results with those of Kaufman et al.[11] allows the conclusion that the cutaneo-cardiac acceleration reflexes observed after non-noxious rubbing, cooling and warming of the skin are entirely due to the activation of mechano- and thermo-receptive units with Group III afferent fibers[1]. This is a remarkable finding and certainly a clear reflection of the specificity of the various cutaneo-sympathetic reflexes, since Group II cutaneous afferents do induce such reflexes in other sympathetic subsystems[26].

Very consistent increases in heart rate were always seen when repetitive Group IV cutaneous afferent volleys were elicited. This tachycardia was observed irrespective of whether stimuli subthreshold for Group IV did or did not evoke changes in heart rate; but it was most obvious if, due to the animals' condition or the stimulus parameters chosen, there was no heart rate change from the myelinated fibers at all.

These findings are well in line with those obtained when painfully pinching the skin of rats and cats[11,27]. It is suggested that these results are all due to the activation

278   A. Sato et al.

of nociceptive afferent units causing an alarming reaction. It is, however, appreciated that the skin contains various types of non-nociceptive afferent units with unmyelinated fibers. But their contribution to the cutaneo-cardiac reflexes cannot be evaluated at present.

Heart Rate Changes Induced by Afferent Volleys in Muscle Nerves

Group I afferent volleys from muscle spindles and Golgi tendon organs do not induce heart rate changes at all, just as volleys in these afferents do not seem to have any action on other sympathetic subsystems[26]. Similarly, volleys in Group II muscle afferents evoked no changes in heart rate, or they had at best very slight and variable effects. Also, in our experiments, selective chemical activation of Group I and II muscle spindle afferent units by succinylcholine[7,18] was equally ineffective.

More than in any other fiber group, the volleys in Group III fibers from muscle induced variable responses both in the bradycardic and in the tachycardic direction. There was no way to predict whether either one of these responses would occur at the beginning of a recording session, despite rigorous efforts to keep the conditions of successive experiments as constant as possible. If there was a bradycardic response to start with, it usually decreased in amplitude in the course of an experiment, and in some cases changed to a tachycardic one. If acceleratory responses were present from the beginning of the recording session they usually remained unchanged throughout the experiment except for some eventual small increase or decrease in amplitude.

The variable effects of muscle Group III volleys are well matched by the effects of these fibers on other sympathetic efferent systems. For instance, in experiments of other authors checking for the "pressor" or "depressor" characteristics of these fibers it was also found that the blood pressure responses upon their activation were difficult to predict, and various experimental parameters have been held responsible for this finding[5,6,10,14,15,17]. But in those, as in the present, experiments no entirely satisfactory explanation of the response diversity was possible.

Just like the cutaneous Group IV volleys, those from muscle Group IV afferents invariably and very consistently induced remarkable increases in heart rate, irrespec-

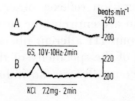

Fig. 1.   Changes in heart rate induced by activity in fine muscle afferent fibers. In A the gastrocnemius-soleus muscle nerve was stimulated by electrical square pulses (10 V, 0.5 msec, 10 Hz, for two min). The bar below the record indicates the period of stimulation. In B, 7.2 mg of KCl in 0.3 ml solution were injected via a catheter in the arteria articularis genu suprema into the gastrocnemius-soleus muscle. The injection started just after the occlusion of the femoral artery and vein at the beginning of the underbar. Two minutes later, at the end of the bar, the vessels were reopened (from[22]).

tive of the action of Group III fibers. A typical example is shown in Fig. 1A. As a rule, the increase in heart rate induced by Group IV muscle volleys was proportional to the stimulus strength, i.e., the number of Group IV afferents being stimulated, reaching a plateau only after all the Group IV fibers were included in the volley. Some occlusion with the effects of Group III volleys was present, but it was not as pronounced as in cutaneous nerves.

Intra-arterial injection of three different algesic chemicals, namely K^+, bradykinin and serotonin, into certain muscles of the lower hind limb (see Methods) was used to mimic the effects of muscle pain on the tonic sympathetic outflow to the heart. Injection of K^+ regularly produced an increase in heart rate (Fig. 1B), and the same was found for the majority of bradykinin injections. But, somewhat to our surprise, in a considerable number of cases injection of bradykinin resulted in a deceleration of the heart rate. Finally, injection of serotonin was rather ineffective in producing heart rate changes, but subsequent injections of either KCl or bradykinin gave rise to enhanced acceleratory responses, i.e., in all probability serotonin produced a temporary sensitization of the muscle nociceptors.

The different responses to various algesic substances are probably due to the different primary afferent response profiles elicited by these substances in Group III and IV fibers. But these are not sufficient to explain why bradykinin injections may evoke acceleration or deceleration of the heart rate. We have to make the additional assumption that within the bradykinin-sensitive units there are at least two subpopulations: one which upon activation elicits acceleration and one which elicits deceleration of the heart rate. If this is so, factors such as the distribution of bradykinin in the muscular tissue or the overall excitability of one or the other type of unit will determine the direction of the heart rate change.

Properties of Somato-cardiac Acceleration Reflexes

With electrical stimulation the latency from the beginning of a near-maximum afferent tetanus to the onset of a just-detectable heart rate change was in the order of five sec for cutaneous and 10 sec for muscle afferent volleys. With chemical stimulation of muscle afferents it was also around 10 sec for K^+ injections but around 20 sec for bradykinin injections. (This difference is entirely due to the longer latency of the peripheral receptor activation by bradykinin[2,4].)

After the onset of a heart rate change it took some 15 to 35 sec to reach its peak following both electrical and chemical afferent stimulation (Fig. 1). With electrical stimulation the reflex acceleration responses often exceeded 50 beats/min. On the average, the reflex responses to chemical stimulation were somewhat smaller, but altogether they were on the same order of magnitude (compare A with B in Fig. 1).

After reaching its peak value the heart rate started to return to its control level even in those experiments where peripheral stimulation continued (Fig. 1). Often under such conditions there was an original rather rapid decline from the peak value to a kind of "plateau" about halfway between the peak and the control level. At the end of the stimulation the heart rate always returned fully to its control value, usually in less than one min.

Single maximum Group IV volleys do not evoke an increase in heart rate.

The minimum frequency of tetanic stimulation to elicit a definite heart rate increase was 0.5 Hz but occasionally even at 0.25, 0.13 or 0.11 Hz (i.e., at stimulus intervals of four, eight or nine sec, respectively) heart rate increases have been observed. Not unexpectedly, their latencies were much longer and their peaks smaller than those elicited by tetani in the best frequency range (six–15 Hz). In this range, about five afferent volleys sufficed to induce a change in heart rate, and near-maximum heart rate changes were usually elicited by a tetanus of a few seconds' duration.

No simple and straightforward relations between heart rate responses and blood pressure changes have been seen, although at first slight increases in heart rate seem to be coupled to pressor responses and decreases to depressor ones. However, there was every possible exception to this pattern, particularly with weak or short inputs. In quite a few cases heart rate changes were observed without any modifications of the blood pressure. In others definite increases in heart rate were accompanied by depressor or by very mixed responses. These findings further support the viewpoint that blood pressure is only a very indirect and possibly quite an inappropriate way of monitoring the central autonomic effects of somatosensory inputs.

SUMMARY AND CONCLUSIONS

Summing up the outcome of the preceding and present experiments[11,22,24,25,27] on the reflex actions of somatosensory inputs on the sympathetic outflow to the heart as indicated by the changes in heart rate of vagotomized, anesthetized rats and cats, it is pointed out that some of the cutaneous and muscular sensory modalities, especially those in the nociceptive domain, have quite powerful excitatory actions on this particular sympathetic subsystem. Others, namely those from the skin with Group II afferent fibers and those from muscle with Group I and II afferents, have no or little effect. The Group III fibers from muscle seem to subserve modalities with accelerating as well as decelerating reflex effects on the heart rate.

The lack of a clear-cut correlation between the reflex effects of somatosensory input on the heart and those on blood pressure adds a further piece of evidence to the already existing ones that Hunt's (1895)[8] concept of "pressor" and "depressor" primary afferent fibers is now considered to be false and should no longer be used as a hypothesis for future experiments.

The somato-cardiac acceleration reflexes offer a quick and reliable way to increase the heart rate at times where, as in sudden fight and flight, a rapid increase in cardiac output is urgently needed. They are an example of the great number of specialized reflex connections which probably exist between the somatosensory and the autonomic nervous system to ensure appropriate adjustments of the autonomic effector organs in response to animals' motor activities and sensory experiences.

Financial supports from the Ministry of Education of Japan and Japan Heart Foundation (to A. Sato), the Japan Society for the Promotion of Science and the Deutsche Forschungsgemeinschaft (to R. F. Schmidt) are gratefully acknowledged.

REFERENCES

1 Burgess, P. R. and Perl, E. R., Cutaneous mechanoreceptors and nociceptors. In: A. Iggo (Ed.), *Handbook of Sensory Physiology, Vol. II, Somatosensory System*, Springer-Verlag, Berlin—Heidelberg—New York, 1973, pp. 29–76.

2 Fock, S. and Mense, S., Excitatory effects of 5-hydroxytryptamine, histamine and potassium on muscular group IV afferent units: A comparison with bradykinin, *Brain Res.*, 105 (1976) 459–469.

3 Foreman, R. D., Schmidt, R. F. and Willis, W. D., Effects of mechanical and chemical stimulation of fine muscle afferents upon primate spinothalamic tract cells, *J. Physiol.* (Lond.), 286 (1979) 215–231.

4 Franz, M. and Mense, S., Muscle receptors with group IV afferent fibers responding to application of bradykinin, *Brain Res.*, 92 (1975) 369–383.

5 Gordon, G., The mechanism of the vasomotor reflexes produced by stimulating mammalian sensory nerves, *J. Physiol.* (Lond.), 102 (1943) 95–107.

6 Gordon, G., The concept of relay nuclei. In: A. Iggo (Ed.), *Handbook of Sensory Physiology, Vol. II, Somatosensory System*, Springer-Verlag, Berlin—Heidelberg—New York, 1973, pp. 137–150.

7 Granit, R., Skoglund, St. and Thesleff, St., Activation of muscle spindles by Succinyl-choline and Decamethonium. The effect of Curare, *Acta physiol. scand.*, 28 (1953) 130–160.

8 Hunt, R., The fall of blood pressure resulting from the stimulation of afferent nerves, *J. Physiol.* (Lond.), 18 (1895) 381–410.

9 Jänig, W., Reciprocal reaction patterns of sympathetic subsystems with respect to various afferent inputs. This volume, pp. 263–274.

10 Johansson, B., Circulatory responses to stimulation of somatic afferents, *Acta physiol. scand.*, 57, Suppl. 198 (1962) 1–91.

11 Kaufman, A., Sato, A., Sato, Y. and Sugimoto, H., Reflex changes in heart rate after mechanical and thermal stimulation of the skin at various segmental levels, *Neuroscience*, 2 (1977) 103–109.

12 Kniffki, K.-D., Mense, S. and Schmidt, R. F., Responses of Group IV afferent units from skeletal muscle to stretch, contraction and chemical stimulation, *Exp. Brain Res.*, 31 (1978) 511–522.

13 Kumagai, Y., Norman, J. and Whitwam, J. G., The sympathetic contribution to increase in heart rate evoked by cutaneous nerve stimulation in the dog, *J. Physiol.* (Lond.), 252 (1975) 37 P–38 P.

14 Laporte, Y., Bessou, P. and Bouisset, S., Action réflexe des différents types de fibres afférentes d'origine musculaire sur la pression sanguine, *Arch. ital. Biol.*, 98 (1960) 206–221.

15 Laporte, Y. and Montastruc, P., Rôle des différents types de fibres afférentes dans les réflexes circulatoires généraux d'origine cutanée, *J. Physiol.* (Paris), 49 (1957) 1039–1049.

16 McDowall, R. J. S., *The Control of Circulation of the Blood*, W. W. Dawson and Sons, Ltd., London, 2nd Edition, 1956.

17 McLennan, H., On the response of the vasomotor system to somatic afferent nerve stimulation, and the effect of anesthesia and curare thereon, *Pflügers Arch.*, 273 (1961) 604–613.

18 Mense, S., Nervous outflow from skeletal muscle following chemical noxious stimulation, *J. Physiol.* (Lond.), 267 (1977) 75–88.

282   A. Sato et al.

19 Mense, S. and Schmidt, R. F., Activation of group IV afferent units from muscle by
    algesic agents, *Brain Res.*, 72 (1974) 305–310.
20 Norman, J. and Whitwam, J. G., The effect of stimulation of somatic afferent nerves on
    sympathetic nerve activity, heart rate and blood pressure in dogs, *J. Physiol.* (Lond.),
    231 (1973a) 76 P–77 P.
21 Norman, J. and Whitwam, J. G., The vagal contribution to changes in heart rate
    evoked by stimulation of cutaneous nerves in the dog, *J. Physiol.* (Lond.), 234 (1973)
    89 P–90 P.
22 Sato, A., Sato, Y. and Schmidt, R. F., Autonomic reflexes elicited by stimulation of
    muscle afferent nerves in the cat, *Proceedings of the 18th International Congress of Neuro-*
    vegetative Research, (1977) 106–108.
23 Sato, A., Sato, Y. and Schmidt, R. F., Somatic afferents and their effects on bladder
    function. This volume, pp. 309–318.
24 Sato, A., Sato, Y. and Schmidt, R. F., Heart rate changes reflecting modifications of
    cardiac sympathetic outflow by cutaneous and muscle afferent volleys, (1979) in
    preparation.
25 Sato, A., Sato, Y. and Schmidt, R. F., Changes in heart rate and blood pressure due to
    the chemical activation of nociceptors in skeletal muscle, (1979) in preparation.
26 Sato, A. and Schmidt, R. F., Somatosympathetic reflexes: Afferent fibers, central
    pathways, discharge characteristics, *Physiol. Rev.*, 53 (1973) 916–947.
27 Sato, A., Sato, Y., Shimada, F. and Torigata, Y., Varying changes in heart rate produced
    by nociceptive stimulation of the skin in rats at different temperatures, *Brain Res.*, 110
    (1976) 301–311.

CHAPTER 20

BARORECEPTOR CONTROL OF VAGAL PREGANGLIONIC ACTIVITY

K. M. Spyer

Department of Physiology, The Medical School, Vincent Drive,
Birmingham, England

INTRODUCTION

The importance of vagal efferent activity in cardiac control has been underlined by numerous experimental studies on several species. In particular, much of the baroreceptor control of the heart is mediated by these efferent fibers[10], but even though this mechanism appears to function in the decerebrate animal, the basic circuitry for baroreceptor-vagal interaction has remained unresolved. Indeed it is only the results of studies during the last five years that have resolved the location of cardiac vagal neurons in the medulla.

The localization of cardiac vagal neurons in the medulla has concerned anatomists and physiologists for a century. The vagus is known to have two motor nuclei in the medulla of mammals: a dorsal nucleus (the dorsal motor nucleus, DMN) and a ventral nucleus (the nucleus ambiguus, NA). By the 1950's it had become generally accepted that the DMN contained those vagal neurons innervating unstriated muscle and the NA those cells which innervated the striated muscle of the respiratory tract[35]. This conclusion rested on evidence from studies looking at the degenerative changes produced in these nuclei after transections of the vagus and its various peripheral branches[35], but ignored or disregarded contradictory evidence from similar experiments by a large number of other investigators (see, for e.g.,[22]). Equally, Szentagothai[41] who placed restricted lesions in the NA and DMN and searched the vagus and its peripheral branches for signs of wallerian degeneration, concluded that vagal cardio-inhibitory fibers, at least in the cat, originated from cells in the NA rather than in the DMN. This demonstration was largely disregarded on the basis that such lesions would not distinguish between damage to fibers *en passant* and cell bodies[35]. The neurophysiological literature is similarly confusing with rival claims on the basis of electrical stimulation experiments that cardio-inhibitory neurons are located in the NA, the DMN, or both[4,5,8,42]. Lesion experiments point, however, to their location in the NA as electrolytic destruction of the DMN is ineffective in abolishing vagally-mediated bradycardia following several procedures[3,18,19], a conclusion that has since been confirmed and extended in the cat by neurophysiological experiments that will be described later[29,30,32,33].

The absence of a definitive description of the location of vagal cardiac neurons (CVM's) in the medulla has not prevented the demonstration of the importance of this cardiac innervation. It is established that the vagal efferents exerting negative chronotropic changes are B fibers[34]. Such neurons in both the cervical vagus and cardiac branches of cats and dogs have been shown to be excited by electrical stimulation of the sinus nerve[14,15,25] or natural baroreceptor stimulation[6,14,16,17,23]. In addition they have usually shown a profound respiratory related discharge, firing primarily during expiration[6,14,16,23]. Since their identification as cardio-inhibitory neurons has mainly rested on their baroreceptor (or sinus nerve, SN) input, it is not surprising that a relatively direct neural pathway linking the baroreceptors to CVM's has been suspected. The complexity of the pathway has been inferred from measuring the latency of the response of these efferent fibers to SN stimulation[23], while in the dog, latencies from 60–120 msec were described to the cardiac branches[12] and 50–100 msec to the cervical vagus[13]. These provide a measure of reflex time, but whether it is possible to infer the central delay as efferent conduction time is unknown. This is exacerbated by the concomitant activation of baroreceptor and chemoreceptor afferents on sinus nerve stimulation. Alternatively, the natural baroreceptor input has been used to obtain a value for the reflex time. These have ranged from 55–240 msec in the dog[14,16] and around 100 msec in the cat[16] and were obtained by timing the discharge of cervical vagal efferent fibers with respect to the arterial pulse wave form. Here unfortunately both the timing of the baroreceptor afferent volley with respect to the arterial pulse (and hence vagal discharge) and efferent conduction time were unknown.

Allowing then that baroreceptor input to CVM's is one of the most important determinants of their activity, studies have shown that the effectiveness of this input is markedly affected by respiration[6,9,17,20,21,26,37]. This was first illustrated in 1960 by Koepchen and his colleagues[20,21] who showed that baroreceptor control of the heart mediated by the vagus was markedly influenced by respiration. A brief stimulus applied to the carotid sinus would evoke cardiac slowing only if timed to occur during expiration; an equivalent stimulus delivered during inspiration was ineffective. This effect has since been confirmed by numerous studies[6,9,17,26,37], and effects on vagal efferent fibers in the dog consistent with this have been illustrated[6]. Such effects do not seem to be restricted to vagally-mediated control of the heart but extend also to the sympathetic arm of the baroreceptor reflex[7]. These observations have led to the belief that the baroreceptor reflex is "gated" by respiratory activity[21,26]. In this context it is significant that sinus arrythmia, the fluctuations in heart rate related to respiration, are mediated primarily by changes in vagal efferent activity[1,2]. These changes are considered to result from two main processes, one related to central respiratory activity[2], the second involving an inhibitory input onto CVM's from afferent vagal receptors excited by lung inflation[1]. Accordingly, vagal efferent fibers fire in expiration, and the question arises at once whether there is a need to imply a respiratory-related gating of the baroreceptor reflex, or whether the effectiveness of this input is determined simply by the excitability of the final common pathway in cardiac control, the CVM.

This brief review leads immediately to three questions: (1) Where are the vagal preganglionic neurons located, (2) how complex is the pathway between the baro-receptors and CVM's and (3) what determines their pattern of response to baro-receptor input during the respiratory cycle? Over the last few years in collaboration with Robin McAllen, I have attempted to obtain information on these three points.

RESULTS

The Location of Cardiac Preganglionic Vagal Neurons in the Medulla

The ambiguities in the conclusions derived from both the neuroanatomical and neurophysiological studies described above led McAllen and me to investigate directly the problem of the location of the cells of origin of vagal cardio-inhibitory fibers. We were aware, and our own observations confirmed, that cardio-inhibitory fibers are B fibers[30]. Accordingly, we placed stimulating electrodes around branches of the thoracic vagus previously shown to slow the heart and searched the medulla for units driven antidromically on stimulating these vagal branches[29,30]. From a detailed study in the cat, we reported that neurons relaying in the cardiac branches, with B fiber axons, were found only in the NA at levels rostral to the obex (see Fig. 1). The absence of such neurons in the DMN did not appear to be a consequence of biased sampling. The DMN extends laterally as a relatively thin group of neurons so that each penetration passing vertically through the medulla would pass through relatively few cells, but in a parallel study we sampled a wide population of DMN efferent neurons, backfiring them from the cervical vagus, before asking whether they relayed to thoracic branches of the vagus. We found no neurons in the DMN with B fiber axons

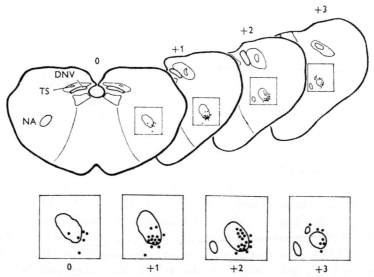

Fig. 1.   Location. The positions of 46 cardiac efferent neurons are shown on four standard sections of the medulla taken at obex level, and at one mm intervals rostrally. Inserts, two mm square, show details of their relationship to the structure of the nucleus ambiguus. TS: tractus solitarius; DNV: dorsal motor nucleus of the vagus; NA: nucleus ambiguus. Reproduced with permission from McAllen and Spyer, 1976.

relaying in the cardiac branches of the right vagus, although three neurons with C fiber axons did relay to these branches[30].

There are, however, at least two other classes of vagal efferent with B fiber axons, bronchomotor and oesophageal motor[14], and so it was necessary to have physiological criteria to confirm (or contradict) our conclusions. We had convincing evidence that the cardiac branches did not contain oesophageal efferents and as we had removed the upper lobe of the right lung in order to expose the cardiac vagal branches, it was perhaps not surprising that stimulating these branches produced no change in airway resistance. Since we often saw small filaments running from the cardiac branches to the excised stump of the lung we considered bronchomotor neurons the most likely contaminants of our sample. It appears that cardiac and bronchomotor efferents may have different properties[14] but unfortunately few vagal efferent neurons identified as above were either spontaneously active or reflexly excitable[30].

In more recent studies we have left these cardiac branches intact so as to observe efferent effects and have used double-barrelled micropipettes so as to apply iontophoretically the excitant amino acid DL-homocysteic acid (DLH) onto antidromically-identified neurons[31-33]. In this way we have been able to adjust the excitability of these neurons and so assess otherwise subliminal inputs that affect them while observing the efferent effects of their induced discharge. Our inferences have been drawn from an analysis of firing patterns, either spontaneous or DLH-induced. In addition we have placed similar electrodes around pulmonary-projecting vagal branches so as to identify neurons relaying to these branches from the NA[32]. It appears that two populations of vagal efferent neurons can be distinguished in the NA. The first, relaying only the cardiac branches, which we consider equivalent to that described in our original study[30], was normally silent, but in the presence of DLH fired during expiration (the period of phrenic silence; all animals had open chests and were artifically ventilated, lung inflation being desynchronized from central respiratory activity). The neurons were shown to have a cardiac rhythm of baroreceptor origin[32,33] and their DLH-evoked activity was able to produce cardiac slowing[31,32]. The second population of efferent neurons, with axons in either cardiac or pulmonary branches of the vagus, were almost always spontaneously active, firing with an inspiratory rhythm. They appear to have similar properties to the vagal efferent fibers recorded by Widdicombe in open-chest cats[43,44] which he considered bronchoconstrictor in function. The activity of these neurons showed no cardiac rhythm and exciting them iontophoretically with DLH produced no cardiac slowing. Evidence was obtained that laryngeal stimulation could excite this group of inspiratory-firing neurons, underlining their probable bronchoconstrictor function. They tended to be located more rostrally within the NA than CVM's, extending into the nucleus retrofascialis[32].

In conclusion, in the cat we have considerable evidence in favor of CVM's being located in the NA[30,32]. There remains, however, the possibility that in other mammalian species CVM's are located in the DMN. Schwaber and Schneiderman[33] describe five neurons in the DMN of the rabbit whose B fiber axons relayed in the cervical vagus and which were excited at short latency from the aortic nerve. Recent experiments in my own laboratory in the rabbit confirm this finding (Khalid, M. E. M., Jordan, D. and Spyer, K. M., unpublished observations).

Baroreceptor Input to CVM's

A major factor in our definition of a CVM was that its discharge was modulated by inputs from the arterial baroreceptors, particularly those of the carotid sinus[32,33]. In a series of experiments on aortic-debuffered cats we have shown that the cardiac rhythm of CVM's depends on an input from the baroreceptors of the carotid sinus, as it was abolished reversibly by bilateral carotid occlusion (see Fig. 2). We also monitored the baroreceptor afferent discharge from the sinus nerve ipsilateral to the CVM under investigation during these studies, processing this discharge in the same manner as the CVM discharge (i.e., producing pulse-triggered histograms of SN and CVM activity). Measuring the time between the pulse-related peaks in SN and CVM activity, the "reflex time" was measured and found to lie between 20–110 msec[33]. It appeared that this latency, which approximates the central delay of the reflex, fell into two peaks (values were also included from experiments in animals with aortic nerves intact, and from which the timing of the SN volley was inferred from the femoral pulse wave) suggesting the possibility of two pathways between barore-ceptors and CVM's (see Fig. 3a). The overall range of values we obtained is not dis-similar to those previously reported for the sinus nerve input to presumed cardiac efferent fibers in the cardiac branches[12,23] and cervical vagus[13] or values for the baroreceptor effects on cervical vagal fibers[14,16,17]. Our values, however, do not include an unknown efferent conduction time and we have an exact record of the afferent volley, two factors previously uncontrolled which may have contributed to the absence of double-peaked distribution of "reflex time" in former studies. This is borne out by Fig. 3b, which shows the effect of adding efferent conduction (i.e., antidromic latency) to the values of "reflex time" measured for the units illustrated in Fig. 3a. These values of central delay to natural baroreceptor stimulation are

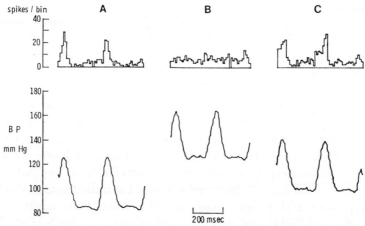

Fig. 2.   Aortic debuffered cat. Upper trace: pulse triggered histogram of CVM activity
(256 cycles superimposed, bin width 10 msec). Lower trace is the averaged femoral
pulse wave form (bin width 10 msec). Unit firing in response to 12 nA DLH. In A
and C the carotid arteries are open, in B the common carotids are occluded beneath
the carotid sinus.

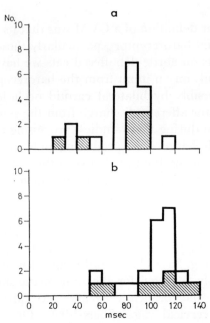

Fig. 3. (a) Histogram of the central delay of CVM's to natural baroreceptor stimulation. Hatched values refer to values measured from sinus nerve volley, open bars to data inferred from pulse wave form. (b) Histogram of reflex time to heart obtained by adding antidromic latency to the values of central delay shown in (a).

likely to be of greater physiological significance than those obtained by electrical stimulation of the SN, which involves concomitant activation of chemo- and baro-receptor afferents, as well as evoking a synchronous afferent volley. In our own study electrical stimulation of the SN evoked excitation of CVM's with a minimal latency of 20–50 msec, latencies which were always significantly shorter than the values determined for the physiological input[33]. Notwithstanding this, the data obtained is particularly revealing as it suggests a surprisingly long central delay in the baro-receptor-CVM reflex.

An exact measurement of central delay would require intracellular recordings from individual CVM's while providing a graded activation of baroreceptor afferents, individual afferents having different thresholds and conduction velocities. In the absence of such data, our measurements of reflex time to CVM's provide a valuable measure of the effective central delay at physiological pressure levels. If the distribution into two peaks can be accepted it suggests the involvement of two pathways between the baroreceptors of the carotid sinus and CVM's. Even the fastest, however, does not necessarily represent a disynaptic pathway. We know that baroreceptor afferents terminate in the NTS[11,24,28] and that the NTS projects to the NA[25,36], but even the synaptic connections in the pathway within the NTS may be complex[11,27,28]. Certainly, for the longer latency responses there is sufficient time for long circuited pathways which may well involve the hypothalamus[39].

The Influence of Respiration on Baroreceptor-vagal Reflexes

It is now well documented that the efficacy of the baroreceptor reflex is markedly affected by respiratory activity. Jordan and I have investigated whether the excitability of the sinus nerve afferent terminals are modulated during the central respiratory cycle, on the basis that a phasic change in terminal excitability might provide the respiratory "gate" of the baroreceptor (and chemoreceptor) reflex[15]. We were unable to find any indication that central respiratory activity evoked a presynaptic control of these afferent terminals in the NTS. This observation does not, however, rule out a postsynaptic mechanism elsewhere in the reflex pathway. McAllen and I were, however, able to test the existence of such a gate with our ability to control the activity of CVM's using iontophoretically applied DLH[33]. We had previously shown that in response to low iontophoretic currents, DLH evoked expiratory firing in CVM's[32] but at higher currents they could sometimes be induced to fire during inspiration as well, although at a lower rate than during expiration[33]. By constructing pulse-triggered histograms of CVM activity during inspiration and expiration separately, we have shown that they receive a baroreceptor input in both phases of respiration although the magnitude of pulse rhythm is smaller during inspiration than expiration[33,40]. This is illustrated in Fig. 4 which shows that the pulse rhythm of a CVM is maintained during inspiration. Similarly, SN stimulation evokes an excitatory response in CVM's in both inspiration and expiration[33]. These observations make it impossible to invoke an all-or-none respiratory "gate" in the baroreceptor reflex pathway. Rather, these

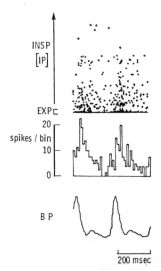

Fig. 4. The influence of respiration on the cardiac rhythm of a CVM. The upper record shows a photographic record of the activity of a CVM as a series of dots triggered from the femoral pressure wave, the sweep being raised by phrenic nerve activity (IP: integrated phrenic nerve activity). The second trace shows the cummulative pulse triggered histogram of CVM activity during this period, and the lower trace the averaged femoral pulse waveform (128 cycles superimposed, bin width 10 msec). The CVM fired throughout the respiratory cycle in response to 60 nA DLH.

data imply that the excitability of CVM's determines whether or not they respond to the baroreceptor input. They normally only fire during expiration and even in silent CVM's, the use of DLH has revealed the subliminal respiratory fluctuations in excitability of CVM's, low currents of DLH evoking discharge only during expiration[32,33]. We consider that this phasic fluctuation in CVM excitability synchronous with respiratory activity is likely to be the result of a powerful inhibitory control of CVM activity exerted by brain stem inspiratory neurons[35,40]. Indeed, although as yet only a preliminary observation, we have evidence that this inhibitory influence involves a cholinergic mechanism as it can be blocked by the iontophoretic application of atropine, and ACh powerfully inhibits CVM's when given iontophoretically (Jordan, D. and Spyer, K. M., unpublished observations). This suggestion is supported by other observations on a central action of atropine evoking bradycardia and vagal activity[17].

CONCLUSION

At this stage in our investigation we have evidence for an excitatory baroreceptor input into CVM's over a polysynaptic pathway[33] and an indication of an inhibitory input from medullary inspiratory neurons[33,40]. These must represent just two of the many inputs that affect the activity of CVM's but they indicate that these neurons must be a site of interaction of inputs, which underlines their integrative function in the control of the heart.

The original work described in this paper resulted from a collaborative study with Dr. R. M. McAllen. This work was supported by a program grant from the MRC.

REFERENCES

1 Anrep, G. V., Pascual, W. and Rössler, R., Respiratory variations of the heart rate. I. The reflex mechanism of the respiratory arrhythmia, *Proc. R. Soc.* B., 119 (1936a) 191–217.

2 Anrep, G. V., Pascual, W. and Rössler, R., Respiratory variations of the heart rate. II. The central mechanism of respiratory arrythmia and the inter-relationships between central and reflex mechanisms, *Proc. R. Soc.* B., 119 (1936b) 218–230.

3 Borison, H. L. and Domjan, D., Persistence of the cardio-inhibitory response to brain stem ischaemia after destruction of the area postrema and the dorsal vagal nuclei, *J. Physiol.* (Lond.), 211 (1970) 263–277.

4 Calaresu, F. R. and Pearce, J. W., Effects on heart rate of electrical stimulation of medullary vagal structures in the cat, *J. Physiol.* (Lond.), 176 (1965) 241–251.

5 Chiarugi, E. and Mollica, A., Contributo alla localizzazione der centro vagale cardio-inhibitore, *Archo Fisiol.*, 54 (1954) 249–267.

6 Davidson, N. S., Goldner, S. and McCloskey, D. I., Respiratory modulation of baroreceptor and chemoreceptor reflexes affecting heart rate activity and cardiac efferent nerve activity, *J. Physiol.* (Lond.), 259 (1976) 523–530.

7 Davis, A. L., McCloskey, D. I. and Potter, E. K., Respiratory modulation of baroreceptor and chemoreceptor reflexes affecting heart rate through the sympathetic nervous system, *J. Physiol.* (Lond.), 272 (1977) 691–705.

8 Gunn, C. G., Sevelius, G., Puiggari, M. S. and Myers, F. K., Vagal cardiomotor mechanisms in the hindbrain of the dog and cat, *Amer. J. Physiol.*, 214 (1968) 258–262.

9 Haymet, B. T. and McCloskey, D. I., Baroreceptor and chemoreceptor influences on heart rate during the respiratory cycle in the dog, *J. Physiol.* (Lond.), 245 (1975) 699–712.

10 Heymans, C. and Neil, E., *Reflexogenic Areas of the Cardiovascular System*, Churchill, London, 1958.

11 Humphrey, D. R., Neuronal activity in the medulla of the cat evoked by stimulation of the carotid sinus nerve. In: P. Kezdi (Ed.), *Baroreceptor and Hypertension*, Pergamon Press, New York, 1967, pp. 131–168.

12 Iriuchijima, J. and Kumada, M., Efferent cardiac vagal discharge of the dog in response to electrical stimulation of sensory nerves, *Jap. J. Physiol.*, 13 (1963) 599–605.

13 Iriuchijima, J. and Kumada, M., Activity in single vagal efferent fibres to the heart, *Jap. J. Physiol.*, 14 (1964) 479–487.

14 Jewett, D. L., Activity in single efferent fibres in the cervical vagus of the dog with special reference to possible cardioinhibitory fibres, *J. Physiol.* (Lond.), 175 (1964) 321–357.

15 Jordan, D. and Spyer, K. M., The excitability of sinus nerve afferent terminals during the respiratory cycle, *J. Physiol.* (Lond.), 277 (1978) 66P.

16 Katona, P.G., Poitras, J., Barnett, O. and Terry, B., Cardiac vagal efferent activity and heart period in the carotid sinus reflex, *Amer. J. Physiol.*, 218 (1970) 1030–1037.

17 Katona, P. G., Lipson, D. and Dauchot, P. J., Opposing central and peripheral effects of atropine on parasympathetic cardiovascular control, *Amer. J. Physiol.*, 232 (1977) H146–151.

18 Kerr, F. W. L., Function of the dorsal motor nucleus of the vagus, *Science*, 157 (1967) 451–452.

19 Kerr, F. W. L., Preserved vagal visceromotor function following destruction of the dorsal motor nucleus, *J. Physiol.* (Lond.), 202 (1969) 755–769.

20 Koepchen, H. P., Lux, H. D. and Wagner, P. H., Untersuchungen über zeitbedauf und zentrale verabeitung des presso receptorischen herzreflexes, *Pflügers Arch.*, 273 (1961) 413–430.

21 Koepchen, H. P., Wagner, P. H. and Lux, H. D., Uber die znsammehange zwischenzentraler erregbarkeit, reflektorischen tonns und atemrhythms bei der nervösen steuerung der herzfrequenz, *Pflügers Arch.*, 273 (1961) 443–465.

22 Kosaka, K., *Neurol. Cbl.*, 28 (1909) 406–1 cited in ref. 35.

23 Kunze, D. L., Reflex discharge patterns of cardiac vagal efferent fibres, *J. Physiol.* (Lond.), 222 (1972) 1–15.

24 Lipski, J., McAllen, R. M. and Spyer, K. M., The sinus nerve and baroreceptor input to the medulla of the cat, *J. Physiol.* (Lond.), 251 (1975) 61–78.

25 Loewy, A. D. and Burton, H., Nuclei of the solitary tract: Efferent projections to the lower brain and spinal cord of the cat, *J. comp. Neurol.*, 1978, in press.

26 Lopes, O. U. and Palmer, J. F., Proposed respiratory "gating" mechanism for cardiac slowing, *Nature*, 264 (1976) 454–456.

27 McAllen, R. M., Projections of the carotid sinus baroreceptors to the medulla of the cat, PhD. Thesis, University of Birmingham, 1973.

28 McAllen, R. M., Jordan, D. and Spyer, K. M., The carotid baroreceptor input to the cat's brain—Where is the first synapse? In: H. P. Koepchen, S. M. Hilton and A. Trzebski (Eds.), *Central Interaction between Respiratory and Cardiovascular Control Systems*, Springer-Verlag, Heidelberg, 1979, in press.

29 McAllen, R. M. and Spyer, K. M., The origin of cardiac vagal efferent neurones in the medulla of the cat, *J. Physiol.* (Lond.), 244 (1975) 82–83P.

30 McAllen, R. M. and Spyer, K. M., The location of cardiac vagal preganglionic moto-neurones in the medulla of the cat, *J. Physiol.* (Lond.), 258 (1976) 187–204.

31 McAllen, R. M. and Spyer, K. M., Bradycardia produced by iontophoretic activation of preganglionic vagal motoneurones, *J. Physiol.* (Lond.), 269 (1977) 40P.

32 McAllen, R. M. and Spyer, K. M., Two types of vagal preganglionic motoneurons projecting to the heart and lungs, *J. Physiol.* (Lond.), 282 (1978) 353–364.

33 McAllen, R. M. and Spyer, K. M., The baroreceptor input to cardiac vagal moto-neurones, *J. Physiol.* (Lond.), 282 (1978) 365–374.

34 Middleton, S., Middleton, H. H. and Grundfest, H., Spike potentials and cardiac effects of mammalian vagus nerve, *Amer. J. Physiol.*, 162 (1950) 553–559.

35 Mitchell, G. A. G. and Warwick, R., The dorsal vagal nucleus, *Acta anat.*, 25 (1955) 371–395.

36 Morest, D. K., Experimental study of the nucleus of the tractus solitarius and area post-rema in the cat, *J. comp. Neurol.*, 130 (1967) 277–299.

37 Neil, E. and Palmer, J. F., Effects of spontaneous respiration on the latency of reflex cardiac chronotropic responses to baroreceptor stimulation, *J. Physiol.* (Lond.), 247 (1975) 16 P.

38 Schwaber, J. and Schneiderman, N., Aortic nerve activated cardio-inhibitory neurons and interneurons, *Amer. J. Physiol.*, 229 (1975) 783–789.

39 Spyer, K. M., Organization of baroreceptor pathways in the brain stem, *Brain Res.*, 87 (1975) 221–226.

40 Spyer, K. M. and McAllen, R. M., The interaction of central and peripheral inputs onto vagal cardiomotor neurones. In: H. P. Koepchen, S. M. Hilton and A. Trzebski (Eds.), *Central Interaction between Respiratory and Cardiovascular Control Systems*, Springer-Verlag, Heidelberg, 1979, in press.

41 Szentagothai, J., The general visceral efferent column of the brain stem, *Acta morph. hung.*, 2 (1952) 313–328.

42 Thomas, M. R. and Calaresu, F. R., Localization and function of medullary sites mediating vagal bradycardia, *Amer. J. Physiol.*, 226 (1974) 1344–1349.

43 Widdicombe, J. G., Action potentials in parasympathetic efferent fibers to the lungs of the cat, *Arch. Exp. Path. Pharm.*, 241 (1961) 415–432.

44 Widdicombe, J. G., Action potentials in parasympathetic and sympathetic fibres to trachea and lungs of dogs and cats, *J. Physiol.* (Lond.), 186 (1966) 56–88.

CHAPTER 21

DIFFERENTIAL RESPONSES IN REFLEX ACTION; THE QUESTION OF BLOOD VOLUME AND PRESSURE CONTROL

Kiyomi Koizumi, Hiroshi Yamashita, Mark Kollai and Chandler McC. Brooks

Department of Physiology, State University of New York,
Downstate Medical Center, Brooklyn, New York, USA

INTRODUCTION

The maintenance of homeostasis and execution of responses of the body to a stimulus generally involve the total organism. It has been stressed in the last decades that autonomic and somatic systems interact with each other[14,24]. More recently interactions between the autonomic and neuroendocrine systems have been a focus of our attention, especially those caused by excitation of receptors in the cardiovascular system.

It is well known that, in conditions such as hemorrhage or shock, the loss of blood and/or reduction of blood pressure bring about chains of reactions which endeavor to maintain blood volume and pressure. There are cardiovascular changes due to shifts in autonomic nervous system activities, there are changes in ADH liberation from the neuroendocrine system and there are alterations in angiotensin production which together alter urine volume production and other body functions. An analysis of reactions simultaneously occurring in both sympathetic and parasympathetic nerves and in hypothalamic neurosecretory neurons, during extication of various receptors in the cardiovascular system, has not been made previously. In addition, the significance of these reactions to the maintenance of homeostasis has not been well evaluated; the important objective is not simply to find out what occurs but to recognize significances and the meaning of the observed phenomena relative to body functions.

We have chosen to use three cardiovascular system receptors in our initial studies of autonomic and neuroendocrine system reactions. They are the sinus and aortic baroreceptors, arterial chemoreceptors and receptors of both atria; the latter being considered by some to be components of the "volume receptors" located in low pressure areas[10].

Although the literature is filled with studies of cardiovascular reactions in response to excitation of baroreceptors and chemoreceptors, not many papers exist which deal with changes in blood ADH level in such reactions (see[27]). Only a few papers have appeared which report studies of neurosecretory cell activities evoked by baro- or chemoreceptor excitation[2,3,6,12,29]. The role of atrial receptors in control of blood volume through the cardiovascular as well as through the hypothalamo-neurohypophysial system is still controversial. Certainly, many studies have shown that stimulation of atrial receptors produces changes in the heart rate as well as in blood ADH levels, but the results are conflicting[10,11]. Moreover, opinion is divided as to the functional significance of such reactions and the contribution of atrial receptors to the maintenance of blood volume[11].

The aim of the studies to be reported was to find out: 1) How these three types of receptors affect the pattern of autonomic activity, whether the receptors exert differential control or generalized control of the sympathetic system, whether there is reciprocal action between the sympathetic and parasympathetic systems; 2) How these receptors affect neurosecretory neurons in the hypothalamus which control ADH secretion, i.e., neurons in the supraoptic (SON) and paraventricular nuclei (PVN).

METHODS

Alpha-chloralose (70 mg/kg) or nembutal (35 mg/kg) anesthetized cats and dogs were used. Figure 1 shows experimental arrangements schematically. Preparations differed depending on the objectives of the experiments, and detailed methods have been reported elsewhere[18-22,29,30]. Stimulation of baroreceptors in the carotid sinus was accomplished by distension of an "isolated" carotid sinus preparation or by inflation of a small latex balloon inserted into the sinus. Baroreceptors in the arch of the aorta were activated by occluding the descending aorta. Chemoreceptors were stimulated by perfusion of carotid sinus with CO_2-saturated Ringer's solution or by injection of lobeline or NaCN into the carotid sinus through a cannula in a lingual artery or into the aorta through the subclavian artery. Receptors situated in the atria were excited by pulling a thread attached to the appropriate area, i.e., sinoatrial region on the right and pulmonary vein-atrial junction on the left.

Extracellular recordings from neurons in SON and PVN were done using glass capillary electrodes filled with 4M NaCl. Neurosecretory neurons were identified by antidromic potentials evoked by stimulation of the posterior lobe of the pituitary or the stalk[17,18]. A "collision technique" was also used[19,30]. Recordings were made from fibers of the cardiac sympathetics, muscle branches of vertebral nerves (forearm vasoconstrictors), renal nerves, as well as from cardiac branches of the vagi. Phrenic nerve recording was done in most cases, particularly when the experiments involved open-chest preparations or use of chemoreceptor excitations. Systemic blood pressure and cardiac rate were monitored throughout the experiment, end-expired CO_2 was checked and rectal temperature was maintained between 37.5–38.5°C.

Action potentials were recorded and displayed in the conventional manner. For quantitative assessment of neuron and nerve activities, the rates of firing of single hypothalamic neurons and single-fiber preparations were counted and integrated; action potentials recorded from whole sympathetic nerves were integrated by area

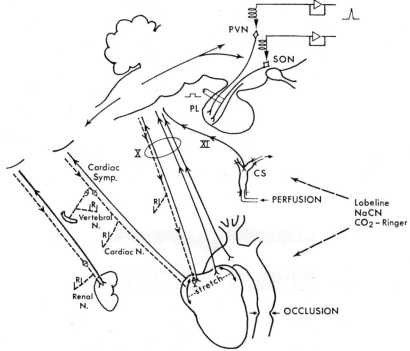

Fig. 1. Schematic diagram of experimental methods. SON: supraoptic nucleus; PVN: paraventricular nucleus; PL: posterior lobe of the pituitary gland; CS: carotid sinus; R: designates recording sites.

integrator. All activities monitored together with blood pressure and heart rate were simultaneously recorded on the same polygraph.

Varied combinations of stimulations and recordings were done in each experiment, but in all cases cardiovascular changes were monitored so that effective and selective stimulations of one set of receptors could be carried out.

RESULTS

1. Stimulation of Baroreceptors

It has been shown repeatedly that the baroreceptor reflex involves inhibition of sympathetic discharges to the heart as well as to blood vessels. Although it is generally assumed that there is reciprocal action between sympathetic and parasympathetic systems in baroreceptor reflexes, surprisingly, no clear demonstration of this relationship by recording from the two nerves has been previously reported. In our studies of cardiac reflexes[22] in which simultaneous recordings were done from both cardiac sympathetic and vagal efferents, we showed that this reciprocal action indeed existed between the two systems innervating the heart in the carotid sinus reflex; distension of carotid sinus inhibited cardiac sympathetic discharges and augmented the activity of

K. Koizumi et al.

cardiac vagal fibers (see Fig. 9 in[23]). Stimulation of baroreceptors of the carotid sinus also inhibited the activity of neurosecretory cells in SON.

As shown in Fig. 2A, distension of the carotid sinus by inflation of a balloon produced complete inhibition of SON neuron activity. The same result was obtained by increasing the sinus pressure in an "isolated" sinus preparation[30]. By applying graded stimulation of baroreceptors by changing the sinus pressure, the inhibitory effect on SON could be graded. It was found that the relationship between stimulus intensities and the effects was almost linear, as seen in Fig. 2B. It is interesting to note that the threshold for myelinated afferent discharge in the sinus nerve is said to be at a sinus pressure of 45 mmHg, while unmyelinated afferents begin to be activated when pressure reaches 135 mmHg (see[13]). As seen in Fig. 2B, the inhibitory effect of baroreceptors on SON neurons reached its maximum at 110–120 mmHg. Therefore, we

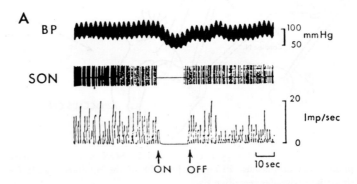

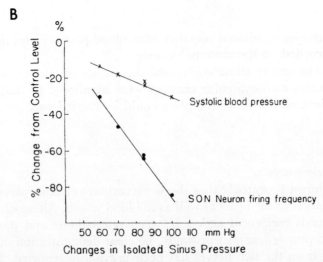

Fig. 2. A: Effects of baroreceptor stimulation on SON neuron activity and on blood pressure. Baroreceptors were stimulated by inflation of a balloon inserted into the left carotid sinus. B: Relationship between stimulus intensities of baroreceptors (an increase in sinus pressure) and degree of inhibitory effects on SON neuron activity and on blood pressure. (Taken from[30].)

can conclude that the baroreceptor influence on SON neurons is transmitted mainly by myelinated fibers in the sinus nerve. The graph also shows that response of blood pressure to baroreceptors appears to be similar to that of SON neurons. Although the slope of the two curves is different, the threshold and the maximum sensitivity of blood pressure response in the baroreceptor reflex seem to occur at a similar level of sinus pressure as in SON neurons.

The effects produced by baroreceptor excitation on SON neurons disappeared when the sinus nerve was cut, indicating that the inhibitory effects were conducted through the sinus afferents. Excitation of baroreceptors in the arch of the aorta also produced an effect on SON neurons quite similar to the effect on carotid sinus[30].

2. *Chemoreceptor Excitation*

The action of chemoreceptors is primarily on respiration but it is recognized that chemoreceptors influence the autonomic system as well as exciting the ADH-producing neurosecretory cells[20,21,29]. Unlike baroreceptors, excitation of chemoreceptors evoked differential action in the sympathetic system. Muscle vasoconstrictors were excited, resulting in a pressor response, at the same time sympathetic cardiac nerves were generally inhibited. The latter phenomenon was complicated by two factors. One

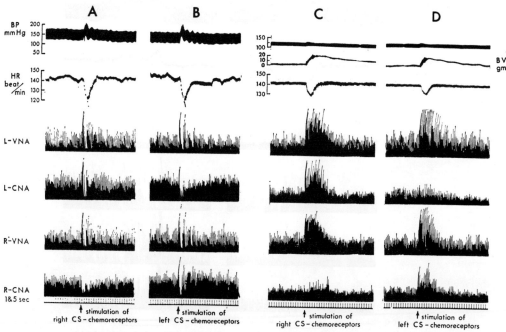

Fig. 3.   Effects of right and left chemoreceptor stimulation on the activity of vertebral nerve (VNA) and cardiac sympathetics (CNA) of both sides. Ten μg of lobeline was injected into the carotid sinus at arrow. A and B: Baroreceptors and vagi intact. C and D: The same test was done under stabilization of systemic blood pressure. Note the almost constant blood pressure. The second tracings (BV) indicate movement of blood (in grams) from the circulatory system to the reservoir. (Taken from[21].)

is the influence of the secondary counteracting baroreceptor reflex evoked by an increase in blood pressure; the other is the laterality in response of cardiac sympathetic fibers to chemoreceptors. Figure 3A shows that the right carotid chemoreceptor stimulation had an inhibitory effect on the cardiac nerve activity of the ipsilateral side but augmented discharge on the contralateral side as well as bilateral vertebral nerve activity. Stimulation of the left chemoreceptors produced the opposite effect (Fig. 3B). When the blood pressure was stabilized to prevent a pressor response from occurring during the chemoreceptor reflex, the excitatory effect of chemoreceptors on the sympathetic system became more prominent because of the lack of counteraction by the baroreceptor reflex. The result was not only a large augmentation of bilateral vertebral nerve and contralateral cardiac nerve activity, but also a loss of inhibition in ipsilateral cardiac nerve; the nerve activity was very slightly augmented or hardly affected (Fig. 3C and D). Thus, the differential action observed by chemoreceptor excitation was originally not qualitative but only quantitative. It is important to emphasize that the secondarily-evoked baroreceptor reflex actually augmented the differential action between bilateral cardiac nerves.

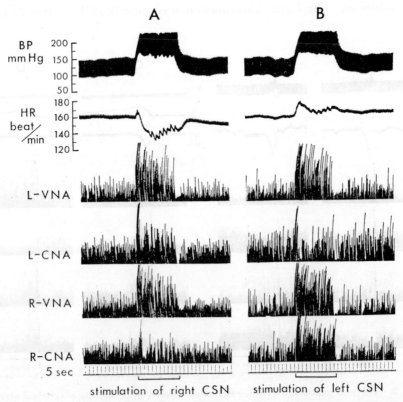

Fig. 4. Effects produced in left and right vertebral (VNA) and cardiac nerve discharges (CNA) by stimulation of carotid sinus nerves (CSN). The stimulus parameters were such that mainly chemoreceptor afferents were activated. Vagotomized Preparation. Note the difference in effects on heart rate obtained from the right and left sinuses. (Taken from[21].)

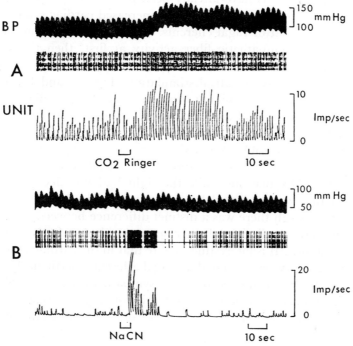

Fig. 5. Effects of stimulating carotid chemoreceptors on the activity of SON neurons. Chemoreceptors were stimulated by infusion of "isolated" sinus with CO_2-saturated Ringer solution (A) and by injection of NaCN (B). From top to bottom: systemic blood pressure; action potentials of an SON neuron; integrated record showing its rate of firing every second. (Taken from[29].)

Cardiac vagal fiber action also must be augmented since in vagi-intact animals bradycardia was the general rule, regardless of cardiac sympathetic discharges. In vagotomized animals, however, heart rate usually followed the activity of the right cardiac nerve, since the right sympathetic nerve has dominant action in controlling the heart rate; right chemoreceptor stimulation produced bradycardia, while left stimulation evoked tachycardia (Fig. 4).

Just as in the autonomic nervous system, chemoreceptor excitation caused an increase in the firing rate of SON neurons[29]. This is illustrated in Fig. 5A and B. SON neuron activity increased following perfusion of the "isolated" sinus with CO_2-saturated Ringer solution or by injection of NaCN or lobeline into the sinus. This occurred regardless of the pressor response simultaneously produced. Of course, the respiration increased in naturally-breathing animals, and in artificially-ventilated animals phrenic discharges were found to be greatly augmented.

3.   Excitation of Receptors of the Right and the Left Atria

Stimulation of stretch receptors in the right and the left atria also evokes reflex changes in the autonomic system as well as in SON neurons. We have recently shown that there are some differences between distension of the two atria on the autonomic system reactions[22]; the results have already been presented in a previous chapter by Nishi and Brooks[23]. Briefly, right atrial stretch increased cardiac sympathetic activity and mildly augmented that of vagal efferents. Left atrial stretch, on the other hand, inhibited both cardiac sympathetic fiber activity at first, then this inhibition was replaced by gradual augmentation of activity. Discharges of cardiac vagal efferents were somewhat increased by left atrial stimulation (Fig. 6A and B). The effects on renal nerve activity were very similar to those observed on cardiac nerves[15]. Thus, changes in heart rate were found to differ depending on whether the right or the left atrium was stretched.

Neurosecretory cells in SON and PVN were affected by left, but not by right, atrial distension[19]. As seen in Fig. 6C and D, left atrial receptors evoked a strong inhibitory effect on SON neurons while the right had no effect on these neurons, though the heart rate was increased by the stimulus. The left atrial receptors also affected heart rate, though there was a distinct difference between the two responses. Bilateral vagotomy always eliminated the response evoked in SON by stimulation of atrial receptors (Fig. 6E). It is interesting to note that in the cardiac reflex most effects on the autonomic nerves were mediated by vagal afferents, particularly the inhibitory action evoked by the left atrial receptors on sympathetic fibers, cardiac as well as renal. The cardiac reflexes depend on the integrity of vagal afferents, though cardiac sympathetic nerves also contain some afferents from the heart. Afferents carried by

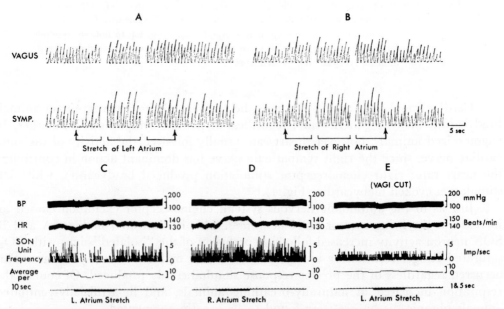

Fig. 6. A and B: Effects of stretch of left and right atria on the activity of cardiac vagus and sympathetic fibers. Integrated records. Breaks in records represent approximately 10 sec. Note the early inhibition of cardiac sympathetic activity in A and its absence in B. C to E: Effects of atrial stretch on SON neuron activity, blood pressure and heart rate. Note differences in effects on SON neuron and heart rate produced by stimulation of left or right atrium.

the sympathetic trunks seem to cause only excitatory reaction in the sympathetic system[16].

4. Interaction Evoked by Receptors

In previous studies we selectively activated only one set of receptors, but in the body more than one receptor is normally activated simultaneouly or successively. For example, in hemorrhage baroreceptors, chemoreceptors as well as atrial receptors must be stimulated. It was, therefore, thought important to find out the relative strength and significance of receptor involvement in various reactions.

It has been known that action of baroreceptors on the sympathetic system is more powerful than that of chemoreceptors, as illustrated in Fig. 7A and B. When both receptors were activated the augmenting action of chemoreceptors on cardiac, vertebral and renal nerves was blocked and the inhibitory action of baroreceptors dominated. Similar results were obtained when competitive effects on neurosecretory cells in SON were examined. As seen in Fig. 7C and D, although neuron discharges were augmented by excitation of chemoreceptors, successive stimulation of baroreceptors inhibited the SON neuron nearly completely, indicating that the powerful inhibitory action of baroreceptors could reverse and overcome the action of chemoreceptors.

The relative importance of the dominance of each receptor, however, is not necessarily similar in the control of autonomic system and neuroendocrine functions. Combination of atrial stretch and baro- or chemoreceptors showed that the action of left atrial receptors was not as strong as that of the other two receptors on SON neuron activity. Figure 8A–C shows that the augmenting effect of baroreceptor deactivation (carotid occlusion) on SON activity could not be reduced below the control level by atrial stretch. Also, a large increase in the firing rate of SON neurons produced by chemoreceptor activation was not at all affected by the inhibitory action of left atrial stretch (Fig. 8D and E). In contrast, it was found that in the control of autonomic system activity cardiac receptors were relatively powerful. The cardiac acceleration produced by right atrium stretch could break through the inhibitory action of the carotid baroreceptors and raise the rate above control values even though it started from subnormal levels (see Fig. 9 of[23]). This power of the atrial accelerator reflex is contributed to by the action of the vagus in potentiating autoregulatory action[5].

Although it has been claimed that in hemorrhage atrial receptors play a larger role than do baroreceptors in effecting the observed increase on ADH in the blood, our findings indicate that baroreceptors are very important in the control of SON neuron activity. Both receptors must participate in all phases of the compensatory reactions to hemorrhage. We have no evidence of any positive excitatory action of atrial or baroreceptors on ADH output; their role in hemorrhage must be that of disinhibition. Our inclination is to think that disinhibition cannot be as important to the release of ADH from the SON as is the probable concurrent excitatory action of chemoreceptors. A low blood flow or oxygen supply to the chemoreceptors certainly can occur in hemorrhage and this, more than pressure reduction, could be the augmenting drive in ADH output.

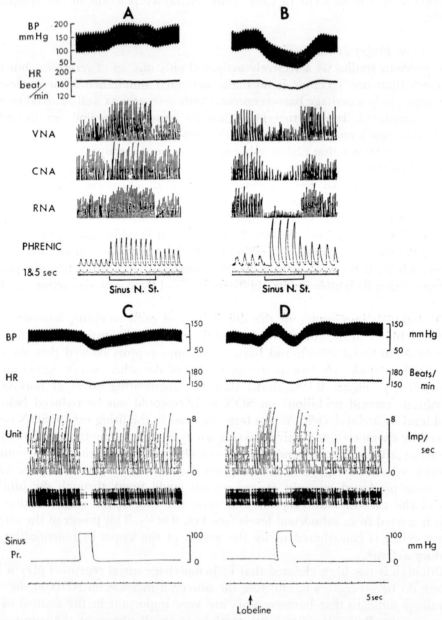

Fig. 7. Autonomic and neuroendocrine responses to combined stimulation of baro- and
chemoreceptors. A and B: Effects of carotid sinus nerve stimulation on the activity
of vertebral (VNA), cardiac sympathetic (CNA), renal (RNA) and phrenic nerves
as well as on blood pressure and heart rate. In A, carotid sinus nerve was stimulated
with a low intensity sufficient to excite chemoreceptor afferents. In B, a stronger
stimulus was applied to excite both baro- and chemoreceptor afferents. C and D:
Changes in SON neuron activity in response to an increase in "isolated" sinus
pressure alone (C) and to a lobeline injection followed by the same baroreceptor
stimulation (D). (C and D taken from[30].)

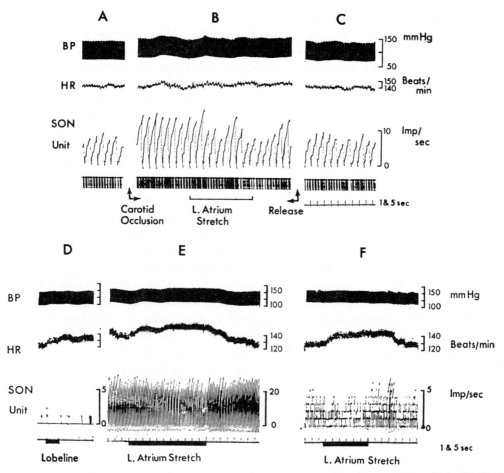

Fig. 8.   Effects of left atrial stretch applied during carotid occlusion (A to C) and during
chemoreceptor stimulation (D to E) on SON neuron activity and cardiovascular
responses. Note that the effects of atrial stretch were small (B) or none (E) when
SON activity was previously increased by carotid occlusion or chemoreceptor
stimulation. In E, calibration for rate of firing of SON neuron is different from that
in D and F. (Taken from[19].)

DISCUSSION

There were two categories of findings in this research which warrant some
discussion.

The first of these is the difference in patterns of response various afferents evoked
from the autonomic system. The baroreceptors of the arch of the aorta and carotid
sinuses have a bilateral asymmetry of action as though serving the total organism and
preserving overall blood pressure homeostasis. The chemoreceptors, on the other
hand, have a stronger contralateral than ipsilateral excitatory action on cardiac
sympathetics although the simultaneous excitatory action on vertebral nerve sympathetic fibers, which are largely vasoconstrictor to muscle vessels, is bilaterally equal.

The significance of this differential action of chemoreceptors and the "discharge as a whole" evoked by other receptors cannot as yet be explained. Analyses of the actions of several receptors are reported in other chapters of this publication.

These observations have been responsible for other realizations. One of these is that differential actions can have a peripheral origin; a reflex sequence can be responsible for something which seemingly might have a central origin. In the chemoreceptor reflex ipsilateral effects on cardiac sympathetics are minimal but not inhibitory. Bradycardia seen when the reflex is evoked in a normal animal is due to vagus involvement which is direct or a result of baroreceptor response to an initial pressor action. This vagus effect dominates ipsilaterally but contralaterally an increase in sympathetic firing may dominate. The baroreceptor involvement is responsible for the ipsilateral inhibition and contralateral excitation usually observed; this is a reciprocal action originating centrally from chemoreceptor stimulation.

Another realization has been that in chemoreceptor- and right atrium stretch-evoked reflexes vagus activity is increased along with cardiac accelerator and some peripheral vasoconstrictor actions. Is this just a matter of inefficiency or a lack of appropriate reciprocal responses from the centers? It can be argued that in a modulatory system the slight augmentation of the vagus effect along with the sympathetic could be useful in that by preventing too great a tachycardia, it protects or assures the increase in cardiac output needed. Analytical studies are thus beginning to indicate that reactions should not be considered singly. The same stimuli that evoke reactions in sympathetic cardiovascular efferents have other actions which are contributory to functional purposes.

The second interest of this paper pertains to the significance of the interaction of these three receptor types (atrial stretch receptors, chemo- and baroreceptors) on control of plasma volume and water balance through action on kidney function, ADH (vasopressin) output and even the renin-angiotensin role in pressure and volume control. Others have spoken of the renin-angiotensin release by sympathetic nerve and epinephrine actions. It is the control of ADH-release which has been our immediate concern.

Activation and deactivation of baroreceptors can significantly affect ADH output from the SON-PVN neurons. Low blood pressure, such as caused by the loss of blood volume in hemorrhage, reduces baroreceptor discharge and by a disinhibition should augment activity in these hypothalamic neurons and increase blood ADH levels. This disinhibition of ADH output associated with a similar disinhibition or release of inhibition of renal vasoconstrictor tone should aid in reducing urine output and restoration of blood volume. Recent evidence also suggests that the hypothalamus is involved in blood pressure response to centrally-administered angiotensin via release of ADH[9]. It can be assumed that in situations such as low blood volume or pressure, the renin-angiotensin system is activated due to augmented sympathetic discharges. This leads to stimulation of SON neurons, the response which compliments the direct excitatory action produced by reduced baroreceptor afferent impulses. Moreover, the role of ADH on the peripheral vasculature seems to be more important than hitherto believed. ADH (arginine vasopressin) is the most powerful pressor peptide in the blood and, for example, mesenteric resistence vessels are said to be far more sensitive to ADH than to angiotensin. ADH constricts not only aortic and mesenteric arterioles but, also, muscular venules are much affected. Such action can be produced by physiological concentration of ADH[1]. It has been stated that the very large increase in blood ADH which occurs under stress is a result of changes in baro- and chemoreceptor activities. Above a certain level ADH has little additional effect on water conservation; its major influence seems to be upon the vascular system, the microcirculation, etc.[8]. In severe hemorrhagic shock it has been found that vasoconstriction of the mesenteric vascular bed is almost absent or attenuated in the absence of ADH or angiotensin[7]. ADH acts in cooperation with autonomic system vasoconstrictors to restore peripheral resistence and blood pressure to normal levels after some accident causes hypotonia.

In the baroreceptor reflex there is an inhibition of sympathetic nerve activity and excitation of vagal fibers; this is accompanied by an inhibition of SON neurons. As stated before, reduction of blood ADH (vasopressin) aids in the lowering of blood pressure by reducing vasoconstriction. The question is how significant is the contribution of ADH to the adjustive reactions which occur under physiological conditions. Although there is no convincing evidence to clarify this point, a partial answer is provided by the findings that baroreceptors are tonically active. Denervation of all baroreceptors creates at least a temporary hypertension; denervation not only raises blood pressure and heart rate, but also blood ADH levels. There is also an accompanied antidiuresis which is reduced or abolished by hypophysectomy[4,25,26]. These findings can be interpreted to mean that baroreceptors must play a role in maintaining the blood pressure as well as ADH concentration within physiological ranges.

The chemoreceptors have a very strong excitatory action on the SON and PVN neurons which is accompanied by an increase in ADH levels in the blood. Very low blood pressure, deficient blood flow and even deoxygenation following hemorrhage would certainly excite the chemoreceptors and their action on the hypothalamic neurons would be unopposed by baroreceptor inhibitions. This would constitute a positive reaction toward restoration of volume and reestablishment of blood pressure homeostasis.

The left atrial receptors, according to our results, although some controversy still remains relative to their role, also play a role in volume-pressure control through an inhibitory action on SON and PVN neurons and ADH release. We agree with those who think that these are important receptors which are significantly involved in volume regulation[10,27,28]. Others have expressed doubt as to whether atrial stretch, such as applied experimentally, occurs under "normal" conditions and thus doubt that atrial control of ADH release has any physiological significance[11]. It is difficult to accept such an adverse argument since we have found a clear difference in effects produced by the left and right atria on neurosecretory neurons of the SON and PVN. Our results have indicated, also, that changes in urine volume or in blood ADH produced by the left atrial stretch are not due to hemodynamic changes or inaccurate ADH assay methods.

In conclusion, we wish again to emphasize that afferent stimuli act through autonomic neurons and the neuroendocrine system to maintain normal blood pressures, vascular volume and water balance.

SUMMARY

This was a study of the reactions initiated by three receptor types: chemo-receptors, baroreceptors and receptors of the atria of the heart which are sensitive to stretch. Their actions on cardiac, vasomotor nerves and the neurons of SON and PVN which release ADH-vasopressin were determined. It was found that the baro-receptors evoke a reciprocal action between parasympathetic and sympathetic nerves; they have a bilaterally equal effect and the power to cause the sympathetic system to react much as a whole; they inhibit SON-PVN neurons. Chemoreceptors tend to cause some vagus excitation in association with increased activity in vasomotor and cardiac sympathetics; action on cardiac sympathetics is asymmetrical—contralateral responses being stronger; they excite SON-PVN neurons. Receptors of the right atria excite cardiac and vasomotor sympathetics bilaterally while inducing a minor aug-mentation of activity in the vagi; they have no effect on the two ADH-releasing hypo-thalamic nuclei. Left atria receptors evoke a momentary reciprocal action of vagi (increase) and cardiac sympathetics (decrease); this is followed by a late dominance of sympathetic activity; the neurons of SON-PVN are inhibited. The peripheral responses observed are contributed to by reflex interactions and patterns of responses are not dictated exclusively by centers. These receptor types act together in regulating pressure and plasma volume; neuroendocrine as well as peripheral neuronal actions on effector tissues are involved.

The work was supported by grants from USPHS (NS-00847), NSF (OI P74–19337) and from the New York Heart Association.

REFERENCES

1   Altura, B. M. and Altura, B. T., Vascular smooth muscle and neurohypophyseal hor-mones, *Fed. Proc.*, 36 (1977) 1853–1860.
2   Barker, J. L., Crayton, J. W. and Nicoll, R. A., Supraoptic neurosecretory cells: Auto-nomic modulation, *Science*, 171 (1971) 206–207.
3   Barker, J. L., Crayton, J. W. and Nicoll, R. A., Antidromic and orthodromic responses of paraventricular and supraoptic neurosecretory cells, *Brain Res.*, 33 (1971) 353–366.
4   Bond, G. C. and Trank, J. W., Effect of bilateral aortic nerve section on plasma ADH titer, *Physiologist*, 13 (1970) 152.
5   Brooks, C. McC. and Lange, G., Interaction of myogenic and neurogenic mechanisms that control heart rate, *Proc. nat. Acad. Sci. USA*, 74 (1977) 1761–1762.
6   Dreifuss, J. J., Harris, M. C. and Tribollet, E., Excitation of phasically firing hypothalamic supraoptic neurons by carotid occlusion in rats, *J. Physiol.* (Lond.), 257 (1976) 337–354.
7   Errington, M. L. and Rocha e Silva, M., Jr., On the role of vasopressin and angiotensin in the development of irreversible hemorrhagic shock, *J. Physiol.* (Lond.), 242 (1974) 119–141.
8   Forsling, M. L., *Anti-diuretic Hormone*, Eden Press, Montreal, 1976.
9   Ganten, D., Fuxe, K., Phillips, M. I., Mann, J. F. E. and Ganten, U., The brain isorenin-angiotensin system: Biochemistry, localization, and possible role in drinking and blood

pressure regulation. In: W. F. Ganong and L. Martini (Eds.), *Frontiers in Neuroendocrinology*, Vol. 5, Raven Press, New York, 1978, pp. 61–99.

10 Gauer, O. H. and Henry, J. P., Neurohormonal control of plasma volume. In: A. C. Guyton and A. W. Cowley (Eds.), *International Review of Physiology, Cardiovascular Physiology* II, Vol. 9, University Park Press, Baltimore, 1976, pp. 145–190.

11 Goetz, K. L., Bond, G. C. and Bloxham, D. D., Atrial receptors and renal function, *Physiol. Rev.*, 55 (1975) 157–205.

12 Harris, M. C., Dreifuss, J. J. and Legros, J. J., Excitation of phasically firing supraoptic neurones during vasopressin release, *Nature*, 258 (1975) 80–82.

13 Kirchheim, H. R., Systemic arterial baroreceptor reflexes, *Physiol. Rev.*, 56 (1976) 100–176.

14 Koizumi, K. and Brooks, C. McC., The integration of autonomic system reactions, *Ergebn. Physiol.*, 67 (1972) 1–68.

15 Koizumi, K., Ishikawa, T., Nishino, H. and Brooks, C. McC., Cardiac and autonomic system reactions to stretch of the atria, *Brain Res.*, 87 (1975) 247–261.

16 Koizumi, K., Nishino, H. and Brooks, C. McC., Centers involved in the autonomic reflex reactions originating from stretching of the atria, *Proc. nat. Acad. Sci. USA*, 74 (1977) 2177–2181.

17 Koizumi, K. and Yamashita, H., Studies on neurosecretory cells in the mammalian hypothalamus. In: F. F. Kao, K. Koizumi and M. Vassalle (Eds.), *Research in Physiology, A Liber Memorialis in Honor of Professor C. McC. Brooks*, Aulo Gaggi, Bologna, 1971, pp. 607–623.

18 Koizumi, K. and Yamashita, H., Studies of antidromically identified neurosecretory cells of the hypothalamus by intracellular and extracellular recordings, *J. Physiol. (Lond.)*, 221 (1972) 683–705.

19 Koizumi, K. and Yamashita, H., Influence of atrial stretch receptors on hypothalamic neurosecretory neurons, *J. Physiol. (Lond.)*, 285 (1978) 341–358.

20 Kollai, M. and Koizumi, K., Differential responses in sympathetic outflow evoked by chemoreceptor activation, *Brain Res.*, 138 (1977) 159–165.

21 Kollai, M., Koizumi, K. and Brooks, C. McC., Nature of differential sympathetic discharges in chemoreceptor reflexes, *Proc. nat. Acad. Sci. USA*, 75 (1978) 5239–5243.

22 Kollai, M., Koizumi, K., Yamashita, H. and Brooks, C. McC., Study of cardiac sympathetic and vagal activity during reflex responses produced by stretch of the atria, *Brain Res.*, 150 (1978) 519–532.

23 Nishi, K. and Brooks, C. McC., Receptors in the heart and the integrative role of cardiac reflexes. This volume, pp. 111–130.

24 Sato, A. and Schmidt, R. F., Somatosympathetic reflexes: Afferent fibers, central pathways, discharge characteristics, *Physiol. Rev.*, 53 (1973) 916–947.

25 Schreier, R. W. and Berl, T., Mechanism of the antidiuretic effect associated with interruption of parasympathetic pathways, *J. clin. Invest.*, 51 (1972) 2613–2620.

26 Share, L., Extracellular fluid volume and vasopressin secretion. In: W. F. Ganong and L. Martini (Eds.), *Frontiers in Neuroendocrinology*, Oxford Univ. Press, New York, 1969, pp. 183–210.

27 Share, L., Blood pressure, blood volume, and the release of vasopressin. In: E. Knobil and W. H. Sawyer (Eds.), *The Pituitary Gland and its Neuroendocrine Control, Handbook of Physiology*, Sec. 7, Vol. 4, Part I, American Physiological Society, Washington, D. C., 1974, pp. 243–255.

28 Share, L., Role of cardiovascular receptors in the control of ADH release, *Cardiology*, 61 (Suppl. 1) (1976) 51–64.

29 Yamashita, H., Effect of baro- and chemoreceptor activation on supraoptic nuclei
    neurons in the hypothalamus, *Brain Res.*, 126 (1977) 551–556.
30 Yamashita, H. and Koizumi, K., Influence of carotid and aortic baroreceptors on
    neurosecretory neurons in supraoptic nuclei, *Brain Res.*, 168 (1979) in press.

CHAPTER 22

SOMATIC AFFERENTS AND THEIR EFFECTS ON BLADDER FUNCTION

A. Sato*, Y. Sato* and R. F. Schmidt**

*2nd Department of Physiology, Tokyo Metropolitan Institute of Gerontology,
Tokyo, Japan, and
**Physiologisches Institut der Universität Kiel,
Kiel, Fed. Rep. Germany*

INTRODUCTION

Normal micturition is influenced by the interaction of autonomic and somatic reflexes. The bladder is innervated by parasympathetic pelvic and sympathetic hypogastric nerves. The external sphincter muscle and the urethral mucosa are innervated by the somatic pudendal nerves. Pelvic and pudendal nerves come out of the sacral spinal cord, while the hypogastric nerves emerge from the lumbar spinal cord. Stimulation of the efferent components of the pelvic nerve evokes vesical contractions while stimulation of the efferents of the hypogastric nerve may have some inhibitory effect on bladder contraction. Afferents of both pelvic and hypogastric nerves provide signal transmission paths for vesical stretch information to the central nervous system. The neural mechanisms of micturition reflexes involving these pelvic, hypogastric and pudendal nerves have been investigated in detail[2,3,11], but somatic afferent contributions from skin or muscles to the micturition complex have been studied only sparsely. In this contribution, recent studies of the neural mechanisms of the somato-vesical reflexes will be discussed.

The electrophysiological analysis of the somato-sympathetic reflexes is well advanced and propriospinal as well as supraspinal reflex components have been identified[24]. However, there is still a great gap between the detailed results of these studies at the neuronal level and those at the visceral effector organ level. For example, it is well known that cutaneous stimulation of the perineal area evokes micturition in chronic spinal patients and animals[1,5,6,13]. This cutaneo-vesical excitatory reflex response, however, has not been previously studied systematically in animals with intact spinal cords. It was recently found that stimulation of the perineal skin of CNS-intact rats[22] and cats[23], whose bladders were only slightly expanded, evoked vesical contractions in association with a reflex increase in the efferent discharge rate of the pelvic nerve. These results in cats will be discussed first.

Electrophysiological studies of the expanded bladder in cats[4,5], in dogs[16,17] and in rats[22] showed that stimulation of perineal skin usually inhibited the large rhythmic micturition contractions of the bladder by inhibiting the rhythmic-burst efferent discharges of the vesical pelvic nerves. Further studies have now revealed that these micturition contractions were inhibited not only by perineal skin stimulation but also by cutaneous stimulation of the abdomen and chest, suggesting that the reflex is organized through a supraspinal pathway, although it was also indicated that this reflex is subject to a strong segmental organization. These results by Sato et al.[23] will be discussed subsequently.

Thirdly, there will be a report on the neural mechanisms of musculo-vesical reflexes. In the motor nervous system, physiological functions of the thick, myelinated group I and II muscle afferent nerves have been well analyzed as the afferent components of the motor reflex control system. The physiology of the thin, myelinated group III and unmyelinated group IV muscle afferents have not been sufficiently analyzed to reveal all of their probable functions, although these thin muscle afferents have been shown to affect respiratory and cardiovascular functions[12,18]. In this paper, the effects of group III and IV muscle afferent stimulation on vesical functions[18,19,20] will be discussed in detail.

Finally, the most recent information about the neural mechanism of the excitatory and inhibitory effects of hind limb afferent volleys on vesical functions in acute[18,19] and chronic spinal cats[21] will be introduced.

METHODS

The experiments were performed on adult cats anesthetized i.p. with chloralose (50–60 mg/kg) and urethane (0.1–0.12 g/kg). The general methods of experimentation including the adjustment of the artificial respiratory condition, the administration of additional anesthesia, the recording and maintaining of the blood pressure, the control and regulation of the body temperature and the mechanical stimulation of the various skin areas, were the same as described previously[10]. The surgical procedures for approaching the urinary bladder, for measuring and recording the intravesical pressure with the balloon method, for collecting urine during the experiment and for recording and counting the efferent activity of the vesical branches of the pelvic and hypogastric nerves were the same as those described by Sato et al.[22].

In addition to natural stimulation of the skin, various cutaneous and muscular afferent nerves of a hind limb were electrically stimulated as described elsewhere[18,19]. In some cases, hind limb muscle afferents were stimulated by i.a. injection of algesic or other chemical substances into hind limb muscles as reported elsewhere[18,20].

Chronic spinal cats were prepared by transecting the spinal cord at the T8–12 level nine to 19 months before the experiments. In the experiments on chronic spinal cats, a rubber endotracheal catheter with a cuff was inserted into the trachea under Ketamine (50–100 mg/kg, i.m.) anesthesia. After recovery from the Ketamine effect, we studied the spinal somato-vesical reflexes without and with chloralose-urethane anesthesia, as described by Sato et al.[21].

RESULTS AND DISCUSSION

Cutaneo-vesical Reflexes
1. *Excitatory and inhibitory reflex responses of the bladder to perineal skin stimulation*

Noxious mechanical stimulation. Sato et al.[23] demonstrated that the noxious mechanical stimulation of pinching the perineal skin caused either an excitatory or an inhibitory reflex response in anesthetized cats depending on the condition of the bladder at the time of stimulation.

When the intravesical pressure was kept low (around 50 mmH$_2$O) with small intravesical balloon volume, the bladder was usually quiescent. When the intravesical pressure was raised to as high as 100–150 mmH$_2$O by expanding the intravesical balloon, the bladder showed large, slow, rhythmic micturition contractions at frequencies of one to three per min, and with peak pressure wave amplitudes of about 400–1000 mmH$_2$O. These large, rhythmic micturition contractions were produced by rhythmic burst discharges of the vesical pelvic efferent nerves as described by de Groat and Ryall[5].

In general, when the bladder was quiescent perineal stimulation induced an excitatory vesical reflex response, but when the bladder displayed rhythmic micturition contractions, an inhibitory reflex response was obtained. Figure 1A is an example of the excitatory response: The bladder was quiescent before perineal stimulation, and both vesical pressure and vesical efferent discharge activity of the pelvic nerve increased when the perineal skin was pinched for 20 sec. Figure 1B shows a typical example of the inhibitory response: The bladder had large, rhythmic micturition contractions before perineal stimulation, and both the micturition contractions and the corresponding rhythmic burst discharges of the vesical pelvic efferent nerve activity were inhibited by pinching the perineal skin for 30 sec. These inhibitions were followed by subsequent increases (rebound) in vesical pressure and in vesical pelvic efferent nerve activity. On the other hand, hypogastric efferent nerve activity was not significantly affected by the stimuli. Occasionally, as shown in C, stimulation during large micturition contractions first elicited a premature contraction of the bladder and corresponding burst discharges in the vesical pelvic nerve followed by the inhibition of vesical contractions and pelvic nerve discharges.

The effect of transection of the pelvic and hypogastric nerves on the cutaneo-vesical reflexes. Neither the excitatory nor the inhibitory cutaneo-vesical reflex described above was affected by bilateral severance of the hypogastric nerves when the pelvic nerves were kept intact. However, bilaterally severing the pelvic nerves completely abolished the rhythmic vesical micturition contractions even when the hypogastric nerves were kept intact, so that only the effect of transection of the pelvic nerves on the excitatory cutaneo-vesical reflex responses for the quiescent bladder could be examined. In cats whose hypogastric nerves were kept intact, the excitatory cutaneo-vesical reflex was completely abolished after bilateral severance of the pelvic nerves.

The results of severing the vesical autonomic nerves and the recording of their discharges indicate that the essential efferent pathways for both the excitatory and inhibitory cutaneo-vesical reflexes are in the vesical pelvic nerves. The hypogastric

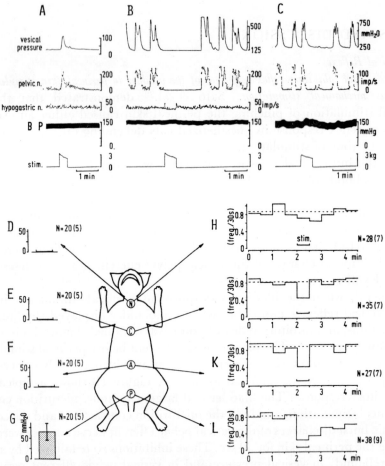

Fig. 1. Cutaneo-vesical reflexes in anesthetized cats with intact neuraxis. A–C: Changes
of the vesical pressure and the vesical autonomic efferent nerve activity upon pinching the perineal skin. A and B were obtained in the same cat; the results in C were
obtained from a different cat. A, B and C show simultaneous recordings of intravesical
pressure (top traces), pelvic efferent nerve activity (2nd traces from top), hypogastric
efferent nerve activity (3rd traces from top, not recorded in C), blood pressure (BP)
and intensity of pinching (20 sec in A; for 30 sec in B and C, bottom traces). In B
high vesical pressure records were clipped off by polygraph pen limitation. Conditions for recording and counting nerve discharge rates were identical for A and B.
D–L: effect on bladder of pinching various skin areas. D and H stimulation of neck;
E and J, chest stimulation; F and K, abdominal stimulation; G and L, perineal
stimulation. D–G: reflex changes in peak amplitude of vesical pressure after pinching
skin while bladder was quiescent. Shaded column and vertical line are mean ±S. D.
Number of trials indicated by N; number of animals used in parentheses. H–L:
poststimulus time histograms of large, rhythmic micturition contractions, compiled
from N trials. Each original contraction record was divided into 30 sec addresses
before and after the start of stimulation and the number of onsets of large contractions
were counted within each address to obtain each histogram. Pinching was administered to various skin areas at random with respect to the phase of large micturition
contraction waves. Abscissae: time in min. Ordinates: frequencies of onset of large
micturition contractions per 30 sec per trial. Horizontal broken lines in poststimulus
time histograms (H–L) show mean frequency during two min period before stimulation. A contraction was added to the histograms only if its amplitude was 33% or
more of the maximal amplitude of the preceeding four or five contractions. Horizontal bar in each histogram: 30 sec periods of stimulation (modified from[23]).

efferent contribution to these reflexes is not clear[23]. All results in cats mentioned above are essentially similar to those in rats[22].

Non-noxious mechanical stimulation. The excitatory vesical reflex of the quiescent bladder was produced by rubbing the perineal skin (non-noxious mechanical stimulation) in cats as has been reported in rats[22]. However, the inhibitory reflex effect on the vesical micturition contractions produced by non-noxious mechanical stimulation was not clearly demonstrated in cats as reported for rats[22].

Thermal stimulation. The vesical reflex effects of thermal stimulation of the perineal skin at different temperatures for one min duration were examined. The results showed that noxious thermal stimulation, for example temperatures above 45°C or below 7°C, was more effective in producing both excitatory and inhibitory reflexes than non-noxious thermal stimulation at temperatures between 13°C and 43°C[23].

McPherson[13] reported a decrease in the peak pressures of rhythmic vesical contractions and a shortening of the intervals between them after applying ice to the hind paws for more than two to five min in anesthetized cats. But he did not see any effects on the bladder when the fore and hind paws were placed in water at 45°C for 15 min, or when the skin of the hind limbs was pinched vigorously for three min. In the present experiments, either excitatory or inhibitory responses of the bladder was observed when either noxious or non-noxious thermal stimulation was applied to the skin of the perineal area. The period of thermal stimulation for these experiments was one min, which was considerably shorter than the two to five min which Mc-Pherson found necessary to produce vesical changes. Such differences may be due to the greater effectiveness of perineal skin stimulation in producing vesical reflex responses.

Kaufman et al.[10] found that noxious mechanical or thermal stimulation of the skin was much more effective than non-noxious stimuli in producing a cardiac acceleration reflex in anesthetized cats. Similar differences in the stimulation effects on the vesical functions were found for noxious and non-noxious cutaneous stimulation in the present experiments in anesthetized cats. Thus, in view of these results, it can be concluded that the central connections between nociceptive cutaneous afferents and autonomic efferents are much stronger than those between non-nociceptive cutaneous afferents and autonomic efferents.

2. Changes in vesical function after pinching various skin areas of the trunk

The effect on the bladder produced by pinching the skin of areas other than the perineum, e.g., neck, chest and abdomen, was also examined in anesthetized cats by Sato et al.[23]. The results are summarized in Fig. 1D–L showing excitatory (G) and inhibitory (J–L) reflexes and no effects (D–F, H). While the bladder was quiescent (D–G), significant excitatory responses were obtained only by perineal stimulation, but not by stimulation of any other skin area tested (neck, chest and abdomen). While the bladder was undergoing large micturition contractions(H–L), these contractions were inhibited by pinching the skin of the perineum, abdomen and chest with the degree of efficacy of stimulation being in this order.

3. Effect of electrical stimulation of hind limb cutaneous afferents on bladder functions

In anesthetized cats, repetitive stimulation of the group III and IV cutaneous afferents of the hind limb resulted in a reflex increase in the tonus of the quiescent bladder, and in inhibition of the rhythmic micturition contractions of the expanded bladder[18,19]. The neural mechanisms of these cutaneo-vesical reflexes are similar to those of the musculo-vesical reflexes, and these results will be mentioned in the next chapter.

Musculo-vesical Reflexes

1. *Effects of electrical stimulation of hind limb muscle afferents on bladder function*

The effects on the vesical function of electrical stimulation of muscle hind limb afferent fibers such as the afferents in the gastrocnemius and soleus muscle nerves (GS) and in the peroneal plus deep peroneal muscle nerve group (PDP) were tested by Sato et al.[18,19]. Repetitive electrical stimulation of the group III and IV muscle afferents had an excitatory effect on the quiescent bladder and an inhibitory effect on the bladder during the large, rhythmic micturition contractions (Fig. 2A), whereas the stimulation of group I and II afferents was ineffective. When the stimulus intensity was increased gradually, excitatory and inhibitory effects appeared in the range in which group III afferents were excited, and became more dominant in the range in which group IV afferent stimulation occurred. The excitatory effects of PDP afferent stimulation was statistically significant, while that of GS stimulation was not significant. On the other hand, the inhibitory effects of PDP and GS afferent stimulation were about the same, both being significant.

2. *Chemical stimulation of muscle afferents*

Stimulation of hind limb muscles by algesic chemical substances such as KCl or bradykinin excited quiescent bladders and inhibited rhythmically contracting bladders, whereas stimulation of the muscles by succinylcholine (excitant of group I and II muscle afferent units) or Tyrode solution did not affect bladder functions. Figure 2B demonstrates that an injection of KCl solution (7.2 mg in 0.3 ml) into the left hind limb artery to the triceps sural and peroneal muscles of two min duration produced an inhibition of micturition contractions of the bladder. Bradykinin (26 μg) also caused inhibition of the micturition contractions.

KCl or bradykinin injected into the hind limb muscle artery is known to excite the thin myelinated group III and unmyelinated group IV muscle afferents[7,8,9,14,15]

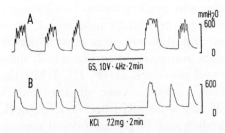

Fig. 2.   Musculo-vesical reflexes in anesthetized cats with intact neuraxis and rhythmic micturition contractions of bladder. A: Gastrocnemius-soleus muscle nerve was stimulated by electrical square pulses (10 V, 0.5 ms, 4 Hz for two min). Period of stimulation indicated by underbar. B: 7.2 mg of KCl (in 0.3 ml solution) was injected into arteria articularis genu suprema within two to three sec after occlusion of femoral artery and vein. Occlusion period (two min) indicated by underbar (from[18]).

and to cause a painful sensation, judging from the animal's behavior[25]. Thus, the observed effects of chemical stimulation of muscle afferents on the vesical functions probably correspond to the effects of electrical stimulation of the group III and IV muscle afferents on the vesical functions. These thin muscle afferents have been shown also to reflexly affect respiratory and cardiovascular functions[12,18].

On the other hand, 5-hydroxytryptamine (135 μg), which is known to excite group III and IV muscle afferents, did not produce any change in vesical functions. This may indicate that there are at least two different types of group III and IV muscle afferents: one which produces bladder reflexes and another which does not.

Stimulation of the group I and II hind limb muscle afferents either electrically or chemically (with succinylcholine) did not produce any change in the vesical functions, indicating that group I and II hind limb muscle afferents are not responsible for producing the vesical reflexes.

Somato-vesical Reflexes in Spinal Cats

1. Results in acute cats

Acute spinal transection at the cervical level resulted in complete disappearance of the rhythmic micturition contractions of the bladder. In these acutely spinalized cats, however, pinching the perineal skin produced reflex vesical contractions. For this spinal reflex, the vesical pelvic efferent nerves were shown to be the major efferents of the reflex arc[23].

2. Results in chronic spinal cats

In chronic spinal cats whose spinal cords were transected nine to 19 months before the experiments, the effects on vesical functions of electrical stimulation of cutaneous or muscle hind limb afferents were examined by Sato et al.[21] before and after application of anesthesia (chloralose-urethane mixture).

When the bladder was quiescent, repetitive stimulation of hind limb afferents increased the pelvic and hypogastric efferent nerve activity (Fig. 3A). Denervation experiments demonstrated that the reflexly increased pelvic efferent nerve activity caused vesical reflex contraction but not the reflexly increased hypogastric efferent

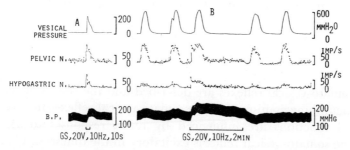

Fig. 3. Musculo-vesical reflexes in chronic spinal cats. A, B: Effect of electrical repetitive stimulation of the GS nerve at Group IV stimulus strength (20 V, 10 Hz, 0.5 ms). Vesical pressure: top traces. Pelvic efferent nerve activity: second traces. Hypogastric efferent nerve activity: third traces. Blood pressure: bottom traces. A: quiescent bladder, tetanus duration 10 sec. B: expanded bladder having large, rhythmic micturition contractions, tetanus duration two min (from[21]).

nerve activity. The vesical reflex contractions were larger and the threshold for evoking such contractions by afferent stimulation was lower (in the range of the group II afferents) in the non-anesthetized condition than in the anesthetized condition (in the range of the group III afferents).

When the vesical volume was expanded to 10–20 ml, there were spontaneous, large, rhythmic micturition contractions of the bladder with a frequency of one to two per min. It has been thought since Barrington[2], that the center for generation of these rhythmic contractions is in the brain stem. The vesical micturition contractions in chronic spinal cats, however, were produced by rhythmic burst discharges mediated by pelvic efferent nerves just as in spinal intact cats. In chronic spinal cats, repetitive stimulation of hind limb afferents produced a transient increase in pelvic efferent nerve activity, which caused transient vesical contractions. Continued stimulation abolished the rhythmic burst discharges of the pelvic efferent nerve activity, and this resulted in an inhibition of the rhythmic micturition contractions (Fig. 3B). This indicates that the inhibitory effect of hind limb somatic afferent stimulation, on the pelvic rhythmic burst discharges related to micturition contractions, can be organized within the spinal cord after it has been separated from the higher central nervous system for a long time. In the case of hind limb afferent stimulation, the degree of inhibition of micturition contractions was less and the threshold intensity for its inhibitory effect was higher in the non-anesthetized condition than in the anesthetized condition.

It is interesting that some anesthetics such as a chloralose-urethane mixture depressed the excitatory somato-vesical reflex seen in the quiescent bladder, whereas they augmented the inhibitory somato-vesical reflex seen in the rhythmically contracting bladder. In both cases, anesthetics seemed to depress the excitability of the pelvic efferent neurons within the spinal cord.

In conclusion, the existence of the somato-vesical reflexes has been confirmed and their neural mechanisms have been analyzed in detail. The physiological significance of the somato-vesical reflexes remains unclear at this moment, but this study suggests possible clinical applications of these reflexes in control of the vesical functions, to either excite or inhibit by proper use of somatic afferent stimulation, especially for those patients who suffer from some kind of micturition problem, a common geriatric occurrence.

SUMMARY

Various somato-vesical reflexes are described and the results of recent investigations into the neural mechanisms of these somato-vesical reflexes in cats are discussed.

1.   Vesical functions are influenced by reflex responses to somatic afferent stimulation. The somato-vesical reflex is excitatory in the quiescent bladder, but during micturition afferent activity inhibits the rhythmically contracting bladder. For both reflexes, the vesical pelvic nerves form the main efferent pathway of the reflex arcs while any contribution of the vesical hypogastric efferent nerves to the reflexes seems to be unimportant.

2.   Stimulation of various skin areas (neck, chest, abdomen and perineum) of

the trunk were performed to determine their effect on the vesical functions. The perineum was the most effective skin area for producing both excitatory and inhibitory reflexes. The abdomen and chest were effective areas for producing an inhibitory reflex effect, but not for excitation.

3. The thin myelinated group III and unmyelinated group IV hind limb skin or muscle afferents were found to be the active afferents in these reflexes.

4. In chronic spinal cats, both excitatory and inhibitory somato-vesical reflexes were observed both in the non-anesthetized and the anesthetized state.

5. The physiological significance and the possible clinical applications of these somato-vesical reflexes are discussed.

This work was supported by grants from the Ministry of Education of Japan and Daiwa Health Foundation (to A. Sato) and also from the Deutsche Forschungsgemeinschaft (to R. F. Schmidt).

REFERENCES

1 Barrington, F. J. F., The nervous mechanism of micturition, *Q. J. exp. Physiol.*, 8 (1914) 33–71.

2 Barrington, F. J. F., The effect of lesions of the hind- and mid-brain on micturition, *Q. J. exp. Physiol.*, 15 (1925) 81–102.

3 Barrington, F. J. F., The central nervous control of micturition, *Brain*, 51 (1928) 209–220.

4 de Groat, W. C., Nervous control of the urinary bladder of the cat, *Brain Res.*, 87 (1975) 201–211.

5 de Groat, W. C. and Ryall, R. W., Reflexes to sacral parasympathetic neurones concerned with micturition in the cat, *J. Physiol.* (Lond.), 200 (1969) 87–108.

6 Denny-Brown, D. and Robertson, E. G., The state of the bladder and its sphincters in complete transverse lesions of the spinal cord and cauda equina, *Brain*, 56 (1933) 397–463.

7 Fock, S. and Mense, S., Excitatory effects of 5-hydroxytryptamine, histamine and potassium ions on muscular group IV afferent units: A comparison with bradykinin, *Brain Res.*, 105 (1976) 459–469.

8 Franz, M. and Mense, S., Muscle receptors with group IV afferent fibers responding to application of bradykinin, *Brain Res.*, 92 (1975) 369–383.

9 Hiss, E. and Mense, S., Evidence for the existence of different receptor sites for algesic agents at the endings of muscular group IV afferent units, *Pflügers Arch.*, 362 (1976) 141–146.

10 Kaufman, A., Sato, A., Sato, Y. and Sugimoto, H., Reflex changes in heart rate after mechanical and thermal stimulation of the skin at various segmental levels in cats, *Neuroscience*, 2 (1977) 103–109.

11 Kuru, M., Nervous control of micturition, *Physiol. Rev.*, 45 (1965) 425–495.

12 McCloskey, D. I. and Mitchell, J. H., Reflex cardiovascular and respiratory responses originating in exercising muscle, *J. Physiol.* (Lond.), 224 (1972) 173–186.

13 McPherson, A., The effects of somatic stimuli on the bladder in the cat, *J. Physiol.* (Lond.), 185 (1966) 185–196.

14 Mense, S., Nervous outflow from skeletal muscle following chemical noxious stimulation, *J. Physiol.* (Lond.), 267 (1977) 75–88.

15 Mense, S. and Schmidt, R. F., Activation of group IV afferent units from muscle by algesic agents, *Brain Res.*, 72 (1974) 305–310.

16 Okada, H. and Yamane, M., Nervous control of the bladder (in Japanese), *Clin. Physiol.*, 3 (1973) 366–374.

17 Okada, H. and Yamane, M., Effects of cutaneous stimulation on the parasympathetic outflow to the bladder in the dog, *The Autonomic Nervous System*, 13 (1976) 57–65.

18 Sato, A., Sato, Y. and Schmidt, R. F., Autonomic reflexes elicited by stimulation of muscle afferent nerves in the cat, *Proceedings of the 18th International Congress of Neurovegetative Research*, (1977) 106–108.

19 Sato, A., Sato, Y. and Schmidt, R. F., Changes in vesical functions by electrical stimulation of hind limb cutaneous and muscle afferent nerves in anesthetized cats, (in preparation).

20 Sato, A., Sato, Y. and Schmidt, R. F., The effects on reflex bladder activity of chemical stimulation of small diameter afferents from skeletal muscle in the cat, *Neuroscience Letters*, 11 (1979) 13–17.

21 Sato, A., Sato, Y., Schmidt, R. F. and Torigata, Y., Electrophysiological studies of somato-vesical reflexes in chronic spinal cats, (in preparation).

22 Sato, A., Sato, Y., Shimada, F. and Torigata, Y., Changes in vesical function produced by cutaneous stimulation in rats, *Brain Res.*, 94 (1975) 465–474.

23 Sato, A., Sato, Y., Sugimoto, H. and Terui, N., Reflex changes in the urinary bladder after mechanical and thermal stimulation of the skin at various segmental levels in cats, *Neuroscience*, 2 (1977) 111–117.

24 Sato, A. and Schmidt, R. F., Somatosympathetic reflexes: Afferent fibers, central pathways, discharge characteristics, *Physiol. Rev.*, 53 (1973) 916–947.

25 Taira, A., Nakayama, K. and Hashimoto, K., Vocalization response of puppies to intra-arterial administration of bradykinin and other algesic agents, and mode of actions of blocking agents, *Tohoku J. exp. Med.*, 96 (1968) 365–377.

CHAPTER 23

THE TRIGEMINAL DEPRESSOR RESPONSE AND ITS ROLE IN THE CONTROL OF CARDIOVASCULAR FUNCTIONS

Mamoru Kumada**, Donald J. Reis*, Naohito Terui** and Roger A. L. Dampney*

*Laboratory of Neurobiology, Department of Neurology, Cornell University Medical Center, New York, USA, and **Institute of Basic Medical Sciences, University of Tsukuba, Ibaraki, Japan*

INTRODUCTION

Stimulation of somatic receptors will elicit cardiovascular responses closely coupled to somato-motor reflexes[18]. In the past the analysis of somato-autonomic interactions has largely been directed towards analysis of the responses mediated by inputs to the spinal cord[17,26]. Such studies have distinguished between a number of different somato-autonomic reflexes including cardiovascular responses by characterization for each of: (a) the nature of the adequate stimulus and of the relevant receptors[14,18,27]; (b) the composition of afferent fibers transmitting the responses[14,19,26]; (c) spinal and supraspinal pathways and their interactions[11,19,24,25,28]; and finally (d) a detailed analysis of the peripheral cardio- and hemodynamic responses[14].

Far less is known with respect to cardiovascular responses regulated by the trigeminal sensory system. In the past only three reflexes have been identified[20]: the diving response and the nasopharyngeal and oculocardiac reflexes. Both the diving response, initiated in diving and non-diving vertebrates by submersion of the face[2,9,12], and the nasopharyngeal reflex elicited by noxious stimulation of the nasal mucosa[3,13,30] consist of bradycardia, intensive peripheral vasoconstriction and apnea. The oculocardiac reflex, a response less frequently studied, appears to consist of a comparable reflex pattern[4,13]. Changes in arterial pressure in these responses are either absent or small[20]. Thus these three reflexes appear to share comparable mechanisms characterized by sympathetic activation coupled with excitation of the cardiac vagus, although the relative contribution of sympathetic and parasympathetic components may differ among individual responses.

We have recently discovered in the rabbit a previously unrecognized response mediated by the trigeminal system and elicited by electrical stimulation within portions of the spinal trigeminal complex or branches of the trigeminal nerve[21,22]. In this paper the spinal trigeminal tract and its nuclei are collectively called the "spinal trigeminal complex". The electrically-evoked response, which we have termed the trigeminal depressor response (TDR), is characterized by a powerful inhibition of ongoing sympathetic vasomotor activity and a consequent fall of arterial pressure, thereby distinguishing the TDR from the other trigeminal responses with which it shares bradycardia and hypopnea or apnea[2,3,13]. The TDR appears to share a comparable response pattern with arterial baroreceptor reflexes[23]; however, it is mediated within the brain by a different anatomical substrate[22]. The magnitude of the sympathetic inhibition suggests it may be of importance in cardiovascular control.

In this paper we shall review present knowledge of the TDR, describing its general characteristics, cardiovascular features, comparability to baroreceptor reflexes and analysis of the rate of its control over the discharge rate of sympathetic neurons innervating the kidney.

RESULTS

General Characteristics of the TDR

The TDR elicited by electrical stimulation of the spinal trigeminal complex or of branches of the trigeminal nerve consists of a fall of arterial pressure, bradycardia and expiratory apnea (Fig. 1). Associated with it is an increase in gastric motility. The fall of arterial pressure, often as great as 80 mmHg, occurs with a latency of approximately

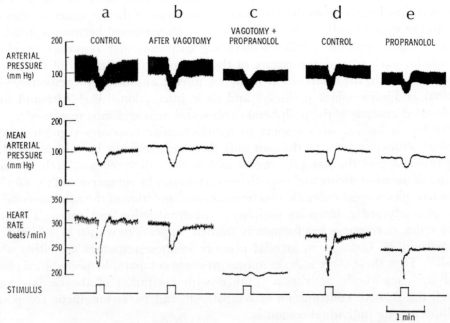

Fig. 1. Effect of vagal and cardiac sympathetic blockade, alone or combined, on trigeminal depressor response. The nucleus caudalis was electrically stimulated in anesthetized, paralyzed rabbits (0.5 msec pulse duration, five Hz, 12 sec train duration at 100 μA). a: control; b: five min after vagotomy; c: 10 min following administration of propranolol (1 mg/kg, i.v.) (vagi intact). Note that both vagal and sympathetic blockade are required to abolish bradycardia while hypotension is unaffected. (Reprinted from Kumada et al.[22], with permission.)

three sec and is sustained during the stimulus train. The bradycardia, often greater than 60 beats/min, has a comparable latency but is not sustained. Low intensity stimulation elicits tachypnea with decreased tidal volume which, with increasing stimulus strength, converts to expiratory apnea. The respiratory responses occur in advance of the cardiovascular response, thereby demonstrating they are not secondary.

The TDR is optimally elicited by electrical stimulation of the brain or peripheral nerves at low frequencies. The optimal frequency lies between five and 10 Hz, both centrally and peripherally. The lowest frequency for eliciting the TDR centrally is 0.3–0.6 Hz. It is slightly higher peripherally at 0.5–1.0 Hz. As the stimulus frequency is increased, the magnitude of the response declines. At frequencies higher than 50 Hz the depressor response may reverse and become pressor.

The threshold for the TDR elicited by a 12 sec train at optimal frequency is 10 μA or less. The response is graded with respect to stimulus intensity up to three to six times the threshold.

Cardiovascular Effects

Arterial pressure. The hypotension of the TDR is primarily due to inhibition of sympathetic vasoconstriction with an associated fall of total peripheral resistance. It

Table 1. Changes in cardiovascular dynamics associated with electrical stimulation of spinal trigeminal complex (trigeminal depressor response) or aortic nerve (aortic depressor reflex).

	N	Trigeminal depressor response			Aortic depressor reflex		
		Control	Trigeminal stimulation	Change (%)	Control	Aortic stimulation	Change (%)
Systemic arterial pressure (mmHg)							
Systolic pressure	43	152 ± 3	103 ± 3	-32***	151 ± 3	104 ± 3	-31***
Diastolic pressure	43	97 ± 2	58 ± 2	-40***	99 ± 3	61 ± 3	-38***
Mean pressure	43	117 ± 2	75 ± 2	-36***	116 ± 2	77 ± 3	-34***
Pulse pressure	43	55 ± 2	46 ± 2	-16***	53 ± 2	43 ± 2	-19***
Cardiodynamics, total peripheral resistance and venous pressure							
Heart rate (beat/min)	30	293 ± 6	255 ± 6	-13***	289 ± 6	259 ± 5	-10***
Cardiac output (ml/min)	12	353 ± 30	336 ± 29	-5***	335 ± 32	308 ± 26	-8**
Stroke volume (ml/beat)	12	1.39 ± 0.12	1.47 ± 0.12	$+6$**	1.34 ± 0.14	1.35 ± 0.13	$+1$ns
Total peripheral resistance (mmHg, min/ml)	12	0.342 ± 0.025	0.224 ± 0.015	-35***	0.378 ± 0.036	0.259 ± 0.022	-31***
Venous pressure (H_2O)	9	3 ± 0	3 ± 0	0ns	3 ± 0	3 ± 0	0ns
Regional blood flow (ml/min)							
Femoral artery	13	11.2 ± 1.1	9.9 ± 0.8	-12*	11.0 ± 1.4	9.6 ± 1.0	-13*
Superior mesenteric artery	9	38.3 ± 3.9	30.2 ± 3.4	-16*	34.4 ± 3.3	29.3 ± 3.2	-15***
Renal artery	11	32.2 ± 2.2	25.6 ± 2.0	-20***	29.4 ± 1.9	22.4 ± 1.9	-24***
Regional vascular resistance (mmHg, min/ml)							
Femoral artery	13	12.0 ± 1.7	8.1 ± 0.7	-32**	12.7 ± 1.9	8.8 ± 1.1	-31**
Superior mesenteric artery	9	3.5 ± 0.3	2.7 ± 0.3	-23**	3.6 ± 0.4	2.7 ± 0.2	-25**
Renal artery	11	3.8 ± 0.2	3.2 ± 0.2	-16***	4.2 ± 0.3	3.4 ± 0.3	-19**

Trigeminal stimulation delivered with stimulus current 5× threshold. Aortic stimulation delivered with stimulus current 10× threshold. All values expressed as mean±S. E. of mean. Significnace (P<0.05); *P<0.05; **P< 0.01; ***P<0.001. ns=not significant. See Methods for method of statistical analysis.

is not due to a reduction of cardiac output; the reduction of cardiac output is disproportionately small during the response (Table 1) and hypotension persists after the bradycardia is abolished (Fig. 1c). On the other hand, the hypertension can be entirely blocked by α-adrenergic blockade with phentolamine without any associated changes in heart rate[22].

The pattern of reduction in sympathetic vasoconstriction is differentiated in the TDR. The greatest fall of resistance occurs in the femoral artery, the least in the renal artery and the reduction of resistance in the mesenteric artery falls in between (Table 1).

Heart rate. The bradycardia associated with the TDR is due to excitation of cardiac vagal neurons and in combination with inhibition of cardiac sympathetic nerves. Thus the bradycardia of the TDR is attenuated but not abolished by bilateral cervical vagotomy, or administration of atropine or β-adrenergic blockade with propranolol (Fig. 1b, e). Both vagal and sympathetic blockades are required for complete elimination of the bradycardia (Fig. 1c).

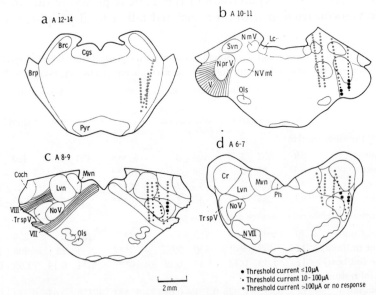

Fig. 2. Localization of sites in the spinal trigeminal complex of the rabbit from which a depressor response is elicited by electrical stimulation. Coronal sections of brain stem at 12–14 mm anterior (a), 10–11 mm anterior (b), 8–9 mm anterior (c), 6–7 mm anterior (d), 4–5 mm anterior (e), 2–3 mm anterior (f), 0–1 mm anterior (g), 1–2 mm posterior (h), and 3–4 mm posterior (i) to the obex. The brain stem was briefly stimulated every 250 μm with a 12 sec train of square-wave pulses (0.5 msec pulse duration, five Hz) and the threshold current was determined at each site. Each line of circles represents an electrode track. Thresholds for responses are represented by large and small filled circles and small open circles. Data were obtained from 22 anesthetized rabbits. Abbreviations: V, trigeminal nerve; VII, facial nerve; VIII, stato-acoustic nerve; Ant horn, anterior horn; Brc, superior cerebellar peduncle (brachium conjunctivum); Brp, middle cerebellar peduncle (brachium pontis); Cgs, central gray

Distribution of Active Sites

Areas of the trigeminal complex from which a depressor response can be elicited with low threshold stimuli (no greater than 10μA) are shown in Fig. 2. These points, called active sites, are restricted to selected portions of the spinal trigeminal complex including the entering rootlets (Fig. 2b) and are found throughout the entire course of the spinal trigeminal tract (Fig. 2c–i). Within the tract, particularly in its rostral portions, the active sites lie dorsally. Active sites are also found within the two caudal nuclear subdivisions of the nucleus of the spinal tract of V, and the nuclei caudalis and interpolaris (Fig. 2g–i). Few responses, on the other hand, are elicited from within the principal sensory nuclei and none at all from within the mesencephalic and motor nuclei of the Vth nerve (Fig. 2b). No responses, or only very minimal ones, can be elicited at sites rostral to the entering trigeminal nerve, or from rostral portions of the nucleus tractus solitarii (Fig. 2d–f) into which entering rootlets of the IXth and Xth cranial nerves enter after traversing the spinal trigeminal complex[1,8,16]; nor from sites medial or lateral to the spinal trigeminal complex. Thus the TDR is most likely due

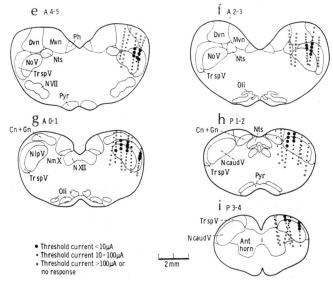

substance; Cn+Gn, nucleus cuneatus and nucleus gracilis; Coch, cochlear nucleus; Cr, inferior cerebellar peduncle (restiform body); Dvn, inferior vestibular nucleus; LC, locus coeruleus; Lvn, lateral vestibular nucleus; Mvn, medial vestibular nucleus; NVmt, motor nucleus of trigeminal nerve; N VII, nucleus of facial nerve; N XII, nucleus of hypoglossal nerve; N caud V, nucleus caudalis of trigeminal nerve; N ip V, nucleus interpolaris of trigeminal nerve; NmX, dorsal motor nucleus of vagus; NoV, nucleus oralis of trigeminal nerve; N pr V, nucleus principalis of trigeminal nerve; Nts, nucleus of solitary tract; Oli, inferior olive; Ols, superior olive; Ph, nucleus praepositus hypoglossi; Pyr, pyramidal tract; Svn, superior vestibular nucleus; Tr sp V, spinal tract of trigeminal nerve. Note that the sites with lowest thresholds are within the spinal trigeminal complex. (Reprinted from Kumada et al.[22], with permission.)

to stimulation of fibers mostly of trigeminal origin, while descending through the tract to synapse with or pass through caudal sensory nuclei of the spinal trigeminal complex.

The TDR can be elicited by stimulation of branches of the trigeminal nerve including the supraorbital, infraorbital, inferior alveolar and lingual nerves, although the response is smaller than that elicited by stimulation of the brain. It should be noted that these are representative branches of the three major divisions of the trigeminal nerve.

Comparison with Baroreceptor Reflexes

The autonomic components of the TDR are almost identical to those elicited by baroreceptor stimulation[23]. As shown in Table 1, the cardiovascular responses elicited by electrical stimulation of the left aortic depressor nerve with stimuli producing equivalent reduction in arterial pressure resulted in changes in cardiac and hemodynamic variables of almost identical magnitudes. Furthermore, in experiments in which both the TDR and the aortic depressor responses of various magnitudes were elicited in the same animal, the regression lines obtained by plotting percent decrease in heart rate, total peripheral resistance or regional resistance, against the percent fall in arterial pressure were similar: There was no significant difference in the slope or Y-intercept of the regression line between the TDR and aortic depressor response for all of the hemodynamic variables[23]. Such observations indicate more directly that the pattern of hemodynamic changes of the TDR is identical with that of baroreceptor reflexes.

Neuronal Mechanisms of the TDR

To further analyze the interaction of the TDR with sympathetic nerve activity we have studied the effects of stimulation of the spinal trigeminal complex on the discharge of postganglionic sympathetic neurons recorded in the renal nerve. Such efferent renal nerve discharge almost exclusively reflects vasoconstrictor activity[6,7].

A single stimulating pulse delivered to the spinal trigeminal complex results in inhibition of efferent renal nerve discharge (Fig. 3). The inhibition, lasting more than 500 msec after a single pulse, can be elicited by stimulation of the ipsi- or contralateral spinal trigeminal complex and is usually not preceeded by sympathetic excitation. The threshold current for sympathetic inhibition is five–40 μA, a stimulus intensity comparable to that required for producing hypotension. As with the arterial pressure response, the magnitude of sympathetic inhibition is graded and directly related to stimulus intensities from three to seven times the threshold.

The effect of the frequency of the stimulus delivered to the spinal trigeminal complex on renal sympathetic nerve activity is strikingly similar to that on the arterial pressure response of the TDR. Figure 3 illustrates renal sympathetic activity averaged over 50 successive trains of stimulation in response to stimulation of the spinal trigeminal complex with a two sec train of rectangular pulses with frequencies ranging from one–333 Hz. At frequencies lower than two Hz (Fig. 3c, d) renal nerve activity is inhibited following each pulse. However, the inhibition is only transient and the corresponding fall in arterial pressure is small. At frequencies of five and 10 Hz (Fig. 3e, f) trigeminal stimulation causes total inhibition of sympathetic activity

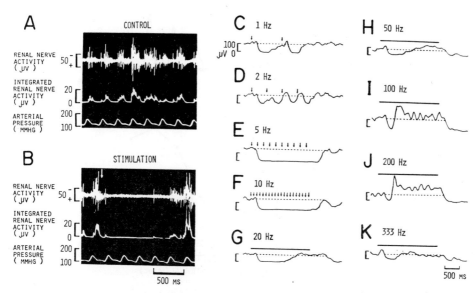

Fig. 3. Renal sympathetic activity, recorded from the left renal nerve, and its inhibition by stimulation of the spinal trigeminal complex. A: a single sweep record of spontaneous renal sympathetic discharges. B: inhibition of spontaneous renal sympathetic discharges by a single pulse (100 μA, 0.5 msec) applied to the left spinal trigeminal complex at the time indicated by an arrow. C–K: averaged response of the renal sympathetic discharges to a two-second train of electrical stimulation (100 μA, 0.5 msec) to the left spinal trigeminal complex at different stimulus frequencies shown at each specimen record. Renal sympathetic discharges are rectified, integrated and averaged for 64 successive sweeps repeated at a rate of once every 10 sec to obtain each recording. Stimulation is applied at the time indicated by an arrow, corresponding to each stimulating pulse, in C–F, or by a solid line above recordings, indicating the period of two-sec stimulation, in G–K. Broken line in C–K signified pre-stimulus level of the renal sympathetic activity.

eliciting a silent period which lasts over the entire period of the two sec stimulation. The maximal sympatho-inhibitory effect corresponds to the period of greatest hypotension of the TDR at these frequencies[22]. At frequencies at or above 50 Hz (Fig. 3h–k) sympathetic excitation becomes greater than sympathetic inhibition. The net result is sympathetic excitation which corresponds to the hypertension seen with trigeminal stimulation at the same frequencies. Thus it appears that sympathetic nerve activity and the changes in arterial pressure elicited by stimulation of the trigeminal complex are comparable.

Trigeminal stimulation not only suppresses tonic sympathetic activity but also inhibits reflexly elicited discharge of the renal sympathetic nerve. The latter effect can be demonstrated by delivering a pair of pulses, i.e., conditioning and test stimuli, with varying time intervals between them. When the test stimulus is delivered through an electrode placed in the medullary pressor area within the nucleus parvocellularis reticularis, a powerful sympathetic excitation is elicited (Fig. 4). However, this sympathetic excitation is inhibited by the conditioning stimulus delivered to the spinal

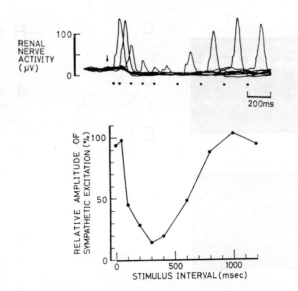

Fig. 4.   Inhibitory curve of trigeminal depressor response. A single pulse (100 μA, 0.5 msec)
is given to the spinal trigeminal complex as conditioning stimulus. The test stimulus
consists of two pulses (200 μA, 0.5 msec, separated by five msec between two pulses)
applied to the medullary pressor area within the nucleus parvocellularis reticularis
at six mm anterior to the obex. The interval between conditioning and test stimuli
was varied up to 1,200 msec. The upper drawing consists of superimposed tracings
of renal nerve activity elicited by test stimuli given a tintervals indicated by small
dots. In the lower drawing, the decrease in renal nerve activity is plotted as a function of time interval.

trigeminal complex 50–1,000 msec prior to the test stimulus. At a stimulus interval of
300 msec sympathetic excitation is diminished to 15% of control values by the conditioning stimulus. Complete recovery of sympathetic excitation occurs about one sec
after trigeminal stimulation (Fig. 4). A similar suppression of reflexly elicited sympathetic excitation by the trigeminal system is seen when sympathetic excitation is
produced by electrical stimulation of the fastigial nucleus of the cerebellum or by
stimulation of the periaqueductal gray in the mesencephalon. These findings therefore
demonstrate that the basic neuronal mechanism of the TDR is inhibition of both tonic
and reflexly elicited sympathetic vasoconstrictor discharge.

Effects of Lesions on the TDR: Comparison with Baroreceptor Mechanisms
    The cardiovascular responses to electrical stimulation of rostral portions of the
spinal trigeminal complex or of the trigeminal nerve are abolished by lesions ipsilateral
to the stimulus and placed within the spinal trigeminal tract and nuclei near the obex.
Such lesions fail to impair the reflex vasodepressor response elicited by electrical
stimulation of the aortic depressor nerve or the reflex bradycardia elicited by the
administration of pressor agents. In contrast, lesions of the nucleus tractus solitarii
(NTS) selectively abolish baroreceptor reflexes without affecting the TDR.
    Of considerable interest, also, is the observation that vasodepressor responses

elicited by stimulation of the main trunk of the vagus nerve distal to the aortic depressor nerve, or of the glossopharyngeal trunk distal to the carotid sinus branch, are eliminated by lesions of the spinal trigeminal tract but not by lesions of the nucleus tractus solitarii[22].

These observations demonstrate that the depressor responses, mediated not only by the trigeminal nerve but also by as yet unidentified branches of the IXth and Xth cranial nerves, other than those arising from arterial baroreceptors, are independent of the nucleus tractus solitarii, but rather depend upon the integrity of the spinal trigeminal complex. Conceivably, the responses from the cranial nerves IX and X, other than arterial baroreceptors, are mediated by branches which split off, upon entering the brain stem, from the main rootlets of IX and X to descend within the spinal trigeminal tract[5,15,29].

DISCUSSION

The Trigeminal System

The TDR represents a heretofore unrecognized reflex mediated by the trigeminal system. While, like the three recognized autonomic reflexes of trigeminal origin, the diving response and the nasopharyngeal and oculocardiac reflexes, it consists of hypopnea and bradycardia; it differs in that the TDR is characterized by a profound fall in arterial pressure due to an inhibition of sympathetic vasoconstrictor activity. The TDR, on the other hand, is in its cardiovascular components identical with those of the arterial baroreceptor reflexes. It differs, however, in that arterial baroreceptor reflexes are mediated by the nucleus tractus solitarii, although the TDR depends entirely upon the spinal trigeminal tract and probably the nucleus caudalis. The trigeminal system not only mediates the depressor response of Vth nerve origin, but also appears to be essential to the processing of vasodepressor responses, arising from branches of the IXth and Xth nerves other than arterial baroreceptor. Thus, the trigeminal system may represent a parallel vasodepressor system, with the arterial baroreceptor reflex mediating responses arising from receptors in the head and neck and from viscera, and possibly sharing a common spinal pathway beyond the trigeminal or solitary relays with the arterial baroreceptor responses.

Functional Considerations

Although the functional significance of the TDR remains as yet unknown, our findings enable us to comment on some of its basic functional characteristics. First, since the TDR can be evoked from all branches of the trigeminal nerve, it is unlikely to arise from any single cranial organ (e.g., the eyes or teeth) nor from areas innervated by only a specific division of the Vth nerve; it is probable it arises from exteroceptive but not from proprioceptive receptors. Second, the TDR can be elicited from stimulation of the supra- and infraorbital nerves (which are cutaneous and thus do not innervate joints or muscle), but not by stimulation of the mesencephalic nucleus of the Vth nerve. Third, the fact that the distribution of receptors for the response are widespread, that the TDR is almost identical with the vasodepressor responses elicited from stimulation of group III afferents in muscle[14] and probably tooth pulp[10] and the threshold for elicitation of the response by electrical stimulation of the trigeminal nerve is within the range for eliciting evoked responses from A-delta fibers[22] all suggest that the TDR may be related to pain mechanisms. Our finding that the spinal trigeminal complex modulates arterial pressure and heart rate adds a new facet to the evidence that the trigeminal system may serve to link the somatic and autonomic nervous systems.

SUMMARY

1.   The TDR represents a new and powerful vasodepressor reflex associated with the trigeminal system. The TDR is characterized by marked decreases in arterial pressure, heart rate, and total peripheral resistance and by a small decrease in cardiac output. Vasodilatation, a result of inhibition of the tonic sympathetic vasoconstrictor activity, is not uniform in the different vascular beds.

2.   Although the hemodynamic pattern of the TDR is strikingly similar to that of the arterial baroreceptor reflex, the two responses are, at least in part, separately organized within the brain: Complete abolition of the arterial baroreceptor reflex by bilateral electrolytic lesions of the nucleus tractus solitarii fail to alter the TDR, whereas caudal lesions of the spinal trigeminal complex abolish the TDR without altering the baroreceptor reflex.

3.   The TDR is most effectively elicited by low frequency electrical stimulation of a selected portion of the spinal trigeminal complex. Stimulation of various branches of the Vth nerve also causes the TDR, although it is much smaller in magnitude. A single shock stimulation of the spinal trigeminal complex can totally eliminate the renal sympathetic vasoconstrictor discharges (the silent period). The duration of the silent period is directly related to the magnitude of hypotension. During the silent period, the sympathetic excitation evoked by stimulation of the medullary pressor area is also suppressed. Thus, the hypotension produced in the TDR is a result of inhibition of both tonic and evoked sympathetic vasoconstrictor discharges.

4.   We conclude that the TDR represents a heretofore unrecognized vasodepressor response dependent upon the spinal trigeminal complex which is at least in part anatomically distinct from pathways subserving the arterial baroreceptor and somatic vasodepressor reflexes. The TDR can be reflexly elicited from widely distributed but yet unidentified receptors innervated by branches of the Vth and of the IXth and Xth cranial nerves other than those innervating arterial baroreceptors. The TDR is of unknown function, but may be related to pain mechanisms.

Supported by Grants HL 18974 and NSG 2259, and a grant from the Ministry of Education of Japan.

REFERENCES

1   Allen, W. F., Origin and destination of the secondary visceral fibers in the guinea pig, *J. comp. Neurol.*, 35 (1923) 275–311.
2   Anderson, J. T., Physiological adaptation in diving vertebrates, *Physiol. Rev.*, 46 (1966) 212–243.

3 Angell-James, J. E. and Daly, M. De B., Reflex respiratory and cardiovascular effects of stimulation of receptors in the nose of the dog, *J. Physiol.* (Lond.), 220 (1972) 673–696.

4 Aschner, B., Über einen bisher noch nicht beschriebenen Reflex vom Auge auf Kreislauf und Atmung Verschwinden des Radialimpulses bei Druck auf Auge, *Wien. Klin.Wschr.*, 21 (1908) 1529–1530.

5 Bonvallet, U. and Sigg, B., Etude electrophysiologique des afferences vagals au niveau de leur penetration dans le bulbe. *J. Physiol.* (Paris), 50 (1958) 63–74.

6 Christensen, K., Lewis, E. and Kuntz A., Innervation of the renal blood vessels in the cat, *J. comp. Neurol.*, 95 (1951) 373–385.

7 Concha, J. H. and Norris, B., Studies on renal vasomotion, *Brit. J. Pharmacol.*, 34 (1968) 277–290.

8 Cottle, M. K. W., Degeneration studies of primary afferents of IXth and Xth cranial nerves in the cat, *J. comp. Neurol.*, 122 (1964) 329–345.

9 Daly, M. de B., Elsner, R. and Angell-James, J. E., Cardiorespiratory control by carotid chemoreceptors during experimental dives in the seal, *Amer. J. Physiol.*, 232 (1977) H 508–516.

10 Dellow, P. G. and Morgan, M. J., Trigeminal nerve input and central blood pressure change in the cat, *Arch. Oral Biol.*, 14 (1969) 295–300.

11 Evans, M. H., The spinal pathways of the myelinated and the nonmyelinated afferent nerve fibers that mediate reflex dilatation of the pupils, *J. Physiol.* (Lond.), 158 (1961) 560–572.

12 Feigl, E. and Folkow, B., Cardiovascular responses in 'diving' and during brain stimulation in ducks, *Acta physiol. scand.*, 57 (1963) 99–110.

13 Gandevia, S. C., McCloskey, D. I. and Potter, E. K., Reflex bradycardia occurring in response to diving, nasopharyngeal stimulation and ocular pressure, and its modification by respiration and swallowing, *J. Physiol.* (Lond.), 276 (1978) 383–394.

14 Johansson, B., Circulatory responses to stimulation of somatic afferents, *Acta physiol. scand.*, 57, Suppl. 198 (1962) 1–91.

15 Kerr, F. W. L., Facial, vagal and glossopharyngeal nerves in the cat. Afferent connections, *Archs Neurol.* (Chicago), 6 (1962) 264–281.

16 Kimmel, D. L., Development of the afferent components of the facial glossopharyngeal and vagus nerves in the rabbit's embryo, *J. comp. Neurol.*, 74 (1941) 447–471.

17 Koizumi, K. and Brooks, C. McC., The integration of autonomic reflexes, their control and their association with somatic reaction, *Ergebn. Physiol.*, 67 (1972) 1–66.

18 Koizumi, K. and Brooks, C. McC., The autonomic nervous system and its role in controlling visceral activities. In: V. B. Mountcastle (Ed.), *Medical Physiology*, 13th ed., Mosby, St. Louis, 1974, pp. 783–812.

19 Koizumi, K., Sato, A., Kaufman, A. and Brooks, C. McC., Studies of sympathetic neuron discharges modified by central and peripheral excitation, *Brain Res.*, 11 (1968) 212–224.

20 Kumada, M., Sensory receptors and afferent mechanisms; somatic receptors. In: O. Kukel, M. N. Levy and A. L. Mark (Eds.), *Second Draft Report of the Neural Control of the Circulation Subgroup to the Hypertension Task Force*, National Heart, Lung and Blood Institute, 1978, pp. 28–31.

21 Kumada, M., Dampney, R. A. L. and Reis, D. J., The trigeminal depressor response: A cardiovascular reflex originating from the trigeminal system, *Brain Res.*, 92 (1975) 485–489.

22 Kumada, M., Dampney, R. A. L. and Reis, D. J., The trigeminal depressor response: A novel vasodepressor response originating from the trigeminal system, *Brain Res.*, 119 (1977) 305–326.

23 Kumada, M., Dampney, R. A. L., Whitnall, M. H. and Reis, D. J., Hemodynamic similarities between the trigeminal and aortic vasodepressor responses, *Amer. J. Physiol.*, 234 (1978) H 67–73.

24 Ranson, S. W. and Hess, C. L. V., The conduction within the spinal cord of the afferent impulses producing pain and vasomotor reflexes, *Amer. J. physiol.*, 38 (1915) 128–152.

25 Sato, A., Kaufman, K., Koizumi, K. and Brooks, C. McC., Afferent nerve groups and sympathetic reflex pathways, *Brain Res.*, 14 (1969) 575–587.

26 Sato, A. and Schmidt, R. F., Somatosympathetic reflexes: Afferent fibers, central pathways, discharge characteristics, *Physiol Rev.*, 53 (1973), 916–947.

27 Skoglund, C. R., Vasomotor reflexes from muscle, *Acta physiol. scand.*, 50 (1960) 311–327.

28 Smith, A. O., Jr., Anatomy of the central neural pathways mediating cardiovascular function. In: W. C. Randall (Ed.), *Nervous Control of the Heart*, Williams & Wilkins, Baltimore, 1965, pp. 34–53.

29 Torvik, A., Afferent connections to the sensory trigeminal nuclei, the nucleus of the solitary tract and adjacent structure, *J. comp. Neurol.*, 106 (1956) 51–141.

30 White, S. W. and McRitchie, R. J., Nasopharyngeal reflexes: Integrative analysis of evoked respiratory and cardiovascular effects, *Aust. J. exp. Biol. med. Sci.*, 51 (1973) 17–31.

SECTION V

CENTRAL INTERACTIONS AND CONTROL
OF THE AUTONOMIC OUTFLOW

Central control of blood pressure and other autonomic reactions has been under study for over one hundred years, at least from the time of Dittmar (1870) and Owsjannikow (1871). Periodically, the matter has been reviewed in special symposia and in Annual Reviews of Physiology (1975, 1976), but there is still much that is unknown. Therefore, it is important that newly devised techniques be used in the study of anatomical substrates for autonomic action. This has been done and reports to follow do present recent accomplishments. Unquestionably, a hierarchy of excitatory and inhibitory centers control the level of tonic discharge, mediate reflexes and organize the patterns of response of the autonomic system evoked by a variety of stimuli.

The special aspects of this very large field which have been our major concern are: anatomical projections and the interconnections that provide pathways through which higher centers exert their control over somato-autonomic reactions; central interactions between the sympathetic and parasympathetic divisions of the autonomic complex; the origins and control of tonic activity in autonomic pre- and postganglionic neurons.

Ideally, one would like to know exactly what happens centrally. Does an afferent branch stimulate multiple "centers" or does activation of one center automatically affect others through field effects, humoral emissions or anatomical interconnections? We are sure central respiratory action affects cardiac reflex actions and imposes a rhythm on the autonomic system. Similarly, cardiac reflexes affect respiration. Nociceptive stimuli affect respiration and cardiovascular actions simultaneously. This is made difficult because "centers" for this are not discrete—possibly intermeshing networks. "Centers" have a role in mediating somatic, visceral and neuroendocrine reactions all together.

In the chapters which follow are analyses of what we now know concerning somato-autonomic reactions and their higher control, inhibitory projections from higher centers and anatomical substrates for hypothalamic control of the autonomic nervous system. Our ultimate objective has not yet been attained but we are moving toward it.

Centers have responsibilities beyond the correlating of incoming signals and the organization of responses. They must deal with the maintenance of states; they are continuously active in organizing behavior and states. States of activity in the cardio-vascular system and in the viscera and states of sensitivity of receptors are set by tonic autonomic system activity. The study of origin of tonic activity, its state in health and disease and what factors determine its level is an important one. Some of the chapters of this section are devoted to discussion of this aspect of the autonomic system's function.

CHAPTER 24

ANATOMICAL SUBSTRATES FOR THE HYPOTHALAMIC CONTROL OF THE AUTONOMIC NERVOUS SYSTEM

Clifford B. Saper

Departments of Medicine and Anatomy and Neurobiology, Washington University School of Medicine, St. Louis, Missouri, USA*

INTRODUCTION

Since the pioneering experiments of Karplus and Kriedl[15], it has been known that electrical stimulation of the hypothalamus can elicit a variety of autonomic responses. However, it was Bard[1,2] who first demonstrated that brain stem transections caudal to the posterior hypothalamic area could abolish the sympathetic "sham rage" which Cannon and Britton[4] had shown to follow decortication. This observation provided the most convincing evidence that the hypothalamus contains a system of cells, normally under cortical inhibition, that is capable of causing a coordinated autonomic activation.

Numerous investigators have since attempted to elucidate the pathways by which the hypothalamus exerts its influence over the autonomic nervous system. Ranson and Magoun and their colleagues[14,22,23] traced a descending projection from the hypothalamus to the sympathetic preganglionic cells of the spinal cord, using electrophysiologic techniques. However, several attempts at identifying a corresponding fiber pathway using axonal degeneration methods[3,40] produced inconsistent results which did not fit well with the physiologic data, and remained unconfirmed. Thus, after reviewing the relevant literature in 1969, Nauta and Haymaker[27] expressed the opinion that no cells in the hypothalamus had been found to project caudally beyond the midbrain, and that one or more relays must be established in the brain stem reticular formation to account for the hypothalamic control of the autonomic nervous system. Similarly, despite considerable evidence that hypothalamic neurons are sensitive to various visceral (and other extrinsic) afferent inputs[8,16,41,46] Nauta and Haymaker could find no evidence for any known pathway by which these influences might reach the hypothalamus.

Within the last few years a number of experiments utilizing the sensitive neuro-

* Present address: Dept. of Neurology, New York Hospital, Conell Medical Center, New York, N. Y. 10021.

anatomical techniques based on the retrograde transport of the histochemically demonstrable enzyme marker horseradish peroxidase (HRP) and the anterograde transport of tritium-labelled proteins have begun to provide evidence for both direct and polysynaptic pathways through which the hypothalamus may influence the autonomic nervous system.

RESULTS AND CONCLUSIONS

Direct Hypothalamo-autonomic Connections

In 1975 Kuypers and Maisky[18] showed that certain neurons in the hypothalamus can be retrogradely labelled by injections of HRP into the spinal cord. Since this was the first clear evidence that the hypothalamus may project directly to the spinal cord, my co-workers and I set out to repeat their experiments. After multiple injections of HRP into the spinal cords of rats, cats and monkeys, or after single injections into the dorsomedial medulla (involving the nucleus of the solitary tract and dorsal motor nucleus of the vagus nerve) in cats and rats, a remarkably similar system of neurons was consistently labelled in the hypothalamus[34]. The largest number of cells was located in the paraventricular nucleus, but smaller numbers of neurons were scattered caudally behind this nucleus in the zona incerta, the lateral hypothalamic area and in the posterior hypothalamic area. In addition some cells in the central gray and Edinger-Westphal nucleus were also found to be labelled. Injections of tritiated amino acids were then made into the hypothalamus in all three species; these succeeded not only in labelling the neurons responsible for the medullary and spinal cord projections, but also in outlining the pathways involved. In these brains descending fibers were found from the hypothalamus through a wide cross-section of the midbrain and pons, including, interestingly, the lateral part of the parabrachial nucleus (see below). Further caudally, the labeled hypothalamic fibers were located along the ventrolateral surface of the medulla, from which one group turned dorsomedially to innervate the nucleus ambiguus, the dorsal motor nucleus of the vagus nerve and the nucleus of the solitary tract, while the remainder passed caudally in the lateral funiculus of the spinal cord to bilaterally innervate the intermediolateral cell column in the thoracic segments of the spinal cord (see Saper, et al.)[34].

The involvement in this proportion of the paraventricular nulceus, almost all of whose cells contain either oxytocin or ADH and have been previously shown to project to the posterior lobe of the pituitary gland[39,42], was of special interest to my colleagues. Swanson[43] has used antibodies directed against oxytocin, ADH and their neurophysin carrier proteins to establish that a group of oxytocin-containing neurons in the paraventricular nucleus, in both rats and monkeys, sends axons along essentially the same path as was outlined by the autoradiographic method. It is not certain, but it seems likely, therefore, that at least some hypothalamo-autonomic axons are collaterals of axons that project to the neurohypophysis, and that they may utilize oxytocin as their transmitter agent. The exact organization of the hypothalamo-autonomic projection is currently under investigation in our laboratory.

A Direct Visceral Afferent Input to the Hypothalamus

Although Morest[24], using the Nauta degeneration method, could only find projections from the nucleus of the solitary tract extending as far forward as the dorsal tegmental nucleus and although Norgren[28,29,30] could only trace "taste afferents" from the nucleus of the solitary tract as far rostrally as the parabrachial nucleus of the pons, Loewy and Burton[21] and Richardo and Koh[32] have found that some neurons in the commissural part of the nucleus of the solitary tract project forward to both the hypothalamus and the thalamus. The thalamic fibers end in the medial part of the ventrobasal complex, while the hypothalamic projection appears to innervate the lateral hypothalamic area and the paraventricular nucleus. Thus, it seems that the hypothalamo-autonomic neurons not only have a direct projection to, but also may receive a direct input from, the primary autonomic nuclei.

Polysynaptic Pathways Which May Connect the Hypothalamus with the Autonomic Nervous System

Considerable date have also come to light in recent years which implicate several structures in the amygdala, septum and pons in modulating the hypothalamic control of the autonomic nervous system. Care should be taken in any such analysis to avoid the assumption that neuroanatomical evidence for connections between two nuclei implies a concomitant degree of physiological interdependence. Certainly only the application of electrophysiological techniques to the data presented here will establish the degree to which this highly-interrelated system is significant in the control of the autonomic nervous system. However, the impressive interconnectivity in this system suggests that the parts have some modulating influence on one another, and provides the best approximation to date for polysynaptic neuroanatomical substrates by which the hypothalamus might influence the autonomic nervous system. Of equal importance is the high degree of connectivity within the hypothalamus[35,36,37,38] so that while certain projections appear to originate from or end upon only discrete portions of the hypothalamus, the potential exists for many other hypothalamic structures to play a role in the ultimate processing of information.

The nucleus of the solitary tract. The nucleus of the solitary tract has, in addition to its hypothalamic projection, a number of other rostral projections to structures which appear to be closely connected to the hypothalamic autonomic system[21,32]. Figure 1 is a series of circuit diagrams which seeks to provide a representation of the connectivity of this system. While this figure is undoubtedly incomplete, it is based upon the most recent information available and certainly provides a good starting point for understanding the connectivity of the central autonomic nervous system.

As Norgren noted[28,29,30], a major terminal region for solitary axons is the parabrachial nucleus, whose medial portion seems primarily concerned with taste afferents from the rostral part of the solitary nucleus, but the lateral part of which appears to be a major relay point for ascending visceral afferent information[21,32]. The further projections of this structure and of the central nucleus of the amygdala and the bed nucleus of the stria terminalis—which also receive direct projections from the nucleus of the solitary tract—will be discussed below. It should also be noted that Loewy and Burton[21]

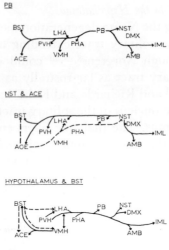

PB

NST & ACE

HYPOTHALAMUS & BST

amygdala—hypothalamus—pons——medulla—spinal cord

Fig. 1. Summary diagram illustrating the great degree of interconnectivity of the central autonomic control system. The upper diagram demonstrates connections pertaining to the parabrachial nucleus; the middle diagram relates to the nucleus of the solitary tract and central amygdaloid nucleus; and the lowest diagram relates to the hypothalamus and bed nucleus of the stria terminalis. ACE: central nucleus of the amygdala; AMB: nucleus ambiguus; BST: bed nucleus of the stria terminalis; DMX: dorsal motor nucleus of the vagus nerve; IML: intermediolateral column of the spinal cord; LHA: lateral hypothalamic area; NST: nucleus of the solitary tract; PHA: posterior hypothalamic area; PVH: paraventricular nucleus; VMH: ventromedial nucleus of the hypothalamus; PB: parabrachial nucleus.

have demonstrated a direct projection from the nucleus of the solitary tract to the intermediolateral cell column of the spinal cord.

The parabrachial nucleus. The parabrachial nucleus stands as a pivotal structure because it is in receipt of projections from virtually every level of this system. It is a primary terminal field for axons from the nucleus of the solitary tract, but it also receives inputs from the lateral hypothalamic area[37] and the central nucleus of the amygdala[13,17]. Recent experiments by Saper and Loewy[33] and by Ricardo and Koh[32] have shown that the lateral (visceral afferent) portion of the parabrachial nucleus, in turn, sends axons rostrally to the lateral hypothalamic area, the paraventricular and ventromedial hypothalamic nuclei, the central nucleus of the amygdala and the bed nucleus of the stria terminalis, in a pattern similar to that demonstrated by Norgren[28,29,30] for the medial parabrachial nucleus. We have also shown, however, that the ventrolateral part of the parabrachial nucleus (i.e., the Kölliker-Fuse nucleus) sends fibers to the intermediolateral column of the spinal cord.

The central nucleus of the amygdala and bed nucleus of the stria terminalis. These structures are considered together because they are both essentially "amygdaloid", the bed nucleus of the stria terminalis being located in the septum and preoptic area along the path of the amygdaloid tract, the stria terminalis, from which it receives many fibers and with which it projects to the hypothalamus. The central nucleus seems to project to the lateral hypothalamic area primarily via the ventral amygdalofugal bundle, and is reciprocally related to the lateral part of the bed nucleus by the stria terminalis[17,45]. The stria terminalis ends in part in the anterior and lateral hypothalamic areas[11], as well as in the capsule of the ventromedial nucleus[44,45] while fibers from the bed nucleus terminate in a similar distribution. The central nucleus, in addition, projects to the parabrachial nucleus[13,17] and to the nucleus of the solitary tract (Schwaber, personal communication).

The lateral part of the bed nucleus and the core of the central nucleus receive direct projections not only from the nucleus of the solitary tract[21,32], but also from the parabrachial nucleus[33,34]. The medial part of the bed nucleus and the capsule of the central nucleus receive projections from the ventromedial nucleus of the hypothalamus[35].

The central tegmental fields.   The central tegmental fields consist of the reticular formation of the midbrain surrounding the red nucleus and dorsal to the substantia nigra. This region receives a substantial input from the parabrachial nucleus[34] as well as the ventromedial nucleus[35] and lateral hypothalamic area[37]. Although information concerning its projection is sparse, Loewy et al.[20] have found a pupillodilator pathway which appeared to originate in the central tegmental fields in the cat, and whose course essentially duplicated that of the hypothalamo-autonomic pathway. Whether efferents from the central tegmental fields augment the descending hypothalamo-autonomic pathway remains to be investigated.

The ventrolateral medulla.   The region along the ventrolateral surface of the medulla through which the hypothalamo-autonomic axons pass, and which Loewy et al.[20] found could, upon electrical stimulation, elicit a variety of profound autonomic responses, also includes the catecholamine-containing A1 and A5 cell groups[5]. Recent experiments applying glycine, an inhibitory neurotransmitter to the A1 region, have shown a marked fall in blood pressure[9,10], as if the activity of cells in these areas, contributing to vascular tone, was inhibited[17]. Further suggestion of the possible contribution of A1 and A5 neurons to autonomic control comes from experiments in which, after ablation of the locus coeruleus, bilaterally, the norepinephrine projection to the intermediolateral column, ostensibly from the A1 and A5 cell groups, is preserved[31]. The A1 and A5 cell groups may receive hypothalamic afferents and, in turn, relay the hypothalamic influence to the vasomotor regions of the spinal cord.

DISCUSSION

The pathways I have recounted and their physiologic significance will, of course, require confirmation by means of electrophysiologic methods. However, they do afford a starting place for the investigation of the central, and especially the hypothalamic, control of the autonomic nervous system.

Of particular interest is the close correlation between these central autonomic nuclei and pathways and certain physiologic observations which have already been made. For example, it has been known since the experiments of Karplus and Kriedl[15] that bilateral autonomic activation could be obtained from unilateral hypothalamic stimulation, even in animals in which the contralateral spinal cord had been hemisected as far caudally as the C8 level. The fact that the direct hypothalamo-autonomic pathway and Loewy's midbrain autonomic pathways both cross to the contralateral intermediolateral cell column at thoracic spinal levels provides an anatomic basis for this observation. A review of the electrophysiologic experiments of Ranson and Magoun and their co-workers[14,22,23] shows that the great majority of their observations are explainable by the pathways outlined here.

Of special interest with reference to this analysis is the correspondence of the hypothalamic-amygdaloid connections with several electrophysiologic observations noted by other authors in this volume. Hilton[12] has compiled considerable information concerning the hypothalamic defense reaction which appears to be elicited along the dorsolateral edge of the ventromedial nucleus as well as along a pathway roughly comparable to the ventral amygdalofugal bundle which connects the ventromedial nucleus with the central nucleus of the amygdala (see Fig. 2). Interestingly, Lisander[19] has, on the other hand, described an inhibitory area in which electrical stimulation is capable of inhibiting the defense reaction. This inhibitory area is anatomically comparable to the region in which the stria terminalis passes through its bed nucleus.

Murphy and Renaud and their co-workers[6,7,25,26] have determined electrophysio-

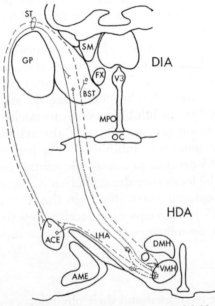

Fig. 2. Schematic diagram of certain hypothalamo-amygdaloid connections which may underlie the phenomena of the hypothalamic defense reaction and the inhibition of this response. The upper figure shows the bed nucleus of the stria terminalis and preoptic area at the level of the defense inhibitory area (DIA) while the lower figure illustrates the ventromedial nucleus of the hypothalamus and central nucleus of the amygdala at the level of the hypothalamic defense area (HDA). ACE: central amygdaloid nucleus; AME: medial amygdaloid nulceus; BST: bed nucleus of the stria terminalis; DMH: dorsomedial nucleus of the hypothalamus; FX: fornix; GP: globus pallidus; LHA: lateral hypothalamic area; MPO: medial preoptic area; OC: optic chiasm; SM: stria medullaris; ST: stria terminalis; V3: third ventricle; VMH: ventromedial nucleus of the hypothalamus.

logically that the input of the ventral amygdolofugal projection and the stria terminalis to the ventromedial nucleus is inhibitory. Furthermore, the inhibitory nature of the strial input seems primarily due to the fact that the fibers of the stria terminalis end in the capsule of the ventromedial nucleus, especially just along its dorsolateral edge, where they synapse upon inhibitory interneurons[6,7,25,26]. These inhibitory interneurons then synapse upon other neurons located more ventrally and laterally in the nucleus[6,7,25,26]. The ventromedial nucleus itself is known to have an inhibitory input to the lateral hypothalamic area[35], which also receives both strial and ventral amygdalofugal inputs, as well as fibers from the bed nucleus of the stria terminalis[38]. The lateral hypothalamic area may play a role in the defense reaction by means of its participation in the direct hypothalamo-autonomic projection[34], by its projection to the parabrachial nucleus[37], or by means of its inhibitory input to the ventromedial nucleus[37]. This latter structure, of course, projects to both the bed nucleus and the capsule of the central nucleus[35]. An understanding of the anatomic substrate which underlies both the defense reaction and the inhibitory region is essential to unravelling the physiologic significance of each.

This work was supported by NIH Grants MH-24604, NS-03777, NS-10943, GM-02016, NS-12751 and American Heart Grant 77-797.

REFERENCES

1 Bard, P., A diencephalic mechanism for the expression of rage with special reference to the sympathetic nervous system, *Amer. J. Physiol.*, 84 (1928) 490–515.

2 Bard, P., The central representation of the sympathetic system as indicated by certain physiologic observations, *Archs Neurol. Psychiat.* (Chicago), 22 (1929) 230–246.

3 Beattie, J., Brow, G. R. and Long, C. N. H., Physiological and anatomical evidence for the existence of nerve tracts connecting the hypothalamus to spinal sympathetic centres, *Proc. R. Soc. B.*, 106 (1930) 253–275.

4 Cannon, W. B. and Britton, S. W., Studies on the conditions of activity in endocrine glands, *Amer. J. Physiol.*, 72 (1925) 283–294.

5 Dahlström, A. and Fuxe, K., Evidence for the existence of monoamine-containing neurons in the central nervous system. I. Demonstration of monoamines in the cell bodies of brain stem neurons, *Acta physiol. scand.*, 62 (Suppl. 232) (1964) 1–55.

6 Dreifuss, J. J. and Murphy, J. T., Convergence of the impulses upon single hypothalamic neurons, *Brain Res.*, 8 (1968) 167–176.

7 Dreifuss, J. J., Murphy, J. T. and Gloor, P., Contrasting effects of two identified amygdaloid efferent pathways on single hypothalamic neurons, *J. Neurophysiol.*, 31 (1968) 237–248.

8 Grizzle, W. E., Johnson, R. M., Schramm, L. P. and Gann, D. S., Hypothalamic cells in area mediating ACTH release respond to right atrial stretch, *Amer. J. Physiol.*, 228 (1975) 1039–1045.

9 Guertzenstein, P. L., Hilton, S. M., Marshall, J. M. and Timms, R. J., Experiments on the origin of vasomotor tone, *J. Physiol.* (Lond.), 275 (1978) 78–79.

10 Guertzenstein, P. G. and Silver, A., Fall in blood pressure produced from discrete regions of the ventral surface of he medulla by glycine and lesions, *J. Physiol.* (Lond.), 242 (1974) 489–503.

11 Heimer, L. and Nauta, W. J. H., The hypothalamic distribution of the stria terminalis in the rat, *Brain Res.*, 13 (1969) 284–297.

12 Hilton, S. M., The defense reaction as a paradigm for cardiovascular control. This volume, pp. 443–449.

13 Hopkins, D. A., Amygdalotegmental projections in the rat, cat and rhesus monkey, *Neuroscience Letters*, 1 (1975) 263–270.

14 Kabat, H., Magoun, H. W. and Ranson, S. W., Electrical stimulation of points in the forebrain and midbrain. The resultant alterations in blood pressure, *Archs Neurol. Psychiat.* (Chicago), 34 (1935) 931–955.

15 Karplus, J. P. and Kreidl, A., Gehirn und sympathicus. I. Zwischenhirn basis und halssympathicus, *Pflügers Arch.*, 129 (1909) 138–144.

16 Kastella, K. G., Spurgeon, H. A. and Weiss, G. K., Respiratory-related neurons in anterior hypothalamus of cat, *Amer. J. Physiol.*, 227 (1974) 710–713.

17 Krettek, J. E. and Price, J. L., Amygdaloid projections to subcortical structures within the basal forebrain and brainstem in the rat and cat, *J. comp. Neurol.*, 178 (1978) 225–254.

18 Kuypers, H. G. J. M. and Maisky, V. A., Retrograde axonal transport of horseradish peroxidase from spinal cord to brain stem cell groups in the cat, *Neuroscience Letters*, 1 (1975) 9–14.

19 Lisander, B., Somato-autonomic reactions and their higher control. This volume, pp. 385–395.

20 Loewy, A. D., Araujo, J. C. and Kerr, F. W. L., Pupillodilator pathways in the brain stem of the cat: Anatomical and physiological identification of a central autonomic pathway, *Brain Res.*, 60 (1973) 65–91.

21 Loewy, A. D. and Burton, H., Nuclei of the solitary tract: efferent projections to the lower brain stem and spinal cord of the cat, *J. comp. Neurol.*, (1978) in press.

22 Magoun, H. W., Descending connections from the hypothalamus, *Res. Publ. Ass. Res. nerv. ment. Dis.*, 20 (1940) 270–285.

23 Magoun, H. W., Ranson, S. W. and Hetherington, A., Descending connections from the hypothalamus, *Archs Neurol. Psychiat.* (Chicago), 39 (1938) 1127–1149.

24 Morest, D. K., Experimental study of the projections of the nucleus of the tractus solitarius and the area postrema in the cat, *J. comp. Neurol.*, 130 (1967) 277–300.

25 Murphy, J. T. and Renaud, L. P., Mechanisms of inhibition in the ventromedial nucleus of the hypothalamus, *J. Neurophysiol.*, 32 (1969) 85–102.

26 Murphy, J. T., Dreifuss, J. J. and Gloor, P., Resonses of hypothalamic neurons to repetitive amygdaloid stimulation, *Brain Res.*, 8 (1968) 153–166.

27 Nauta, W. J. H., and Haymaker, W., Hypothalamic nuclei and fiber connections. In: W. Haymaker, E. Anderson and W. J. H. Nauta (Eds.), *The Hypothalamus*, Charles C. Thomas, Springfield, Ill., 1969, pp. 136–209.

28 Norgren, R., Gustatory afferents to ventral forebrain, *Brain Res.*, 81 (1974) 285–295.

29 Norgren, R., Taste pathways to hypothalamus and amygdala, *J. comp. Neurol.*, 166 (1976) 17–30.

30 Norgren, R., and Leonard, C. M., Ascending central gustatory connections, *J. comp. Neurol.*, 150 (1973) 217–238.

31 Nygren, L. G. and Olson, L., A new major projection from locus coerulus: The main source of noradrenergic nerve terminals in the ventral and dorsal columns of the spinal cord, *Brain Res.*, 132 (1977) 93–95.

32 Ricardo, J. A. and Koh, E. T., Anatomical evidence of direct projections from the nucleus of the solitary tract to the hypothalamus, amygdala, and other forebrain structures in the rat, *Brain Res.*, 153 (1978) 1–26.

33 Saper, C. B. and Loewy, A. D., Efferent connections of the parabrachial nucleus of the pons in the rat, *Neurosci. Abst.*, (1978).

34 Saper, C. B., Loewy, A. D., Swanson, L. W. and Cowan, W. M., Direct hypothalamo-autonomic connections, *Brain Res.*, 117 (1976) 305–312.

35 Saper, C. B., Swanson, L. W. and Cowan, W. M., The efferent connections of the ventro-medial nucleus of the hypothalamus of the rat, *J. comp. Neurol.*, 169 (1976) 409–442.

36 Saper, A. D., Swanson, L. W. and Cowan, W. M., Some efferent connections of the rostral hypothalamus in the squirrel monkey (*Saimiri sciureus*) and cat, *J. comp. Neurol.*, 184 (1979) 205–242.

37 Saper, C. B., Swanson, L. W. and Cowan, W. M., An autoradiographic study of the efferent connections of the lateral hypothalamic area in the rat, *J. comp. Neurol.*, 183 (1979) 689–706.

38 Saper, C. B., Swanson, L. W. and Cowan, W. M., The efferent connections of the anterior hypothalamic area in the rat, cat and monkey, *J. comp. Neurol.*, 182 (1978) 575–600.

39 Sherlock, D. A., Field, P. M. and Raisman, G., Retrograde transport of horseradish peroxidase in the magnocellular neurosecretory system of the rat, *Brain Res.*, 88 (1975) 403–414.

40 Smith, O. A., Anatomy of central neural pathways mediating cardiovascular function. In: W. C. Randall (Ed.), *Control of the Heart*, Williams and Wilkins, Baltimore, 1965, pp. 34–53.

41 Spyer, K. M., Baroreceptor sensitive neurones in the anterior hypothalamus of the cat, *J. Physiol.* (Lond.), 224 (1972) 245–257.

42 Swaab, D. F., Nijveldt, F. and Pool, C. W., Distribution of oxytocin and vasopressin in the cat supraoptic and paraventricular nucleus, *J. Endocrinol.*, 67 (1975) 461–462.

43 Swanson, L. W., Immunohistochemical evidence for a neurophysin-containing autonomic pathway arising in the paraventricular nucleus of the hypothalamus, *Brain Res.*, 128 (1977) 346–353.

44 Swanson, L. W. and Cowan, W. M., Hippocampo-hypothalamic connections: Origin in subicular cortex, not Ammon's horn, *Science*, 189 (1975) 303–304.

45 Swanson, L. W. and Cowan, W. M., Autoradiographic studies of the development and connections of the septal area in the rat. In: J. F. DeFrance (Ed.), *The Septal Nuclei*, Plenum, New York, 1974, pp. 37–63.

46 Thomas, M. R. and Calerasu, F. R., Responses of single units in the medial hypothalamus to electrical stimulation of carotid sinus nerve in the cat, *Brain Res.*, 44 (1972) 49–62.

CHAPTER 25

TONIC ACTIVITY OF THE AUTONOMIC NERVOUS SYSTEM: FUNCTIONS, PROPERTIES, ORIGINS

Canio Polosa, Allan Mannard and Wendy Laskey

Department of Physiology, McGill University, Montreal, Quebec, Canada

INTRODUCTION

A prominent feature of the autonomic nervous system is the presence of a continuous flow of impulses from the central and peripheral neurons of this system to the effector organs. This is the "tonic" or "background" activity of autonomic neurons, and these terms, as used here, refer to all patterns of unevoked, repetitive action potential discharge recorded from these neurons under a particular set of control conditions. Many types of neurons, other than autonomic, also exhibit tonic activity[11]. Investigations of this property, in a particular neuron population, can be directed towards answering a number of general questions. What is the functional significance of tonic activity? What are the characteristics of tonic activity in single neurons and how is this related to the activity of the neuron population? How is tonic activity generated and how is it distributed to effector organs?

Recent neurophysiological studies on autonomic neurons have provided sufficient data to partially answer some of these questions for the tonic activity of sympathetic and of parasympathetic, pupilloconstrictor and cardioinhibitor, neurons. This review presents a synthesis of old and new data relating to the tonic activity of these three types of autonomic neurons.

FUNCTIONS OF AUTONOMIC TONE

Several main functions can be attributed to autonomic tone. First, autonomic tone contributes to the maintenance of a required level of activity in autonomic effector cells. For example, normal systemic arterial pressure is maintained at a level greater than that determined by the properties of the blood vessels themselves by the contraction of vascular smooth muscle evoked by tonically active sympathetic postganglionic neurons. Second, the tonic activity of autonomic neurons and effector cells provides them with the capability for "bidirectional" responses, i.e., for increase as well as decrease in activity. This capability is of obvious importance for homeostasis. Third, neurogenic tone "primes" effector cells, so that neurally-mediated adjustments in their activity can be made without the lag inherent in building up a response in quiescent tissue. In a similar manner, tonic activity of pre- and postganglionic neurons and their antecedents enhances propagation of activity in neural networks of which they are components and contributes to an increased responsiveness to changing conditions. Fourth, the sensitivity (i.e., the response to a particular change in input activity) of autonomic effector cells is set by the level of neurogenic tone. Since the relation between effector cell response and level of neural activity is, in general, probably sigmoidal[19], the response of the effector cell to a change in autonomic nerve activity is highly dependent on the pre-existing level of nerve activity.

Additional advantages in the control of effector systems result from combining tone from the sympathetic and parasympathetic components of the autonomic nervous system. Effector systems with dual antagonistic innervation may be expected to be inherently stable, i.e., to show minimal effects from widespread perturbations of neuronal activity which alter the activity of the two components in the same direction, such as may occur due to the action of central nervous system stimulants or depressants. On the other hand, the same effector systems should be highly sensitive to any factor which increases the difference between the activity levels of its sympathetic and parasympathetic innervation, as in the case, for example, of the effects of changes in baroreceptor input on heart rate.

THE TONIC ACTIVITY OF SYMPATHETIC NEURONS

Evidence of Tonic Activity in the Sympathetic Nervous System

Tonic activity of pre- and postganglionic sympathetic neurons has been directly documented in the neural recordings obtained by a number of investigators (see list in reference[47]). Of particular interest are the intracellular recordings from tonically active ganglionic[50] and preganglionic (Coote and Westbury, unpublished observations) neurons. Remarkable technical achievements of recent years have been the recording of tonic activity from postganglionic axons in conscious humans[26] and in the unanaesthetized, freely-moving cat[39,53,63]. Indirect evidence of the existence of tonic activity in sympathetic nerves to various effector organs is the fall in systemic arterial pressure resulting from ganglionic blockade[21] or from ventral root block[25], the fall in heart rate after sympathectomy or β-adrenergic blockade[60], the miosis of Horner's syndrome[5] and the disappearance of electrodermal potentials after denervation[71].

Properties of Tonic Activity of Preganglionic Neurons

One-fourth to one-fifth of all sympathetic preganglionic neurons (SPN's) are tonically active in the CNS-intact, anesthetized cat[34,57]. The proportion seems uniform at all spinal cord levels[34] (also Jänig and Szulczyk, unpublished observations). Since the total number of SPN's has been estimated[28] at 4×10^4, tonic activity, in the anesthetized, CNS-intact cat should involve approximately 10^4 neurons. Which ones among the SPN's are active is likely to be determined by: 1) neuron excitability, possibly inversely related to soma size[27]; 2) number and efficacy of synaptic connections; and 3) types of synaptic connections. Concerning the latter factor, the work of Jänig and collaborators[23,30,33] on sympathetic neurons supplying the cat's hind limb has shown that tonic activity is distributed among sympathetic ganglionic neurons (SGN's) according to the nature of their target cells and that a similar pattern of distribution is observed among SPN's. According to these authors, tonic activity is prominent among vasoconstrictor neurons to skin and muscle, very weak among sudomotor neurons and absent among pilomotor and vasodilator neurons.

Mean firing rates of SPN's in CNS-intact, anesthetized or decerebrate, unanesthetized cats are consistently low, with values ranging from 1.2 to 2.1 Hz in various studies[37,47,65]. Jänig and Schmidt[34] reported different mean firing rates for SPN's with myelinated (1.7 Hz) and unmyelinated (2.9 Hz) axons. On the assumption that neurons with smaller diameter axons have smaller cell bodies, this difference could be explained on the basis of the size principle[27], i.e., SPN's with smaller cell bodies and higher input resistance are more excitable than larger cells and hence fire at higher rates, even though both types of cells may be receiving a similar input.

The number of active upper thoracic SPN's and their mean firing rates are highest in preparations with intact CNS (or midcollicular decerebrate), become less when the spinal cord is separated from the brain stem and become very small when, in the acute spinal animal, the dorsal roots are cut[47]. This relationship between the amount of neural connections available to the SPN and the activity level of the SPN suggests that the activity is mainly generated by synaptic input. A pacemaker property of the SPN or a direct action of the physico-chemical environment of the neuron may account for the persistence of tonic activity in a few upper thoracic SPN's in the isolated spinal cord with sectioned dorsal roots[1,55,57]. However, the role of ventral root afferents, hypoxia and cord temperature in determining this residual activity has not been evaluated. It is interesting to mention that in a similar preparation tonic activity persists in some γ-motoneurons[70]. The tonic activity of sympathetic neurons innervating the colon seems, on the contrary, to be entirely generated by local (spinal) mechanisms, since their level of activity is unchanged after spinal cord section and dorsal rhyzotomy[15].

Origin of the Synaptic Input Responsible for the Tonic Activity of SPN's

The SPN is connected to a set of sensory systems and central neuron groups. The input(s) responsible for the generation of tonic activity must come from this set. Among the former we can list skeletal muscle and skin afferents, visceral afferents, baroreceptor afferents[41], central[45] and peripheral[29] chemoreceptors, vestibular afferents[69], visual afferents[56] and central temperature receptors[68]. The SPN is also connected with CNS structures like the nuclei of the brain stem reticular formation, nuclei of the hypothalamus and cerebellum and areas of the cerebral cortex[12]. Since resting discharge is a widespread property of sense organs[22] and of CNS neurons[11,64], it is likely that background synaptic activity will be generated on the SPN membrane as a result of connections with these neuron systems. While all these inputs must be considered as potentially important in contributing tonic excitatory and inhibitory influences to the SPN, demonstrations showing that they have a role has been given only for a few. So far, it has been shown that removal of baroreceptor input causes tone to increase[29], thus indicating the tonic inhibitory action of this input. It has also been shown that sympathetic tone can be reduced by removal of peripheral chemoreceptor input in conditions of hypoxia[29], by bilateral ablation of the lateral reticular nucleus of the medulla[24] and by elimination of central chemoreceptor activity by low CO_2[44] or by cooling chemoreceptive area S of the ventral surface of the medulla[45].

Discharge Patterns of SPN's

Most tonically-firing SPN's fire irregularly, i.e., the timing of spikes cannot be predicted from previous activity. In about half of them, in the CNS-intact or decerebrate cat, this basic mode of firing is rhythmically modulated at the rate of the heart beat (cardiac modulation), at the rate of the central respiratory activity (Traube-Hering or respiratory modulation) and at a three minute repetition rate (Mayer or slow modulation). The appearance of the latter modulation seems to be favored by experimental conditions departing from normal[59] and therefore will not be discussed further. Respiratory modulation occurs frequently, being found in about half of the units in the upper thoracic cord[58]. It is due to a periodic facilitation of the neurons during inspiration. This modulation results in burst firing of the SPN which is reminiscent of the firing of motoneurons of respiratory muscle. During the burst, relatively high instantaneous firing frequencies can be reached (e.g., 20–40 Hz). Cardiac modulation, which has been found in both thoracic and lumbar SPN's[65], varied in incidence in different studies, ranging from 15% in some[47,65] to 60% in others (Jänig and Szulczyk, unpublished observations). It is due to a depression of the neurons during part of each cardiac cycle.

SPN Firing Mechanism During Tonic Activity

The SPN is the site of convergence of synaptic pathways originating from afferent systems and from nuclei at all levels of the neuraxis (see above). The continuous resting discharge of neurons in these pathways is the likely source of the background synaptic input to the SPN. The pooling (or superposition) on the SPN membrane of the synaptic effects of the spike trains arriving from all these sources should result in a random sequence of PSP's[47]. The irregular background spike emission by the SPN would then arise from this random series of EPSP's through transformation by SPN processes (EPSP summation and refractoriness). Rhythmic firing (respiratory and cardiac modulation) would arise if the probability of SPN discharge was, in addition, periodically modulated. Concerning the role of EPSP summation, on the assumption that the response of a small unit to a given synaptic current is large because of its high total membrane resistance, EPSP's in SPN's should be large in size, so that few EPSP's may be required for reaching the firing threshold. Intracellular measurements by Coote and Westbury (unpublished observations) confirm this prediction. This high sensitivity to the input might help explain why small cells like SPN's and γ-motoneurons retain their discharge in the isolated spinal cord. Rhythmically-modulated discharge (cardiac and respiratory modulation) could appear as a result of either periodic synchronization (excitatory or inhibitory) of presynaptic neurons (i.e., a modulation of the tendency for coincident PSP arrival) or periodic fluctuation in excitability of the SPN. Concerning refractoriness, the period of reduced excitability lasting 50–100 msec after a discharge[48], would result in a smaller probability of firing than expected for a random process for this duration of time after a spike.

Physiological Significance of the Rhythmic Modulation of SPN Firing

The respiratory and cardiac modulating mechanisms, in addition to being the expression of a periodic facilitatory and inhibitory input to the SPN, respectively, have the interesting property of synchronizing the activities of all the SPN's they influence. This synchronization, in turn, is likely to result in enhancement of transmission at ganglionic synapses by spatial summation. Enhancement of transmission at neuroeffector junctions by spatio-temporal summation is also likely to result. In other words, by means of this synchronizing process, greater ganglion cell and effector organ activity may be obtained than if the same number of spikes per sec in the same number of preganglionic axons were unsynchronized. The high frequency firing within the bursts, typical of respiratory modulated discharge, may lead to increased acetylcholine synthesis in SPN terminals[7] which should also increase the probability of transmission through the ganglia.

Chemical Transmitters Involved in Tonic Activity of SPN's

At the present time little is known about the neurotransmitters involved in the generation of tonic activity in SPN's. Iontophoretic studies have indicated some of the putative transmitters to which the SPN is sensitive[16], and alterations of tonic and reflex activity of SPN's have been produced by chemical activation of monoaminergic pathways by "precursor loading"[46]. De Groat and Ryall[16] found that 80% of the SPN's tested were excited by serotonin (5-HT) and 40% were depressed by norepinephrine (NE) applied by iontophoresis. Acetylcholine was without effect, while glutamate, as usual, excited all cells. It is possible, therefore, that 5-HT is the mediator of some excitatory processes underlying tonic activity, while NE could be the mediator of tonic inhibition. Precursor "loading" is a procedure by which the amount of transmitter synthesized, stored and released by nerve terminals can be increased[10]. Several studies on the effects of monoamine precursors on the SPN's have been made. L-3, 4-dihydroxyphenylalanine (L-DOPA), a precursor of dopamine, NE and epinephrine, depresses tonic and reflex activity of the SPN[14,2]. These results seem consistent with the previous iontophoretic data. Franz et al.[20], however, found mixed depressant and excitatory effects from L-DOPA injection, and attributed the former to 5-HT displaced from serotonergic terminals and the latter to NE newly synthesized in adrenergic terminals. A depressant effect of DL-5-hydroxytryptophan (DL-5-HTP, precursor of 5-HT) on the tonic and reflex firing of the SPN has also been found[14,20]. L-5-HTP, however, excites SPN's in spinal cats[2]. Clearly these studies with precursors, although contributing interesting and controversial new data, have not yet produced any definitive evidence concerning the nature of the chemical transmitters involved in tonic activity.

Properties of Tonic Activity of Ganglionic Neurons

The spike trains generated by SPN's represent the source of the tonic activity of SGN's. Tonic activity of SGN's disappears after elimination of their preganglionic input[50]. Analysis of the main features of tonic activity of the SGN allows inferences concerning what modifications tonic activity undergoes by transmission through the ganglion.

Fraction of the neuron pool having tonic activity. The fraction of the neuron population which has tonic activity seems much higher for the SGN than for the SPN. For the cat hind limb, Horeyseck and Jänig[30] found that 92% of postganglionic axons in cutaneous nerves and all those in muscle nerves are active. When the postganglionic axons are examined with reference to their effector destination, it was found that while vasoconstrictor, sudomotor and pupillodilator axons have tonic activity, pilomotor and vasodilator[23,55] axons do not. Sudomotor neurons fire at a much lower frequency than vasoconstrictor neurons[33].

Mean firing rates. Mean firing rate also seems higher for the SGN than for the SPN. Mirgorodski and Skok[50] found a mean rate of 3.4 Hz for a large sample of cells of the superior cervical ganglion in cats and rabbits anaesthetized with chloralose or urethane. In cats with chloralose anaesthesia, Jänig and Schmidt[34] found a mean rate of 4.0 Hz for postganglionic axons of the cervical nerve. It is interesting to comment here on the indirect method of estimating firing rates of SGN's during their tonic activity by finding the frequency of repetitive supramaximal stimulation of sectioned peripheral nerve trunks at which the activity level of the effectors equals the presection level[19]. This method is likely to give an underestimate of the true firing rate, because electrical stimulation results in a synchronous efferent volley, which is likely to have a greater synaptic efficacy than the natural, largely asynchronous activity of SGN's.

Discharge patterns. The discharge patterns of SGN's appear similar to those of the SPN's. Chalazonitis and Gonella[13] have described, for neurons of the stellate ganglion, irregular firing and firing modulated at the cardiac and respiratory rate but have not given figures on the relative proportion of these. For neurons of the superior cervical ganglion, Mirgorodski and Skok[50] report that 48% of the tonically active neurons are respiratory modulated, while cardiac modulation was observed in only a few units. Respiratory and cardiac modulation has also been described in recordings of human postganglionic axons[26] and of postganglionic axons in the hind limb of the cat[33].

The "amplification" of tonic activity in the ganglia. The higher incidence of tonic activity in ganglionic neurons as compared with preganglionic is likely due to divergence and convergence of the excitatory input from tonically active SPN's, and to the high safety factor for transmissions at ganglionic synapses. Physiological evidence of convergence of several active preganglionic axons on a single SGN has been given by Mirgorodski and Skok[51] who showed, with a reversible anodal block, that tonically active preganglionic axons greatly different in threshold and conduction velocity contributed to the EPSP activity recorded in single SGN's. Anatomical data[6,17] show that each SPN connects with 300–400 SGN's and that each SGN is innervated by about 25 SPN's. On the average, five of these will have tonic activity. Taking mean firing rate of SPN's as two spikes/sec, mean frequency of EPSP arrival will be 10/sec for the average SGN. EPSP's in SGN's are known to be large relative to neuron threshold[9]. These facts seem capable of explaining both the greater proportion of tonically active SGN's than of SPN's and their greater firing rate. Since there are more SGN's than SPN's (17:1 ratio according to Foley and Schnitzlein[18]) there should be more than half a million tonically active SGN's as compared with the 10,000 active SPN's.

In summary, tonic activity of SPN's seems to be generated both by sensory input and by input from within the CNS. The large amplifying capability of the ganglia makes it possible for the tonic activity of a relatively small number of SPN's to maintain the neurogenic tone of organs with sympathetic innervation.

THE TONIC ACTIVITY OF PARASYMPATHETIC NEURONS

Pupilloconstrictor Parasympathetic Neurons

Preganglionic pupilloconstrictor neurons, located in the rostral extension of the oculomotor nerve nucleus, innervate the sphincter muscle of the iris via the neurons of the ciliary ganglion, whose axons travel in the short ciliary nerves. These neurons are one of the two efferent limbs of the light reflex, which regulates the amount of light incident on the retina by appropriate alterations of pupil size.

Sillito and Zbrozyna[66], using extracellular microelectrodes, have recorded the tonic activity of orthodromically-identified pupilloconstrictor preganglionic neurons in the midbrain of cats with cervical sympathetic nerve section. These units were identified as pupilloconstrictor because they were excited by light stimulation of the retina, which constricted the pupil, and were inhibited by stimulation of the hypothalamic defense area, which dilated the pupil. The tonic activity of these neurons, in the absence of light stimulation of the retina, consists of remarkably regular spike trains at frequencies of six to 10 Hz. These firing rates are high when compared with those of other autonomic neurons and should be associated with a nearly full response of the effector cells[66].

Recordings from postganglionic axons in the short ciliary nerves[54] show that the regularity and frequency of the preganglionic spike discharge are preserved in the discharge of the ganglionic neurons. In addition, ganglion cells fire synchronously[54], an observation suggesting that the preganglionic discharges must also be synchronized. Neither preganglionic nor postganglionic pupilloconstrictor neurons show cardiac or respiratory modulation of their firing patterns.

It would seem reasonable to consider the retina as a possible source of the excitation underlying the background firing of pupilloconstrictor neurons. The retina is functionally coupled to these neurons through the afferent limb of the pupillary light reflex. Retinal ganglion cells show background firing in darkness[42] and this dark activity initiates spike trains in units of the lateral geniculate nucleus[8]. The dark discharge in optic nerve and lateral geniculate nucleus is abolished by chemical destruction of retinal receptors, and this abolition is associated with full dilatation of the pupil[61]. Whether this dilatation is due to suppression of the tonic activity of the pupilloconstrictor neurons or to other mechanisms is not known. Other studies, however, have shown that deafferentation of pupilloconstrictor neurons does not affect the rate or regularity of their tonic firing. Nisida and Okada[54] found that transections of the midbrain above and below the oculomotor nerve nuclei and section of the nerve supply of the extrinsic eye muscles leaves the tonic activity of postganglionic pupilloconstrictor neurons unchanged. This finding is supported by the data of Keller[38] who found that animals chronically deafferented by similar sections displayed constricted pupils that could be dilated by atropine.

The limited evidence available suggests therefore that tonic activity of the pupilloconstrictor preganglionic neurons originates within the midbrain itself. The remarkable regularity of their firing patterns suggests that these neurons are either driven by non-neurogenic sources (e.g., pCO_2, pH, temperature), have pacemaker activity of their own or are driven by a very stable neuronal oscillator. The latter possibility is favored by the observation that pupilloconstrictor postganglionic neurons often fire synchronously[54].

Cardiac Vagal Preganglionic Neurons

The cell bodies of parasympathetic preganglionic neurons supplying the heart, which were once thought to be in the dorsal motor nucleus of the vagus[52], are actually located in the nucleus ambiguus of the medulla[49]. Their axons run in the vagus nerve and make synaptic connections with ganglion cells in the cardiac muscle itself. A continuous release of acetylcholine from the cardiac ganglion cells occurs in response to the tonic activity of the preganglionic neurons. This is inferred from the fact that section of the cervical vagus nerve or administration of atropine usually results in an increase in heart rate. The magnitude of this increase can be used as an indicator of the pre-existing level of vagal tone. The level of vagal tone varies greatly with the animal's species, age, physiological condition and the presence of drugs such as anesthetics[36].

A relatively pure population of cardio-inhibitory preganglionic axons is found in the cardiac branches of the vagus nerve[49] and their tonic activity has been recorded extracellularly at this site[43]. Antidromic activation of cardiac vagal branches has been used to locate the soma of the preganglionic neurons in the medulla, and information on the tonic activity of these cells has been obtained by microelectrode recording[67]. Other criteria which characterize cardio-inhibitory neurons are: an inverse relationship between their discharge frequency and heart rate, pulse and respiratory modulation in their firing patterns, and their excitation by baroreceptor activation. These criteria for identification have been used in studies of cardiac vagal efferents isolated from the cervical vagus nerve[32,35,36].

The proportion of tonically active neurons varies greatly with the experimental conditions, as might be predicted from data based on indirect assessment of cardiac vagal tone. Spyer and McAllen[67] found that only 28% of antidromically-identified cardiac vagal preganglionic neurons were tonically active in the chloralose-anesthetized cat. These authors noted the marked effect of variations in end-tidal pCO_2 on tonic activity: Hyperventilation, used in their experiments to suppress the firing of neighboring respiratory neurons, also depressed the tonic firing of cardiac vagal neurons. Kunze[43], in cats under chloralose, found no tonic activity in units isolated from cardiac vagal branches at mean arterial blood pressures below 150 mmHg. These animals, however, were also hyperventilated and had an end-tidal pCO_2 of 2%. These two sets of findings seem consistent with the knowledge that cats have a low level of vagal tone[36]. In contrast, Iriuchijima and Kumada[32], in morphine-chloralose anesthetized dogs, found 54 tonically active units in a population of 58 vagal efferent fibers excited by electrical stimulation of the carotid sinus nerve.

The spike trains of active cardiac vagal neurons show marked cardiac and respiratory modulation. Concerning the cardiac modulation, it is well known that increases in systemic arterial pressure above normal levels excite cardio-inhibitory neurons and that this effect depends on the integrity of baroreceptor afferent pathways[29]. In addition, Kunze's observations[43] show that baroreceptor afferents are a major source of the tonic activity of cardiac vagal preganglionic neurons. In chloralose-anesthetized cats, sequential section of the carotid sinus and aortic nerves leads to a progressive loss of tonic activity in this neuron pool. Complete baroreceptor deafferentation abolishes all activity. The intensity of the baroreceptor input determines the firing rate of individual neurons[35] as well as the proportion of active units in the pool[43]. The modulation of baroreceptor firing by the arterial pressure pulse is reflected in the markedly pulse-modulated firing pattern of the cardio-inhibitory neurons[32,35,36,43,67]. The baroreceptor input is probably distributed to all cardiac vagal neurons. The presence of subliminal excitatory input from this source in silent cardio-inhibitory neurons has been demonstrated by the observation that excitatory responses of these cells to iontophoretically-applied glutamate are pulse-modulated[67].

The latency of the baroreceptor-mediated reflex excitation of cardiac vagal neurons, when measured as the time between peak aortic pressure and onset of the increased firing rate, is greater than 50 msec and as long as 240 msec[35,36,43]. Estimates of central delay, made from the data of Jewett[35], give values of at least 40 msec. Such long central delays are quite common for synaptic pathways controlling autonomic neurons.

While baroreceptors seem to provide the main excitatory input for the maintenance of cardiac vagal tone, the observation that in dogs with denervated carotid sinus and aortic arch, sinus arrythmia not attributable to modulation of sympathetic tone, reappears during sleep[62] suggests that other inputs must also contribute to the maintenance of vagal tone under these experimental conditions.

Nearly all tonically active cardiac vagal preganglionic neurons generate spike trains with a respiratory periodicity characterized by a reduction in firing rate during inspiration. Often the neurons are silent in inspiration. This firing pattern has been described in cats[43,67], and dogs[32,35,36]. When silent cardiac vagal preganglionic neurons are made to fire by iontophoresis of excitant amino acids, the evoked firing also occurs mainly during expiration[67]. Thus, all cardiac vagal neurons, whether tonically active or silent, receive this respiration-synchronous input. Although there is evidence that cardiac vagal preganglionic neurons are directly influenced by pulmonary stretch receptor afferents[3], the persistence of respiratory modulation in the firing of these neurons in vagotomized animals[67] indicates that the modulation must be generated within the CNS. Assuming then that cardiac vagal neurons receive an input from brain stem respiratory neurons, which periodically alters their firing rate, this input could cause either an inhibition occurring during inspiration or an excitation occurring during expiration. When activity of brain stem respiratory neurons is abolished by hypocapnia, tonic activity of cardiac vagal neurons is maintained, but respiratory modulation of their firing is lost[36,43]; this finding is consistent with the hypothesis of an inspiration-synchronous inhibition. McAllen and Spyer[67], on the basis of their observations on silent cardiac vagal neurons activated by excitant amino acids, also consider it likely that respiratory modulation results from inhibition of activity during inspiration and suggest an input from the medullary inspiratory neurons of the lateral group as the source of the modulation. Consequences of this respiratory modulation of tonic activity of cardiac vagal neurons are the cardiac respiratory arrythmia[4] and the striking respiratory fluctuation in responsiveness of the heart to baro- and chemoreceptor input[40].

In summary, the tonic activity of cardiac parasympathetic preganglionic neurons seems to be generated mainly by activity in arterial baroreceptor afferents and modulated by central inspiratory activity. While these neurons have been shown to have connections with other afferent inputs, e.g., peripheral chemoreceptors[36,43] and somatic afferents[31], data concerning the role of these inputs in the generation of tonic activity are not presently available.

The experimental work by the authors was supported by the Medical Research Council of Canada and the Quebec Heart Foundation. The authors are grateful to Drs. Coote, Jänig, and Spyer for providing much appreciated unpublished data.

REFERENCES

1　Alexander, R. S., The effects of blood flow and anoxia on spinal cardiovascular centers, *Amer. J. Physiol.*, 143 (1945) 698–708.

2　Amicarella-Boyle, R. and Polosa, C., An investigation of the effects of L-dopa and 5-HTP on sympathetic preganglionic neurones, *Fed. Proc.*, 35 (1976) 509.

3　Anrep, G. V., Pascual, W. and Rössler, R., Respiratory variations of the heart rate. I. The reflex mechanism of the respiratory arrhythmia, *Proc. R. Soc. B.*, 119 (1936) 191–217.

4　Anrep, G. V., Pascual, W. and Rössler, R., Respiratory variations of the heart rate. II. The central mechanism of the respiratory arrhythmia and the inter-relations between the central and the reflex mechanisms, *Proc. R. Soc. B.*, 119 (1936) 218–230.

5　Bernard, C., *Leçons sur la Physiologie et la Pathologie du Systeme Nerveux*, Bailliere, Paris, 1858.

6　Birks, R. I., The relationship of transmitter release and storage to fine structure in a sympathetic ganglion, *J. Neurocytol.*, 3 (1974) 133–160.

7　Birks, R. I., A long-lasting potentiation of transmitter release related to an increase in transmitter stores in a sympathetic ganglion, *J. Physiol.* (Lond.), 271 (1977) 847–862.

8　Bishop, P. O., Levick, W. R. and Williams, W. O., Statistical analysis of the dark discharge of lateral geniculate neurones, *J. Physiol.* (Lond.), 170 (1964) 598–612.

9　Blackman, J. G., Function of autonomic ganglia. In: J. Hubbard (Ed.), *The Peripheral Nervous System*, Plenum, New York, 1974.

10　Burn, J. H. and Rand, M. J., The effect of precursors of noradrenaline on the response to tyramine and sympathetic stimulation, *Brit. J. Pharmacol.*, 15 (1960) 47–55.

11　Burns, B. D., The Mammalian Cerebral Cortex. Arnold, London, 1958.

12　Calaresu, F. R., Faiers, A. A. and Mogenson, G. J., Central neural regulation of heart and blood vessels in mammals, *Progr. Neurobiol.*, 5 (1975) 1–35.

13　Chalazonitis, A. and Gonella, J., Activite electrique spontanee des neurones du ganglion stellaire du chat. Etude par microelectrode extracellularie, *J. Physiol.* (Paris), 63 (1971) 599–609.

14　Coote, J. H. and MacLeod, V. H., The influence of bulbospinal monoaminergic pathways on sympathetic nerve activity, *J. Physiol.* (Lond.), 241 (1974) 453–475.

15　De Groat, W. C., Booth, A. M., Krier, J., Milne, R. J., Morgan, C. and Nadelhaft, I., Neural control of the urinary bladder and large intestine. This volume, pp. 50–67.

16 De Groat, W. C. and Ryall, R. W., An excitatory action of 5-Hydroxytryptamine on sympathetic preganglionic neurons, *Exp. Brain Res.*, 3 (1967) 299–305.

17 Elfvin, L. G., The ultrastructure of the superior cervical sympathetic ganglion of the cat, *J. Ultrastr. Res.*, 8 (1963) 441–476.

18 Foley, J. O. and Schnitzlein, H. N., The contribution of individual thoracic spinal nerves to the upper cervical sympathetic trunk, *J. comp. Neurol.*, 108 (1957) 109–120.

19 Folkow, B., Impulse frequency in sympathetic vasomotor fibres correlated to the release and elimination of the transmitter, *Acta physiol. scand.*, 25 (1952) 49–76.

20 Franz, D. N., Hare, B. D. and Neumayr, R. J., Reciprocal control of sympathetic pre-ganglionic neurons by monoaminergic bulbospinal pathways and a selective effect of clonidine. In: P. Milliez and M. Safar (Eds.), *Recent Advances in Hypertension*, Vol. I. Boehringer, Reims, 1975.

21 Goodman, L. S. and Gilman, A., *The Pharmacological Basis of Therapeutics*, 4th ed., McMillan, 1970, p. 594.

22 Granit, R., *Receptors and Sensory Perception*, Yale University Press, New Haven, 1955, Chapter 3.

23 Grosse, M. and Jänig, W., Vasoconstrictor and pilomotor fibres in skin nerves to the cat's tail, *Pflügers Arch.*, 361 (1976) 221–229.

24 Guertzenstein, P. G. and Silver, A., Fall in blood pressure produced from discrete regions of the ventral surface of the medulla by glycine and lesions, *J. Physiol.* (Lond.), 242 (1974) 489–503.

25 Guyton, A. G., *Textbook of Medical Physiology*, 5th ed., Saunders, Philadelphia, 1976, p. 259.

26 Hagbarth, K. E. and Vallbo, A. B., Pulse and respiratory grouping of sympathetic impulses in human muscle nerves, *Acta physiol. scand.*, 74 (1968) 96–108.

27 Henneman, E., Somjen, G. and Carpenter, D. O., Functional significance of cell size in spinal motorneurons, *J. Neurophysiol.*, 28 (1965) 560–580.

28 Henry, J. L. and Calaresu, F. R., Topography and numerical distribution of neurons of the thoraco-lumbar intermediolateral nucleus in the cat, *J. comp. Neurol.*, 144 (1972) 205–213.

29 Heymans, C. and Neil, E., *Reflexogenic Areas of the Cardiovascular System*, Churchill, London, 1958.

30 Horeyseck, G., Jänig, W., Kirchner, F. and Thämer, V., Activation and inhibition of muscle and cutaneous postganglionic neurones to hind limb during hypothalamically-induced vasoconstriction and atropine-sensitive vasodilation, *Pflügers Arch.*, 361 (1976) 231–240.

31 Iriuchijima, J. and Kumada, M., Efferent cardiac vagal discharge of the dog in response to electrical stimulation of sensory nerves, *Jap. J. Physiol.*, 13 (1963) 599–605.

32 Iriuchijima, J. and Kumada, M., Activity of single vagal fibers efferent to the heart, *Jap. J. Physiol.*, 14 (1964) 479–487.

33 Jänig, W. and Kümmel, H., Functional discrimination of postganglionic neurones of the cat's hind paw with respect to the skin potentials recorded from the hairless skin, *Pflügers Arch.*, 371 (1977) 217–225.

34 Jänig, W. and Schmidt, R. F., Single unit responses in the cervical sympathetic trunk upon somatic nerve stimulation, *Pflügers Arch.*, 314 (1970) 199–216.

35 Jewett, D. L., Activity of single efferent fibres in the cervical vagus nerve of the dog, with special reference to possible cardio-inhibitory fibres, *J. Physiol.* (Lond.), 175 (1964) 321–357.

36 Katona, P. G., Poitras, J. W., Barnett, G. O. and Terry, B. S., Cardiac vagal efferent

activity and heart period in the carotid sinus reflex, *Amer. J. Physiol.*, 218 (1970) 1030–1037.

37   Kaufman, A. and Koizumi, K., Spontaneous and reflex activity of single units in lumbar white rami. In: F. F. Kao, K. Koizumi and M. Vassalle (Eds.), *Research in Physiology. A Liber Memorialis in Honor of Professor Chandler McCuskey Brooks*, Aulo Gaggi, Bologna, 1971, pp. 469–481.

38   Keller, A. D., The striking inherent tonus of the deafferented central pupilloconstrictor neurons, *Fed. Proc.*, 5 (1966) 55.

39   Kirchner, F., Spontaneous activity of the renal sympathetic nerve in the unanaesthetized cat, *Acta physiol. pol.*, 24 (1973) 129–134.

40   Koepchen, H. P., Wagner, P. H. and Lux, H. D., Über die Zusammenhang zwischen zentraler Erregbarkait, reflectorischentous und atemrhythmus bei der nervösen Steuerung der Herzfrequenz, *Pflügers Arch.*, 273 (1961) 443–465.

41   Koizumi, K. and Brooks, C. M., The integration of autonomic system reactions: A discussion of autonomic reflexes, their control and their association with somatic reactions, *Ergebn. Physiol.*, 67 (1972) 1–68.

42   Kuffler, S. W., Fitzhugh, R. and Barlow, H. B., Maintained activity in the cat's retina in light and darkness, *J. Gen. Physiol.*, 40 (1957) 683–702.

43   Kunze, D. L., Reflex discharge patterns of cardiac vagal efferent fibres, *J. Physiol.* (Lond.), 222 (1972) 1–15.

44   Lioy, F., Hanna, B. and Polosa, C., CO_2-dependent component of the neurogenic vascular tone in the cat, *Pflügers Arch.*, in press.

45   Lioy, F. and Hanna, B., Cardiovascular effects of medullary chemoreceptors, *Fed. Proc.*, 37 (1978) 744.

46   Lundberg, A., Integration in the reflex pathway. In: R. Granit (Ed.), *Muscular Afferents and Motor Control.*, Wiley, New York, 1966.

47   Mannard, A. and Polosa, C., Analysis of background firing of single sympathetic preganglionic neurons of cat cervical nerve, *J. Neurophysiol.*, 36 (1973) 398–408.

48   Mannard, A., Rajchgot, P. and Polosa, C., Effect of post-impulse depression on background firing of sympathetic preganglionic neurons, *Brain Res.*, 126 (1977) 243–261.

49   McAllen, R. M. and Spyer, K. M., The location of cardiac vagal preganglionic motoneurones in the medulla of the cat, *J. Physiol.* (Lond.), 258 (1976) 187–204.

50   Mirgorodsky, V. N. and Skok, V. I., Intracellular potentials recorded from a tonically active mammalian sympathetic ganglion, *Brain Res.*, 15 (1969) 570–572.

51   Mirgorodsky, V. N. and Skok, V. I., The role of different preganglionic fibres in tonic activity of the mammalian sympathetic ganglion, *Brain Res.*, 22 (1970) 262–263.

52   Mitchell, G. A. G. and Warwick, R., The dorsal vagal nucleus, *Acta Anat.*, 25 (1955) 371–395.

53   Ninomiya, I. and Yonezawa, Y., Sympathetic nerve activity, aortic pressure and heart rate in response to behavioral stimuli. This volume, pp. 433–442.

54   Nisida, I. and Okada, H., The activity of the pupilloconstrictor centers, *Jap. J. Physiol.*, 10 (1960) 64–72.

55   Nisida, I., Okada, H. and Kakano, O., The activity of the cilliospinal centers and their inhibition in pupillary light reflex, *Jap. J. Physiol.*, 10 (1960) 73–84.

56   Passatore, M. and Pettorossi, V. E., Efferent fibers in the cervical sympathetic nerve influenced by light, *Exp. Neurol.*, 52 (1976) 66–82.

57   Polosa, C., Spontaneous activity of sympathetic preganglionic neurons, *Can. J. Physiol. Pharmacol.*, 46 (1968) 887–896.

58   Polosa, C., Gerber, U. and Schondorf, R., Central mechanisms of interaction between

354   C. Polosa et al.

      sympathetic preganglionic neurons and the respiratory oscillator, *Proc. Symp.* "*Central interaction between Respiratory and Cardiovascular Control Systems*", Berlin, July 12–15, 1977.

59   Preiss, G. and Polosa, C., Patterns of sympathetic neuron activity associated with Mayer waves, *Amer. J. Physiol.*, 226 (1974) 724–730.

60   Randall, W. C., *Neural Regulation of the Heart*, Oxford University Press, New York, 1977, pp. 63–64.

61   Rodjeck, R. W., Maintained activity in cat retinal ganglion cells, *J. Neurophysiol.*, 30 (1967) 1043–1071.

62   Samaan, A. and Heymans, C., La frequence cardiaque du chien en differentes conditions experimentales d'activite et de repos, *Cr. Sco. Biol. Paris*, 115 (1934) 1383–1388.

63   Schad, H. and Seller, H., A method for recording autonomic nerve activity in unanaesthetized, freely moving cats, *Brain Res.*, 100 (1975) 425–430.

64   Schlag, J., *L'activite Spontanee des Cellules du Systeme Nerveux Central*, Arscia, Bruxelles, 1959.

65   Seller, H., The discharge pattern of single units in thoracic and lumbar white rami in relation to cardiovascular event, *Pflügers Arch.*, 343 (1973) 317–330.

66   Sillito, A. M. and Zbrozyna, A. W., The activity characteristics of the preganglionic pupilloconstrictor neurones, *J. Physiol.* (Lond.), 211 (1970) 767–779.

67   Spyer, K. M. and McAllen, R. M., The interaction of central and peripheral inputs onto vagal cardiomotor neurones, *Proc. Symp.: Central Interaction between Respiratory and Cardiovascular Control Systems*, Berlin, July 12–15, 1977, in press.

68   Ström, G., Central nervous regulation of body temperature. In: J. Field, H. W. Magoun and V. E. Hall (Eds.), *Handbook of Physiology, I. Neurophysiology* II, American Physiological Society, Washington, D. C., 1960, pp. 1173–1196.

69   Tang, P. C. and Gernandt, B. E., Autonomic responses to vestibular stimulation, *Exp. Neurol.*, 24 (1969) 558–578.

70   Voorhoeve, P. E., Autochtonous activity of fusimotor neurones in the cat, *Acta physiol. pharmacol. neerl.*, 9 (1960) 1–43.

71   Wang, G. H., *The Neural Control of Sweating*, University of Wisconsin Press, Madison, Wis., 1964, p. 14.

CHAPTER 26

ORIGINS OF TONIC ACTIVITY IN HYPERTENSION

Juro Iriuchijima

Department of Physiology, Faculty of Medicine, University of Tokyo, Tokyo, Japan

INTRODUCTION

Although some patients with primary hypertension have increased plasma catecholamines which may reflect increased sympathetic nerve tonicity, the role of the autonomic nervous system in human arterial hypertension in general is still a subject of controversy. As far as the spontaneously hypertensive rat (SHR), a genetic hypertensive rat strain isolated by Okamoto and Aoki[8], is concerned, however, the neurogenicity of its hypertensive state has been advocated by different groups of scientists[1,2,6,9], using different methods.

In 1967 Okamoto et al.[9] studied the effects of section and pithing of the central nervous system on the arterial pressure of SHR. The hypertension was maintained after transection above the pons (cerveau isolé) in an experiment under artificial respiration with gallamine, with or without chloralose. When transection was made between the medulla and the spinal cord (encéphale isolé), however, the arterial pressure was decreased to such an extent that there was no significant difference in arterial pressure between hypertensive rats and normotensive controls. Okamoto et al. also recorded action potentials from the splanchnic nerve in SHR's and normotensive control rats under chloralose anesthesia. Impulse frequency was much higher in the former. From these findings they have concluded that the hypertensive state in SHR is maintained principally by an increase in the sympathetic tone, the origin of which is located in the medullary cardiovascular centers.

The increase in splanchnic discharge in SHR's was confirmed by a different method[2]. Splanchnicectomy was performed on SHR's and normotensive control rats under pentobarbital anesthesia. After arterial pressure had stabilized at a new lower level, the peripheral cut end of the splanchnic nerve was stimulated electrically with a train of supramaximal pulses to determine the frequency needed to restore arterial pressure to the level before splanchnicectomy. The frequency, which is assumed to represent the average discharge rate of sympathetic vasoconstrictor fibers in the splanchnic nerve, was significantly higher in SHR's than in normotensive control rats. After bilateral splanchnicectomy, the difference in arterial pressure between the groups was no longer significant.

However, it is possible that the neurogenicity of hypertension is an apparent phenomenon which is observable in an acute experiment under anesthesia only. If SHR's were kept alive after bilateral splanchnicectomy, hypertension recurred in one week. Even total abdominal sympathectomy plus bilateral stellatumectomy could not impede the recurrence of hypertension. Arterial pressure fell precipitously as soon as these sympathectomized SHR's were anesthetized with pentobarbital[4].

The present study was undertaken to investigate whether the increase in sympathetic impulses originating in the medullary cardiovascular centers was the sole cause of the hypertensive state in SHR's and neurogenic hypertensive rats prepared by sinoaortic denervation without anesthetics. The spinal cord was transected in hypertensive and control rats so that the connection between the medullary centers and the thoracolumbar segments were interrupted. Arterial pressure was compared between hypertensive and control rats after the effect of ether employed at the time of cord section was eliminated.

METHODS AND RESULTS

Cord Section in SHR's[5]

SHR's and normotensive control rats were anesthetized with ether. The femoral artery was cannulated for direct measurement of mean arterial pressure. A venous catheter was inserted into a femoral vein.

The effect of spinal cord section on arterial pressure of an SHR is presented in Fig. 1. At the arrow transection was performed between vertebrae C7 and Th 1 and ether anesthesia was terminated. Consciousness appeared to be restored in several minutes. Arterial pressure first dropped precipitously after cord section, then recovered gradually and reached a steady level in about an hr.

The time course of change in the mean $\pm$SD of arterial pressure after cord section is plotted in Fig. 2 for groups of SHR's (filled circles) and normotensive control rats (open circles). In this figure, pressure in neurogenic hypertensive rats is also included (crosses, see below). For the first several min the arterial pressure of SHR's and

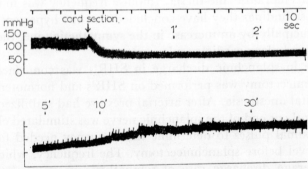

Fig. 1.   The effect of spinal cord section (arrow) between C7 and Th 1 vertebrae on arterial pressure in an SHR. The rat was anesthetized with ether until transection. The lapse of time since cord section is entered in the figure in min. Note that sweep speed was reduced to 1/10 in the lower panel[5].

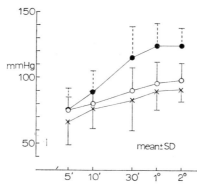

Fig. 2. Time course of change of arterial pressure after cord section. Filled circles: SHR's; open circles: normotensive control rats; crosses: neurogenic hypertensive rats. There were significant differences between SHR's and normotensive control rats 30, 60 and 120 min after cord section at P<0.025, 0.005 and 0.001, respectively.

normotensive control rats were similar but gradually diverged. Thirty min after transection and thereafter the SHR arterial pressure was significantly higher than that of normotensive control rats. Heart rates in the two groups were the same.

Cord Pithing in SHR's[5]

It is possible that, after cord section, tonic activity in the so-called spinal sympathetic centers, separated from the higher centers, is more frequent in SHR's than in normotensive control rats to maintain a higher pressure level in the former. To eliminate this kind of sympathetic nervous activity, the spinal cord below the level of vertebra Th 1 was destroyed by advancing a steel rod two mm in diameter into the spinal canal in SHR's and normotensive control rats under ether anesthesia, which was terminated as soon as cord pithing was completed.

When the rod was advanced into the spinal canal, arterial pressure was irregularly elevated for a brief period. Subsequently, the pressure fell rather rapidly and then gradually recovered, as after cord section, reaching a new steady level within about 30 min.

Two hr after cord section the mean arterial pressure $\pm$SD from 10 SHR's was 81.3$\pm$8.62 mmHg while that from nine normotensive rats was 70.1$\pm$5.56 mmHg. The difference was significant at P<0.005 by the t-test.

Ganglion blockade with hexamethonium bromide induced a marked decrease in arterial pressure both in SHR's and normotensive control rats after cord section. After cord pithing, however, intravenous injection of hexamethonium bromide (30 mg/kg) did not decrease arterial pressure but slightly increased it (Fig. 3B). Subsequent anesthesia with pentobarbital (30 mg/kg, i.v.) decreased arterial pressure in both SHR's and normotensive control rats to the same level (Fig. 3C). Pentobarbital also abolished the significant difference in pressure between the groups after cord section.

Cord Section in Neurogenic Hypertensive Rats

Neurogenic hypertension is produced in Wistar rats by a sinoaortic denervation

J. Iriuchijima

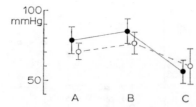

Fig. 3. The effect of hexamethonium and pentobarbital on arterial pressure of SHR's
(filled circles, n=12) and normotensive control rats (open circles, n=10) after cord
pithing. Mean±SD. A: 2 hr after cord pithing. The difference in pressure between
the groups was significant at P<0.025. B: After hexamethonium bromide 30 mg/kg,
i. v. (P<0.025). C: After pentobarbital 30 mg/kg, i.v. (P>0.5).

according to Krieger[7]. Cord section experiments were performed on these rats as on
SHR.

The time course of the mean arterial pressure ±SD from six neurogenic hypertensive rats in the first 2 hr after cord section is plotted in Fig. 2 (crosses). It was not
significantly different from that in normotensive control rats (open circles). These
neurogenic hypertensive rats were all male and 23±6.7 (mean ±SD) weeks of age.
Sinoaortic denervation had been performed 9.5±3.3 weeks before. The mean blood
pressure measured at the tail in the conscious state prior to the cord section experiment
was 179±11.1 mmHg. The recovery of pressure to a higher level as observed in SHR's
30–120 min after cord section was not observed in neurogenic hypertensive rats.

DISCUSSION

Under anesthesia, the hypertensive state in SHR's appears to be maintained largely by an increased sympathetic nerve activity with its origin in the medullary
cardiovascular centers[1,2,3,9]. An increase in sympathetic nerve activity is present in
unanesthetized SHR's also[6]. However, this is not the sole hypertensive factor in this
kind of experimental hypertensive animal. Since arterial pressure was significantly
higher in SHR's than in normotensive rats after high spinal cord section, the hypertensive factors in the former are not confined to medullary cardiovascular centers.
Arterial pressure in SHR's was still higher than that in normotensive control rats even
after destroying the thoracolumbar spinal segments by cord pithing. The difference in
pressure after cord pithing was unaffected by hexamethonium but abolished by pentobarbital. These findings indicate the presence of non-neural hypertensive factors in
SHR's which is susceptible to pentobarbital.

On the other hand, the hypertensive state in neurogenic hypertensive rats seems
to be maintained principally by an increase in sympathetic nerve activity with its
origin in the medullary cardiovascular centers, since the hypertension disappeared
when the thoracolumbar segments were separated from the higher centers by cord
section.

SUMMARY

Under pentobarbital anesthesia the hypertensive state in spontaneously hypertensive rats (Okamoto strain) appears to be maintained principally by an increase in sympathetic nerve tone originating from the medullary cardiovascular centers. However, non-neural hypertensive factors also exist, since the arterial pressure in SHR's was higher than that in normotensive control rats in the conscious state after cord section or cord pithing. However in chronic neurogenic hypertensive rats prepared by sinoaortic denervation, the hypertension seems purely neurogenic, as its name denotes, since interruption between the medullary cardiovascular centers and the thoracolumbar segments by cord section lowered the arterial pressure to the same level as that in cord-sectioned normotensive control rats.

REFERENCES

1 Iriuchijima, J., Cardiac output and total peripheral resistance in spontaneously hypertensive rats, *Jap. Heart J.*, 14 (1973) 267–272.

2 Iriuchijima, J., Sympathetic discharge rate in spontaneously hypertensive rats, *Jap. Heart J.*, 14 (1973) 350–356.

3 Iriuchijima, J., Effect of clonidine on sympathetic discharge rate of spontaneously hypertensive rats, *Jap. Heart J.*, 15 (1974) 401–406.

4 Iriuchijima, J. and Numao, Y., Hypotensive effects of pentobarbital and diuretics on sympathectomized spontaneously hypertensive rats, *Arch. int. Pharmacodyn. Thér.*, 226 (1977) 149–155.

5 Iriuchijima, J. and Numao, Y., Effects of cord section and pithing on spontaneously hypertensive rats, *Jap. J. Physiol.*, 27 (1977) 801–809.

6 Judy, W. V., Watanabe, A. M., Henry, D. P., Besch, H. R., Murphy, W. R. and Hockel, G. M., Sympathetic nerve activity role in regulation of blood pressure in the spontaneously hypertensive rat, *Circulation Res.*, 38 (1976) Supp. II, 21–29.

7 Krieger, E. M., Neurogenic hypertension in the rat, *Circulation Res.*, 15 (1964) 511–521.

8 Okamoto, K. and Aoki, K., Development of a strain of spontaneously hypertensive rats, *Jap. Circul. J.*, 27 (1963) 282–293.

9 Okamoto, K., Nosaka, S., Yamori, Y. and Matsumoto, M., Participation of neural factor in the pathogenesis of hypertension in the spontaneously hypertensive rat, *Jap. Heart J.*, 8 (1970) 168–180.

CHAPTER 27

BRAIN STEM REGIONS MEDIATING THE CEREBRAL ISCHEMIC AND CUSHING RESPONSES: RELATIONSHIP TO THE TONIC VASOMOTOR CENTER OF THE MEDULLA

Donald J. Reis, Roger A. L. Dampney, Nobutaka Doba and Mamoru Kumada

Laboratory of Neurobiology, Department of Neurology,
Cornell University Medical College, New York, USA

INTRODUCTION

The lower brain stem, comprising the lower pons and medulla, plays an important role in the regulation of arterial pressure. The observation that the basal level of arterial pressure is unchanged after removal of the brain stem rostral to the middle of the pons, but falls to minimal levels after subsequent transection of the spinal medullary junction, suggests that the region contains intrinsic neurons, presumably continuously active, which exert background drive to spinal vasomotor neurons[1,44]. These findings have led to a view that the lower brain stem functions as a "tonic vasomotor center" whose integrity is essential for the maintenance of normal levels of blood pressure.

Exploration of the lower brain stem by electrical stimulation has demonstrated that the area contains anatomically segregated zones from which sympathetic vasomotor neurons can be excited or inhibited resulting, respectively, in an elevation or reduction of the arterial pressure[2,12,13,19,27,28,52,54]. These zones, often referred to in functional terms as "pressor" or "depressor" centers, have also been shown to: (a) mediate vasomotor reflexes arising from somatic or visceral receptors; (b) integrate neural activity descending from suprabulbar regions with reflex cardiovascular responses mediated at the segment; and (c) serve as a principal, but not exclusive[48], relay stations between the cardiovascular representation in brain and the sympathetic outflow to spinal cord.

Despite advances in knowledge of the organization of cardiovascular function within the lower brain stem, the distribution of neurons which function in maintaining tonic levels of arterial pressure is unknown. The fact that bilateral lesions placed within a variety of areas of the pons and medulla including the pressor areas[12,25,28,33,36,37,41] do not result in a collapse of arterial pressure comparable to that produced by spinal transection suggests that such neurons may be dispersed[33].

Recent investigations in our laboratory[14,15,25,30,45] into the central organization of two circulatory reflexes, the cerebral ischemic response (the pressor response elicited by rendering the brain ischemic)[3,6,17,23,24,38,39,47,50], and the Cushing response (the rise of arterial pressure and the bradycardia elicited by acute elevation of intracranial pressure)[4,5,7,8,11,15,20,21,25,26,32,43,44], have provided new insights into the organization of the lower brain stem in circulatory control. Our studies have demonstrated that these two reflexes are initiated by direct stimulation of the brain, appear comparable in their pattern of cardiovascular responses and are mediated by a highly restricted region of the dorsal medulla. Of particular interest is the observation that lesions restricted to portions of this region not only abolish the ischemic and Cushing reflexes but invariably result in a reduction of arterial pressure to levels comparable with those elicited by transection of the spinal cord. Our findings therefore suggest that this particular region of the medulla may be identical with the so-called tonic vasomotor center, and as such, possesses interesting reflex functions. In this paper we shall review some of these studies.

THE CEREBRAL ISCHEMIC REFLEX

Cardiovascular Components

The cerebral ischemic response consists of an elevation of arterial pressure, bradycardia and apnea, elicited by interrupting the blood supply to the head[3,6,17,23,34,38,39,47,50]. In our studies the cardiovascular components of the cerebral ischemic response have been analyzed in detail in rabbits, usually paralyzed and artificially ventilated. Cerebral ischemia was elicited by the technique of Miyakawa[39], a method by which the vertebral arteries are permanently occluded and the ischemic response elicited by briefly clamping the carotid arteries. Blood flow was measured by electromagnetic flow meters.

The integrated cerebral ischemic response (i.e., elicited in animals with baroreceptors intact) consists of the well-known triad of hypertension, bradycardia and, in spontaneously breathing animals, apnea (Table 1). The elevation of arterial pressure is due to an increase in total peripheral resistance. This leads to ventricular overload and a fall in cardiac output (as reflected by the fall of blood flow in the ascending aorta, Table 1). The reduction in cardiac output and the hypertension can be reversed by α-adrenergic blockade.

The increase in total peripheral resistance is associated with a stereotyped and differentiated pattern of vasoconstriction greatest in the renal, intermediate in the mesenteric and least in the femoral arteries (Table 1). Vasoconstriction in all three beds is largely mediated by sympathetic nerves: Surgical sympathectomy entirely abolishes the vasoconstriction in renal and mesenteric arteries and converts vasoconstriction to vasodilatation in the femoral artery. The observation that the persistent vasoconstriction or vasodilatation disappears after adrenalectomy demonstrates that cerebral ischemia liberates adrenal catecholamines.

The reflex bradycardia elicited by ischemia disappears and in fact is often converted to tachycardia by transection of the vagi or administration of atropine. The reflex tachycardia appearing after vagotomy is blocked by β-adrenergic antagonists

Table 1. Cardiovascular responses associated with the cerebral ischemic and cushing responses.

	Cerebral ischemia (Rabbit)			Cushing response (Cat)			
	Control	Ischemia[a] % of control	Elect. Stim.[b] % of control	Control	Probe[c] % of control	Micro-[d] injection % of control	Elect. Stim.[e] % of control
BP$_m$ (mmHg)	105±2.3 (10)	175***(10)	166***(7)	105.2 (49)	164***(49)	151**(17)	168**(58)
HR (beats/min)	318±18 (10)	54**(10)	(barodenervated)	220±4 (49)	80**(49)	81*(17)	69***(58)
Ascending Aortic Flow (ml/min)	293±2.9 (4)	43**(4)	—	—	—	—	—
TPR (mmHg/min/ml)	.358±.079 (4)	417***(4)	—	—	—	—	—
Fem. Flow (ml/min)	11.1±0.8 (9)	78**(9)	83***(4)	10.6±0.3 (45)	91ns(45)	70ns(16)	71***(69)
Mes. Flow (ml/min)	63.8±10.8 (5)	86**(5)	—	30.5±17.2 (19)	56**(19)	65**(5)	43**(8)
Renal Flow (ml/min)	31.6±8.3 (5)	10.1***(5)	9***(4)	21.1±1.3 (18)	87ns(18)	98ns(6)	98ns(6)
Common Carotid Flow (ml/min)	—	—	—	21.8±1.1 (15)	144***(15)	28*(9)	152*(6)
Fem. Res. (mmHg/ml/min)	9.8±.58 (4)	200***(4)	204***(4)	10.3±0.3 (45)	231***(45)	222***(16)	290***(69)
Mes. Res. (mmHg/ml/min)	1.43±.13 (9)	230***(9)	—	3.3±0.1 (19)	315*(19)	241*(5)	467*(8)
Renal Res. (mmHg/ml/min)	3.05±.85 (15)	1822***(5)	1874***(4)	5.0±0.1 (8)	248***(8)	—	181***(6)
Common Carotid Res. (mmHg/ml/min)	—	—	—	5.1±0.3 (15)	127ns(15)	119ns(9)	115ns(6)
Respiration	Eupnea	Apnea	Tachypnea	Eupnea	Apnea	—	Apnea

(n) = number of animals.

Significance: (p<0.5): * p<.02; ** p<.01; *** p<.001; ns=not significant.

(a) Ischemia produced for 30–50 sec.

(b) Electrical stimulation by square wave pulses of 0.5 msec for 12 sec at 50 Hz, 100 μA.

(c) Distortion of 150–300 mmHg (2–4 g/mm²).

(d) Rapid infusion of 1–3 μ artificial CSF at pressures, usually 10 cm H$_2$O.

(e) Stimulus as in (b) except magnitude set at 3 X the threshold, usually 40 μA.

but persists after adrenalectomy. These observations indicate that cerebral ischemia coactivates both cardiac vagal and sympathetic nerves, the vagal effect predominating.

After the abolition of baroreceptor reflexes by transection of the aortic depressor and carotid sinus nerves, the bradycardia elicited by cerebral ischemia is profoundly reduced. Thus, prior to denervation, ischemia reduced the heart rate on the average to 54% of control; after baroreceptor denervation (which by itself did not alter heart rate) ischemia resulted in a slowing of heart rate to 89% of control (n=10; P<.001). Baroreceptor denervation, on the other hand, had no effect on the elevation of arterial pressure or pattern of the reflex changes in regional blood flows and resistances. Thus, baroreceptors contribute substantially to the bradycardia elicited by cerebral ischemia without influencing the vasomotor components.

The Effects of Brain Stem Transections and Deafferentation on the Cerebral Ischemic Response as Elicited from the Brain

The vasomotor and respiratory components of the cerebral ischemic response persist after transection of the brain stem at the level of the VIIth cranial nerve and/or after transection of cranial nerves IX–XI; however, they are abolished by subsequent transection of the spinal cord[14,45] at C1. The bradycardia also persists after pontine section, is abolished by transection of the IX–XIth cranial nerves (presumably because of interruption of vagal efferents) and persists after spinal section at C1. Thus the cerebral ischemic response originates entirely from receptors lying within the medulla oblongata, and not from receptors lying within the cranium but outside the brain.

Localization of Sites in the Medulla Possibly Mediating the Cerebral Ischemic Response

To localize the regions within the lower brain stem from which the cerebral ischemic response could be elicited, we undertook a strategy with two objectives: First, we sought to identify regions of the lower brain stem from which a response with cardiodynamic characteristics identical to those elicited by cerebral ischemia could be simulated by focal electrical stimulation. Second, having identified such a region(s), we examined the effects on the reflex of placement of bilateral electrolytic lesions within it.

Simulation by electrical stimulation.   Electrical stimulation of low intensity, restricted to small areas of the brain stem, elicited an elevation of arterial pressure with changes in peripheral flow which qualitatively and quantitatively were similar to those of ischemia. In animals with baroreceptors intact, stimulation elicited bradycardia; with baroreceptors interrupted, bradycardia was usually absent.

The region from which a rise of arterial pressure and bradycardia were elicited with stimuli of low intensity is shown in Fig. 1. The positive region was largely confined to dorsal portions of the medullary reticular formation from the level of the middle of the inferior olivary nucleus to the level of the facial nerve nucleus. The positive region did not conform to any single nucleus of the reticular formation. Rather, it primarily overlapped two reticular nuclei identified by Meesen and Olszewski[35] as the nucleus reticularis parvocellularis and dorsal portions of the nucleus gigantocellularis, particularly at the level corresponding to the medial and caudal portions of the facial nucleus, the site from which the largest responses were obtained.

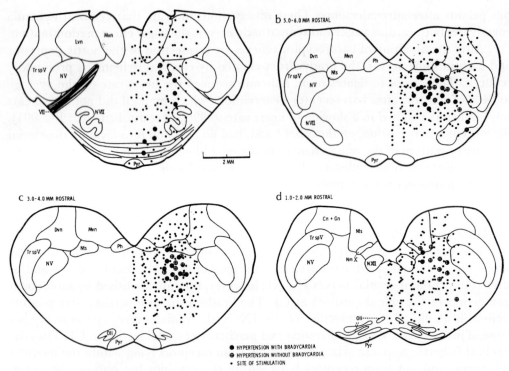

Fig. 1.   Distribution of sites in the brain stem of nine rabbits from which a simulated cerebral
          ischemic response was elicited by electrical stimulation (12 sec train, 50 Hz, 100 μA).
          All points are grouped on four representative sections taken at different levels anterior
          (rostral) to the obex. Large solid circles mark points where the pressor response
          was associated with bradycardia, while the crossed circles mark points where the
          pressor response was accompanied by little change in heart rate, or a slight brady-
          cardia. Small filled circles are negative sites.
              Abbreviations: VII: facial nerve; Cn: nucleus cuneatus; Dvn: descending vestibular
          nucleus; Gn: nucleus gracilis; Lvn: lateral vestibular nucleus; Mvn: medial ves-
          tibular nucleus; NV: nucleus of trigeminal nerve; N VII: nucleus of facial nerve;
          N XII: nucleus of hypoglossal nerve; NmX: dorsal motor nucleus of vagus; Nts:
          nucleus of solitary tract; Oli: nucleus of the inferior olive; Ph: nucleus praepositus
          hypoglossi; Pyr: pyramidal tract; Rgc: nucleus reticularis gigantocellularis; RP:
          nucleus reticularis pontis; Rpc: nucleus reticularis parvocellularis; Tr spV: spinal
          tract of the trigeminal nerve.

Effects of focal brain stem lesions on the cerebral ischemic response.   Bilateral electrolytic
lesions were placed in 24 rabbits within the same regions of the dorsal medulla from
which electrical stimulation (prior to placement of the lesion) elicited a simulated ischemic response (Table 2; Fig. 2). In four animals (Group A) the lesions: (a) almost
completely abolished the vasopressor component of the ischemic response; (b) resulted
in a profound and sustained fall of the arterial pressure to approximately 25–40 mmHg;
and (c) did not abolish the reflex bradycardia. In these animals the complete collapse
of blood pressure could not, for two reasons, be attributed to secondary ischemic
damage of the brain or spinal cord: first, the persistence of the bradycardia indicated

Table 2. Effects of bilateral lesions of rabbit brain stem on pressor response to cerebral ischemia.

Group	Animal # (Experiment #)	% of Response remaining[a] after lesion $\dfrac{\text{CIR* after lesion}}{\text{CIR before lesion}} \times 100$	Areas damaged[b] (Minor damage in parentheses) (Figure of lesion in brackets)	Rostro-caudal site of major damage (mm Rostral to Obex)
Group A:	Lesion at pressor site:			
	Remaining pressor response <10%			
	1 (24)	3	Rpc (Rgc, Mvn, Nts) [Fig. 3]	3
	2 (17)	5	Rpc (Rgc, Mvn) [Figs. 1, 3]	3
	3 (23)	5	Rpc (Rgc, Mvn, Nts) [Fig. 3]	3
	4 (19)	7	Rpc (Rgc, Mvn) [Fig. 3]	3
Group B:	Lesion at pressor site:			
	Remaining pressor response between 10% and 79%			
	5 (21)	25	Rgc [Fig. 4b]	3
	6 (14)	44	Rgc (Rpc, Mvn)	3
	7 (22)	67	Rpc (Rgc)	3
	8 (20)	67	Rpc [Fig. 4a]	3
Group C:	Lesion at pressor site:			
	Remaining pressor response >80%			
	9 (10)	82	Rgc	3
	10 (4)	89	Rpc	5
	11 (7)	95	Rpc (Rgc, Mvn) [Fig. 4c]	6
	12 (2)	95	Rgc	3
	13 (12)	100	N VII (Rpc, Rlat)	5
	14 (8)	100	Rgc (Mvn)	3
	15 (6)	112	Rpc (Rgc, NV, Tr spV)	6
Group D:	Controls: Lesion outside of area from which CIR is elicited (ref. [5])			
	Remaining pressor response >80%			
	16 (16)	82	Nts (Dvn)	1
	17 (13)	85	Oli (Rgc, Pyr)	2
	18 (3)	88	Dvn (Mvn)	3
	19 (9)	90	Mvn	3
	20 (1)	90	NV (TrspV)	3
	21 (11)	95	Nts [Fig. 4d]	1
	22 (16)	96	Lvn (Mvn)	7
	23 (5)	96	NV (Tr spV, Rpc)	0
	24 (25)	100	Rlat	3

a Mean arterial pressure.

b For abbreviations see legend to Fig. 1.

* CIR: Cerebral ischemic response (here denoting only the rise in arterial pressure).

that the brain stem was still viable; and second, a pressor response could be elicited at any time after the lesion by electrically stimulating sites in the medulla caudal to the lesion.

In four animals (Group B) lesions only partially (to 25–75% of control) reduced the response to ischemia. In these animals the blood pressure fell, but to a lesser degree. Bradycardia persisted.

In the remaining seven animals (Group C) thel esion did not reduce the pressor

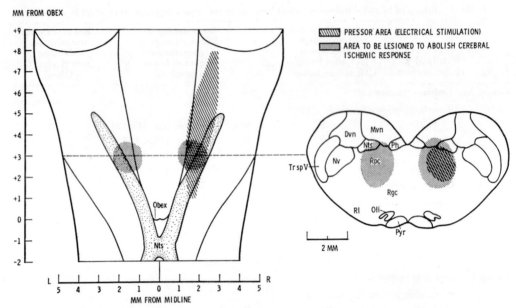

Fig. 2.   Localization of area mediating the vasomotor component of the cerebral ischemic
response in rabbit brain stem. Left: Dorsal view of floor of IVth ventral. The distribution of points from which the vasomotor component can be elicited by electrical
stimulation of the brain stem is indicated by the elongated crosshatched area which,
although bilateral, is only shown on the right. The area in which lesions abolished
the response is represented bilaterally as a round dotted area. The lightly shaded
strips on both sides of the drawing descending behind the obex represents the distribution of the nucleus tractus solitarii. Right: Cross section of medulla three mm rostral
to obex, showing critical zone. Abbreviations as in Fig. 1.

response to ischemia by less than 20%, a value close to the change in response in nine
operated controls (Group D). Animals of group D had lesions placed outside of the
dorsal medulla; such lesions did not change the response or resting blood pressure.

The lesions effective in abolishing the pressor response to ischemia in animals of
Group A were always restricted to caudal portions of the area of the medulla from
which electrical stimulation elicited a pressor response (Fig. 2). This zone was about
three mm rostral to the obex (the A3 level), lying close to the rostral pole of the
inferior olive. The effective lesion had to damage three nuclei of the medullary reticular
formation: portions of the nucleus parvocellularis, the dorsal part of the nucleus
gigantocellularis and the ventro-medial portion of the medial vestibular nucleus. The
lesions in animals of Group B, while also restricted to the A3 level, were smaller and
often encompassed only one of the three reticular nuclei. Lesions in Group C, when at
the A3 level, were considerably ventral to the effective site or, when they included the
three nuclei, were substantially more rostral, lying approximately five to six mm rostral
to the obex (A6).

Central Integration of the Cerebral Ischemic Reflex

Our results, therefore, indicate that the pressor component of the cerebral ischemic response depends upon the integrity of a critical area of the dorsal medullary reticular formation. It is from this area that the integrated vasomotor response can be elicited by electrical stimulation and abolished by focal lesions. The fact that the bradycardia produced by electrical stimulation of the area was substantially reduced by baroreceptor denervation, and that the reflex bradycardia persisted when lesions abolished the vasopressor responses, suggest that the vasomotor and cardiovagal components are mediated by separate regions of the brain stem, the latter possibly resulting from ischemic excitation of cardiovagal neurons within the nucleus ambiguus[6].

Whether the adequate stimulus for the cerebral ischemic response is hypoxia, ischemia or reduction in perfusion pressure is not yet certain. However, in the rabbit many neurons in the critical area of the dorsal medulla, which increase their discharge in response to ischemia, also respond in a comparable manner to systemic hypoxia[29]. This observation suggests that hypoxia is the principal stimulus for the ischemic response.

THE CUSHING RESPONSE

The Cushing Reflex in Cats in Response to Increased Intracranial Pressure

The Cushing response consists of an elevation in arterial pressure, bradycardia and apnea elicited by increasing the intracranial pressure[4,5,7,8,11,20,21,25,26,32,43,44]. In our laboratory we have studied the physiology of the Cushing response in cats anesthetized with chloralose and usually paralyzed and ventilated[15,25]. Cardiovascular activity was measured by conventional methods with measurements of regional blood flow by electromagnetic flow meters.

The Cushing response can be elicited in cats by acutely increasing the intracranial pressure by rapid inflation of an epidural balloon to 50–200 mmHg[25]. The response, similar in its general properties to that reported in other species[4,5,7,8,11,20,21,36,43,44] consists of a rapid rise of arterial pressure of approximately 30–50 mmHg mean pressure, bradycardia, and a small reduction of blood flow with a substantial elevation of resistance (to 155–205% of control) in the femoral, renal, and mesenteric arteries. There is also an increase of blood flow without change of resistance in the common carotid artery, suggesting a passive increase of pressure within the cerebral circulation.

The Cushing Response as a Reflex Response to Direct Stimulation of the Medulla

The Cushing response elicited by elevation of the intracranial pressure by a balloon persists in cats in which the brain stem has been transected at midpons, the cerebellum removed and all cranial nerves transected[25]. It is, however, abolished by subsequent transection of the brain stem at the spinal-medullary junction. Thus, the response is elicited by direct stimulation of neurons in the lower brain stem.

That the responsive area is anatomically restricted can be demonstrated in two ways: First, an elevation of arterial pressure and bradycardia (Table 1) can be elicited by directly pressing on the brain stem[15,25], in our studies with a probe one mm in diameter. The response has a threshold, usually at or just over 150 mmHg, is graded with respect to the force of the stimulus, has a brief latency (usually less than eight sec) and

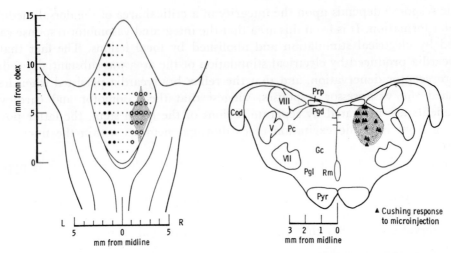

Fig. 3. Left: A dorsal view of cat brain stem showing on the right side of the drawing the positive sites from which the Cushing response was evoked by local probe pressure (open circles), and projected onto the surface of the brain, the region from which microinjection evoked a similar response (stippled). On the left side of the drawing are depicted the locations of electrode tracts from which the response was evoked by electrical stimulation (closed circles). The small solid circles indicate sites from which no response was evoked by any of the three types of stimulation. Right: The distribution of sites (solid triangles) from which the Cushing response was elicited by microinjection of one to three μl of mock CSF in anesthetized cat in 17 experiments. The section is taken at the level of the facial nucleus. The shaded area represents the general distribution of portions of the reticular formation from which the response could be elicited by electrical stimulation.

   Abbreviations (modified from Taber, 1961): Cod: nucleus cochlearis dorsalis; Gc: nucleus gigantocellularis; Pc: nucleus parvocellularis; Pgd: nucleus paragigantocellularis dorsalis; Pgl: nucleus paragigantocellularis lateralis; Prp: nucleus prepositus hypoglocci; Pyr: tractus pyramidalis; Rm: nucleus raphe magnus; V: nucleus tractus spinalis trigemini; VII: nucleus nervi facialis.

can only be evoked from a small paramedial strip running along the floor of the IVth ventricle (Fig. 3). Comparable elevations of arterial pressure cannot be elicited by distortion of any other region, dorsal or ventral, of the pons and medulla.

   Second, a rise of arterial pressure and slowing of heart rate can also be elicited by rapid microinjection of a one μl bolus of artificial CSF into specific sites of the brain stem (Table 1, Fig. 3)[15]. The stimulus threshold for eliciting a substantial response is approximately seven to 23 mmHg (around 10 cm H_2O), or 10% of the magnitude of the pressure required to elicit the response by pressing on the floor of the IVth ventricle. The areas from which injections elicited a response lie just below the sensitive regions on the ventricular floor. The adequate stimulus of microinjection appears to be distortion, since varying the temperature, pH or prolonging the duration of an equal volumetric injection fails to elicit any response. These observations suggest that distortion of the ventricular surface elicits its reflex effects by transmission to regions lying at a distance from the ventricular surface.

   Electrical stimulation within the distortion-sensitive areas of the cat can also elicit a hemodynamic pattern identical to that of the Cushing response (Table 1, Fig. 3). The region with the lowest threshold lies directly under the responsive paramedian zone of the IVth ventricle and corresponds almost exactly to that from which the microinjection of CSF elicits a response.

Cardiovascular Responses of the Cushing Reflex

The cardiovascular responses elicited by local distortion of the floor of the IVth ventricle by probe, by microinjection of artificial CSF into the brain, or by electrical stimulation, are all qualitatively equivalent to the response elicited by directly increasing intracranial pressure. The responses consist (Table 1) of an elevation of systemic arterial pressure, apnea and bradycardia. Associated with these is a variable reduction in blood flow and an invariable increase of peripheral resistance in the mesenteric, renal and femoral arteries, the decrease in flow being greatest in the mesenteric bed. There is an increase of flow without change of resistance in the common carotid artery.

The bradycardia elicited by distortion or by electrical stimulation of the dorsal medulla is dependent upon the vagus nerves: Transection abolishes the response, sometimes converting it to tachycardia. Like the cerebral ischemic response, the bradycardia elicited by electrical stimulation appears largely due to a secondary baroreflex: Interruption of the baroreceptor reflex centrally by the placement of lesions in the nucleus tractus solitarii[16,37] abolishes the bradycardia produced by electrical stimulation of the dorsal medulla. This observation indicates, therefore, that much of the bradycardia is secondary to the reflex rise of arterial pressure. Like the cerebral ischemic response, the Cushing response is also associated with a substantial release of adrenal medullary catecholamines.

Localization of Regions Mediating the Cushing Reflex in the Cat

The region of the dorsal medulla from which the Cushing response can be evoked in cats does not correspond to any specific nuclear group within the reticular formation. The responsive areas partially overlap several nuclei, including the more dorsal portion of the nucleus reticularis gigantocellularis, the nucleus reticularis parvocellularis, small portions of the nucleus reticularis pontocaudalis[10] and a nucleus designated the nucleus paragigantocellularis dorsalis by Taber[49]. It is evident, therefore, that the region from which the Cushing response is elicited in cats is comparable in its distribution to that from which the cerebral ischemic response can be elicited in the rabbit.

Effects of Lesions on the Cushing Response

The Cushing response, when elicited by electrical stimulation of the brain, persists after small transecting lesions are placed rostral, lateral or medial to the stimulating electrode. A small lesion, however, transecting the most caudal portions of the zone from which the Cushing response can be elicited (corresponding to the A3 zone of the ischemic area in rabbits) influences both the magnitude of the response and the resting level of the arterial pressure. With a lesion placed contralaterally to the stimulating electrode, the response and magnitude of arterial pressure is reduced by about half. An ipsilateral lesion will virtually abolish the Cushing response and will also result in a reduction of arterial pressure to about 50% of control. Bilateral lesions in this caudal zone result in complete abolition of the Cushing response as well as the reduction of arterial pressure to levels comparable to those produced by spinal transections. The results suggest that, like the cerebral ischemic response, the regions mediating the Cushing reflex and those necessary for maintaining arterial pressure at normal levels are coextensive.

What is the Adequate Stimulus for the Cushing Response?

The nature of the stimulus evoking the Cushing response and the identity of the receptive elements are unknown. The adequate stimulus, however, is unlikely to be ischemia and/or hypoxia alone, in view of: (a) the very short latency of the response[24]; (b) the direct dependence of the response upon the rate at which tissue pressure is altered within the receptive area[15]; and (c) the very low pressures required in the tegmental area to produce a pressor response i.e., <10 cm H_2O. It seems more likely that the adequate stimulus, as others have suggested[24,51,55], is mechanical distortion occurring within or transmitted into the receptive area in the medullary tegmentum.

COMPARISON OF THE CEREBRAL ISCHEMIC AND CUSHING RESPONSES

It is evident, therefore, that while the cerebral ischemic and Cushing responses differ with respect to their adequate stimuli, hypoxia or distortion respectively, they share many characteristics. In our studies, although the responses were analyzed in two different species and under slightly different experimental conditions, the similarities between the features of the responses are striking in five respects:

(a) First, the autonomic components (Table 1) of the two responses are very similar. Both consist of hypertension due to differentiated vasoconstriction in peripheral vessels, a vagal bradycardia which is largely secondary to baroreceptor reflex mechanisms and apnea. While the pattern of vasoconstriction differed between the cerebral ischemic and Cushing responses (renal arterial constriction was maximal in the former, minimal in the latter), the differences most likely are either species-dependent or related to variations in the manner in which the animals were prepared. This conclusion is based on the fact that while the patterning of the response differed between the two species, yet within the same species the response was consistent irrespective of whether it was elicited by electrical or natural stimulation.

(b) Second, both the cerebral ischemic and Cushing responses are elicited by direct excitation of the brain. The receptive regions for the vasomotor component of both responses are localized primarily to dorsal portions of rostral medulla.

(c) Third, the patterning of the cardiovascular components of the responses can be simulated by electrical stimulation within comparable areas of the medulla oblongata. Both responses appear to be elicited primarily from the nucleus parvocellularis reticularis and the dorsal part of nucleus gigantocellularis.

(d) Fourth, it is only bilateral lesions restricted to the caudal portion of the electrically excitable zone which result in an abolition of both responses.

(e) Finally, lesions which effectively abolish the reflex pressor responses always result in a fall of arterial pressure to levels comparable to those produced by transections of the spinal cord at C1.

RELATIONSHIP BETWEEN THE REGIONS MEDIATING THE CUSHING AND ISCHEMIC RESPONSES AND TONIC VASOMOTOR CENTERS OF THE BRAIN

This study, therefore, has identified a region of the dorsal medulla from which focal distortion, hypoxia or electrical stimulation will elicit an elevation of arterial pressure, differentiated with respect to the distribution of organ blood flow, and within which lesions will result in a fall of arterial pressure to levels similar to that produced by transection of the spinal cord. The area is contained in, but is not coextensive with, the so-called pressor area of the reticular formation, i.e., the area from which others have produced elevations of arterial pressure by punctate-electrical stimulation[2,12,13,19,27,28,52,54]. Functionally and anatomically, however, it is distinct from those portions immediately adjacent which mediate the cardiovascular components of the defense reaction[13]. The region, while not lying precisely within the confines of any single nucleus, is centered largely on the nucleus reticularis parvocellularis and the dorsal part of the nucleus gigantocellularis. It is from the former that Trouth et al.[52] elicited the most powerful pressor response by focal electrical stimulation in the brain stem and from which Gootman and Cohen[22] found the shortest latency between medullary stimulation and evoked potentials in the splanchnic nerve. It is also a region into which baroreceptor afferents project[36]. The active area lies within the distribution of the central tegmental tract, a major associative pathway within the brain stem which contains ascending projections from brain stem noradrenergic neurons[53], and which in itself is probably of importance in cardiovascular control.

The collapse of arterial pressure elicited by lesions of this area and this area alone strongly suggests that it may function as the elusive tonic vasomotor center of the medulla. Although it has been recognized for over a century that the integrity of the medulla oblongata is essential for maintenance of normal levels of arterial pressure, the localization of this region has never been established. For example, bilateral lesions placed in a number of nuclei of the medulla in cats, rats or rabbits have failed to lower arterial pressure. The regions include the nucleus tractus solitarii[16,19,30,36,37], inferior olivary nuclei, nucleus gigantocellularis, lateral reticular nuclei, and paramedian reticular nuclei[36,37], the spinal trigeminal system[28] and large areas of the medullary dorsal reticular formation, including the vestibular nuclei[12,19,33]. Indeed, such negative data led to the view that the representation of tonic vasomotor function is diffuse. Indeed, the only study to our knowledge in which a comparable fall of arterial pressure was produced by small bilateral lesions was that of Fallert and Bucher[19] who demonstrated that lesions placed in roughly comparable regions of the rabbit brain stem resulted in an immediate and profound fall of arterial pressure.

Thus, our observations suggest that the region of the medulla necessary for the maintenance of normal levels of blood pressure is restricted to and coextensive with the area mediating the cerebral ischemic response. These considerations therefore contradict the view that the Cushing and ischemic responses, which heretofore had been primarily viewed as emergency responses, are due to activation of neural areas normally quiescent. Rather, these observations suggest that there is an increase in the activity of an area of the brain already tonically active and essential for driving sympathetic vasomotor fibers. Both the cerebral ischemic and Cushing responses, therefore, merely represent exaggerated but otherwise normal inputs to an intrinsic neural network in the lower brain stem which continuously drives the sympathetic nervous system.

If indeed this area is necessary in providing normal background drive onto the spinal preganglionic outflow, the question arises as to what keeps this area tonically active? One possibility relates to the fact that small distorting pressures within this area, in the range of 10 cm of H_2O, can produce substantial elevations of arterial pressure. This distorting force is comparable in magnitude to the normal pressure transients measured interstitially in the brain from reflected arterial and respiratory pulses[9,42]. Thus, the neurons in these regions are sensitive to the small distorting forces radiating from blood vessels and undoubtedly from movements of the brain during normal posture. In addition, small fluctuations in pO_2 in the terminal capillary bed may also provide some background drive. Thus, medullary neurons in the dorsal medulla may be kept in a state of tonic activity in response to processes inextricably linked to the life process itself: the beat of the heart and respiration.

SUMMARY

We have analyzed the central neural organization of the cerebral ischemic response in anesthetized rabbits and Cushing response in anesthetized cats. The autonomic components of the ischemic response (elicited by rendering the brain ischemic) and the Cushing response (elicited by increasing intracranial pressure diffusely, or by focal distortion of the brain stem) are very similar. Both responses consist of: (a) arterial hypertension; (b) a differentiated vasoconstriction, mostly neurogenic, in renal, femoral and mesenteric arteries; (c) vagal bradycardia largely secondary to the baroreflex initiated by the rise of arterial pressure; and (d) apnea. Both responses are elicited by direct stimulation of the medulla, the ischemic response principally by hypoxia, the Cushing response primarily by distortion. The vasomotor responses can be simulated by punctate-electrical stimulation of a region of the dorsal medulla, largely restricted to the parvocellular and gigantocellular reticular nuclei. Bilateral electrolytic lesions of caudal portions of this zone abolish the reflex vasomotor responses and invariably result in a collapse of arterial pressure to levels comparable to that produced by spinal cord transection. We conclude that the vasomotor components of the cerebral ischemic and Cushing responses are due to direct stimulation of receptors in highly restricted areas of the dorsal medullary reticular formation. These areas represent a subdivision of the so-called pressor centers of the medulla and are anatomically coextensive with an area functionally serving as the so-called tonic vasomotor center. Tonic activity of neurons in this region may be maintained by small, naturally occurring fluctuations of interstitial pressures, pO_2, and distortion of brain associated with head movements and postural changes.

This research was supported by grants from NHLBI (HL 18974) and NASA (NSG 2259).

REFERENCES

1 Alexander, R. S., Tonic and reflex functions of medullary sympathetic cardiovascular centers, *J. Neurophysiol.*, 9 (1946) 205–217.

2 Amoroso, E. C., Bell, F. R. and Rosenberg H., The relationship of the vasomotor and respiratory regions in the medulla oblongata of the sheep, *J. Physiol.* (Lond.), 126 (1954) 86–95.

3 Anrep, G. V. and Segall H. N., The central and reflex regulation of the heart rate, *J. Physiol.* (Lond.), 211 (1970) 263–277.

4 Berman, I. R. and Ducker, T. B., Pulmonary, somatic and splanchnic circulatory responses to increased intracranial pressure, *Ann. Surg.*, 169 (1969) 210–216.

5 Berman, I. R. and Ducker, T. B., Changes in pulmonary, somatic and splanchnic perfusion with increased intracranial pressure, *Surg. Gyn. Obstet.*, 128 (1969) 8–14.

6 Borison, H. L. and Domjan, D., Persistence of the cardio-inhibitory responses to brainstem ischaemia after destruction of the area postrema and the dorsal vagal nuclei, *J. Physiol.* (Lond.), 211 (1970) 263–277.

7 Brashear, R. E. and Ross, J. C., Hemodynamic effects of elevated cerebrospinal fluid pressures alterations with adrenergic blockade, *J. clin. Invest.*, 49 (1970) 1324–1333.

8 Brashear, R. E. and Ross, J. C., Circulating beta-adrenergic stimulator during elevated cerebrospinal fluid pressure, *Arch. int. Med.*, 127 (1971) 748–753.

9 Brock, M., Winkelmuller, W., Poll W., Marakakus, E. and Dietz, H., Measurement of brain-tissue pressure, *Lancet* II (1972) 595–596.

10 Brodal, A., *The Reticular Formation of the Brainstem: Aspects and Functional Correlations*, Thomas, Springfield, Ill., 1957, pp. 8–12.

11 Brown, F. K., Cardiovascular effects of acutely raised intracranial pressure, *Amer. J. Physiol.*, 185 (1956) 510–514.

12 Chai, H. I. and Wang, C. Y., Localization of central cardiovascular control mechanism in lower brain stem of the cat, *Amer. J. Physiol.*, 202 (1962) 25–30.

13 Coote, J. H., Hilton, S. M. and Zbrozyna, A. W., The pontomedullary area integrating the defense reaction in the cat and its influence on muscle flow, *J. Physiol.* (Lond.), 229 (1973) 257–274.

14 Dampney, R. A. L., Kumada, M. and Reis, D. J., Localization of brainstem regions mediating the cerebral ischemic reflex, *Neurosciences Abstracts*, Society for Neurosciences, 5th Annual Meeting, New York City (1975).

15 Doba, N. and Reis, D. J., Localization of the lower brain stem of a receptive area mediating the pressor response to increased intracranial pressure (the Cushing response), *Brain Res.*, 47 (1972a) 487–491.

16 Doba, N. and Reis, D. J., Acute fulminating neurogenic hypertension by brainstem lesions in rat, *Circulation Res.*, 32 (1973) 584–593.

17 Downing, S. E., Mitchell, J. H. and Wallace, A. G., Cardiovascular responses to ischaemia, hypoxia and hypercapnia of the central nervous system, *Amer. J. Physiol.*, 204 (1963) 881–887.

18 Evan, J. P., Espey, F. F., Kristoff, R. V., Kimbell, F. D. and Ryder, H. W., Experimental and clinical observations on rising intracranial pressure, *Arch. Surg.*, 63 (1951) 107–114.

19 Fallert, M. and Bucher, V. M., Localisation eines blutdruckaktiven. Substrats in des Medulla oblongata des Kaninchens, *Helv. Physiol. Acta*, 24 (1966) 139–163.

20 Faulhauer, K., Herrmann, H. D. and Harbauer, G., Cardiovascular response to slowly increased intracranial pressure, *Acta Neurochirurgica*, 24 (1971) 63–70.

21 Gonzales, N. C., Overman, J. and Maxwell, J. A., Circulatory effects of moderately and severely increased intracranial pressure in the dog, *J. Neurosurg.*, 36 (1972) 721–727.

22 Gootman, P. M. and Cohen, M. I., Evoked splanchnic potentials produced by electrical stimulation of medullary vasomotor regions, *Exp. Brain Res.*, 13 (1971) 1–14.

23 Guyton, A. C., Acute hypertension in dogs with cerebral ischemia, *Amer. J. Physiol.*, 154 (1948) 45–54.

24 Hoff, J. T. and Mitchell, R. A., The effect of hypoxia on the Cushing response. In: M. Brock and H. Dietz (Eds.), *Intracranial Pressure*, Springer-Verlag, New York, 1972, pp. 205–209.

25 Hoff, J. T. and Reis, D. J., Localization of regions mediating the Cushing response in CNS of cat, *Arch. Neurol.*, 23 (1970) 228–240.

26 Johnston, I. H., Rowan, J. O., Harper, A. M. and Jennett, W. B., Raised intracranial pressure and cerebral blood flow. I. Cisterna magna infusion in primates, *J. Neurol. Neurosurg. Psychiat.*, 35 (1972) 285–296.

27 Kahn, N. and Mills, E., Centrally evoked sympathetic discharge: A functional study of medullary vasomotor areas, *J. Physiol.* (Lond.), 191 (1967) 339–352.

28 Kumada, M., Dampney, R. A. L. and Reis, D. J., The trigeminal depressor response: A novel vasodepressor response originating from the trigeminal system, *Brain Res.*, 119 (1978) 305–326.

29 Kumada, M., Dampney, R. A. L. and Reis, D. J., Unpublished observations.

30 Kumada, M., Dampney, R. A. L. and Reis, D. J., Profound hypotension and abolition of the vasomotor component of the cerebral ischemic response produced by restricted lesions of medulla oblongata: Relationship to the so-called tonic vasomotor center, *Circulation Res.*, (1978), in press.

31 Levy, M. N., Ng, M. L. and Zieske, H., Cardiac response to cephalic ischemia, *Amer. J. Physiol.*, 215 (1968) 169–175.

32 Lloyd, T. C., Jr., Effect of intracranial pressure on pulmonary vascular resistance, *J. appl. Physiol.*, 35 (1973) 332–335.

33 Manning, J. W., Cardiovascular reflexes following lesions in medullary reticular formation, *Amer. J. Physiol.*, 208 (1965) 283–288.

34 McDowell, R. J. S., Chemical control of heart rate, *Q. J. exp. Physiol.*, 23 (1933) 269–276.

35 Meesen, H. and Olszewski, J., *A Cytoarchitectonic Atlas of the Rhombencephalon of the Rabbit*, Karger, Basel, 1949.

36 Miura, M. and Reis, D. J., Blood pressure response from fastigial nucleus and its pathway in brainstem, *Amer. J. Physiol.*, 219 (1970) 1330–1336.

37 Miura, M. and Reis, D. J., Role of the solitary and paramedian reticular nuclei in mediating cardiovascular reflex responses from carotid baro- and chemoreceptors, *J. Physiol.* (Lond.), 223 (1972) 525–548.

38 Miyakawa, K., A method of complete interception of the blood supply to the brain of the rabbit, *Med. J. Shinshu Univ.*, 11 (1966) 105–112.

39 Miyakawa, K. (Ed.), *A Blood Pressure Oscillation*, Shinshu University, 1972.

40 Myers, R., Systemic vascular and respiratory effects of experimentally induced alterations in intracranial pressure, *J. Neuropath. exp. Neurol.*, 1 (1942) 241–264.

41 Nathan, M. A. and Reis, D. J., Chronic labile hypertension produced by lesions of the nucleus tractus solitarii in the cat, *Circulation Res.*, 40 (1977) 72–81.

42 Poll, W., Brock, M., Marakakis, E., Winkelmuller, W. and Dietz, H., Brain tissue

pressure. In: M. Brock and H. Dietz (Eds.), *Intracranial Pressure*, Springer-Verlag, New York, 1972, pp. 188–194.

43 Richardson, T. Q., Fermoso, T. D. and Pugh, G. O., Effect of acutely elevated intracranial pressure on cardiac output and other circulatory factors, *J. Surg. Res.*, 5 (1965) 318–322.

44 Reis, D. J., Central neural mechanisms governing the circulation with particular reference to the lower brainstem and cerebellum. In: *Neural and Psychological Mechanisms in Cardiovascular Disease*, "Il Ponte", Milan, 1972, pp. 255–280.

45 Reis, D. J., Dampney, R. A. L., Doba, N. and Kumada, M., Central control of blood pressure: A proposed localization of the "tonic vasomotor center" of the medulla. In: *Arterial Hypertension*, Excerpta Medica, Amsterdam, 1977, pp. 19–23.

46 Rodbard, S. and Saiki, H., Mechanisms of the pressor response to increased intracranial pressure, *Amer. J. Physiol.*, 168 (1952) 234–244.

47 Segawa, K., Ross, J. M. and Guyton, A. C., Quantitation of cerebral ischemic pressor response in dogs, *Amer. J. Physiol.*, 200 (1961) 1164–1168.

48 Saper, C. B., Loewy, A. D., Swanson, L. W. and Cowan, W. M., Direct hypothalamo-autonomic connections. *Brain Res.*, 117 (1976) 305–312.

49 Taber, E., The cytoarchitecture of the brain stem of the cat, *J. comp. Neurol.*, 116 (1961) 17–69.

50 Takeuchi, T., Ushiyama, Y. and Miyakawa, K., Undulatory change of oxygen tension around the bulbar vasomotor center during system blood pressure oscillation in rabbits, *Med. J. Shinshu Univ.*, 14 (1969) 353–383.

51 Thompson, R. K. and Malina, S., Dunamic axial brain stem distortion as a mechanism explaining the cardiorespiratory changes in increased intracranial pressure, *J. Neurosurg.*, 16 (1959) 664–675.

52 Trouth, C. O., Loeschcke, H. N. and Berndt, J., Topography of the circulatory responses to electrical stimulation in the medulla oblongata. Relationships to respiratory responses, *Pflügers Arch.*, 339 (1973) 185–201.

53 Ungerstedt, U., Stereotaxic mapping of the monoamine pathways in the rat brain, *Acta physiol. scand.*, 82, Suppl. 367 (1971) 1–48.

54 Wang, S. C. and Ranson, S. W., Autonomic responses to electrical stimulation of the lower brain stem, *J. comp. Neurol.*, 71 (1939) 437–455.

55 Weinstein, J. D., Langfitt, T. W., Bruno, L., Zaren, H. A. and Jackson, J. L. F., Experimental study of patterns of brain distortion and ischemia produced by an increased mass, *J. Neurosurg.*, 28 (1968) 513–521.

CHAPTER 28

BULBOSPINAL INHIBITORY INFLUENCES ON SYMPATHETIC PREGANGLIONIC NEURONS

K. Dembowsky, J. Czachurski, K. Amendt and H. Seller

I. Physiologisches Institut, University of Heidelberg, Heidelberg, Federal Republic of Germany

INTRODUCTION

The first indication of the existence of a spinal descending sympatho-inhibitory system was given in a report by Lim, Wang and Yi in 1938[23]. These authors recorded a reduction in blood pressure during electrical stimulation of the dorsolateral funiculus of the spinal cord at the level of T_4. In the last few years systematical analysis with recordings of blood pressure and activity in various pre- and postganglionic sympathetic nerves have revealed two different sympatho-inhibitory pathways: one in the dorsolateral and one in the ventrolateral funiculus[3,14-16]. It has been shown that stimulation of these pathways can reduce tonic background activity as well as the spinal component of the somato-sympathetic reflex[1,3,13,18,29].

In recent years a number of investigations have been performed in order to describe the origin and the functional relationship of these descending sympatho-inhibitory pathways. Especially, the involvement of baroreceptors in the inhibition of sympathetic activity at the spinal level has been questioned[1,2,4,5,11,12,17,18,22,29,30,32]. Contrary results have been obtained relative to baroreceptor action on the cord when the spinal somato-sympathetic reflexes were taken as indications of an inhibitory action at the spinal level. Some investigators did not find any change in spinal reflex amplitude[2,17,22] but others reported a 20–30% reduction during baroreceptor stimulation[1,4].

Besides the involvement of the baroreceptors, however, another inhibitory effect on the sympathetic background and reflex activity of supraspinal origin has to be taken into consideration; this is the so called "postexcitatory depression" or "silent period"[19,27]. This silent period appears after stimulation of the hypothalamus[24], the carotid sinus nerve[6] and various somatic afferents[19,27]. Use of the term "postexcitatory depression" to describe this phenomenon, however, is rather misleading because this inhibition may also occur without any prior excitation[18,20,21]. On the basis of this finding a separate inhibitory and excitatory process—both activated by somatic afferents—has been suggested[21].

The present investigation was designed to get more information about the functional significance and relationship of the descending sympatho-inhibitory pathways.

The following questions were investigated in particular: 1) Are the sympatho-inhibitory pathways tonically active? 2) Does baroreceptor denervation alter the effects of the inhibitory pathways? 3) Is the origin of these inhibitory pathways in the medulla oblongata or at higher levels of the central nervous system? 4) What is the mechanism of the inhibitory effect on the spinal somato-sympathetic reflex elicited by electrical stimulation of the carotid sinus nerve?

METHODS

The experiments were performed on 37 adult cats (2–2.5 kg) of either sex. The cats were anesthetized with α-chloralose (60–70 mg/kg, i.v.) after induction with ether. The femoral vein and artery were catheterized and a tracheotomy was performed. Cats were paralyzed with hexacarbacholine and artificially ventilated. The end-tidal CO_2 was kept at 3.5–4.0 Vol. %. Rectal temperature was maintained at 37–38°C.

The white ramus at the third thoracic segment (WR-T_3) was isolated retro-pleurally on the left side and cut before it joined the sympathetic trunk ganglion. The nerve was freed from its connective tissue and placed on a bipolar platinum electrode. The nerve activity was amplified (Tektronix AM 502, 0.02 to 3 kHz) and displayed on an oscilloscope (Tektronix 7603). The output of the amplifier was also connected to an averager (Nicolet 1072) and 16 consecutive reflex responses were averaged. The fourth thoracic intercostal nerve, the carotid sinus nerve and the hypoglossal nerve were also prepared from the left side. They were peripherally cut and placed on bipolar silver electrodes for electrical stimulation. A single pulse or two pulses at an interval of three msec, 0.6–2.0 V for 0.5 msec was generally used for stimulation of the intercostal nerves. The interval between each stimulation was three to four sec.

A reversible blockade of all descending and ascending spinal pathways was performed by cooling the spinal cord between the second and third cervical segment. A hollow metal ring was placed around the spinal cord after section of the C_2 and C_3 dorsal and ventral roots. The metal ring was perfused with cold ethanol. The temperature of the metal ring at the surface of the spinal cord was measured by a small thermistor probe and it was kept at 4–6°C during blockade by adjustment of the perfusion rate. In control experiments the temperature inside the spinal cord was measured with a needle thermistor. There was a maximal difference in temperature between the surface and the middle of the spinal cord of 3°C. Stimulation of the dorsal funiculus cranial during the cold block and recording of the activity caudal to it revealed that all conduction of activity was blocked at temperatures below 10°C at the surface of the cord.

Denervation of the baroreceptors was carried out by transection of both carotid sinus nerves and both vagal nerves close to the nodose ganglion. The completeness of the baroreceptor denervation was always tested. A sure proof of complete denervation was unchanged background activity in the white ramus in noradrenaline-induced blood pressure increase.

RESULTS

A reversible blockade of all ascending and descending tracts by cooling the spinal cord between C_2 and C_3 to temperatures of 4–6°C produced a decrease of the mean arterial pressure to 40–50 mmHg. To exclude any influence of this low blood pressure on the transmission of the spinal component of the somato-sympathetic reflex, blood pressure was kept at control levels by continuous infusion of angiotensin or noradrenaline during the cooling period.

The background tonic activity in the white ramus at T_3 (WR-T_3) was markedly reduced during spinal cord blockade. A quantitative analysis of the reduced activity during the blockade was performed by means of impulse counting in multifiber strands. With this method it could be shown that 10–20% of the tonic discharges were still present during the blockade.

If the T_4 intercostal nerve was stimulated, an early spinal and a late supraspinal reflex could be recorded in the WR-T_3. The supraspinal reflex was completely abolished during the cooling period (Fig. 1) while the amplitude of the spinal reflex was increased to 150–400% of the control (Figs. 1 and 2). The latency of the spinal reflex was 13.4 ± 2.5 msec before and it was reduced by one to three msec during the blockade. The increase of the reflex amplitude was persistent during the whole dura-

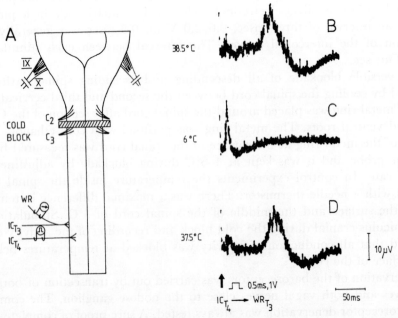

Fig. 1. A: Schematic graph of the experimental procedure. B, C and D: Averaged reflex responses in the T_3 white ramus after stimulation of T_4 intercostal nerve before (B), during (C) and after (D) spinal cold blockade. Note the significant increase of the early spinal reflex and the extinction of the late supraspinal reflex during the cold blockade.

tion of the blockade and it declined to control levels within a few minutes after the end of the blockade (Fig. 2).

In order to resolve the question of the origin of this descending inhibitory action on the spinal somato-sympathetic reflex, a series of experiments was performed with spinal blockade before and after baroreceptor denervation. From these experiments one example is shown in Fig. 2. After baroreceptor denervation there was neither a significant change in the amplitude of the spinal reflexes with intact spinal cord nor a difference in the increase of the reflexes during spinal blockade.

In another series of experiments the increase in spinal reflex amplitude during cold blockade was tested before and after midcollicular decerebration. These experiments also indicated no difference in the effect of the blockade on the spinal reflex after decerebration.

The possibility of baroreceptor influence on the spinal somato-sympathetic reflex was additionally tested by two procedures, i.e., adequate stimulation of the baroreceptors and electrical stimulation of the carotid sinus nerve. For strong, adequate, pulsatile stimulation of all baroreceptors a blood pressure increase up to 200 mmHg was produced by an infusion of noradrenaline (Fig. 3). During the period of increased blood pressure the amplitude of the averaged spinal reflexes was never altered to values beyond the range of the spontaneous variations (Fig. 3). This variation was always 20–30% of the mean value and it occurred both with intact and denervated baroreceptors. The supraspinal reflex was always completely abolished during the first minutes and recovered to 10–15% of the control during the period of high blood pressure.

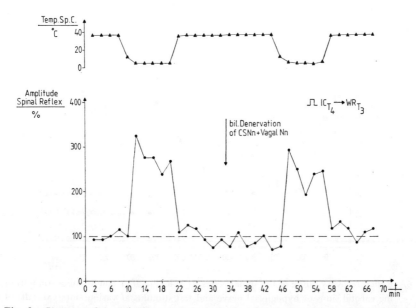

Fig. 2.   Increase of the spinal somato-sympathetic reflex during spinal cold blockade before and after baroreceptor denervation. Upper trace: temperature at the surface of the spinal cord at C_2–C_3. Carotid sinus and vagal nerves were prepared before this recording period and cut at the marking arrow.

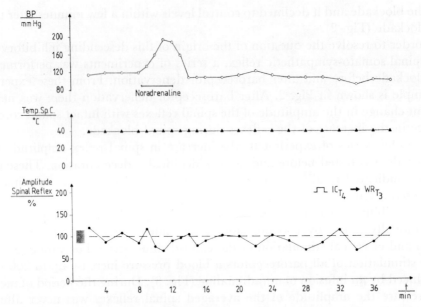

Fig. 3.   Mean arterial pressure, temperature of the spinal cord at the cooling device and
          amplitude of the spinal reflex of the T₃ white ramus before, during and after infusion
          of noradrenaline (10 μg, i.v., per min). The hatched area at 100% of the spinal
          reflex indicates the standard deviation.

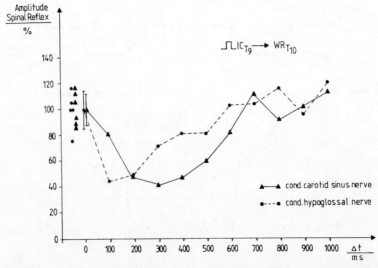

Fig. 4.   Reflex recovery curve of the spinal reflex at WR-T₁₀ after conditioning stimulus of
          the carotid sinus or hypoglossal nerve and test stimulus at various intervals (Δt) of
          the T₉ intercostal nerve. The sequence of the interval between the conditioning and
          testing stimuli was unsystematically varied. (Stimulus parameters for carotid sinus
          and hypoglossal nerve: three impulses 100 Hz, 0.5 msec, 7 V; intercostal nerve:
          one impulse, 0.5 msec, 0.6 V).

The only results which might indicate a baroreceptor inhibition of the spinal somato-sympathetic reflex to a greater degree than attained in spontaneous variations were obtained with electrical stimulation of the carotid sinus nerve[4,5]. We have performed identical experiments to investigate the possibility that mechanisms other than the baroreceptor inhibitory mechanism are involved in this reduction of the spinal reflex. In these experiments activity in the white ramus at T_{10} was recorded and the intercostal nerve at T_9 was stimulated. The sinus nerve was stimulated (three impulses, 0.5 msec, 100 Hz, five to seven V) at various intervals (100–1000 msec) before the stimulation of the intercostal nerve. With this procedure a reduction of the spinal reflex amplitude was obtained which was significant within a range of 100 to 600 msec of the conditioning-testing stimulus interval (Fig. 4). The maximal reduction to 40% of the control amplitude occurred at an interval of 300 msec (Fig. 4). If the response to the sinus nerve stimulation itself was tested a clear reflex with a latency between 40–50 msec could be recorded in the T_{10} white ramus. The reflex response could also be recorded, although with smaller amplitude, if the intensity of the sinus nerve stimulation was lowered to 0.05 msec and 0.5 V.

To prove that this process is completely independent of the baroreceptor inhibition we stimulated another cranial nerve, the hypoglossal nerve, without any depressor or sympatho-inhibitory function. If this stimulation was used as a conditioning stimulus a similar response curve was obtained (Fig. 4). The conditioning stimulus also produced a reflex response in the white ramus.

DISCUSSION

These results indicate that a tonic bulbospinal inhibition of the transmission of the spinal somato-sympathetic reflex pathway exists under these experimental conditions. This inhibition acts independently of baroreceptor input.

During cold blockade of the spinal cord there is also a strong reduction of tonic background activity in the white rami and it can be argued that the background activity may limit the spinal reflex response in the intact spinal cord because of the refractory period of the preganglionic neurons. This argument can be refuted by the following findings: 1) The discharge frequency of single preganglionic neurons is only one to two per sec[19,28] and the refractory period measured with the technique of paired antidromic stimulation is 11–15 msec[10,25]. From these facts and from the finding that only a small percentage of tonically active preganglionic neurons at the thoracic level do exhibit a spinal reflex[28] it is improbable that the refractory period is a limitation of the amplitude of the spinal reflex in the whole white ramus when the intercostal nerve is stimulated every three to four sec. 2) Variations of the background activity by other means than the blockade of descending pathways, for example increase during asphyxia and after baroreceptor denervation or decrease during baroreceptor activation, do not significantly alter the spinal reflex amplitude.

From these experiments it is impossible to draw any conclusion relative to the site of inhibitory action at the spinal level. It cannot be stated whether this inhibition acts directly on the preganglionic neurons and in this way also reduces the tonic background activity or whether it is acting only on the interneurons of the spinal reflex pathway. A similar tonic bulbospinal inhibition, however, has been demonstrated for the transmission of visceromotor and somatomotor reflexes[7,8]. The inhibition by this so-called dorsal reticulospinal system has been shown to take place at the interneurons of the spinal reflex pathway[8,9]. This inhibitory system of flexor reflexes is also present after decerebration and its descending pathway is in the dorsolateral funiculus which is identical with the region of the main descending sympatho-inhibitory pathway[3,14,15]. This leads to the suggestion that the tonic inhibition of sympathetic and motor reflexes is probably one uniform system which acts on interneurons of all polysynaptic reflexes.

It has been clearly demonstrated in these experiments that the baroreceptors do not support this bulbospinal inhibition. As has been shown before[2,17,22,29] it was also impossible to produce a significant reduction of the spinal somato-sympathetic reflex by adequate baroreceptor activation. Contradictory results by other authors[1,4] who have described a small reduction of the spinal reflex with the same method cannot be explained. From our experiments, however, we cannot conclude that baroreceptor inhibition is not taking place to some degree at the spinal level. First there is the possibility that this inhibition acts only on those preganglionic neurons which do not exhibit a spinal reflex. The only way to prove this possibility is the demonstration of IPSP's with intracellular recordings of preganglionic neurons after baroreceptor activation. Secondly a spinal baroreceptor inhibition may act at an interneuron within a descending sympatho-excitatory pathway. There is much evidence for this possibility brought up by experiments using stimulation of sympatho-excitatory pathways and adequate baroreceptor activation[1,12,30,32]. Gebber and McCall[11] have recorded activity in spinal sympathetic interneurons which were inhibited by baroreceptor activation. This mode of baroreceptor inhibition at the spinal level is not contrary to our finding of the inefficacy of baroreceptors on the early spinal somato-sympathetic reflex.

The effect of electrical stimulation of the carotid sinus nerve on the spinal sympathetic reflex finds an easy explanation for its action by other than the baroreceptor mechanism. Another mechanism is evident because the reduction of the spinal reflex is much greater during electrical stimulation than during adequate activation of the baroreceptors[4] and it can also be produced to the same degree by stimulation of the hypoglossal nerve. The stimulus strength which has been used by Coote and Macleod[4] and in our experiments is far above the threshold for excitation of chemoreceptor afferents[6]. This stimulation of the carotid sinus nerve or hypoglossal nerve leads to an excitatory response in various pre- and postganglionic sympathetic nerves[6,31]. This excitation, however, leads to the well-known phenomenon of "postexcitatory depression" or the "silent period"[6,19,27]. This term is generally used for all inhibitory processes after a sympathetic reflex response is induced by somatic or visceral afferents. This "postexcitatory depression", however, can be subdivided into different spinal and supraspinal components[26]. A strong inhibitory influence on the spinal reflex pathway from the brain stem level is included in this "postexcitatory depression". This action is different from that of baroreceptors and similar to that of tonic descending inhibition. Therefore it may be speculated that excitation of somatic or visceral afferents leads to a short-lasting activation of the tonic bulbospinal inhibitory system.

SUMMARY

In chloralose anesthetized cats sympathetic reflexes in thoracic white rami were induced by stimulation of an intercostal nerve. A complete blockade of the spinal cord by cooling at C_2–C_3 produced an increase of the early spinal reflex to 150–400% and a complete extinction of the late supraspinal reflex. The increase of the spinal reflex during cold blockade was also present after baroreceptor denervation and/or midcollicular decerebration. Baroreceptor activation did not produce any significant change in the spinal reflex. A conditioning stimulus of the carotid sinus nerve elicited first an excitation in the white ramus and subsequently a marked reduction of the spinal test reflex at conditioning-testing intervals of 100–600 msec. Stimulation of the hypoglossal nerve gave similar results. From these findings it is concluded that: 1) A strong tonic bulbospinal inhibition on the transmission of the spinal somato-sympathetic reflex is present in the anesthetized cat. This inhibition is not supported by baroreceptors. 2) Adequate baroreceptor activation does not significantly influence the transmission of the spinal reflex. 3) The reduction of the spinal reflex after electrical stimulation of the carotid sinus nerve or the hypoglossal nerve is caused by the "postexcitatory depression".

These studies were supported by the German Research Foundation within the SFB 90 "Cardiovasculäres System".

REFERENCES

1 Barman, S. M. and Wurster, R. D., Interaction of descending spinal sympathetic pathways and afferent nerves, *Amer. J. Physiol.*, 234 (1978) H223–H229.

2 Coote, J. H., Downman, C. B. B. and Weber, W. V., Reflex discharges into thoracic white rami elicited by somatic and visceral afferent excitation, *J. Physiol.* (Lond.), 202 (1969) 147–159.

3 Coote, J. H. and MacLeod, V. H., The influence of bulbospinal monoaminergic pathways on the sympathetic nerve activity, *J. Physiol.* (Lond.), 241 (1974) 453–475.

4 Coote, J. H. and MacLeod, V. H., Evidence for the involvement in the baroreceptor reflex of a descending inhibitory pathway, *J. Physiol.* (Lond.), 241 (1974) 477–496.

5 Coote, J. H. and MacLeod, V. H., The effect of intraspinal microinjections of 6-Hydroxydopamine on the inhibitory influence exerted on spinal sympathetic activity by the baroreceptors, *Pflügers Arch.*, 371 (1977) 271–277.

6 De Groat, W. C. and Lalley, P. M., Reflex sympathetic firing in response to electrical stimulation of the carotid sinus nerve in the cat, *Brain Res.*, 80 (1974) 17–40.

7 Downman, C. B. B. and Hussain, A., Spinal tracts and supraspinal centres influencing visceromotor and allied reflexes in cats, *J. Physiol.* (Lond.), 141 (1958) 489–499.

8 Engberg, I., Lundberg, A. and Ryall, R. W., Reticulospinal inhibition of transmission in reflex pathways, *J. Physiol.* (Lond.), 194 (1968) 201–223.

9 Engberg, I., Lundberg, A. and Ryall, R. W., Reticulospinal inhibition of interneurones, *J. Physiol.* (Lond.), 194 (1968) 225–236.

10 Fernandez De Molina, A., Kuno, M. and Perl, E. R., Antidromically-evoked responses from sympathetic preganglionic neurones, *J. Physiol.* (Lond.), 180 (1965) 321–335.

11 Gebber, G. L. and McCall, R. B., Identification and discharge patterns of spinal sympathetic interneurons, *Amer. J. Physiol.*, 231 (1976) 722–733.

12 Gebber, G. L., Taylor, D. G. and Weaver, L. C., Electrophysiological studies on organization of central vasopressor pathways, *Amer. J. Physiol.*, 224 (1973) 470–481.

13 Illert, M., Effects upon the somato-sympathetic reflex transmission in spinalized cats, *Pflügers Arch.*, 332 (1972) R65.

14 Illert, M. and Gabriel, M., Mapping the cord of the spinal cat for symapthetic and blood pressure responses, *Brain Res.*, 23 (1970) 274–276.

15 Illert, M. and Gabriel, M., Descending pathways in the cervical cord of cats affecting blood pressure and sympathetic activity, *Pflügers Arch.*, 335 (1972) 109–124.

16 Illert, M. and Seller, H., A descending sympatho-inhibitory tract in the ventrolateral column of the cat, *Pflügers Arch.*, 313 (1969) 343–360.

17 Kirchner, F., Sato, A. and Weidinger, H., Bulbar inhibition of spinal and supraspinal sympathetic reflex discharges, *Pflügers Arch.*, 326 (1971) 324–333.

18 Kirchner, F., Wyszogrodski, I. and Polosa, C., Some properties of sympathetic neuron inhibition by depressor area and intraspinal stimulation, *Pflügers Arch.*, 357 (1975) 349–360.

19 Koizumi, K. and Brooks, C. McC., The integration of autonomic system reactions: Discussion of autonomic reflexes, their control and their association with somatic reactions, *Ergebn. Physiol. Biol. Chem. exptl. Pharmacol.*, 67 (1972) 1–68.

20 Koizumi, K. and Sato, A., Reflex activity of single sympathetic fibres to skeletal muscle produced by electrical stimulation of somatic and vago-depressor afferent nerves in the cat, *Pflügers Arch.*, 332 (1972) 283–301.

21 Koizumi, K., Sato, A., Kaufman, A. and Brooks, C. McC., Studies of sympathetic neuron discharges modified by central and peripheral excitation, *Brain Res.*, 11 (1968) 212–224.

22 Koizumi, K., Seller, H., Kaufman, A. and Brooks, C. McC., Pattern of sympathetic discharges and their relation to baroreceptor and respiratory activities, *Brain Res.*, 27 (1971) 281–294.

23 Lim, R. K. S., Wang, S. C. and Yi, C. L., On the question of myelencephalic sympathetic centre. VII. The depressor area a sympatho-inhibitory centre, *Chin. J. Physiol.*, 13 (1938) 61–78.

24 Pitts, R. F. and Bronk, D. W., Excitability cycle of the hypothalamus-sympathetic neurone system, *Amer. J. Physiol.*, 135 (1942) 504–522.

25 Polosa, C., Spontaneous activity of sympathetic preganglionic neurons, *Can. J. Physiol. Pharmacol.*, 46 (1968) 887–896.

26 Sato, A., Spinal and supraspinal inhibition of somatosympathetic reflexes by conditioning afferent volleys, *Pflügers Arch.*, 336 (1972) 121–133.

27 Sato, A. and Schmidt, R. F., Somatosympathetic reflexes: Afferent fibers, central pathways, discharge characteristics, *Physiol. Rev.*, 53 (1973) 916–947.

28 Seller, H., The discharge pattern of single units in thoracic and lumbar white rami in relation to cardiovascular events, *Pflügers Arch.*, 343 (1973) 317–330.

29 Seller, H. and Illert, M., Comparison of two inhibitory influences upon lumbar preganglionic sympathetic activity. In: W. Umbach and H. P. Koepchen (Eds.), *Central Rhythmic and Regulation*, Hippokrates, Stuttgart, 1974, pp. 215–220.

30 Snyder, D. W. and Gebber, G. L., Relationships between medullary depressor region and central vaso-pressor pathways, *Amer. J. Physiol.*, 252 (1973) 1129–1137.

31 Szulczyk, P., Descending spinal sympathetic pathway utilized by somato-sympathetic reflex and carotid chemoreflex, *Brain Res.*, 112 (1976) 190–193.

32 Taylor, D. G. and Gebber, G. L., Baroreceptor mechanisms controlling sympathetic nervous rhythms of central origin, *Amer. J. Physiol.*, 228 (1975) 1002–1013.

CHAPTER 29

SOMATO-AUTONOMIC REACTIONS AND THEIR HIGHER CONTROL

Björn Lisander

Department of Physiology, University of Göteborg, Göteborg, Sweden

INTRODUCTION

During a symposium held in March 1978 we discussed the function and characteristics of the viscermotor system per se and how it is principally controlled. It is, however, well known that this important part of the nervous system is strongly influenced by cortico-hypothalamic levels and what characterizes these particular autonomic effects is their very close linkage to behavioral and endocrine changes. Thus, the highest brain levels, responsible for "cognitive and affective" functions, involve in their expressions all three efferent systems of the body, forming patterns that are designed to cope with the various environmental challenges that the organism has to face in daily life.

The first hints of knowledge concerning some of these patterns are ageold, for example the everyday observations of heart rate, facial color, intestinal movements, etc., in connection with emotions and their more or less vivid expressions. However, knowledge of the precise role of cortico-hypothalamic levels in these reactions has emerged only late and slowly. Early in the century, Karplus and Kreidl[14] performed their studies on electrical hypothalamic stimulation in curarized cats, observing sometimes marked changes in arterial blood pressure. These changes as well as those observed by Ranson and Magoun[22], focused interest upon the autonomic effects induced from the hypothalamus. Cannon[2] realized, however, quite early the importance of the diencephalon also for the integrated expressions of emotionally-colored behavior, although he ascribed the central role to the thalamus, rather than the hypothalamus. It became increasingly clear from the work by Hess[10], Bard[1] and others that the autonomic changes that were induced from the hypothalamus were generally linked to behavioral adjustments and in a way it is even justifiable to state that the main action of the hypothalamus is on overall behavior.

Somatomotor expressions of emotional behavior vary considerably between species but the autonomic and hormonal adjustments appear to differ considerably less. According to MacLean[19], the phylogenetically oldest of three forebrain compartments is the "protoreptilian brain", important for the more stereotyped, species-typical behavior. Later developed is the "paleomammalian brain" or the limbic system which is involved in more complex self- and species-preserving behavior, apparently playing a key role in "instincts" and emotions and the associated patterns of expression. The neocortex, finally, interacts with the older forebrain parts and allows for individualized behavior and can, at least in humans, considerably modify the emotions and more or less completely suppress the somatomotor component of emotional expressions.

To a great extent, the hypothalamus integrates and triggers the final coordinated responses. However, a great variety of complex excitatory and inhibitory inputs, both from the periphery and from higher centers, determines hypothalamic activity, both qualitatively and quantitatively. The brain continually receives information from telereceptors, other exteroreceptors and from interoreceptors as well. Through such connections widespread alerting or inhibitory influences may be exerted on the forebrain compartments mentioned, under the appropriate conditions leading to well-coordinated response patterns, initiated via the hypothalamus.

By now several hypothalamic areas have been identified where topical stimulation causes drastic and often quite specific autonomic changes, which are commonly linked to hormonal and somatomotor adjustments in an integrated fashion. These response patterns, which are usually similar to those occurring in response to certain environmental stimuli in intact organisms, may be termed "push-button patterns". It is thought that these hypothalamic neuron pools, physiologically activated by various influences, can by diverging but precisely organized pathways modulate the three efferent systems of the body.

I would like to discuss some of these hypothalamic patterns. The most well-known of these is the defense reaction which will be presented in detail by professor Hilton, but there are some aspects I would also like to elaborate on.

From other hypothalamic areas can be induced so-called pressor responses with more or less generalized signs of increased sympathetic discharge, but without any activation of the cholinergic sympathetic vasodilator fibers. The functional significance of these adjustments is obscure.

Finally, from other hypothalamic areas can be elicited sympatho-inhibitory responses. Possibly, they are involved in so-called "withdrawal behavior" or even emotional fainting in front of great situational difficulties, where flight or attack are deemed impossible.

PATTERNS OF REACTIONS

Reactions involving alerting or fight or flight are probably the most studied of the "push-button patterns". Topical stimulation in the hypothalamic defense area can induce a complex response pattern with autonomic, hormonal and somatomotor readjustments: the defense reaction.

The question arises whether this fascinating, topically-induced pattern in all respects is similar to the changes taking place in situations provoking fear or rage. Naturally, we have a better knowledge concerning the autonomic changes in animals subject to topical stimulation than we have about the naturally-occurring readjustments.

Some questions may be posed in this connection. It is well known that the vascular effect of an activation of the cholinergic sympathetic vasodilator fibers can only be maintained for a very limited period, in spite of continued stimulation.

One hypothesis is that the neurogenic influence is counteracted by an increased myogenic activity in the vessels[4]. Whatever the cause, suppose that the animal develops an autonomic defense reaction in face of an external threat but makes no immediate muscle movements. Then there would not be the benefit of a neurogenic muscle vasodilatation during somatomotor activity later as the vessels are then refractory to the neurogenic stimulus. From the theleological standpoint, there would be need for a central nervous mechanism inhibiting the cholinergic fibers until somatomotor activity begins.

Zanchetti and co-workers have studied the readjustments taking place in natural aggressive behavior in cats[25]. Some differences between topically-induced behavior and reflex behavior seem to exist. Confrontation without actual fighting is often associated with bradycardia rather than tachycardia and cardiac output can fall rather than increase. Interestingly, confrontation without fighting is accompanied by a neurogenic muscle vasoconstriction rather than a dilatation. The active cholinergic dilatation is elicited first during muscle movements and then in active muscle groups only.

How then can the central computer during the defense reaction limit the vasodilatation to muscle groups in action? I would like to point to one possible mechanism. As is obvious from Fig. 1 cerebellar cortical stimulation can inhibit components of the hypothalamically-induced defense reaction, including cholinergic sympathetic muscle vasodilatation[16].

One attractive hypothesis is that the cerebellar cortex continuously receives in-

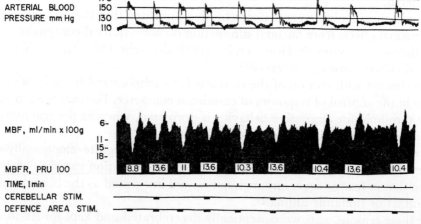

Fig. 1. Chloralosed cat. Defense area stimulations, with and without simultaneous stimulation in the vermal cortex of the anterior cerebellar lobe (both at 50 Hz, one msec, 3 V). MBF and MBFR denote muscle blood flow and muscle blood flow resistance, respectively. Note that the muscle vasodilatation from defense area stimulation is reduced by cerebellar cortical stimulation.

formation concerning somatomotor activity and is thereby also able to suppress components of the defense reaction and thus coordinate somatomotor and visceromotor activity. Possibly, although even more hypothetically, this structure may modulate autonomic activity during exercise.

The cerebellar cortex exerts an inhibitory influence on the underlying nuclei which are, in turn, excitatory in nature. The autonomically active part of the cortex projects on the fastigial nucleus. Stimulation of the rostral part of this nucleus causes marked pressor responses. Dr. Martner in our department has analysed the effects of stimulation in this fastigial pressor area[20]. He has found evidence that this structure can influence a multitude of autonomic reflexes affecting gastrointestinal motility, bladder motility and circulation. The fastigial effects were often modulatory, damping prevailing activity when it was high but exerting a facilitatory influence when activity was low. This type of interaction was generally the case for the gastrointestinal system while the influence on sympathetic activity to the cardiovascular system was mainly facilitatory. In unanesthetized cats, stimulation of the same area caused a stereotype somatomotor pattern with licking and chewing movements or, at higher stimulation intensities, predatory behavior[20,23].

There is evidence for connections between the cerebellum and limbic-hypothalamic levels. Such pathways have been demonstrated both with electrophysiological methods and in histological studies. There is also functional evidence pointing in this direction (see[20]). Notably, in the experiments by Zanchetti and Zoccolini[26], fastigial stimulation could cause sham rage in thalamic cats, an effect which was abolished by acute precollicular decerebration.

The question thus arises via what central structures does the fastigial nucleus elicit its autonomic and behavioral effects. There is a distinct possibility that the observed changes reflect a fastigial action on more rostral levels like the hypothalamus and the limbic system, but also the alternative of facilitation of bulbar relay centers has to be considered.

Experiments involving acute decerebration indicated that the cardiovascular and gastrointestinal effects from fastigial stimulation do not require diencephalic or higher levels of the nervous system[20]. However, in acutely decerebrated cats, the characteristic behavioral effects were not observed[17].

Experiments with section of the neuraxis have emphasized the role of the hypothalamus in the control of responses of emotional character. For example, in thalamic cats, the threshold for aggressive behavior is decreased, whereas the reactivity of the acutely decerebrated animal is drastically lowered[1].

However, infrahypothalamic structures can also integrate emotionally-colored responses. Cats kept for weeks and months after decerebration can display behavior similar to that in fear or rage, although not as well integrated as the behavior patterns seen in intact or thalamic animals[1].

For these reasons, cats were aseptically decerebrated and kept for six to 30 days after the operation[17]. In these animals, fastigial pressor area stimulation could elicit a pattern suggestive of fear or rage. That is, they displayed vocalization, righting of head and shoulders, running movements, protrusion of claws and piloerection and retraction of the nictitating membranes. Immediately after the stimulus, licking and chewing movements regularly occurred. In some cats, this latter "oral" behavior predominated during fastigial stimulation.

Thus, the cerebellum in interaction with subhypothalamic brain stem structures can initiate and modulate integrated behavioral responses of a nature which in the intact animal are usually elicited from limbic-hypothalamic structures. Apparently, there are cerebellar projections to bulbar and mesencephalic neuron pools involved in emotional behavior, in all likelihood the same which can be activated in intact animals or thalamic preparations.

Of interest is that similar behavior, reminiscent of flight or attack, could be induced also by nociceptive stimuli, somatic afferent nerve stimulation or by bilateral common carotid occlusion, suggesting that several types of afferent inputs ultimately converge on lower brain stem neuron pools, integrating emotional behavior.

In some hypothalamic areas pressor responses can be elicited with more or less marked overall signs of sympathetic activation but with no engagement of the vasodilator system. Their functional significance is obscure. But it leads us to a very important question. Is the classical defense reaction the only way that an animal responds in a threatening situation?

One can perform a very simple experiment to elucidate this point. Put a cat in a box and record blood pressure and heart rate. Then, if the box is gently rocked without the animal expecting it, the animal may respond with a bradycardia at a constant or slightly elevated blood pressure. If the rocking is repeated after 15–30 sec there is nearly always a tachycardia and a blood pressure rise (unpublished observation).

In our department a similar approach has been used in the study of spontaneously hypertensive rats (SHR's)[8]. The SHR's and normotensive control rats (NCR's) were placed in a box with two separate chambers where they could be subjected to alerting stimuli in the form of noise, light and vibration during recording of blood pressure and heart rate. Both types of animals responded with a blood pressure rise to the alerting stimulus. The SHR's nearly always displayed a tachycardia. But in the NCR's one-third of the animals showed bradycardia. This response to alerting stimuli was not a reflex adjustment to the blood pressure rise but must have been centrally elicited since it preceded the blood pressure rise in most cases. Consequently, normotensive and even renal hypertensive control rats responded more frequently than SHR's to these types of stressful stimuli with an autonomic pattern that included vagal activation. The SHR's, on the other hand, had more consistently sympathetic excitation, combined with vagal suppression. This suggests that the neurogenic adjustments characterizing the classical defense reaction dominate in the SHR. Furthermore, SHR's appeared to react more vividly in this direction to given alerting stimuli, thus exhibiting a "central hyperreactivity" with respect to such responses.

Concerning gastrointestinal function, the topically-induced defense reaction includes an inhibition of gastric motility[12,15]. We also have here some interesting observations in humans, e.g., by Wolff and Wolf[24]. In a situation of sudden fear, the classical subject Tom displayed a blanching of the mucosa and a decreased acid secretion. But in other situations, characterized by frustration, it is everyday experience that acid secretion can increase and even ulcerations can occur. If the SHR's were immobilized for 12 hours, their blood pressure went up by about 50 mmHg and much more so than in NCR's. After the immobilization they were killed and found to have gastric ulcers but concerning these mainly vagally mediated effects both NCR's and SHR's showed about equal degrees and frequency of lesions[9].

Apparently, there are several autonomic, emotionally colored patterns the organism can choose between in various situations, which if only blood pressure and heart rate are followed may appear as apparently fairly undifferentiated hypothalamic "pressor responses". However, knowing the important role of the hypothalamus in emotionally colored responses, I would like to point to the possibility that they may be part of the claviature the limbic system plays on in various emotionally charged situations.

Stimulation in a region in the dorsolateral hypothalamus causes food intake in the unanesthetized animal. If the same point is stimulated in the anesthetized animal it was observed by Folkow and Rubinstein[6] that there is a moderate pressor response with muscle vasoconstriction, some increase in intestinal blood flow and a vagally mediated increase in gastrointestinal motility. They also studied gastric motility and observed an increased activity in the cholinergic excitatory fibers to the stomach.

To what extent does this autonomic response mimic the changes taking place during natural food intake? What happens to gastric motility during eating?

Since the days of Cannon[3] it has been known that there is a vagally mediated relaxation of the stomach in connection with food intake. Figure 2 is from one of our experiments on this problem[15]. The animals had an esophageal fistula permitting sham feeding and also a gastrostomy so that gastric volume could be recorded with the balloon method. When the animals ate, the stomach relaxed even though the food did not reach the stomach. This relaxation depended on the consistency of the food: the coarser, the bigger the response. Milk or water almost never gave any response. These responses could not be blocked by guanethidine or by atropine. They were, however, abolished by intra-abdominal vagotomy. It thus appears that the noncholinergic, nonadrenergic vagal relaxatory fibers are responsible for the receptive relaxation of the stomach.

Another specialized type of sympatho-excitatory pattern is the diving response which has been observed in a large number of species. This pattern is especially pronounced in habitual divers but it exists also in non-divers, including humans. Submersion leads to a pattern of vasoconstriction and bradycardia, causing a markedly decreased cardiac output and the transformation of the circulation to a heart-brain

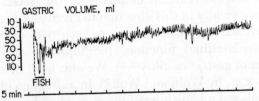

Fig. 2.   Unanesthetized cat with esophagostomy and a gastric fistula. A marked receptive relaxation of the stomach takes place when the animal is sham fed with large pieces of fish.

pump. This response is elicited by a complex interplay between reflex influences elicited from cutaneous receptors, receptors in airways and the thorax and the arterial chemoreceptors. It appears to be basically integrated at lower brain stem levels[21] (see Fig. 3).

But in threatening situations, divers like the seal can display this pattern as an anticipatory response, in other words they may induce it before they plunge into the water. It may also be turned off upon the proper information from the telereceptors. Seals approaching the surface after a dive may show a decrease in the bradycardia. If the animal interrupts the ascent and continues to stay under water, the bradycardia returns (see[21]).

Nothing is known about what central nervous structures may mediate these anticipatory responses but it seems most likely that neocortical or limbic-hypothalamic areas are involved in this complex pattern.

In 1959 Folkow, Johansson and Öberg[5] found an area in the anterior hypothalamus where stimulation caused a marked depression of blood pressure and heart rate. There was a generalized decrease in sympathetic activity as well as an increased vagal tone on the heart. Löfving[18] found that this hypothalamic area participates in a more complex inhibitory system, originating from the anterior cingulate gyrus and acting on a sympatho-inhibitory area in the medulla where the baroreceptor afferents relay.

It was found by Folkow and co-workers that if baroreceptors are unloaded, the effects of inhibitory area stimulation are greatly augmented. This could, of course, be explained by the simple fact that there then was more sympathetic tone to inhibit but there seems to be an interesting interrelationship between the topically induced pattern and the baroreceptor reflexes.

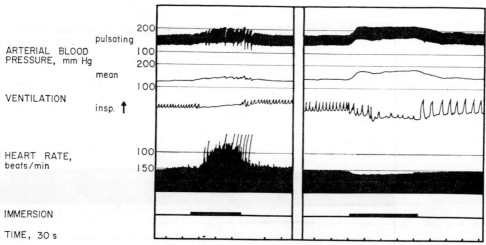

Fig. 3. "Chronically" decerebrate cat, third day postoperative. The brain stem was completely divided in the intercollicular region. During this experiment, the trachea was cannulated and the head was submerged in such a way that the animal could breathe freely through the cannula. Note the respiratory arrest and bradycardia during the simulated dive. After vagotomy in the neck (second panel) no bradycardia occurred.

For quite a long time there has been evidence that the diencephalon may participate in the tonic regulation of blood pressure. Hilton and Spyer[11] found that the effects of baroreceptor activation were decreased if the inhibitory area was destroyed. Baroreceptor activation also caused an increased activity in neurons in this area. Therefore, they envisaged the central relay station for the baroreceptor reflexes as an elongated neuron pool, stretching from the medulla oblongata through the brain stem to the rostral hypothalamus.

Stimulation in this area also affects the gastrointestinal system. There is a marked inhibition of sympathetic tone in the gastrointestinal tract leading to increased motility[12]. There is evidence that the baroreceptor reflexes do not affect gastrointestinal motility, provided that the adrenals are eliminated[7]. This must mean that the inhibitory area subserves more functions than to participate in the baroreceptor reflexes.

Dr. Delbro and I have recently investigated the influence of inhibitory area stimulation on the spinal sympathetic gastrointestino-gastrointestinal reflex. Previous experiments concerning gastric motility were carried out in laparotomized animals where the activity of this reflex could be presumed to be high due to the operative trauma. Possibly, the effect of inhibitory area stimulation would be quite different in nonlaparotomized animals. We therefore performed the experiments on cats with a chronic Thiry Vella loop. When they had recovered from the operation, they were subjected to an acute experiment. In these animals, with no acute abdominal irritation, inhibitory area stimulation had no effect on gastric motility (Fig. 4). But an identical stimulation, carried out when the gastrointestino-gastrointestinal reflex was activated by distension of the intestinal loop[7], caused a marked increase in gastric tone (Fig. 5).

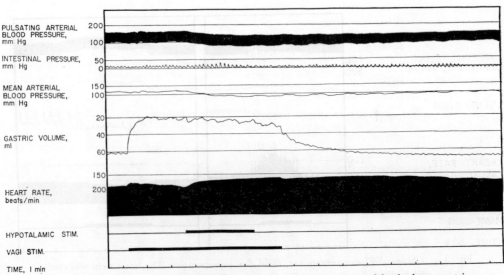

Fig. 4.   Cat with Thiry Vella loop, chloralosed. Pressure was measured in the loop, gastric volume was recorded with the balloon method and the cut vagi were efferently stimulated in the neck. Inhibitory area stimulation causes no change in gastric tone when performed against a background of submaximal efferent vagal stimulation.

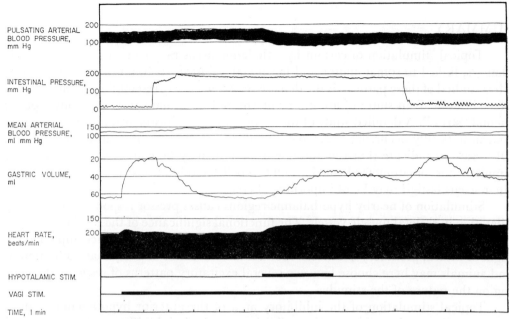

PULSATING ARTERIAL
BLOOD PRESSURE,
mm Hg

INTESTINAL PRESSURE,
mm Hg

MEAN ARTERIAL
BLOOD PRESSURE,
ml mm Hg

GASTRIC VOLUME,
ml

HEART RATE,
beats/min

HYPOTALAMIC STIM.

VAGI STIM.

TIME, 1 min

Fig. 5.   Same animal as in Fig. 4. Distension of the isolated intestinal loop causes a marked
inhibition of vagally elicited gastric tone. In this situation, an identical hypothalamic
stimulation (50 Hz, one msec, 0.2 mA) elicits a decrease in gastric volume.

These data are compatible with a hypothalamic inhibition of the gastrointestino-
gastrointestinal reflex. It is interesting to note that the medullary depressor area, which
was suggested by Löfving[18] as a relay station for the cardiovascular effects both of
central and reflex origin also seems to exert an inhibitory influence on this spinal
reflex[13].

It is unclear whether the adjustments induced from the inhibitory area correspond
to a well-defined behavior. Hypothalamic stimulation in unanesthetized animals has
in our hands not given any clear answer, probably because the area is intermingled
with neurons not functionally related. Löfving[18] performed a limited number of pilot
experiments with stimulation in the anterior cingulate gyrus, observing an inhibition
of behavior and a decreased muscle tone. He suggested that this response was activated
in emotional fainting and also in the so-called "playing dead" reaction exhibited by
animals like the opossum as an important protection behavior. It is certainly true that
both humans and other animals can react with an overall inhibition in the face of some
types of situations, characterized by despair, hopelessness and a feeling of being
"cornered". Whether the inhibitory reaction is involved in this efferent pattern or not
cannot be stated at present.

However, this type of naturally occurring withdrawal response illustrates that
there is a wide spectrum of somato-autonomic reactions that can be initiated by the
higher levels of the central nervous system.

SUMMARY

Topical stimulation of certain hypothalamic areas may cause drastic autonomic changes, linked to somatomotor and hormonal adjustments in an integrated fashion. Most studied of these patterns is the defense reaction, closely resembling changes taking place in animals in states of arousal or alarm and in humans under various types of mental "stress". A detailed study of the cardiovascular adjustments, however, suggests that in naturally occurring behavior the autonomic changes are still more complex. Observations indicate that the autonomic pattern may be constantly modulated by simultaneous somatomotor behavior and cerebellar modulations via the anterior lobe; the nucleus fastigii may be of importance here.

Stimulation of nearby hypothalamic regions causes pressor responses without any dilatation in skeletal muscle vessels. The functional significance of these effects remains obscure. In unanesthetized animals, the pressor responses may be accompanied by flight or attack, predatory behavior or food intake. It is not unlikely that both humans and animals may here choose between several excitatory patterns of response depending on the nature of the stimulus.

Topical stimulation of the inhibitory area of the anterior hypothalamus causes in the cardiovascular system a generalized sympathetic inhibition and an increased vagal tone on the heart. It has been suggested that this response pattern is associated with emotional situations leading to inhibitory responses seen in "mental shock" situations in humans, sometimes escalating into emotional fainting and also with the "playing dead reaction", occurring in some species in certain situations of danger where escape or attack seems impossible.

REFERENCES

1 Bard, P. and Macht, M. B., The behaviour of chronically decerebrate cats. In: G. E. W. Wolstenholme and M. O'Connor (Eds.), *Ciba Foundation Symposium on the Neurological Basis of Behaviour*, J. & A. Churchill Ltd., London, 1958, pp. 55–75.

2 Cannon, W. B., *Bodily Changes in Pain, Hunger, Fear and Rage*, Appleton, New York and London, 1929.

3 Cannon, W. B. and Lieb, C. W., The receptive relaxation of the stomach, *Amer. J. Physiol.*, 29 (1911) 262–273.

4 Djojosugito, A. M., Folkow, B., Lisander, B. and Sparks, H., Mechanism of escape of skeletal muscle resistance vessels from the influence of sympathetic cholinergic vasodilator fibre activity, *Acta physiol. scand.*, 72 (1968) 148–156.

5 Folkow, B., Johansson, B. and Öberg, B., A hypothalamic structure with a marked inhibitory effect on tonic sympathetic activity, *Acta physiol. scand.*, 47 (1959) 262–270.

6 Folkow, B. and Rubinstein, E., Behavioural and autonomic patterns evoked by stimulation of the lateral hypothalamic area in the cat, *Acta physiol. scand.*, 65 (1965) 292–299.

7 Furness, J. B. and Costa, M., The adrenergic innervation of the gastrointestinal tract, *Reviews of Physiology*, 69 (1974) 1–51.

8 Hallbäck, M. and Folkow, B., Cardiovascular responses to acute mental "stress" in spontaneously hypertensive rats, *Acta physiol. scand.*, 90 (1974) 684–698.

9 Hallbäck, M., Magnusson, G. and Weiss, L., Stress-induced ulcer in spontaneously hypertensive rats, *Acta physiol. scand.*, 91 (1974) 6A–7A.

10 Hess, W. R., *Functional Organization of the Diencephalon*, Grune & Stratton, New York, 1957.

11 Hilton, S. M. and Spyer, K. M., Participation of the anterior hypothalamus in the baroreceptor reflex, *J. Physiol.* (Lond.), 218 (1971) 271–293.

12 Jansson, G., Lisander, B. and Martinson, J., Hypothalamic control of the adrenergic outflow to the stomach in the cat, *Acta physiol. scand.*, 75 (1969) 176–186.

13 Johansson, B., Jonsson, O. and Ljung, B., Supraspinal control of the intestino-intestinal inhibitory reflex, *Acta physiol. scand.*, 63 (1965) 442–449.

14 Karplus, J. P. and Kreidl, A., Gehirn und Sympathicus; VII. Mitteilung. Über Beziehungen der Hypothalamuszentren zu Blutdruck und innerer Sekretion, *Pflügers Arch.*, 215 (1927) 667–672.

15 Lisander, B., The hypothalamus and vagally mediated gastric relaxation, *Acta physiol. scand.*, 93 (1975) 1–9.

16 Lisander, B. and Martner, J., Cerebellar suppression of the autonomic components of the defence reaction, *Acta physiol. scand.*, 81 (1971) 84–95.

17 Lisander, B. and Martner, J., Behavioural signs of emotional excitement from fastigial stimulation in "chronically" decerebrate cats, *Acta physiol. scand.*, 95 (1975) 350–352.

18 Löfving, B., Cardiovascular adjustments induced from the rostral cingulate gyrus, *Acta physiol. scand.*, 53, suppl. 184 (1961) 1–82.

19 MacLean, P. D., The triune brain, emotion and scientific bias. In: F. O. Schmitt (Ed.), *The Neurosciences, Second Study Program*, Rockefeller University Press, New York, 1970, pp. 336–349.

20 Martner, J., Cerebellar influences on autonomic mechanisms. An experimental study in the cat with special reference to the fastigial nucleus, *Acta physiol. scand.*, 94, suppl. 425 (1975) 1–42.

21 Martner, J., Wadenvik, H. and Lisander, B., Apnoea and bradycardia from submersion in "chronically" decerebrated cats, *Acta physiol. scand.*, 101 (1977) 476–480.

22 Ranson, S. W. and Magoun, H. W., The hypothalamus, *Ergebn. Physiol.*, 41 (1939) 56–163.

23 Reis, D. J., Doba, N. and Nathan, M. A., Predatory attack, grooming and consummatory behaviour evoked by electrical stimulation of cat cerebellar nuclei, *Science*, 23 (1973) 845–847.

24 Wolf, S. and Wolff, H. G., *Human Gastric Function. An Experimental Study of a Man and his Stomach*, Oxford University Press, New York, 1943.

25 Zanchetti, A., Hypothalamic control of circulation. In: S. Julius and M. D. Esler (Eds.), *The Nervous System in Arterial Hypertension*, C. C. Thomas, Springfield, Ill., 1976, pp. 397–428.

26 Zanchetti, A. and Zoccolini, A., Autonomic hypothalamic outbursts elicited by cerebellar stimulation, *J. Neurophysiol.*, 17 (1954) 475–483.

SECTION VI

HOMEOSTASIS AND THE MAINTENANCE
OF BALANCED STATES

There are three inseparable but somewhat different roles played by the centers which regulate body functions and behavior. The control and integrative action required are carried on primarily by centers of the brain and spinal cord but, as stated previously, some interactions occur peripherally which are also determinant of response patterns. The autonomic system is highly involved in all three of these roles which are: 1) the initiation and control of behavior appropriate to the prevailing situation, 2) the use of recall in the direction of activity and in anticipation and perception of what may be required and 3) the maintenance of required constancies and balances in body states. This latter is the subject of the next section of this publication.

The aspect of the physiology of homeostasis which will be discussed is the interaction which occurs between reflexes, somatic and autonomic systems and the sympathetic and parasympathetic divisions of the autonomic system in the maintenance of certain constancies.

One of the most remarkable constancies observed in humans and other mammals is temperature homeostasis. The entire body is, of course, involved, but the modulatory-controlling activity of the autonomic system is responsible for the great refinements attained.

Homeostasis is not passively maintained. We generally consider reflexes as components of active performance to meet a behavioral need. As soon as one begins to consider maintenance of states, the mechanisms maintaining homeostasis, it becomes apparent that some receptors, at least, can be thought of as detecting imbalances and of initiating corrective reactions. Certainly, chemoreceptors and baroreceptors can be considered from this point of view as has been done in this section.

Those control mechanisms which maintain homeostasis and balanced states, even when the organism is subject to stress or when required to engage in violent activity, act to a large extent through the autonomic system although the somatic system is often extensively involved. The integrative action of the autonomic system is essential.

There is one final point which will be emphasized in this section. Claude Bernard's term, constancy of the internal environment, and Cannon's term homeostasis, convey the concept of fixity. These theoretical constancies are seldom observed. The point is, that there is resistance to imbalances and there are reactions which restore balances. In the course of normal living there is a constant interplay of homeostatic forces rather than maintenance of "locked in" unvaried states.

CHAPTER 30

AUTONOMIC NERVOUS CONTROL OF TEMPERATURE HOMEOSTASIS

W. Riedel* and M. Iriki**

*Max-Planck-Institut für Physiologische und Klinische Forschung, W. G. Kerckhoff-Institut, Bad Nauheim, Federal Republic of Germany, and **Tokyo Metropolitan Institute of Gerontology, Tokyo, Japan*

INTRODUCTION

Homeothermy differentiates certain classes of animals including humans as being "higher animals" and expresses the fact that these living beings maintain a constant internal body temperature despite wide changes in the environmental temperature. Homeothermy is consistent with the idea of a constant "milieu interieur"[4], temperature being one of the constants preserved by regulated physiological processes.

Speculating about the increasing complexity of physiological regulation during the course of evolution, Adolph[1] has indicated that "genetic selection may favor a combination of regulations that reinforce one another. That combination integrates regulation. One can regard such integration as a higher-level regulation. Further, one may imagine that hierarchies of regulation exist".

That this concept particularly characterizes the temperature regulation system has been confirmed by investigations of autonomic mechanisms involved in temperature homeostasis. This system is characterized by multiple representation of thermoregulatory controller functions at different levels of the central nervous axis at which multiple thermal inputs converge and by which multiple effector functions are controlled[60]. Temperature regulation may thus be characterized as a multilevel control system, with the hypothalamus as the highest level of integration[54]. This system has successfully been put into control loop categories by postulating that the signals of multiple peripheral and inner warm and cold sensors converge onto the temperature controlling network at the hypothalamic level. Concepts like those put forward by Bligh[6] and Hammel[26] explain why by local heating or cooling of the skin, the spinal cord or the hypothalamus, qualitatively identical heat loss or heat producing effector responses are elicited.

The autonomic nervous system is essentially involved in temperature regulation but controls many effectors which seem at first glance not related to temperature regulation. However, by "combination of regulations" the autonomic nervous contributions to temperature regulation are linked with various other control functions which mutually influence each other. Under this aspect varying effector responses may occur in response to a particular disturbance of the internal milieu depending on the afferent input profile impinging upon the various levels of the hierarchically-organized controlling system.

Although the integrity of the thermosensitive preoptic-anterior hypothalamic region and the input of the peripheral thermoreceptors are essential for normal thermoregulation, the sensors of this hypothalamic region do not exclusively provide the information needed relative to deep body temperature. Evidence has been presented for existence of medullary[39], spinal[61,62] and extracentral deep body temperature sensors[47,50], by recording their activity or by observing specific thermoregulatory effector responses elicited by their adequate stimulation. Thermoregulatory responses have been obtained from decerebrated[5,12], medullary[13] and spinal animals[68,69]. These findings indicate, in support of Thauer's[65] view, the existence of similar controlling networks operating at different levels of the neuraxis.

The Jacksonian concept of levels of central nervous functions precisely describes the organization of the autonomic nervous system making it but little different from the somatic in this regard[29]. This implies that its organization can be characterized as having a segmental arrangement extending from the spinal level to the brain stem. Particularly, the sympathetic division reflects this principle of organization but also the parasympathetic divison conforms to it though in a less obvious manner. As emphasized by Koizumi and Brooks[34] and Sato and Schmidt[55], the basic functional organization of the autonomic nervous system lies in its reflex arcs. Their intrinsic, segmentally organized control and the suprasegmental pathways converging on it establish the specificity present in the organization of the spinal sympathetic outflow[3]. This principle of organization does not, however, preclude seemingly generalized reactions, for instance those required in emergency situations[9] and others induced by particular experimental conditions.

It seems obvious that the similarity between the multilevel organization of the temperature regulation system and the segmentally arranged autonomic nervous system facilitates their interactions. Thus, a subtle control of complex patterns of autonomic effector functions should be expected in the maintenance of body temperature. On the other hand, generalized and widespread autonomic actions could be mediated under particular conditions of thermal stress as well. Both types of adaptative reactions can be observed in the homeothermic organism when it reacts to changes in its thermal environment.

RESULTS AND DISCUSSION

In an emergency situation of exposure to extreme cold the dominant role in initiating both the heat production and heat conservation mechanisms has been ascribed to the action of catecholamines liberated by the sympatho-adrenal system either locally or systemically[10]. Increased sympathetic discharge to peripheral blood vessels or the piloerectors increases peripheral insulation and consequently decreases heat loss to the environment, while by simultaneous activation of the adrenal medulla adrenaline is liberated[37] providing by its lipolytic and glycogenolytic action for extra thermogenesis; thus it constitutes one of the main hormones for cold defense. In the chronic adaptive and regulatory adjustments to cold, however, the more or less uniform action of the hormone adrenaline seems to be replaced by specific neural control exerted by the sympatho-adrenal system to "influence excessively separate organs or functions"[9], in order to economize the final common effector output according to the specific situation. This can be seen in the selective mobilization of metabolic substrates, in response to energy needs signalled by cold, which is evidently a function of the sympathetic nervous system[7]. Evidence has been presented that adipose tissue cells are innervated by sympathetic noradrenergic fibers[27] and that these efferents can activate in response to cold-specific enzyme reactions in the lipolysis-fatty acid esterification cycle[40]. This refers particularly to brown adipose tissue. The very selective nature of its sympathetic innervation, however, is demonstrated by the finding that simultaneously the vasomotor tone to adipose tissue, acting on α-adrenergic receptors, decreases. Whereas the thermogenetic effect can be abolished by β-blockade, the cold induced increase of blood flow, although reduced, still occurs[8,64]. This finding suggests the existence of functionally different populations of sympathetic fibers. A dual nervous supply has been considered by Derry and co-workers[16]. The action of nerves on adipose tissue during exposure to cold thus demonstrates how, by the integrative action of the autonomic nervous system, the final common effector response is optimized since heat as well as energy substrate flow is increased towards the tissues which demand it.

Whereas sympathetic control of both glucose and lipid mobilization and metabolism is amply documented in temperature regulation, corresponding parasympathetic control functions are highly hypothetical. There exists circumstantial evidence for a reduction of cold induced adrenergic activation of energy metabolism by stimulation of central parasympathetic nuclei[14]. However, direct evidence of cholinergic links in the neural control of lipid metabolism in temperature regulation has not yet been found.

The endocrine pancreas plays a key role in glucose metabolism and is apparently influenced by both the sympathetic and parasympathetic nerves[11,19,38,42,71]. Some nerve fibers enter the pancreatic islets independently of their vasculature supply[28]. On the basis of different effects of α- and β-adrenergic blockers on insulin production, Porte and Robertson[46] concluded that there is a balanced α- and β-adrenergic tone in islet innervation. These authors have shown that hypothermia is associated with a complete inhibition of the insulin response to glucose and glucagon, an effect which could be abolished by α-adrenergic blockade. An increase in blood glucose level which was abolished by splanchnicotomy was found during hypothalamic cooling[2]; it was ascribed to the simultaneously increased adrenaline secretion. However, the concept of a neural control of insulin effects on glucose metabolism has never attracted much interest either in studies of thermoregulation or other metabolic processes.

Considering the constancy of body temperature as the result of balanced heat production and heat loss, it is not surprising that the autonomic nervous system is fundamentally engaged in the control of convective and evaporative heat flow adjustments, making, thereby, the circulatory system the main effector system of body temperature regulation.

The extent to which the core is insulated from the environment depends on the characteristics of blood flow through the shell. Thus, surface circulation is one of the most important and specific thermoregulatory effector systems. Its vascular innervation, whether constrictor or dilator, is predominantly sympathetic. A decrease of cutaneous blood flow represents a cold defense response by reducing heat transfer from the core to the shell while the simultaneous diversion of blood flow to the body core favors heat storage. On exposure to heat, blood flow is diverted from the body core to the shell, increasing heat transfer to the heat-dissipating surfaces which are the skin and, particularly in panting animals, the mucosal surfaces of the upper respiratory tract.

Evidence for a subtle control of circulatory functions by the autonomic nervous system was first indicated by the generation of differential vasomotor response patterns which occur in thermoregulation. This differentiation was found to account for the patterns of antagonistic blood flow adjustments in peripheral and inner vascular beds as shown in Fig. 1. These patterns are the typical circulatory response not only to stimulation of cutaneous thermoreceptors by the environment[48] but also to adequate temperature stimulation of thermoreceptors within the body core, such as those of the central thermodetector regions in the hypothalamus[56,57] or the spinal cord[36]. Figure 1 additionally shows that despite considerable changes in regional blood flow the arterial pressure is not affected. This pattern preserves, by combinations of regulatory actions, not only temperature but also blood pressure homeostasis. The proof of the neural origin of this homeostatic response pattern was contributed by a series of investigations in rabbits in which direct recording of the regional activities of sym-

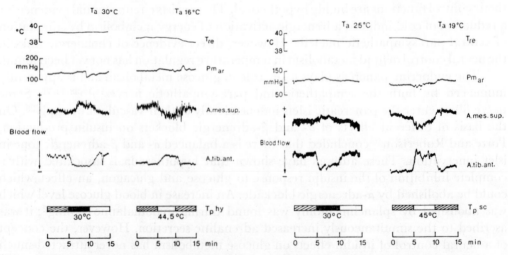

Fig. 1.   Antagonistic blood flow changes in intestine (A. mes. sup.) and skin (A. tib. ant.) of conscious dogs during hypothalamic (left side) and spinal (right side) thermal stimulation. Blood flow values were obtained using electromagnetic flowmeters. T_a: ambient air temperature; T_{re}: rectal temperature; Pm_{ar}: arterial mean pressure; $T_p$hy: hypothalamic perfusion temperature; $T_p$sc: spinal canal perfusion temperature. Cooling (black bar), heating (white bar), perfusion with water at core temperature (hatched bars). (From Schönung et al.[57].)

pathetic efferents was performed during central and peripheral thermal stimulation[30,49,67]. The results have unequivocally and for the first time shown that the entire cardiovascular response pattern is based on the ability of the sympathetic nervous system to differentiate its outflow up to the degree of reciprocal changes occurring in the concurrent activity. The stereotype shape of this integrated cardiovascular response to adequate temperature stimulation of thermosensitive regions so different as the hypothalamus, the spinal cord and the skin makes it unlikely to have been the result of nonspecific reflex activations. This integrated regulatory response conforms to Adolph's[1] concept of a "combination of regulations" and implies that all sections of the sympathetic outflow are involved in the homeostatic function of this thermally induced pattern of differential circulatory adjustment.

Concerning cardiac control in temperature regulation, homeothermic animals including humans respond to a rise of core temperature with an increase in heart rate. Cardiac output rises more steeply with body temperature than does heart rate because both its components, heart rate and stroke volume, increase with body temperature[66]. The conclusion that cardiac sympathetic activity thus changes in a direction opposite to cutaneous sympathetic activity was confirmed by direct simultaneous recording from branches of both sections[31]. In response to spinal heating, cardiac sympathetic total discharge activity increased and decreased during spinal cooling. A corresponding increase or decrease in heart rate could, however, be observed in vagotomized animals only, suggesting that both sympathetic and vagal efferents contribute to the heart rate response.

The involvement of renal innervation in autonomic thermoregulatory adjustments has been disclosed by recording from renal sympathetic efferents simultaneously with recording of preganglionic splanchnic activity. The activity of both efferents increased on peripheral warming and decreased on peripheral cooling. Also in the unanesthetized, freely moving rabbit renal efferent activity increased at warm ambient temperatures while during cold defense activation, either by pyrogen or by external cooling, the activity was lowered and thus responded antagonistically to activity changes occurring in the skin. These results are consistent with findings of Ninomiya and Fujita[43] obtained during peripheral and brain heating and cooling in anesthetized cats. Although at first glance a direct relationship between adjustments of renal sympathetic nerve activity and temperature homeostasis is not obvious, renal participation might contribute to the homeostasis of body fluid under conditions imposed by thermal disturbances.

The obvious homeostatic function of the thermoregulatory pattern of cardiovascular adjustments, by which heat transfer from the body core to the surface is established, has only roughly been disclosed by means of mass discharge recordings which have demonstrated regional differentiation in sympathetic outflow to diverse sections of the cardiovascular system. There is increasing evidence that the sympathetic and probably also the parasympathetic system is able to exert a finer control by selective innervation of structures subserving particular functions within a certain cardiovascular system section or an organ.

A recently disclosed example is the participation of vasodilator fibers in the augmentation of skin blood flow under thermal conditions which supplements the reduction of vasoconstrictor tone, at least in some species. It has been shown that after exclusion of adrenergic and cholinergic transmitter mechanisms by reserpine and atropine, heating the spinal cord in dogs[58] or the hypothalamus or the trunk skin[44] induced an increase of blood flow in the skin, and in the mucosa of the tongue[45]. Electrical stimulation of sympathetic fibers under these conditions elicited a vasodilatation which ganglionic blockade or nervous section abolished. A neurogenic cutaneous vasodilator component in heat stress has also been inferred for humans[17,21,53] and the baboon[25] from hemodynamic studies. Direct support for this hypothesis required the analysis of cutaneous vasomotor innervation by recording single unit activity. Corresponding studies of the innervation of the cat's hind leg have revealed a distinct population of sympathetic fibers that could only be activated by heat and could be clearly distinguished from the vasoconstrictor, pilomotor and sudomotor populations[23]. Their graded response to a spinal heat stimulus together with that of a vasoconstrictor fiber is shown in Fig. 2. It is obvious that both fiber populations are influenced by spinal heat stimulus in a reciprocal manner. Also in the innervation of the rabbit's ear, filaments were found which increased their activity only during spinal heating, whereas spinal cooling was without any effect on their activity despite a fall in ear temperature. From the results presented in Fig. 2 one may conclude that the specifically heat activated vasodilators may operate independently of the vasoconstrictors and the sudomotor population, thus establishing a selective control of heat dissipation at the body's surface.

These findings show that within the vasomotor supply of a given cardiovascular field nonuniformity of vasomotor outflow can be found; its differential activation apparently depends on specific components within the entire afferent input profile. According to this notion, and considering the similarity of the multilevel temperature control system and the segmentally arranged autonomic nervous system, thermal and cardiovascular inputs at different levels of the neuraxis should induce an inhomogeneity of autonomic activity in other sections of the cardiovascular system. This inhomogeneity should vary with the variation of the input profile. Indeed, by combined peripheral and central thermal stimulation under differing circulatory conditions, varying patterns of nonuniformity, up to the degree of reciprocal changing activity, could be found in the innervation of the heart and the kidney in rabbits. Figure 3 demonstrates simultaneously recorded activity of two sympathetic filaments of the right heart during spinal heating in animals held at warm ambient temperatures after sinoaortic denervation and vagotomy. The activity of both filaments was completely depressed by a noradrenaline-induced blood pressure rise prior to denervation. The activity of only one filament (R. ant.) showed a consistent relationship to heart rate when it was increased during spinal heating or decreased during spinal cooling or hypercapnia. The activity of the other filament (R. post.) was diminished during spinal heating but activated during hypercapnia. These reciprocal changes of activity indicate the existence of two functionally different fiber populations of sympathetic efferents in the innervation of the heart. Further analysis by simultaneous records from two single fiber preparations in the vagotomized rabbit revealed that the activity of the cardioaccelerator population was predominantly influenced by central temperature signals causing inhibition by cooling and activation by heating. The activity of the other

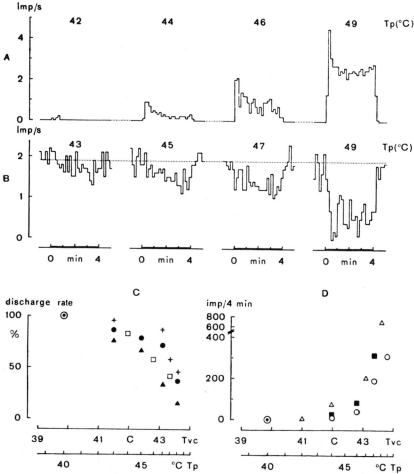

Fig. 2. Quantitative responses of spontaneously active and silent cutaneous postganglionic
neurons to spinal cord heating of variable temperatures. A: Silent postganglionic
neuron to the hairy skin. B: Spontaneously active postganglionic neuron to the hairless
skin. The dotted lines denote the prestimulation activity. C, D: Relation between the
temperature induced by spinal cord heating and activity in four spontaneously
active postganglionic neurons (C) and three silent postganglionic neurons (D).
The ordinate scales indicate the depression of the activity (C) and the excitation (D)
during the four-min stimulation periods. T_p: perfusion temperature; T_{vc}: vertebral
canal temperature close to the thermode as evaluated by Simon and Iriki[62]. (From
Gregor et al.[23].)

fiber population was activated by central warm stimulation at cold ambient temperature but inhibited during central heating at warm ambient temperature. Since under
these conditions cardiac output changed in the same direction as the activity of this
fiber population it may have influenced myocardial function. There are reports[52]
that in humans under conditions of external heat and dehydration the two components
of cardiac output, namely heart rate and stroke volume, change in an inverse relationship unrelated to central venous pressure.

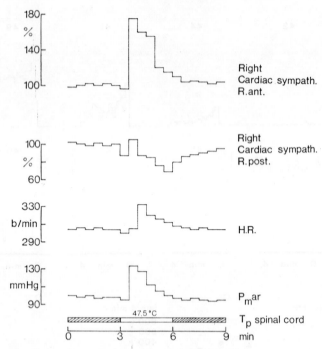

Fig. 3.   Simultaneously recorded activity of two sympathetic filaments (R. ant. and R. post.)
innervating the right heart during spinal heating at warm ambient temperature.
Sinoaortic denervated and vagotomized rabbit. H. R.: heart rate; $P_m$ar: arterial
mean pressure. Thermal stimulation parameters as in Fig. 1.

The same nonuniformity could be found in renal innervation when combined
peripheral and central thermal stimuli were simultaneously applied. Using the single
fiber technique two fiber populations could be discriminated in the sympathetic vasomotor supply to the kidney by their different spike heights and by their different
susceptibilities to vasoactive drugs. Both populations were inhibited by either electrical
baroreceptor stimulation or by a blood pressure rise caused by systemic application of
noradrenaline. However, in response to a similar blood pressure rise caused by systemic
application of angiotensin, one population (A) was considerably activated, whereas
the other (B), the one discharging with larger spikes, was completely depressed.
The same phenomenon of differential sensitivity to these vasoactive drugs was also
observed in preganglionic sympathetic fibers and indicates a central activating action
of angiotensin on a particular population of sympathetic fibers[51]. As shown in Fig. 4
these two fiber populations, A and B, were oppositely influenced by central heat
stimulation. In addition, the direction of the activity change of each population depended on the external thermal condition. The same dependence on or setting by
external thermal conditions was found for the response to spinal cooling, however,
both populations reacted equidirectionally to this stimulus.

The effects of different combinations of thermal inputs on the sympathetic
cardiovascular innervation have elucidated the phenomenon of sympathetic differentiation at two levels of resolution depending on whether mass discharges to different

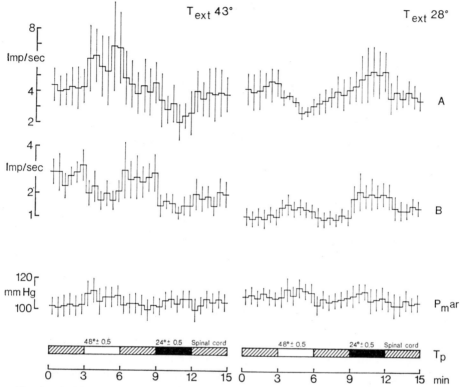

Fig. 4. Activity changes of renal sympathetic efferents (fiber population A and B) and changes of arterial mean pressure (P_mar) as influenced by spinal heating and cooling at warm (left side) and cold ambient temperature (right side). Mean values from eight rabbits with standard deviations. Thermal stimulation parameters as in Fig. 1.

organs or single fiber activity in the supply to a particular organ were analyzed. In the first case it has been shown that the pattern of reciprocal differentiation is, in qualitative respects, largely independent of the site of thermal stimulation. In the second case, changing contributions of fiber populations to the activation of single organs were found when the profile of thermal input was changed.

Considering the similarity between the multilevel temperature regulation system and the segmentally organized sympathetic system, similar degrees of patterning of sympathetic outflow can be expected when the interaction between a given thermal stimulus and varying inputs from the baroceptive afferents of the circulation are investigated. Analysis of mass discharge recordings from sympathetic branches to the skin, heart and intestine after sinoaortic denervation and vagotomy has shown that the differentiated sympathetic response pattern known from the normal animal was qualitatively preserved and was demonstrable by the response to spinal heat stimulus[63]. Hemodynamic studies have further shown that the differentiated response of cardio-vascular innervation to both hypothalamic heating and cooling was not qualitatively changed by sinoaortic denervation and vagotomy[22]. However, loss of blood pressure homeostasis was observed during spinal heating and on spinal cooling not only blood pressure homeostasis was lost, but the response pattern was qualitatively altered in that the splanchnic reaction changed from inhibition to activation. These results suggest two conclusions: First, the pattern of thermally induced sympathetic differentiation is, in principle, generated without essentially involving the baroreflex system. Second, the baroreflex input normally modulates part of the sympathetic outflow in a quantitative manner to preserve pressure homeostasis and the loss of this modulation may, at particular thermal input profiles, even lead to a qualitative change of response in one or more divisions of the cardiovascular innervation. The nature of modulation of sympathetic differentiation by the baroreceptor signal may be that it alters the responsiveness of medullary or spinal sympathetic neurons to thermoregulatory drives or vice versa. This hypothesis has been tested with a method by which baroreceptor response curves of total renal nervous activity were obtained in unanesthetized rabbits during graded variations of the arterial blood pressure by means of aortic and v. cava balloons. Under conditions of cold defense induced either by external cooling or in the initial febrile phase, the slope of the baroreceptor response curve was found to be substantially decreased and its threshold shifted to higher blood pressure values as compared to the slope obtained during external heating. This response has verified that mutual modulations of thermal and baroreflex responses of cardiovascular innervation do, in fact, occur. It may further be inferred that changes of regional sympathetic activity induced by changes of the thermal input profile may be quantitatively modulated by baroreceptor signals, however they are dependent on the actual arterial pressure to an extent which even includes change of direction.

Considering the results of single unit studies under conditions of thermal stimulation, qualitative modulation of the sympathetic outflow by baroreceptor signals might be brought about by influences on only a particular population within the vasomotor outflow or by differential effects on several populations. The same relationship may apply for the other types of afferents constituting the entire receptive cardiovascular input profile. According to Korner and Uther[35] this includes the input from chemoreceptor afferents which, by itself, may induce a pattern of sympathetic differentiation clearly distinct from the induced in thermoregulation[31].

There remain a few special effector systems which supplement the circulatory adjustments of the surface to the benefit of temperature homeostasis in either heat stress or cold defense. Some animals such as cattle, horses, sheep and goats and also humans are able to increase heat transfer from the skin to the environment by evaporation of sweat. The sweat glands have been shown to be under sympathetic control, the transmitter involved, however, has been identified as either acetylcholine[15] or adrenaline[20]. By correlation of neural activity to the skin with the fast, atropine-sensitive skin potential[70] and by observing the responses to thermal stimuli, to various other somatic stimuli and to chemoreceptor stimulation, the sudomotor population can be distinctly discriminated from the vasoconstrictor, vasodilatator and pilomotor population[23,33]. That the neuronal activation of sweat glands may occur independently from the changes of the vasomotor tone in the skin or the local circulatory conditions has been shown by McCook and co-workers[41]. Differential sudomotor and vasomotor responses can be elicited in heated subjects when rapidly shifted from a hot to a cool

environment or vice versa, cutaneous vasodilatation either preceding or following
the onset of sweating.

Erection of hairs in furred animals but also, ineffectively, in humans, and ruffling
of feathers in birds are characteristic responses to cold. It improves insulation by
increasing the amount of air held close to the body surface and is usually accompanied
by postural changes. The reactions are the results of sympathetic fiber discharges to
the piloerector muscles. That these fibers can differentially respond at least with
regard to the sequence of their activation to somatic stimuli and asphyxia has been
shown by Grosse and Jänig[24].

The role of the parasympathetic nervous system in temperature regulation has
garnered much less interest until now, probably because it contributes to only a few
special mechanisms. However, the parasympathetic nervous system may be, in principle, equally important in thermoregulation, although not in the general manner
true for the sympathetic system. As mentioned earlier, vagal efferents are apparently
activated simultaneously with cardiac sympathetic fibers, balancing the control of
heart rate response. Most important, however, is the activation of salivary glands and
the serous glands in the upper respiratory tract by parasympathetic secretory nerves[18]
in panting animals and animals which accomplish evaporative heat dissipation by
saliva spreading. Figure 5 demonstrates the observations of Sharp and Hammel[59]
on salivation and skin blood flow and body temperature of exercising and resting dogs
as influenced by hypothalamic heating and cooling. The positive correlation between
hypothalamic temperature and salivation on the one hand and increased skin blood
flow as estimated by the rise of ear pinna temperature on the other hand are completely
identical with the temperature response relationships found in the components of the
evaporative heat dissipating systems as respiratory rate and blood flow in the mucosa

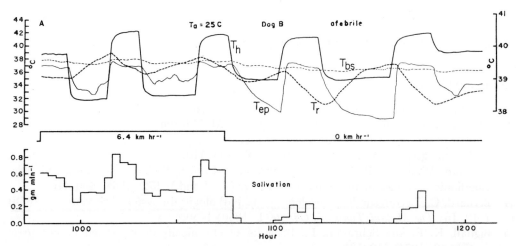

Fig. 5. Salivation rate (cannulated parotid duct), ear blood flow as estimated by ear pinna
temperature (T_{ep}), backskin temperature (T_{bs}) and rectal temperature (T_r) influenced by hypothalamic heating and cooling (T_h) in an afebrile dog at rest and during
exercise at an ambient temperature of 25°C. (From Sharp and Hammel[59].)

of the upper respiratory tract, which altogether constitute the integrated final common effector response of evaporative heat loss.

If one presumes that parasympathetic secretory nerves have mediated the thermoregulatory control of salivation rate, an activation of these nerve fibers has to be assumed under conditions at which there is an increased demand for heat loss. Other sections of the parasympathetic outflow may, however, react differently to the same stimulus as demonstrated by the results of Iriki and Kozawa[32]. Heating the spinal cord in rabbits elicited simultaneously with the typical thermoregulatory response of increased skin blood flow a decrease of activity in visceral vagal filaments. The reverse effect was obtained upon spinal cooling.

From these results it is obvious that the principle of differential efferent control in autonomic homeostatic adjustments, which has been established for the sympatho-adrenal system, is valid also for the parasympathetic system.

CONCLUSION

At different levels of the neuraxis the thermoregulatory control system interacts with the autonomic nervous system defining it a major role in temperature homeostasis. Both the sympathetic and the parasympathetic divisions control a multitude of specific thermoregulatory effector mechanisms. Of more general importance, however, appears the sympathetic system, which mediates in addition the circulatory adjustments required by the activities of the heat producing and the heat dissipating mechanisms. Depending on the entire thermal and cardiovascular input profile both autonomic divisions exhibit typical patterns of regional differentiated efferent outflow. In single fiber preparations functionally different fiber populations have been identified within the innervation of any investigated cardiovascular field. Their differential activation by the integrative action of the autonomic nervous system in thermoregulation enables a selective control of structures subserving particular functions, thus optimizing the final common effector response.

REFERENCES

1   Adolph, E. F., *Origins of Physiological Regulations*, Academic Press, New York, 1968.
2   Andersson, B., Ekman, B., Hökfelt, B., Jobin, M., Olsson, K. and Robertshaw, O., Studies of the importance of the thyroid and the sympathetic system in the defence to cold of the goat, *Acta physiol. scand.*, 69 (1967) 111–118.
3   Beacham, W. S. and Perl, E. R., Background and reflex discharge of sympathetic pre-ganglionic neurones in the spinal cat, *J. Physiol.* (Lond.), 172 (1964) 400–416.
4   Bernard, C., Lecons sur la physiologie et la pathologie du systeme nerveux, 1 (1858) 1–19. In: *The Medical Times and Gazette*, 1 (1860) 1–30.
5   Bignall, K. E. and Schramm, L., Behavior of chronically decerebrated kittens, *Exp. Neurol.*, 42 (1974) 519–531.
6   Bligh, J., Neuronal models of mammalian temperature regulation. In: J. Bligh and R. Moore (Eds.), *Essays on Temperature Regulation*, North-Holland, Amsterdam, 1972, pp. 105–120.
7   Brodie, B. B., Maickel, R. P. and Stern, D. N., Autonomic nervous system and adipose

tissue. In: A. E. Renold and G. F. Cahill, Jr. (Eds.), *Handbook of Physiology, Adipose Tissue*, Amer. Physiol. Soc., Washington, D. C., 1965, pp. 583–600.

8 Brück, K. and Wünnenberg, B., Untersuchungen über die Bedeutung des multilokulären Fettgewebes für die Thermogenese des neugeborenen Meerschweinchens, *Pflügers Arch.*, 283 (1965) 1–16.

9 Cannon, W. B., *Bodily Changes in Pain, Hunger, Fear and Rage*, C. T. Branford, Boston, Mass., 1953.

10 Cannon, W. B., Querido, A., Britton, S. W. and Bright, E. M., The role of adrenal secretion in the chemical control of body temperature, *Amer. J. Physiol.*, 79 (1927) 466–507.

11 Cegrell, L., Adrenergic nerves and monoamine-containing cells in the mammalian endocrine pancreas, *Acta physiol. scand.*, Suppl. 314 (1968) 17–23.

12 Chai, C. Y. and Lin, M. T., Effects of thermal stimulation of medulla oblongata and spinal cord on decerebrate rabbits, *J. Physiol.* (Lond.), (1973) 409–419.

13 Chambers, W. W., Seigel, M. S., Lin, J. C. and Lin, C. N., Thermoregulatory responses of decerebrate and spinal cats, *Exp. Neurol.*, 42 (1974) 282–299.

14 Choinowski, H., Bartsch, P., Rüdiger, W. and Werner, V., Die kalorische Wirkung des Adrenalins unter verschiedenen Umgebungstemperaturen und elektrischer hypothalamischer Reizung, *Acta biol. med. germ.*, 27 (1971) 269–278.

15 Dale, H. H. and Feldberg, W., The chemical transmission of secretory impulses to the sweat glands of the cat, *J. Physiol.* (Lond.), 82 (1934) 121–128.

16 Derry, D. M., Schönbaum, E. and Steiner, G., Two sympathetic nerve supplies to brown adipose tissue of the rat, *Canad. J. Physiol. Pharmacol.*, 47 (1969) 57–63.

17 Edholm, O. G., Fox, R. H. and MacPherson, R. K., The effect of cutaneous anaesthesia on skin blood flow, *J. Physiol.* (Lond.), 132 (1956) 15–16P.

18 Emmelin, N. G., Nervous control of salivary glands. In: C. F. Code (Ed.), *Handbook of Physiology, Alimentary Canal*, Vol. 2, Amer. Physiol. Soc., Washington, D. C., 1967, pp. 595–632.

19 Findlay, J. A., Gill, J. R., Lever, J. D., Randle, P. J. and Spriggs, T. L. B., Increased insulin output following stimulation of the vagal supply to the perfused rabbit pancreas, *J. Anat.*, 104 (1969) 580.

20 Findlay, J. D. and Robertshaw, D., The role of the sympatho-adrenal system in the control of sweating in the ox (Bos taurus), *J. Physiol.* (Lond.), 155 (1965) 72–85.

21 Fox, R. H. and Hilton, S. M., Sweat gland activity as a contributory factor to heat vasodilatation in the human skin, *J. Physiol.* (Lond.), 133 (1956) 68–69P.

22 Göbel, D., Martin, H. and Simon, E., Primary cardiac responses to stimulation of hypothalamic and spinal cord temperature sensors evaluated in anaesthetized paralyzed dogs, *J. Thermal Biology*, 2 (1977) 41–47.

23 Gregor, M., Jänig, W. and Riedel, W., Response pattern of cutaneous postganglionic neurones to the hind limb on spinal cord heating and cooling in the cat, *Pflügers Arch.*, 363 (1976) 135–140.

24 Grosse, M. and Jänig, W., Vasoconstrictor and pilomotor fibers in skin nerves to the cat's tail, *Pflügers Arch.*, 361 (1976) 221–229.

25 Hales, J. R. S., Rowell, L. B. and Strandness, D. E., Active cutaneous vasodilatation in the hyperthermic baboon, *Proc. Austr. Physiol. Pharmacol. Soc.*, 8 (1977) 70P.

26 Hammel, H. T., The set-point in temperature regulation: Analogy or reality. In: J. Bligh and R. Moore (Eds.), *Essays on Temperature Regulation*, North-Holland, Amsterdam, 1972, pp. 121–137.

27 Havel, R. J. and Goldfien, A., The role of the sympathetic nervous system in the metabolism of free fatty acids, *J. Lipid Res.*, 1 (1959) 102–108.

28 Heinzen, B. R., Observations on the innervation of the pancreatic islets, *Arch. Surg.*, 81 (1960) 627–631.

29 Ingram, W. R., Central autonomic mechanisms. In: J. Field, H. W. Magoun and V. E. Hall (Eds.), *Handbook of Physiology, Neurophysiology*, Vol. 2, Amer. Physiol. Soc., Washington, D. C., 1960, pp. 951–978.

30 Iriki, M., Riedel, W. and Simon, E., Regional differentiation of sympathetic activity during hypothalamic heating and cooling in anaesthetized rabbits, *Pflügers Arch.*, 328 (1971) 320–331.

31 Iriki, M., Riedel, W. and Simon, E., Patterns of differentiation in various sympathetic efferents induced by changes of blood gas composition and by central thermal stimulation in anesthetized rabbits, *Jap. J. Physiol.*, 22 (1972) 585–602.

32 Iriki, M. and Kozawa, E., The change of vagal activity evoked by spinal cord thermal stimulation in anesthetized rabbits, *Experientia*, 32 (1976) 1293–1294.

33 Jänig, W. and Kümmel, H., Functional discrimination of postganglionic neurones to the cat's hind paw with respect to the skin potentials recorded from the hairless skin, *Pflügers Arch.*, 371 (1977) 217–225.

34 Koizumi, K. and Brooks, C. McC., The integration of autonomic system reactions: A discussion of autonomic reflexes, their control and their association with somatic reactions, *Rev. Physiol. Biochem. Pharmacol.*, 67 (1972) 1–68

35 Korner, P. I. and Uther, J. B., Reflex autonomic control of heart rate and peripheral blood flow, *Brain Res.*, 87 (1975) 293–303.

36 Kullmann, R., Schönung, W. and Simon, E., Antagonistic changes of blood flow and sympathetic activity in different vascular beds following central thermal stimulation, *Pflügers Arch.*, 319 (1970) 146–161.

37 Leduc, J., Catecholamine production and release in exposure and acclimation to cold, *Acta physiol scand.*, 53, Suppl. 183 (1961) 1–101.

38 Libman, L. J. and Sutherland, S. D., An investigation into the intrinsic innervation of the pancreas, *J. Anat.*, 99 (1965) 420–421.

39 Lipton, J. M., Thermosensitivity of medulla oblongata in control of body temperature, *Amer. J. Physiol.*, 224 (1973) 890–897

40 Masoro, E. J., Effect of cold on metabolic use of lipids, *Physiol. Rev.*, 46 (1966) 67–101.

41 McCook, R. D., Wurster, R. D. and Randall, W. C., Sudomotor and vasomotor responses to changing environmental temperature, *J. appl. Physiol.*, 20 (1965) 371–378.

42 Niijima, A., Studies on the nervous regulatory mechanism of blood sugar levels, *Pharmacol. Biochem. and Behav.*, 3, Suppl. 1 (1975) 139–143.

43 Ninomiya, I. and Fujita, S., Reflex effects of thermal stimulation on sympathetic nerve activity to skin and kidney, *Amer. J. Physiol.*, 230 (1976) 271–278.

44 Peter, W. and Riedel, W., Skin vasodilatation and panting influenced by hypothalamic thermal stimulation in the reserpine-treated dog, *Pflügers Arch.*, Suppl. to 377 (1978) R30.

45 Pleschka, K., Roth, R. and Colaric, F., Neurogenic vasodilatatory component in tongue blood flow control during thermal panting in the dog, *Int. Cong. Physiol. Sci.*, Lille Satellite Symposium, 39 (1977).

46 Porte, D., Jr. and Robertson, R. P., Control of insulin secretion by catecholamines, stress, and the sympathetic nervous system, *Fed. Proc.*, 32 (1973) 1792–1796.

47 Rawson, R. O. and Quick, K. P., Evidence of deep-body thermoreceptor response to intra-abdominal heating of the ewe, *J. appl. Physiol.*, 28 (1970) 813–820.

48 Rein, H., Vasomotorische Regulationen, *Ergebn. Physiol.*, 32 (1931) 28–72.

49 Riedel, W., Iriki, M. and Simon, E., Regional differentiation of sympathetic activity

during peripheral heating and cooling in anaesthetized rabbits, *Pflügers Arch.*, 332 (1972) 239–247.

50 Riedel, W., Siaplauras, G. and Simon, E., Intra-abdominal thermosensitivity in the rabbit as compared with spinal thermosensitivity, *Pflügers Arch.*, 340 (1973) 59–70.

51 Riedel, W. and Peter, W., Non-uniformity of regional vasomotor activity indicating the existence of 2 different systems in the sympathetic cardiovascular outflow, *Experientia*, 33 (1977) 337–338.

52 Rothstein, A. and Towbin, E. J., Blood circulation and temperature of men dehydrating in the heat. In: E. F. Adolph (Ed.), *Physiology of Man in the Desert*, Interscience, New York, 1947, pp. 172–196.

53 Rowell, L. B., Reflex control of the cutaneous vasculature, *J. Invest. Dermatol.*, 69 (1977) 154–166.

54 Satinoff, E., Neural integration of thermoregulatory responses. In: L. V. DiCara (Ed.), *Limbic and Autonomic Nervous Systems Research*, Plenum Press, New York, 1974, pp. 41–83.

55 Sato, A. and Schmidt, R. F., Somatosympathetic reflexes: Afferent fibers, central pathways, discharge characteristics, *Physiol. Rev.*, 53 (1973) 916–947.

56 Schönung, W., Wagner, H., Jessen, C. and Simon, E., Differentiation of cutaneous and intestinal blood flow during hypothalamic heating and cooling in anaesthetized dog, *Pflügers Arch.*, 328 (1971) 145–154.

57 Schönung, W., Jessen, C., Wagner, H. and Simon, E., Regional blood flow antagonism induced by central thermal stimulation in the conscious dog, *Experientia*, 27 (1971) 1291–1292.

58 Schönung, W., Wagner, H. and Simon, E., Neurogenic vasodilatatory component in the thermoregulatory skin blood flow response of the dog, *Naunyn-Schmiedeberg's Arch. Pharmacol.*, 273 (1972) 230–241.

59 Sharp, F. R. and Hammel, H. T., Effects of fever on salivation response in the resting and exercising dog, *Amer. J. Physiol.*, 223 (1972) 77–82.

60 Simon, E., Temperature regulation: The spinal cord as a site of extrahypothalamic thermoregulatory functions, *Rev. Physiol. Biochem. Pharmacol.*, 71 (1974) 1–76.

61 Simon, E., Rautenberg, W., Thauer, R. and Iriki, M., Auslösung thermoregulatorischer Reaktionen durch lokale Kühlung im Vertebralkanal, *Naturwissenschaften*, 50 (1963) 337.

62 Simon, E. and Iriki, M., Sensory transmission of spinal heat and cold sensitivity in ascending spinal neurons, *Pflügers Arch.*, 328 (1971) 103–120.

63 Simon, E. and Riedel, W., Diversity of regional sympathetic outflow in integrative cardiovascular control: Patterns and mechanisms, *Brain Res.*, 87 (1975) 323–333.

64 Smith, R. E. and Horwitz, B. A., Brown fat and thermogenesis, *Physiol. Rev.*, 49 (1969) 330–425.

65 Thauer, R., Der Mechanismus der Wärmeregulation, *Ergebn. Physiol.*, 41 (1939) 607–805.

66 Thauer, R., Circulatory adjustments to climatic requirements. In: W. F. Hamilton and P. Dow (Eds.), *Handbook of Physiology, Circulation*, Vol. 3, Amer. Physiol. Soc., Washington, D. C., 1965, pp. 1921–1966.

67 Walther, O.-E., Iriki, M. and Simon, E., Antagonistic changes of blood flow and sympathetic activity in different vascular beds following central thermal stimulation. II. Cutaneous and visceral sympathetic activity during spinal cord heating and cooling in anesthetized rabbits and cats, *Pflügers Arch.*, 319 (1970) 162–184.

68 Walther, O.-E., Simon, E. and Jessen, C., Thermoregulatory adjustments of skin blood flow in chronically spinalized dogs, *Pflügers Arch.*, 322 (1971) 323–335.

69 Walther, O.-E., Riedel, W., Iriki, M. and Simon, E., Differentiation of sympathetic activity at the spinal level in response to central cold stimulation, *Pflügers Arch.*, 329 (1971) 220–230.
70 Wang, G. H., *The Neural Control of Sweating*, The University of Wisconsin Press, Madison, 1964.
71 Woods, S. C. and Porte, D., Jr., Neural control of the endocrine pancreas, *Physiol. Rev.*, 54 (1974) 596–619.

CHAPTER 31

CENTRAL NERVOUS INTERACTIONS BETWEEN CHEMORECEPTOR AND BARORECEPTOR CONTROL MECHANISMS

M. Iriki* and P. I. Korner**

*Tokyo Metropolitan Institute of Gerontology, Tokyo, Japan, and
**Baker Medical Research Institute, Melbourne, Australia

INTRODUCTION

The last few years have seen many changes in our concepts of the operation of the sympathetic nervous system, since Cannon[2] suggested that it was predominantly a system for uniform mass action to cope with emergencies facing the organism. There is now much evidence, as has been discussed elsewhere in this symposium, that environmental and behavioral stimuli can elicit differentiated autonomic patterns with diverse sympathetic neural responses[5-12,19,26]. Up till recently, however, little attention has been paid to the way in which the autonomic responses to one afferent input can become greatly modified by the lack of activity in another. This is probably due to the fact that in classic "open loop" analysis of cardiovascular reflexes the methods employed have consisted of stimulating one particular group of receptors under carefully controlled conditions while minimizing changes in other inputs. This approach has given rise to the view that circulatory control was through arrays of distinctive reflexes. Since the autonomic responses produced in classic reflex analysis are always the same, we have tended to speak of "reflexes" as though they were invariant entities and have largely ignored the importance of interactions. However, during many circulatory disturbances there are often simultaneous changes in several receptor groups, which vary with the nature of the different disturbances and with their intensity[13-15,17,20,25]. Under these conditions the autonomic effects evoked by unit change in activity of the particular input often become greatly altered[17,23,24,29]. Because of the key role of the input to the central nervous system (CNS) from the arterial baroreceptors in virtually every type of circulatory disturbance, changes in arterial baroreflex properties owing to interactions with other afferents are of particular interest. Under the influence of such afferent interactions a particular autonomic effector can respond quite differently to unit arterial pressure change than under control conditions.

In our laboratories we have studied some of the central nervous interactions involving pathways from the various circulatory baroreceptors (e.g., arterial and cardiopulmonary baroreceptors) and those arising from the arterial chemoreceptors. The present report illustrates the considerable changes in arterial baroreflex properties that occur through such interactions.

METHODS

Baroreceptor-Heart Period Reflex

The "steady-state" properties of the baroreceptor-heart period reflex were studied in unanesthetized rabbits[16,17]. Briefly, the method consisted of raising and lowering intravascular pressures for a period of 30 sec by graded inflation of small balloons placed around the upper part of the descending aorta and the upper part of the inferior vena cava. This produced changes in mean arterial pressure, pulse pressure, right atrial pressure and probably in the other cardiac chambers. This is because the heart and blood vessels are arranged in a closed hydraulic loop, so that any circulatory disturbance will elicit changes in several groups of circulatory baroreceptors. Therefore, in the unanesthetized intact animal it is not only at the arterial baroreceptors where balloon inflation produces changes in the degree of stimulation, but also in atrial and ventricular receptors and in those in the pulmonary artery. However, detailed analysis of the role of the afferents of the carotid sinus nerve, the aortic nerve and of the vagus have suggested that it is the arterial baroreceptors, particularly those of the carotid sinus region, that normally make the greatest contribution to the baroreceptor-heart period reflex[1,16,17].

The mean arterial pressure-heart period (pulse interval) curves are sigmoid in shape (Fig. 1). Each curve has a lower heart period plateau, a part where heart period increases monotonically with rising blood pressure, and an upper heart period plateau. It can be characterized by three parameters[16]: 1) the heart period range (HPR) which is the difference between the upper and lower plateau levels; 2) the median blood pressure (BP_{50}), which is determined after probit transformation of the sigmoid curve, and is the mean arterial pressure at half HPR; 3) the average gain ($\overline{G}$) which is the average slope ($\mathit{\Delta}$ Heart period/$\mathit{\Delta}$ mean arterial pressure) between $+1$ and -1 standard deviations from the mean of the curve[16].

Mean Arterial Pressure-Sympathetic Nerve Activity Reflexes

Most of our studies were performed in anesthetized, paralyzed and artificially ventilated rabbits[7], though recently we have carried out preliminary work in conscious rabbits using the collagen fiber electrode of Ninomiya and associates[27].

Methods of recording from the cardiac, renal, splanchnic and ear sympathetic nerves have been described previously[5-9]. Whole nerve sympathetic activity was recorded with bipolar platinum electrodes. The nerve potentials were fed into a low noise differential amplifier, the amplified potentials were rectified and the area under the curve integrated over two sec intervals, after exclusion of noise.

Baroreflex curves were again obtained by raising and lowering intravascular pressures using perivascular balloons[7]. Before each balloon inflation resting sympathet-

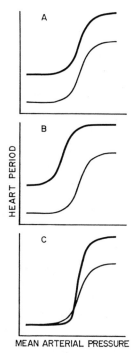

Fig. 1. Schema showing different types of "resetting" of the arterial baroreceptor-heart
period (pulse interval) reflex. This is exemplified by various shifts in arterial pressure-
heart period curve during a disturbance (heavy curve) from its normal control
position (light curve). A: When heart rate neurons are activated through pathways
that are independent of those receiving arterial baroreceptor projections, only the
mean level of the heart period is altered and none of the arterial pressure-dependent
parameters change (i.e., heart period range, gain, median blood pressure and threshold). B: The disturbance has evoked arterial pressure-independent effects with
equal shifts in the two plateau levels; there have also been some effects on part of the
motoneuron pool receiving baroreceptor projections which have resulted in a reduction in the median blood pressure and in threshold pressure. C: The effect of the
disturbance is entirely on parts of the motoneuron pool receiving baroreceptor projections and every parameter of the curve has been altered; the increase in upper
plateau is due to an increase in heart period range. (Reproduced from Korner et al.[17]
with permission from the American Heart Association.)

ic nerve activity (SNA) was averaged over five integration cycles, while the changes
during balloon inflation were averaged over the last five cycles at the end of a 25–30
sec inflation period. Recovery of one to two min was allowed before the start of the
next cycle when blood pressure and resting SNA had fully recovered. Integrated SNA
was determined in 10 mmHg steps at mean arterial pressures ranging from 40 to 130–
140 mmHg. SNA at 60 mmHg, with the rabbit ventilated with air, was expressed as
100 units and SNA at other pressures or during hypoxia was expressed in terms of
this value[7]. The sigmoid curves were characterized by: 1) SNA range from minimum
SNA to the upper curve plateau or to SNA at 40 mmHg when a definite plateau was
absent; 2) median blood pressure (BP_{50}) calculated after probit transformation as the
blood pressure at half SNA range; 3) average gain ($\bar{G}$).

RESULTS AND COMMENTS

Assessment of Reflex Interactions

When a particular reflex is studied under classic "open-loop" conditions, a given change in input A will produce a characteristic response A^1. Similarly the change in another input B will elicit the response B^1. When the two inputs are changed simultaneously the response to (A+B) will only conform to the simple summation model A^1+B^1 if the CNS pathways to the different autonomic motoneuron pools are independent of one another. More commonly, the response will include an interaction term. Thus, the responses to (A+B) will be $A^1+B^1+A^1(A^1B^1)B^1$. The interaction term A^1B^1 signifies that the response is nonlinear and changes in input A will vary with the level of activity of input B.

Baroreceptor-Heart Period Reflex

The effects of different disturbances on the properties of the baroreceptor-heart period reflex have been used to study CNS reflex interactions. Figure 1 illustrates schematically the possible shifts from control which can be induced[17]. The control curve is largely determined by changes in arterial baroreceptor input. In Fig. 1A the other inputs altered by the disturbance shift only the ordinate level of the control curve and have no effect on the arterial pressure-related parameters, i.e., heart period range, BP_{50} and gain. The other inputs involved in the disturbance thus project to neurons not receiving arterial baroreceptor projections. An experimental example of this type of shift is the effect of hyperventilation on the mean arterial pressure-heart period curve in the rabbit which is reflexly mediated through lung inflation afferents[14,17,20].

Figure 1C shows the effects of interactions, with the disturbance changing one or more of the arterial pressure-related curve parameters. In the example shown the inputs associated with the disturbance greatly alter the heart rate response to arterial pressure changes due to interaction with the baroreceptor projections. In the intermediate case of Fig. 1B the inputs associated with the disturbance produce both types of change: 1) "baroreflex-independent" shifts in the two plateau levels and 2) some "baroreflex-dependent" changes in curve properties, with a reduction in BP_{50} and threshold pressure in this particular example.

Acute arterial hypoxia (art. $P_{O_2} < 35$ mmHg) in the conscious rabbit elicited both "baroreflex-independent" and "baroreflex-dependent" changes from control in the mean arterial pressure-heart period curve (Fig. 2). In the first few minutes after induction of hypoxia there was elevation of both plateau levels, and changes in arterial pressure-related curve properties including elevation in heart period range, BP_{50} and threshold pressure and in gain[14,17]. In atropinized rabbits in which only the sympathetic was functioning there was also a baroreflex-independent rise in heart period plateau levels, and elevation in BP_{50} and threshold. The baroreflex-independent effect was thus due to the synergistic effects of vagal excitation and cardiac sympathetic inhibition. On the right-hand side of Fig. 2 are shown the responses of infracollicularly decerebrated pontine preparations[21]. In animals with both effectors intact only the

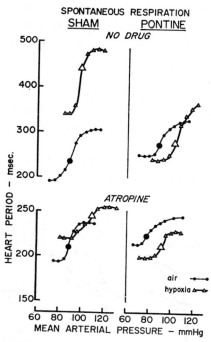

SPONTANEOUS RESPIRATION

Fig. 2. Mean arterial pressure and heart period curves during control period breathing air (filled circles) and during 12 min hypoxia (open triangles) is spontaneously breathing and sham-operated and pontine animals with both vagus and sympathetic nerves intact (top panels), and in atropinized preparations with intact sympathetic nerves (lower panels). Large circles and triangles are resting HP values. (From Korner[14], with permission.)

upper plateau of the curve rose above control level, but the lower plateau remained unchanged. In addition there was elevation in BP_{50} and threshold. By contrast, in pontine atropinized rabbits the baroreflex curve was displaced in the opposite direction, with a lowering of both plateau levels, and an increase in BP_{50}. In a pontine preparation with both effectors functioning the baroreflex-independent component of the response thus consisted of simultaneous excitation of the vagus and cardiac sympathetic, masking any shift in the lower plateau. The pontine animals' response to the disturbance is less well coordinated than that of rabbits with intact suprapontine pathways. The latter appeared necessary for the synergistic responses of the two effectors.

The roles of the various afferent mechanisms responsible for the baroreflex-independent and baroreflex-dependent curve changes have been analyzed in atropinized animals maintained at constant ventilation during both control and hypoxic periods (Fig. 3). The baroreflex-independent rise in plateau levels was larger early in hypoxia (Fig. 3) than in animals ventilating spontaneously (Fig. 2). It was not mediated through vagal afferents but through the carotid sinus and aortic nerves, i.e., through the arterial chemoreceptors. The increase in BP_{50} and threshold occurring early in hypoxia resulted from interactions between the inputs from the arterial

420   M. Iriki and P. I. Korner

baroreceptors and chemoreceptors. As shown in Fig. 3, the "resetting" of the baroreflex curve alters during the latter part of hypoxia. The increase in gain and heart
period range at this time can be seen to be due to cardiopulmonary baroreceptor
(vagal)—chemoreceptor interactions (Fig. 3) with both effects being abolished after
vagotomy.

    We also studied the effects of arterial hypoxia on cardiac SNA baroreflex curves
(Fig. 4)[7,8]. These were studied in anesthetized rabbits and hypoxia inhibited cardiac
SNA at a given arterial pressure; there was reduction in SNA range and in gain,
mainly owing to arterial baroreceptor-chemoreceptor interaction[7]. Cardiac SNA was
no longer inhibited during hypoxia after section of the carotid sinus and aortic nerves.
In decerebrate rabbits "resetting" of the cardiac SNA was in the opposite direction to

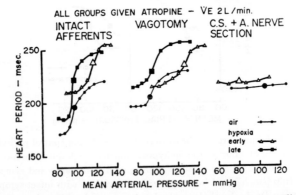

Fig. 3. Mean arterial pressure-heart period curves under control conditions (fine line,
        filled circles), between 1–12 min severe arterial hypoxia (fine line, open triangles)
        and between 33–45 min hypoxia (heavy line, filled squares). Animals studied had
        the CNS intact and included a group with all afferents intact, vagotomized animals
        and animals with section of the carotid sinus and aortic nerves. All animals were
        ventilated at 21 min^{-1} throughout the experiment. (From Korner et al.[17], with
        permission.)

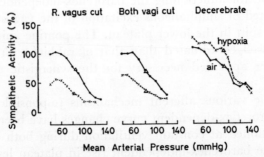

Fig. 4. Average mean arterial-right cardiac SNA curves obtained in anesthetized, artificially
        ventilated rabbits during ventilation with air (solid lines) and during arterial hypoxia
        (dashed lines); the triangle in the middle of each curve represents the mean resting
        values between balloon inflations. Left: animals with right vagus cut (n=5); middle:
        animals with both vagi cut (n=5); right: decerebrate pontine rabbits (n=6).

animals with intact CNS, with an increase in SNA at a given blood pressure (Fig. 4). The conclusions reached were thus broadly similar to those obtained from analyzing mean arterial pressure-heart period curves in the conscious rabbit, though there were some differences. For example, in the baroreflex curves obtained by nerve recording in the anesthetized animals there was no increase in pressure threshold and BP_{50} for cardiac inhibition and the plateau shifts were limited to only one plateau of the sigmoid curve. If some of these effects were mediated through pathways with a relatively high threshold, they would be less obvious under anesthesia than in the conscious rabbit.

Effect of Hypoxia on Regional Sympathetic Constrictor Motoneuron Pools

These studies were performed in sodium pentobarbitone anesthetized, paralyzed rabbits, ventilated artificially[7-9]. Baroreflex curves were obtained under control conditions and during severe arterial hypoxia ($Pa_{O_2} < 35$ mmHg) in the renal, splanchnic and ear sympathetic nerves. Recording was made of only a single sympathetic outflow in any one experiment.

Under control normoxic conditions lowering mean arterial pressure below resting by inflating the inferior vena caval balloon increased renal and splanchnic SNA, while increasing blood pressure by inflating the aortic balloon diminished SNA in those outflows. These arterial pressure-related changes were abolished after section of the carotid sinus and aortic nerves, indicating that they were mediated through the arterial baroreceptors[7]. In the ear sympathetic nerve, which in the rabbit supplies mainly the arterio-venous anastomoses of the ear skin, there was no relationship of control SNA to arterial pressure changes, indicating that this particular autonomic outflow was not altered significantly by changes in arterial baroreceptor activity.

Arterial hypoxia "reset" the renal baroreflex curve in the opposite direction to that observed in the cardiac sympathetic (Figs. 4 and 5). In the renal sympathetic there was a shift to the right of the baroreflex curve, so that there was elevation of the upper plateau level and significant increases in BP_{50}, gain and SNA range (Fig. 5, upper left). In the same animals after vagotomy "resetting" of the baroreflex curve in hypoxia was similar but the rise in SNA range was even bigger (Fig. 5, upper middle). The shifts in the renal baroreflex curves depended on the integrity of the aortic and carotid sinus nerves, and were even more marked in vagotomized rabbits[7]. Thus in the intact animal during hypoxia the increased input from the chemoreceptors contributes to the increase in BP_{50} and gain. It also increased SNA range while vagal afferents had a moderating role on this parameter.

We also studied another series of decerebrate rabbits with intact afferents (Fig. 5, upper right)[8]. In these animals the magnitude of the shifts in renal baroreflex curves was considerably smaller than in rabbits with intact CNS pathways, suggesting that suprapontine mechanisms participated in the normal response.

In animals with intact CNS the shifts in the splanchnic baroreflex curve during hypoxia were small and variable and not statistically significant (Fig. 5, middle right)[8]. However, in vagotomized rabbits there was a significant increase in BP_{50}, though no change in gain, during hypoxia (Fig. 5, middle panel). These findings suggest that in the intact anesthetized animal arterial baroreceptor-chemoreceptor

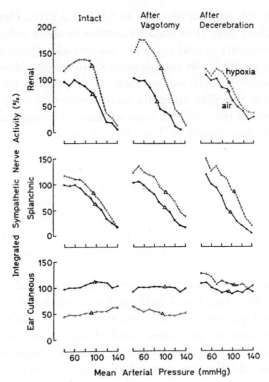

Fig. 5.   Mean arterial pressure-integrated SNA curves in renal (top panels, n=6), splanchnic
(middle panels, n=6) and ear sympathetic (lower panels, n=6) obtained in anesthetized, artificially ventilated rabbits during inhalation of air (solid lines) and during
severe arterial hypoxia (dashed lines). Left column: all afferents intact; middle
column: vagotomized animals; right column: decerebrate rabbits with intact afferents.
Other notations as in Fig. 4.

interactions produce an increase in SNA for a given blood pressure compared with
control, but that these effects are almost completely masked owing to vagal afferent
activity. Moreover, the masking of the arterial baroreceptor-chemoreceptor interaction appears to be mediated at suprapontine CNS sites, since in decerebrate animals
with intact vagi hypoxia elicited a shift of similar magnitude in the splanchnic baroreflex as in vagotomized rabbits with intact CNS.

Under normoxic conditions ear SNA was unaffected by arterial and cardiopulmonary baroreflex influences, and SNA was unaffected by section of the carotid
sinus nerves (Fig. 5, lower panels)[9]. During hypoxia there was marked inhibition of
ear SNA, which was minimally influenced by vagotomy but abolished by section of
the carotid sinus and aortic nerves[9], suggesting that it was chemoreceptor-mediated.
This inhibitory effect was again mediated through suprapontine pathways, since ear
SNA increased during arterial hypoxia in decerebrate rabbits. In hypoxic animals
with intact vagi there was a small, but statistically significant, increase in ear SNA
with rising blood pressure (Fig. 5, lower left), which was not present after vagotomy
(Fig. 5, lower middle). This was considered to be due to a CNS chemoreceptor-
cardiopulmonary baroreflex interaction[9].

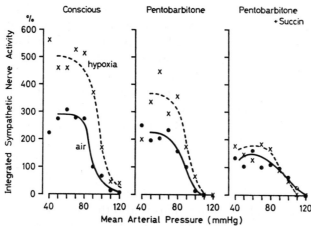

Fig. 6. Renal baroreflex curve obtained during ventilation with air (circles, solid lines) and during arterial hypoxia (crosses, dashed lines) in one rabbit. Left: conscious animal, 48 hours after implanting nerve electrode; middle: anesthesia with pentobarbitone during spontaneous ventilation; right: during anesthesia and paralysis with succinylcholine and constant artificial ventilation. (Iriki, Ninomiya and Korner, unpublished.)

Studies of Renal SNA in Unanesthetized Rabbits

To date we have only performed some preliminary experiments on recording renal SNA in conscious rabbits using the Ninomiya collagen electrode[26]. Figure 6 shows results obtained from one such an experiment. The important point is that under normoxic conditions the baroreflex gain is considerably greater and the "resetting" during hypoxia is more pronounced than under pentobarbitone and pentobarbitone +succinylcholine. The findings suggest, while our conclusions based on findings in anesthetized animals appear in the main to be qualitatively similar to those in unanesthetized animals, quantitative aspects of the responses will require further evaluation.

DISCUSSION

The above analysis suggests that in any given autonomic motoneuron pool some neurons receive projections from specific afferents but not from others, while other neurons receive projections from several sources. Examples of the former include the chemoreceptor and lung inflation receptor-mediated "baroreflex-independent" shifts in plateau levels of the mean arterial pressure-heart period curves in the conscious rabbit, and the chemoreceptor inhibition of ear SNA and ear skin hyperemia[3,9,17,19]. Previous analysis has indicated that the "baroreflex-independent" shifts in the heart period plateau levels are time-dependent and are much more pronounced at the beginning of hypoxia than later on[17]. The reasons for this time-dependence are not entirely clear. One suggestion is that the "heart rate" motoneurons receiving distinctive chemoreceptor projections do so through relatively high threshold pathways, with marked lowering of activity as the peripheral chemoreceptors adapt somewhat to the hypoxia stimulus. This would help to explain why such "baroreflex-independent" responses are only evident in conscious rabbits, but not in anesthetized animals.

The main point has been the demonstration of chemoreceptor-arterial baro-receptor interactions and chemoreceptor-cardiopulmonary baroreceptor interactions affecting the different motoneuron pools. Just as hypoxia elicits a differentiated pattern of resting SNA, so the above interactions result in a differentiated pattern of baroreflex "resetting". Thus renal SNA becomes more responsive to unit arterial pressure change with an increase in the "pressure-dependent" SNA range, while the opposite effects occur in relation to cardiac SNA responses to pressure stimuli. Analysis of the splanch-nic sympathetic baroreflex has shown that the apparent absence of any resetting in the intact anesthetized rabbit is due to the opposing effects of chemoreceptor and cardiopulmonary afferent influences in this particular motoneuron pool.

Comparison of the responses of rabbits with intact CNS and pontine decerebrate rabbits indicate that some of the interactions are mediated through suprapontine as well as through bulbospinal pathways. This is also the case for "baroreflex-independ-ent" effects. Presumably the more divergent sites provide greater opportunity for interaction and a finer type of central control.

It should be emphasized that there are now several other experimental examples demonstrating the importance of baroreceptor-chemoreceptor interactions of the type discussed[4,23,24,29]. Moreover, changes in baroreflex properties also occur during sleep[28] and after administration of drugs such as clonidine which affect central autonomic mechanism[18]. They also occur during electrical stimulation of discrete brain regions such as the defense area, from which it appears to be possible to elicit a differentiated pattern of changes in baroreflex properties of the various regional motoneuron pools[22]. The latter experiments provide models of baroreflex "resetting" by central command mechanisms and during different types of behavior.

The marked changes in baroreflex properties that occur through afferent inter-actions emphasize that "reflexes" are far from invariant entities. Cardiovascular control does not occur through arrays of autonomous reflexes but the system behaves rather like a variable reference servocontrol mechanism where the responses to changes in any one input are greatly modified by the activity of some of the other components of the afferent input profile.

SUMMARY

Analysis of the baroreceptor-heart period reflex and of the renal, splanchnic and ear sympathetic responses to arterial pressure changes has been performed in rabbits under normoxic conditions and during arterial hypoxia. Interactions between arterial baroreceptor-chemoreceptor inputs can greatly alter the various effector responses to arterial pressure stimuli. The changes in properties are not uniform in every sympathetic motoneuron pool with enhanced responsiveness in some (e.g., renal) and diminished responsiveness in others (e.g., cardiac). Many of the interactions are mediated through suprapontine pathways. The analysis demonstrates that the prop-erties of the arterial baroreflex are not invariant but can be greatly altered through changes in the activity of other specific afferents.

REFERENCES

1 Blombery, P. A. and Korner, P. I., Role of aortic and carotid baroreceptors in the baroreceptor-heart rate reflex of unanaesthetized rabbits, *Proc. XXVII Internat. Congr. Physiol. Sci., Paris*, 13 (1977) 82 (abstract).

2 Cannon, W. B., *Bodily Changes in Pain, Hunger, Fear and Rage*, 2nd ed., Appleton, New York, 1929.

3 Chalmers, J. P. and Korner, P. I., Effects of arterial hypoxia on the cutaneous circulation of the rabbit, *J. Physiol. (Lond.)*, 184 (1966) 685–697.

4 Heistad, D. D., Abboud, F. M., Mark, A. L. and Schmid, P. G., Interaction of baroreceptor and chemoreceptor reflexes. Modulation of the chemoreceptor reflex by changes in baroreceptor activity, *J. clin. Invest.*, 53 (1974) 1226–1236.

5 Iriki, M., Riedel, W. and Simon, E., Regional differentiation of sympathetic activity during hypothalamic heating and cooling in anaesthetized rabbits, *Pflügers Arch.*, 328 (1971) 320–331.

6 Iriki, M., Pleschka, K., Walther, O.-E. and Simon, E., Hypoxia and hypercapnia in asphyctic differentiation of regional sympathetic activity in the anaesthetized rabbit, *Pflügers Arch.*, 328 (1971) 91–102.

7 Iriki, M., Dorward, P. and Korner, P. I., Baroreflex 'resetting' by arterial hypoxia in the renal and cardiac sympathetic nerves of the rabbit, *Pflügers Arch.*, 370 (1977) 1–7.

8 Iriki, M., Kozawa, E., Korner, P. I. and Dorward, P., Baroreflex 'resetting' in various regional sympathetic efferents during arterial hypoxia in normal and decerebrated rabbits, *Proc. 18th Internat. Congress of Neurovegetative Research*, Tokyo, 1977, pp. 92–94.

9 Iriki, M., Korner, P. I. and Dorward, P. K., Arterial and cardiopulmonary baroreceptor and chemoreceptor influences and interactions on ear sympathetic nerve discharge in the rabbit (submitted).

10 Kendrick, E., Öberg, B. and Wennergren, G., Extent of engagement of various cardiovascular effectors to alterations of carotid sinus pressure, *Acta physiol. scand.*, 86 (1972) 410–418.

11 Kendrick, E., Öberg, B. and Wennergren, G., Vasoconstrictor fibre discharge to skeletal muscle, kidney, intestine and skin at varying levels of arterial baroreceptor activity in the cat, *Acta physiol. scand.*, 85 (1972) 464–476.

12 Kollai, M. and Koizumi, K., Differential responses in sympathetic outflow evoked by chemoreceptor activation, *Brain Res.*, 138 (1977) 159–165.

13 Korner, P. I., Integrative neural cardiovascular control, *Physiol. Rev.*, 51 (1971) 312–367.

14 Korner, P. I., Central and peripheral 'resetting' of the baroreceptor system, *Clin. exp. Pharmacol. Physiol.*, 2, suppl., 2 (1975) 171–178.

15 Korner, P. I., Problems of integrative cardiovascular control, *Proc. Aust. Physiol. & Pharmacol. Soc.*, 7 (1976) 35–48.

16 Korner, P. I., Shaw, J., West, M. J. and Oliver, J. R., Central nervous system control of baroreceptor reflexes in the rabbit, *Circulation Res.*, 31 (1972) 637–652.

17 Korner, P. I., Shaw, J., West, M. J., Oliver, J. R. and Hilder, R. G., Integrative reflex control of heart rate in the rabbit during hypoxia and hyperventilation, *Circulation Res.*, 33 (1973) 63–73.

18 Korner, P. I., Oliver, J. R., Sleight, P., Robinson, J. S. and Chalmers, J. P., Effects of clonidine on the baroreceptor-heart rate reflex and on single aortic baroreceptor fibre discharge, *European J. Pharmacol.*, 23 (1974) 189–198.

19 Korner, P. I. and Uther, J. B., Dynamic characteristics of the cardiovascular autonomic

effects during severe arterial hypoxia in the unanaesthetized rabbit, *Circulation Res.*, 24 (1969) 671–687.

20 Korner, P. I. and Uther, J. B., Stimulus-cardiorespiratory effector response profile during arterial hypoxia in the unanaesthetized rabbit, *Aust. J. exptl. Biol. Med. Sci.*, 48 (1970) 663–685.

21 Korner, P. I., Uther, J. B. and White, S. W., Central nervous integration of the circulatory and respiratory responses to arterial hypoxemia in the rabbit, *Circulation Res.*, 24 (1969) 757–776.

22 Kumada, M., Schramm, L. P., Altmansberger, R. A. and Sagawa, K., Modulation of carotid sinus baroreceptor reflex by hypothalamic defence response, *Amer. J. Physiol.*, 228 (1975) 34–45.

23 Mancia, G., Influence of carotid baroreceptors on vascular responses to carotid chemoreceptor stimulation in the dog, *Circulation Res.*, 36 (1975) 270–276.

24 Mancia, G., Shepherd, J. T. and Donald, D. E., Interplay among carotid sinus, cardiopulmonary and carotid body reflexes in dogs, *Amer. J. Physiol.*, 230 (1976) 19–24.

25 McRitchie, R. J. and White, S. W., Role of trigeminal, olfactory, carotid sinus and aortic nerves in the respiratory and circulatory response to nasal inhalation of cigarette smoke and other irritants in the rabbit, *Aust. J. exptl. Biol. Med. Sci.*, 52 (1974) 127–140.

26 Ninomiya, I., Irisawa, H. and Nisimaru, N., Non-uniformity of sympathetic nerve activity to the skin and kidney, *Amer. J. Physiol.*, 224 (1973) 256–264.

27 Ninomiya, I., Yonezawa, Y. and Wilson, M. F., Implantable electrode for recording nerve signals in awake animals, *J. appl. Physiol.*, 41 (1976) 111–114.

28 Smyth, H. S., Sleight, P. and Pickering, G. W., Reflex regulation of arterial pressure during sleep in man: A quantitative method for assessing baroreflex sensitivity, *Circulation Res.*, 24 (1969) 109–121.

29 Wennergren, G., Little, R. and Öberg, B., Studies on the central integration of excitatory chemoreceptor influences and inhibitory baroreceptor and cardiac receptor influences, *Acta physiol. scand.*, 96 (1976) 1–18.

CHAPTER 32

HOMEOSTATIC CONTROLS IN THE REGULATION OF AUTONOMIC NERVOUS SYSTEM FUNCTION

A Discussion by
S. K. Manchanda* and Chandler McC. Brooks**

*Department of Physiology, All India Institute of Medical Sciences, New Delhi, India, and
**Department of Physiology, Downstate Medical Center, State University
of New York, Brooklyn, New York, USA

INTRODUCTION

Homeostasis is no longer a new term and as is often the case its meaning has gradually been modified or expanded, if you will, during the half century since its introduction[3]. It is appropriate therefore to mention a few new emphases as the past is reviewed and as we look toward the future.

The maintenance of homeostasis requires integrative activity. The integrative processes directed by the central nervous system and executed by the autonomic system, the endocrine system and the somatic motor neurons control behavior and maintain constancies of body states. It is almost unavoidable to speak of control as purpose-oriented despite frequently heard objections to this concept. If one confines the use of "purpose" to physiology it evidently is acceptable: "Although we all disclaim teleological thinking, in fact we all think in terms of purpose—and ask, 'how does this reflex aid in the preservation of the constancies of the internal environment?' "—Whitteridge[10]. We can say that stimuli of external and internal origin initiate responses which produce change or maintain constancies essential to survival.

The role of the autonomic system in the maintenance of homeostasis is well recognized and a good deal has been written about the types of reactions involved. Claude Bernard's original concept that it "is the fixity of the *milieu interieur* which is the condition of free and independent life" and Cannon's term homeostasis also implies maintenance of constancies characteristic of normal resting states. The body does react to resist changes from the norm and the somatic and autonomic systems do act to restore normality after it has been disturbed. However, during even low levels of behavioral activities body states are changed and some show definite cyclical fluctuations. It is appropriate therefore that we think more of the dynamics of adjustments of body states and possibly even rejuvenate the concepts of "trophotropic" and "ergotrophic" reactions advanced by Hess[2]. These terms were proposed in an effort to avoid the implication that parasympathetic and sympathetic functions are always antagonistic; they also express an endeavor to focus attention on function rather than on concepts which have anatomical confinements. The ergotropic reactions are "coupled with energy expenditure" and control with an "endophylactic-trophotropic" system which "provides for protection and restitution"[4]. Energy balance, protection and restitution cover a rather broad scope but do not emphasize one cardinal feature of homeostasis—that is the concept of balance. To attain that one needs opposing action, such as excitation and inhibition.

HOMEOSTASIS AND THE MAINTENANCE OF BALANCES

There really are two related concepts which should be discussed. They are: 1) the preservation of essential constancies or homeostasis in Cannon's terms "the coordinated physiological processes which maintain most of the steady states in the organism", and 2) the establishment and maintenance of balances in non-normal states which is equally essential. This latter is spoken of as heterostasis (hetero meaning other than usual; stasis meaning position)[8]. The importance of the maintenance of balance and the seriousness of imbalances to health and disease was recognized by the early Greek and Chinese physician-philosophers.

The constancies normally maintained in the body by autonomic and somatic cooperation are quite dissimilar. Body temperature does show diurnal and other fluctuations of about 1.5°C above and below the agreed upon normal mean of 37°C (98.6°F) but in the activities and exposures of daily living it swings way beyond this range (35–40°C; 95.5–104°F). As extremes of internal temperatures are approached counter reactions become stronger and stronger but eventually cease above and below certain limits (106°–80°F). A homeotherm then becomes poikilothermic and the term "poikilostasis" might be useful at times.

The matter of more importance to a consideration of integrative reactions is that set points can shift and individuals can function quite well for long periods at a different level of balance. The term "heterostasis" is appropriate in speaking of maintenance of unusual states by somewhat different patterns of reaction. Presumably one might observe in the same individual maintenance of a normal state (body temperature homeostasis) but accompanied by a special balance in another state (a metabolic heterostasis). This raises the question of the interrelationship of states.

What we define as body states differ remarkably as do their set points and constancies. There is an energy intake-energy output balance and a basal metabolic rate indicative of normality. The variations from the mean which are considered to be within the confines of normality are vastly greater than for body temperature. Blood glucose levels also fluctuate greatly within confines which do not evoke compensatory reactions against hypoglycemia or hyperglycemia. The centers of the nervous system monitor simultaneously many body states each of which has its normal set point, normal variations and thresholds for initiation of compensatory reactions. There is a heterogeneity of states. Our usual custom is to consider only one state at a time but in actuality all are affected together and all are controlled together. It is impossible to change one state without affecting others. A high metabolic activity in tissues creates more heat, depletes blood glucose more quickly and puts some stress on maintenance of acid-base balance. In reality all states are being managed together and this requires a high degree of differential or selective action. Maintenance of certain constancies is more important to survival than is the maintenance of others. Stores can be depleted, debts acquired and even some chronic imbalances tolerated. The central interactions required to relate and adjust balances are still a challenge to our methodologies and our analytical abilities.

There is still another matter of importance and that is the ability of an organism to react in an emergency, react as a whole to meet a threat regardless of what happens to body constancies. This requires what we might consider a decision relative to purpose. Stress is a threat to continuity but of course disturbance of body constancies is a threat requiring reactions to maintain either homeostasis or at least a heterostasis.

REACTIONS TO STRESS: PROTECTION AND RESTITUTION

If one can expand the term "protection" to include resistance to change and "restitution" to include various forms of accommodation, adaptation as well as manufacture of materials required for establishing old or new balances, they do express the autonomic system's reaction to stress.

Not much will be said about the autonomic system's involvement in reactions to stress but the following considerations are pertinent. There are two categories of autonomic involvement; they are reactions which occur in short dramatic emergencies and those which mobilize adjustments to or resistance to chronic stress.

Cannon's concept of the emergency function of the sympatho-adrenal system typifies the quick, short compensatory reactions organized by the autonomic system. The emotional reactions caused by anticipation of injury or which accompany injury and crises are in this category and reveal a total activation of the sympatho-adrenal system. Within this response as a whole there are the reciprocal actions described by Riedel and Iriki (Chapter 30). Many emergencies are threats to stabilities of actual imbalances created by injury, toxicities, hemorrhage, etc. Response to hemorrhage involves shunting of blood, shortened clotting time, release from storage of red cells and plasma proteins and augmented heart action. The parasympathetic division is not completely inhibited by the strong sympatho-adrenal reactions. Vagus action on the heart can actually be considered cooperative with the sympathetic system in increasing cardiac output since by slowing the heart a greater stroke volume and cardiac output is possible than in an unopposed sympathetic-epinephrine-induced tachycardia. Balancing actions are involved immediately in response to emergency but they are most important in terminating reactions to emergencies. Augmentation of autonomic system action required to maintain blood pressure and flow not only causes vasoconstriction but renin-angiotension liberation[6] which affects ADH-vasopressin output from the hypothalamus. If this is not eventually terminated another type of imbalance and chronic stress could result. There is no sharp line of division between response to short- and long-term stress.

In response to long-term stressors the autonomic system also acts but in a different fashion. The endocrines are activated to some degree through autonomic innervations.

Metabolic processes are secondarily augmented and new balances are set for some states while mechanisms maintaining others are strengthened. The hypothalamus, autonomic, thyroid and adrenal control loops are activated in chronic exposure to cold. Stress is evoked by many things and each must be compensated for in special ways. The different types of body reactions to stress have been discussed by Selye in a very interesting way[7].

Two final statements will conclude this discussion. First, it appears that in every reaction initiated in the body or even in tissues there is an element of reversal which is frequently made apparent as an after effect. Accommodation, adaptation and reversals occur. It appears that peripheral, autoregulatory[2,5], as well as central and ganglionic interactions are involved in these diminishing and reversing functions. These interactions contribute to the establishment of balances and the maintenance of steady states or homeostasis. Second, the concept of homeostasis is now being used by those studying behavior and operant conditioning[1,9]. This brings us to the subject matter of the next section of this book—that dealing with the conditioning of autonomic system function.

REFERENCES

1 Bohus, B., Pituitary peptides and adaptive autonomic responses. In: W. H. Gispen, van Wimersma Griedanus, Tj. B., B. Bohus and D. de Wied (Eds.), *Hormones, Homeostasis and the Brain*, Progress in Brain Research, Vol. 42, Elsevier, Amsterdam, 1975, pp. 275–284.

2 Brooks, C. McC. and Lange, G., Interaction of myogenic and neurogenic mechanisms that control heart rate, *Proc. nat. Acad. Sci. USA*, 74 (1977) 1761–1762.

3 Cannon, W. B., Organization for physiological homeostasis, *Physiol. Rev.*, 9 (1929) 399–431.

4 Hess, W. R., *Diencephalon, Autonomic and Extrapyramidal Functions*, Grune and Stratton, New York, 1954.

5 Lange, G. and Brooks, C. McC., Neural influences on cardiac autoregulatory processes, *Amer. J. Physiol.*, submitted.

6 Reid, I. A., Morris, B. J. and Ganong, W. F., The renin-angiotensin system, *Ann. Rev. Physiol.*, 40 (1978) 377–410.

7 Selye, H., Homeostasis and heterostasis. In: C. McC. Brooks, K. Koizumi and J. O. Pinkston (Eds.), *The Life and Contributions of Walter B. Cannon 1871–1945: His Influence on the Development of Physiology in the Twentieth Century*, State University of New York Press, Albany, 1972, pp. 108–112.

8 Selye H., Homeostasis and the Reactions to Stress. In: C. McC. Brooks, K. Koizumi and J. O. Pinkston (Eds.), *The Life and Contributions of Walter B. Cannon 1871–1945: His Influence on the Development of Physiology in the Twentieth Century*, State University of New York Press, Albany, 1972, pp. 89–107.

9 Shapiro, A. P., Redmond, D. P., McDonald, R. H., Jr. and Gaylor, M., Relationships of perception, cognition, suggestion and operant conditioning in essential hypertension. In: W. H. Gispen, Tj. B. van Wimersma Greidanus, B. Bohus and D. de Wied (Eds.), *Hormones, Homeostasis and The Brain*, Progress in Brain Research Vol. 42, Elsevier, Amsterdam, 1975, pp. 299–312.

10 Whitteridge, D., Cardiovascular reflexes initiated from afferent sites other than the cardiovascular system itself, *Physiol. Rev.*, Suppl. 4, 40 (1960) 198–200.

SECTION VII

BEHAVIOR

Behavior is generally equated with activity, active response to stimuli, but in the broader sense it encompasses all aspects of the flow of life processes. This has already been illustrated in previous sections of this volume. The chief concerns of this chapter are the consideration of patterns of behavior which appear to be inherent or unlearned and those behavioral accomplishments which can be learned or conditioned. The autonomic system plays a definite role in both these types of behavior and this is the matter to be emphasized.

One of the important aspects of this section is that the totalities of reactions are emphasized. The analytical approach permits identification of centers essential to particular reaction phenomena but creates a false simplicity and often a distortion of significances. Little by little, however, as is well illustrated in this collection of contributions, analysis has revealed interactions which occur not only centrally but all along the afferent and efferent pathways. It is now recognized by some at least that how the total organism is affected and what it does is the important thing. The study of what happens in cell membranes, at individual synapses or even in special reflex arcs or "centers" is no longer enough.

There is evidence that patterns of response are evoked by stimuli. Some of these appear to be basic and intrinsic in all individuals. It is conceivable that other response patterns are created by conditioning or there is an overlay of learned reactions superimposed upon the primitive inherent performances. These are the considerations treated in the following contributions of this section.

Those who have studied the autonomic system, although fully aware of its role in emotional expression and in behavioral activity, have seldom thought of it as being much involved in the learning or memory functions of the nervous system. Although Pavlov's observations concerning conditioning were made chiefly on organs autonomically innervated, we have always considered the cerebral centers as the only components involved in learning. To be sure, a few have had some realization that the autonomic system is peculiarly involved. This concept, however, has only recently come under close scrutiny by those behaviorists who are now using classical, Pavlovian, procedures and the newly developed operant conditioning methodologies. This represents a new field of autonomic system study.

CHAPTER 33

SYMPATHETIC NERVE ACTIVITY, AORTIC PRESSURE AND HEART RATE IN RESPONSE TO BEHAVIORAL STIMULI

Ishio Ninomiya* and Yoshiharu Yonezawa**

*Department of Cardiac Physiology, Research Institute National Cardiovascular Center, Osaka, Japan, and ** The Department of Electrical Engineering, Hiroshima Institute of Technology, Hiroshima, Japan

INTRODUCTION

It has been observed in every day life that changes in heart rate, arterial blood pressure, cardiac output and other cardiovascular variables occur preceding, simultaneous with or following such behavioral stimuli as exercise, postural changes, fighting, eating and drinking[1,2,4,5,12,14,23-25]. These phenomena suggest that in awake conditions the heart and blood vessels are influenced directly from the higher central nervous system through the autonomic nervous system as well as reflexly from various receptors.

Studies on reflex and central neural regulations of circulation in both anesthetized and unanesthetized animals have been performed mainly by measuring hemodynamic variables[13,18,19,22]. In these studies, considerably larger differences have been noticed in the quality of data obtained from the conscious instrumented animal than obtained from the classical anesthetized animal. It has been suggested that general anesthesia radically alters cardiovascular function and responsiveness by changing the neural signal as well as by a direct action on the heart and vessels.

The majority of experiments designed to study neural signals to the heart and vessels have been carried out in anesthetized animals; also, in these studies the main objective was to analyse the reflex effects of baroreceptor[9,15], volume receptor[3,6,8,11,26], chemoreceptor[7] and thermoreceptor[16]. Only a few experiments have been performed on conscious animals[10,17,20,21]. Continuous measurements, in such conscious animals, of sympathetic nerve activity in response to various behavioral stimuli should provide direct information concerning neural signals from the higher central nervous system controlling the cardiovascular system. The purpose of this study was to provide such information and to analyse the neuro-regulatory mechanisms operating in conscious animals in relation to changes in behavior.

METHODS

Preparation of Animals

The experiments were carried out on cats (2.0–4.3 kg., b.w.) selected carefully from the standpoint of temperament; a well-mannered but spirited cat would tolerate a long-term chronic experiment after implantation surgery. They were anesthetized with sodium pentobarbital (30–35 mg/kg., i.p.) for implantation surgery. No dietary pretreatment was performed, but an antibiotic drug was administered before and after surgery. All experiments were carried out in an air-conditioned room with the temperature maintained between 20 and 25°C.

Implantation of Electrode

Under aseptic conditions, a bundle of nerve fibers from the left renal nerve (1.2–2.2 cm in length) was separated from the renal plexus located near the renal artery and vein. The nerve bundle (about one cm in length) was desheathed carefully at the site of electrode implantation. The details of the size and configuration of the implantable electrode assembly have been described previously[17]. After the nerve bundle was placed in the channel through the slit of the implantable electrode assembly, the slit was closed completely by sutures. The implantable electrode assembly was then sutured to the surrounding connective tissue. The lead cables from the implantable electrodes consisting of a recording electrode and a reference electrode were brought to the body surface and a socket was firmly attached to the skin of the back.

Recording

Renal nerve activity (RNA) was picked up from the recording electrode of the implanted assembly in both anesthetized and unanesthetized cats by using either direct lead wires[10,17,20,21] or a multichannel telemetry system[28].

In conscious cats, it is important to discriminate bioelectrical noise (BEN) consisting of electromyogram (EMG) and electrocardiogram (ECG) from the RNA tracing. Therefore, during the experiments the original RNA and BEN around the recording electrode (i.e., within one mm) were measured simultaneously by the reference electrode in the implanted electrode assembly. The original RNA and BEN were amplified by a differential amplifier with a band pass filter of 60 Hz to two k Hz, rectified by an absolute value circuit and integrated by RC integrators (time constant, 0.02 and one sec). Figure 1 shows a schematic diagram of the recording system. The output signal from the integrator was displayed on a pen recorder. The original RNA, BEN, ECG and simple integrated RNA were monitored by a digital memory scope. An example of the data sampled at 1024 points within a period of 819.2 msec is shown in the right panel of Fig. 1. The original RNA and BEN show different time courses. This indicates the recording system is reliable. If the time courses and spectra of RNA and BEN signals resembled each other, the data were not used. Averaged RNA synchronous with cardiac cycle was measured by a signal processor. The R spike of the ECG was used as an external trigger signal for averaging the RNA.

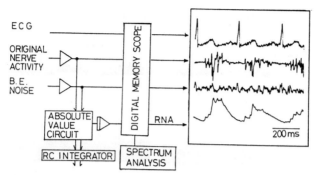

Fig. 1. A schematic diagram of monitoring and recording systems of electrocardiogram (ECG), renal nerve activity (RNA) and bioelectrical noise (BEN) in conscious animals. Original nerve activity and BEN sampled randomly for 819.2 msec were compared. Difference in wave forms of two signals indicates the recording system is reliable.

In all cats studied, teflon-coated silver wires were implanted in both the right and left chest walls for recording ECG's. ECG was measured simultaneously with RNA and BEN by using the telemetry system. The R-R interval of the ECG was continuously measured and displayed on a pen recorder. Heart rate was estimated from the inverse value of the R-R interval.

The left common carotid artery and jugular vein were cannulated for the recording of blood pressure and infusion of solutions. In four cats the aortic blood pressure was recorded by a strain gauge through a cannula.

RESULTS

Discharge Pattern of the Renal Nerve Activity after Implantation Surgery

Immediately after implantation surgery, the cats were still under a moderately anesthetized condition. Discharge patterns of RNA were regular and showed a grouped activity synchronous with the cardiac cycle. This is in good agreement with data reported previously[15,16]. The R-R interval of the ECG was very stable. During light anesthesia, from two to eight hr after surgery, mean and grouped RNA synchronous with cardiac cycle increased gradually. Rhythmic variation in RNA synchronous with respiratory movements tended to appear. In addition, a rhythmic increase was observed frequently in RNA with a period of 20 to 40 sec (Fig. 2, left panel). Heart rate increased further and in turn the cyclic variations tended to disappear.

During the transition period from anesthesia to the conscious state, the cats began to move their forepaws and hind limbs and tried to stand or walk. During such escape responses, RNA and BEN increased significantly and the recording of signals was interrupted frequently.

On the first day after the implantation surgery, the cats became completely conscious. In all cats studied, RNA and heart rate increased nearly to the maximum level during the postoperative experiment days. This increase in RNA and heart rate may partly be related to postsurgical stress including pain, fever and dehydration. On the

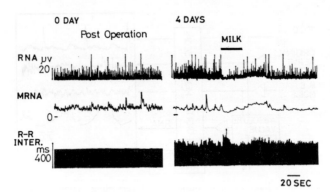

Fig. 2.   Renal nerve activity (RNA), mean renal nerve activity (MRNA) and R-R interval
recorded under slightly anesthetized condition on the day of operation and that
recorded in a conscious condition on the fourth day after operation were compared.
Note a difference in calibration of RNA. See text for details.

second and third days after surgery, RNA, BEN and heart rate varied widely depending on whether the animal was resting, sitting, drinking or excited. Moreover, RNA
and heart rate changed significantly due to emotional stimuli. For example, when a
visitor entered the laboratory, RNA and heart rate often increased suddenly for a few
seconds though the animal was lying down quietly without any observable change in
behavior.

The experiments with the conscious animals were performed not earlier than
48 hours after the end of anesthesia.

Renal Nerve Activity while Drinking Milk and Water

An example of the data sampled on the fourth day after surgery is shown in the
right panel of Fig. 2. During the control periods, absolute magnitude of RNA and
MRNA decreased to approximately half of that obtained on day zero after surgery.
This decreased RNA was partly caused by reduction in the frequency of impulses as
well as by decrease in the amplitude of impulses[10]. An increase in R-R interval from
302 msec to 390 msec coincided with a decrease in heart rate from 198 cpm to 153 cpm
during the resting state.

When a cup containing milk was shown to a cat, the animal became excited and
stood up to drink the milk. RNA fluctuated from eight to 15 sec, while the heart rate
tended to increase with various time courses. When the cat began to drink, RNA was
inhibited rapidly, while R-R interval was prolonged from 320 msec to 510 msec with
an overshoot response and reached the maximum level within five sec. While the cats
was drinking the milk, R-R interval recovered to the control values, but in some
cases no recovery in RNA and heart rate was observed (Fig. 3). On the third day after
electrode implantation RNA, MRNA and R-R intervals of the ECG were measured
simultaneously by the telemetry system. In anticipation of milk, the animal stood up
and walked near the cup containing milk. Heart rate increased significantly, but RNA
only fluctuated during this period. When the cat began to drink the milk, RNA and
MRNA were inhibited immediately and reached a minimum level within five sec.

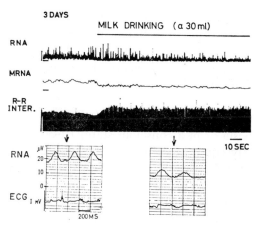

3 DAYS

MILK DRINKING (a 30 ml)

RNA

MRNA

R-R
INTER.

10 SEC

RNA μV
20
10
0

ECG 1 mV

200MS

Fig. 3. While drinking milk, renal nerve activity (RNA), mean renal nerve activity (MRNA) and R-R interval of ECG were recorded on the third day after surgery. Calibration: RNA: 40 μV; R-R interval: 400 msec. RNA and ECG were averaged over 50 cardiac cycles before and during drinking milk. See text for details.

An increase in R-R interval and a decrease in heart rate occurred with a time delay of two to three sec after reduction in RNA and reached a maximum level (480 msec) 15 sec after the cat began to drink. While drinking milk, the inhibition of RNA and bradycardia continued.

In seven other cats studied, RNA and heart rate tended to increase in many trials before drinking milk or water and then they decreased rapidly with or without an undershoot response simultaneous with or following drinking. While drinking milk, the time courses of RNA, MRNA and R-R interval varied significantly among the different trials on a given experiment day in the same animal. MRNA and heart rate reached a minimum level between five and 30 sec after onset of drinking.

In four cats, mean aortic blood pressure was measured by the lead cable method, which restricted the animals' free movement. In all cats aortic blood pressure became elevated slightly prior to drinking milk and then fell rapidly at onset of drinking.

In the conscious state as in the anesthetized condition, a grouped activity synchronous with the cardiac cycle was observed in all cats examined. This is in a good agreement with data reported previously[10,17,20]. The magnitude of grouped activity varied from cycle to cycle under a given condition. To enhance the signal-to-noise ratio and to reduce the cycle variation of the grouping, the integrated RNA were averaged over 50 cardiac cycles, using the R spike of the ECG as a trigger signal. Examples of the data obtained before and during drinking milk are shown at the bottom of Fig. 3. During the control periods, grouped RNA was clearly detected. The time interval between the R spike of the ECG and the peak value of grouped activity ranged from 160 to 200 msec. While the cat was drinking milk, grouped RNA synchronous with cardiac cycle was observed, but tonic RNA was decreased significantly. The time interval between the R spike of the ECG and the peak value of grouped activity was prolonged from 40 to 60 msec as compared with that obtained during control periods.

From the overall data it can be concluded that RNA, heart rate and aortic blood pressure tended to increase prior to drinking milk or water while standing, walking or under emotional stimuli such as anticipation of milk. When the cat began to drink, RNA, heart rate and aortic blood pressure decreased immediately with various time courses including an undershoot response.

Renal Nerve Activity during Infusion of Normal Saline Solution

Under light anesthesia or in a conscious state, 10–30 ml of 0.9% saline solution, which was approximately equal in volume to the milk intake, was injected through the cannula implanted previously. When injection speed was increased, aortic blood pressure tended to elevate and in turn RNA was inhibited reflexly by baroceptor inputs. In such a case, it was difficult to distinguish whether the reduction in RNA during infusion was caused by the baroceptor input or volume receptor input. Therefore, the injection speed was carefully controlled to avoid elevation in aortic blood pressure. As reported previously[21,26] MRNA decreased gradually while aortic blood pressure remained almost constant. This slow reduction in MRNA induced by volume load may be caused reflexly by inputs from the volume receptors.

Renal Nerve Activity during Postural Changes

Effects of postural changes on cardiovascular variables in animals have been studied by many investigators[5,19], but discharge patterns of the sympathetic nerve activity during postural changes have not been described. In this study renal nerve activity (RNA) was measured simultaneously with heart rate in both spontaneous and forced postural changes.

Figure 4 shows an example of the data obtained during various conditions such as sleeping, standing and walking. During sleeping periods RNA and BEN decreased, while the R-R interval was prolonged. When the cat stood up or even jumped up

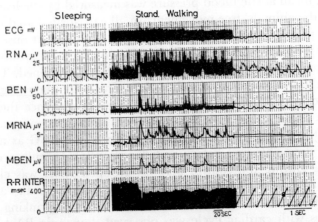

Fig. 4.   Shown are the effects of sleeping, spontaneous standing and walking on the electrocardiogram (ECG), renal nerve activity (RNA), bioelectrical noise (BEN), mean renal nerve activity (MRNA), mean bioelectrical noise (MBEN) and R-R interval of ECG. See text for details.

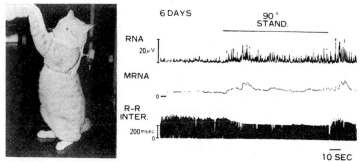

Fig. 5. The effects of postural changes on the renal nerve activity (RNA), mean renal nerve activity (MRNA) and R-R interval. On the sixth day after the operation, a small amount of RNA is observed at control periods, but with forced upright standing position (left pannel) RNA increased significantly with an overshoot response, while the R-R interval decreased.

suddenly from a prone position and then started to walk, significant changes in ECG, RNA, MRNA, MBEN and R-R interval were observed. It was noted that RNA, MRNA and heart rate increased suddenly prior to an increase in BEN. The increase in BEN was always simultaneous with muscular activity due to spontaneous standing. In many chronic cats, along with spontaneous postural change a massive increase in RNA which preceded or occurred simultaneously with the increase in BEN was always recorded. Time course and magnitude of responses varied among the different trials. These results suggest that prior to change in posture the increase in sympathetic nerve activity to the heart and blood vessels was induced directly from the higher central nervous system. During walking periods RNA, BEN and heart rate increased above the resting levels.

The effects of forced upright standing posture (rump angle of 90 degrees) on the heart rate and RNA were studied in seven cats. In Fig. 5, RNA, MRNA and R-R interval were measured before and during forced upright standing posture on the sixth day after surgery. When the cats were made to stand up on their hind legs with heads up, RNA always increased with an overshoot response, while the R-R interval decreased. In contrast to spontaneous standing posture, the increase in RNA and heart rate occurred almost simultaneously with the forced upright standing posture. When the standing position was suspended, RNA responses varied among the different trials.

DISCUSSION

The present study shows that the use of anesthetic drugs masks or even abolishes one of the neuroregulatory mechanisms which operates in conscious animals in response to emotional and behavioral stimuli.

Using chronically implanted flow sensors, it was observed that renal blood flow was very sensitive to mild neurobehavioral stimuli in the laboratory and suggested that changes in renal flow might be mediated from the sympathetic adrenergic fibers[27]. In this study, sympathetic nerve activity to the kidney (RNA) was measured directly using implantable electrodes[17] in conscious cats and it was found that the RNA varied significantly in everyday life in response to emotional and behavioral stimuli.

Classical (i.e., Pavlovian) or operant behavioral conditioning procedures can be used to provide a well defined means for activating the neuroregulatory mechanisms[18], but in this study the experiments were carried out under "natural" circumstances. This was done because it is desirable to record the neural signals responsible for the regulation of circulation during spontaneous behavior. The RNA and probably to the heart was rapidly inhibited at the onset of drinking milk or water. Neural mechanisms responsible for this inhibition of RNA can be explained as follows. It has been recently shown that RNA was reduced by intravenous infusion of isotonic saline or dextran in conscious animals[21] as well as in anesthetized animals[3,8,26]. Similarly, in this study RNA was inhibited during intravenous infusion of normal saline solution. The contribution of volume receptors to the inhibition of RNA during oral uptake of fluids can be considered to be one of the major mechanisms. However, inhibition of RNA observed at the onset of spontaneous oral uptake was faster than that observed at the time of direct intravenous volume loading. This suggests that the initial rapid inhibition of RNA cannot be produced by both baro- and volume receptors in the circulatory system, but might be induced by inputs originating from the higher central nervous system simultaneous with behavior change. The decrease in heart rate and aortic pressure can be explained by the inhibition in sympathetic nerve activity in both spontaneous oral uptake and intravenous injection of fluids.

It is generally accepted that during postural changes the gravitational effect is an initiating factor of change in cardiovascular dynamics[5,19]. During the upright standing posture (rump=90 degrees), a decrease in stroke volume led to a reduction of cardiac output and a fall in arterial blood pressure. The fall in arterial blood pressure reflexly produced an increase in sympathetic nerve activity to various organs[9,22], and in turn caused an increase in heart rate and peripheral resistance. Therefore, the baroceptor reflex system was considered to be the most important regulatory mechanism for readjustment of arterial blood pressure during postural changes.

The present study has demonstrated that at the instant when skeletal muscles became active for standing or even in anticipation of standing, sympathetic nerve activity to the kidney and heart rate increased. This early initial increase in sympathetic nerve activity served to increase peripheral vascular resistance and even before assuming the upright position it tended to prevent the reduction of arterial blood pressure. Furthermore, with spontaneous upright standing posture, the increase in RNA was far greater than that expected from the relationship between arterial blood pressure and sympathetic nerve activity under anesthesia. The results of this experiment have suggested that with a spontaneous postural change a centrally initiating mechanism instead of the baroceptor reflexes is a very important factor for the increase in sympathetic nerve activity, and in turn may induce more rapid adjustment of cardiovascular dynamics during postural changes in conscious animals.

SUMMARY

Using implantable electrodes, sympathetic nerve activity to the kidney (RNA) was measured simultaneously with aortic blood pressure (AP) and electrocardiogram (ECG) under both spontaneous oral uptake of fluids (milk and water) and intravenous injection of normal saline, and during postural changes.

At the onset of oral uptake of fluids RNA, AP and heart rate (HR) decreased with an undershoot response and reached the minimum level within 15 sec. In contrast, when normal saline solution was injected intravenously, RNA always decreased gradually within 40 sec during volume loading (10–30 ml). The initial rapid reduction of RNA observed at the onset of oral uptake of fluids was induced directly by inputs from the higher central nervous system simultaneous with behavioral stimuli rather than by inputs from baro- and volume receptors.

Increase in RNA and HR in response to forced upright standing posture was observed in the conscious state. In some cases, the increase in RNA occurred prior to spontaneous postural changes, suggesting that in conscious animals the cardiovascular system is controlled by both feedforward signals from the central nervous system and feedback signals from the baroceptors during postural changes.

This study was supported in part by research grants from The Asahi Shimbun, Ministry of Health and Welfare, and Ministry of Education, Science and Culture of Japan.

REFERENCES

1 Adams, D. B., Baccelli, G., Mancia, G. and Zanchetti, A., Cardiovascular changes during naturally excited fighting behavior in the cat, *Amer. J. Physiol.*, 216 (1969) 1226–1235.

2 Adams, D. B., Baccelli, G., Mancia, G. and Zanchetti, A., Relation of cardiovascular changes in fighting to emotion and exercise, *J. Physiol.* (Lond.), 212 (1971) 321–335.

3 Clement, D. L., Palletier, C. L. and Shepherd, J. T., Role of vagal afferents in the control of renal sympathetic nerve activity in the rabbit, *Circulation Res.*, 31 (1972) 824–830.

4 Cohen, O. H. and Obrist, P. A., Interactions between behavior and the cardiovascular system, *Circulation Res.*, 37 (1975) 693–706.

5 Gauer, O. H. and Thron, H. L., Postural changes in the circulation. In: W. F. Hamilton (Ed.), *Circulation, Handbook of Physiology*, Sec. 2, Vol. 3, American Physiological Society, Washington, D. C., 1965, pp. 2409–2440.

6 Goetz, K. L., Bond, G. C. and Bloxham, D. D., Atrial receptors and renal function. *Physiol. Rev.*, 55 (1975) 157–205.

7 Iriki, M., Walther, O. E., Pleschka, K. and Simon, E., Regional cutaneous and visceral sympathetic activity during asphyxia in the anesthetized rabbit, *Pflügers Arch.*, 322 (1971) 167–182.

8 Karim, F., Kidd, C., Malpus, C. M. and Penna, P. E., The effects of the left atrial receptors on sympathetic efferent nerve activity, *J. Physiol.* (Lond.), 227 (1972) 243–260.

9 Kirchheim, H. R., Systemic arterial baroceptor reflexes, *Physiol. Rev.*, 56 (1976) 100–176.

10 Kirchner, F., Correlations between changes of activity of the renal sympathetic nerve and behavioral events in unrestrained cats, *Basic Research in Cardiology*, 69 (1973) 243–256.

11 Koizumi, K., Ishikawa, T., Nishino, H. and Brooks, C. McC., Cardiac and autonomic system reactions to strech of the atria, *Brain Res.*, 87 (1975) 247–261.

12 Mancia, G., Baccelli, G. and Zanchetti, A., Regulation of renal circulation during behavioral changes in the cat, *Amer. J. Physiol.*, 227 (1974) 536–542.

13 McCutcheon, E. P., *Chronically Implanted Cardiovascular Instrumentation*, Academic Press, New York, 1976, pp. 357–394.

14 Ninomiya, I. and Wilson, M. F., Cardiac adaptation at the transition phases of exercise in unanesthetized dogs, *J. appl. Physiol.*, 21 (1966) 953–958.

15 Ninomiya, I. and Irisawa, H., Nonuniformity of the sympathetic nerve activity in response to baroceptor inputs, *Brain Res.*, 87 (1975) 313–322.

16 Ninomiya, I. and Fujita, S., Reflex effects of thermal stimulation on sympathetic nerve activity to skin and kidney, *Amer. J. Physiol.*, 230 (1976) 271–278.

17 Ninomiya, I., Yonezawa, Y. and Wilson, M. F., Implantable electrode for recording nerve signals in awake animals, *J. appl. Physiol.*, 41 (1976) 111–114.

18 Randal, D. C., Neural control of the heart in the intact nonhuman primate. In: W. C. Randal (Ed.), *Neural Regulation of the Heart*, Oxford University Press, New York, 1977, pp. 381–408.

19 Rushmer, R. F., *Cardiovascular Dynamics* (4th ed.), Saunders, Philadelphia, 1976.

20 Schad, H. and Seller, H., A method for recording autonomic nerve activity in unanesthetized, freely moving cats, *Brain Res.*, 100 (1975) 425–430.

21 Schad, H. and Seller, H., Reduction of renal nerve activity by volume expansion in conscious cats, *Pflügers Arch.*, 363 (1976) 155–159.

22 Smith, O. A., Reflex and central mechanisms involved in the control of the heart and circulation, *Ann. Rev. Physiol.*, 36 (1974) 93–123.

23 Vatner, S. F., Franklin, D. and Van Citter, R. L., Mesenteric vasoactivity associated with eating and digestion in the conscious dog, *Amer. J. Physiol.*, 219 (1970) 170–184.

24 Vatner, S. F., Patrick, T. A., Higgins, C. B. and Franklin, D., Regional circulatory adjustments to eating and digestion in conscious unrestrained primates, *J. appl. Physiol.*, 28 (1974) 524–529.

25 Vatner, S. F., Effects of exercise and excitement on mesenteric and renal dynamics in conscious, unrestrained baboons, *Amer. J. Physiol.*, 234 (1978) H210–H214.

26 Weaver, L. C., Cardiopulmonary sympathetic afferent influences on renal nerve activity, *Amer. J. Physiol.*, 233 (1977) H592–H599.

27 Wilson, M. F. and Iriuchijima, J., Neural control of peripheral flow distribution, *Circulation*, Suppl 2. (1967) 35–36.

28 Yonezawa, Y., Ninomiya, I. and Nishiura, N., A multichannel telemetry system for recording cardiovascular neural signals and electrocardiography in unrestrained animals, *Amer. J. Physiol.*, in press.

CHAPTER 34

THE DEFENSE REACTION AS A PARADIGM FOR CARDIOVASCULAR CONTROL

S. M. Hilton

Department of Physiology, The University of Birmingham,
The Medical School, Birmingham, England

INTRODUCTION

The study of circulatory control has suffered as much as many others in physiology, and more than most, from the analytical approach that seemed essential for any experimental work in an area of such complexity. This approach had proved extremely fruitful in development of the physical sciences and had only seemed to run into difficulties in the realm of subatomic particles. It is not in any way surprising that the early attempts to put physiology on a firm scientific footing should have proceeded along similar lines. This approach, however, has led to a peculiarly pervasive distortion of reality, according to which the brain stem has been held to be an assembly of regions, each of which controls a single, cardiovascular variable, all such variables being considered as single entities. Arterial blood pressure is one such entity, not because it is the product of a single organ (even of a single system), but simply due to the historical and practical accident that it can be measured by a single, simple instrument. Pressor and depressor "centers" of the medulla could thus be defined, and it was a small and obvious step to lump them together as a "vasomotor center", as every student of physiology will agree. Only add to this account the Cartesian notion of the reflex and all is explained: Appropriate afferent pathways act through this center to elicit appropriate responses. This is the assumed basis of control.

Such a simple, mechanistic approach as just outlined is both comforting and confusing. It comforts because it is easy to understand, and it confuses because it cannot accommodate a wealth of relevant findings. Moreover, it provides little prospect of achieving a rational method of therapeutic control of arterial blood pressure; but those who concentrate on the fashionable study of input-output relationships will naturally continue to work with the traditional ideas, and this may be an important reason why past discussions of the flaws inherent in it have made little impact.

RESULTS AND DISCUSSION

The Defense Reaction

An alternative approach is to identify biologically significant patterns of response and to localize the parts of the brain stem that play an important role in the integration of each of these patterns. This has proved straightforward and useful in the case of the defense reaction. This term (abwehrreaktion) was first proposed by Hess[13]. It was already known that the hypothalamus exerts a measure of control over basic behavior patterns, such as fear and rage[3] but Hess and his colleagues had gone further. In a monumental series of experiments they located regions of the hypothalamus, some of which, on electrical stimulation, elicited alimentary or sexual reactions, and one which elicited the so-called defense reaction. This last is expressed initially as an alerting reaction on threshold stimulation, consisting of pricking of the ears and pupillary dilatation during which the cat may look up and around; while with stronger stimulation, piloerection develops, the claws are unsheathed, the animal hisses and spits and starts running movements which may end in flight or directed attack. Needless to say, this is identical with the reaction which a cat displays in a fully developed form when subjected to a very painful stimulus or confronted by a dog. The early, alerting stage of the reaction is elicited by any sudden stimulus, such as even a moderately loud sound[13].

The defense reaction is a basic behavioral response in all higher animals; the details varying only a little from one species to another. In man, too, the reaction, in a mild form at least, is a frequent occurrence in our daily lives, and though we have learned, more or less successfully, to inhibit our movements of attack or flight, the responses of the internal organs appear to persist, for the most part unchanged. Cannon was the first to make a detailed study of the visceral as well as the somatic components of these reactions. Starting from the premise that the reaction as a whole is adaptive, insofar as it leads, in nature, to the preservation of the organism, he proceeded to show how all the bodily changes then known to occur as components of the reaction could be viewed within the framework of this general concept[4].

There seems every reason to think of the cardiovascular components of the reaction as also contributing to the maximum efficiency of the organism during a period of emergency[14]. These components constitute a pattern which is readily understandable in the context of this hypothesis; for venous reservoirs are mobilized and cardiac output increased, with a redistribution of blood flow, mostly favoring skeletal muscle at the expense of the gastrointestinal tract and skin. Moreover, this whole pattern of change is achieved during the early, alerting stage of the reaction, before the overt movements involved in flight or attack. For this reason it was proposed that the cardiovascular response be designated as a preparatory reflex[2].

In a series of investigations, my colleagues and I have located regions in the hypothalamus, midbrain, pons and medulla, all of which presumably act together in the normal, conscious animal to integrate the full pattern of response—behavioral and visceral, although the cardiovascular components have been the main focus of our attention. This led to the suggestion that such a longitudinal form of anatomical and functional organization along the length of the brain stem might prove to be a characteristic feature of the mode of integration of such patterned responses, in which case studies of the central nervous physiology of defense reactions would give the most valid insight into the fundamental questions of cardiovascular control[15,16]. In the following sections I will deal with three quite different studies in which we have recently been engaged, all of which have led to results pointing to the same conclusion.

Cerebral Cortical Influences on the Cardiovascular System

There have been many reports in the past of changes in arterial blood pressure obtained on stimulation of the motor cortex (cf. review by Hoff, Kell and Carrol[21]) and several reports of muscle vasodilatation mediated by the sympathetic outflow[9,10,29]. The most recent study[7] even indicated such vasodilatation in a single limb, in baboons and monkeys.

When repeating such experiments, in cats under althesin anesthesia, we stimulated the hind limb area of the motor cortex under rigorous experimental control, designed to avoid reflex effects evoked through stimulation of meningeal afferent fibers or stimulus spread to noncortical structures[19,20]. We used althesin, as Timms[26] had shown that it does not seem to depress or distort transmission through the hypothalamus or midbrain, at least so far as the defense reaction is concerned. We then found that the threshold stimulus for a vasodilator effect in the contralateral hind limb was the same as that for muscle contraction, and the magnitude of the one was related to that of the other. Lesions in the medullary pyramid reduced both together, and prevention of the somatic motor response by gallamine or spinal cord section at L_{4-5} (which leaves the sympathetic outflow to the hind limbs intact) led to the abolition of the vascular response. As the muscle vasodilatation was insensitive to atropine and guanethidine except, significantly, in those experiments in which these agents reduced the muscle contraction, we could only conclude that this vasodilatation is simply a post-contraction hyperemia, evoked independently of the sympathetic nervous system.

These negative results led us to ask whether the cerebral cortex can influence the defense reaction elicited from lower parts of the brain. Release of so-called sham-rage on frontal decortication has long been known[5,22] and there is much evidence of inhibitory influences originating in the orbital cortex, so Dr. Timms has recently been exploring the frontal cortical areas of cats under althesin to see if they can affect the defense response, especially its cardiovascular components[27,28].

In these experiments, defense reactions were evoked by electrical stimulation in the amygdala, its projection pathway towards the hypothalamus or the hypothalamus itself. The recorded responses included the well-established increases in respiration, arterial blood pressure, heart rate and hind limb vascular conductance, together with decreased conductance in the mesenteric and renal vascular beds. Sites were then located in the anterior and lateral sigmoid gyri and the rostral part of the orbital gyrus which, though without effect on cardiovascular variables when stimulated alone, caused a significant reduction of an amygdaloid test response evoked simultaneously, and sometimes almost abolished it, the muscle vasodilatation being affected most[27,28]. There is also evidence of a facilitatory region which is not as yet precisely defined, but which is located at the medial aspect of the frontal cortex, projecting possibly in the median forebrain bundle. In no case did stimulation in any of these cortical areas significantly alter a test response evoked from the hypothalamus, which indicates that the main site of interaction is in, or near, the hypothalamus itself. In the few experiments in which they have been tested, defense reactions evoked as a reflex on stimulation of the radial nerve or carotid chemoreceptors have also been similarly modulated.

The Cardiovascular Response to Stimulation of Peripheral Chemoreceptors

In the course of some of our earlier experiments on high decerebrate cats with the hypothalamus intact, we were surprised to find that stimulation of the carotid chemoreceptors could evoke the full defense reaction[17]. Dr. Marshall and I have been following this up more recently in animals with the central nervous system intact. This could only have been done before now in conscious animals, since most of the autonomic components of the defense reaction (and the behavioral features) cannot be elicited under conventional anesthesia. Effectively, we have been reinvestigating the chemoreceptor reflex in cats anesthetized with althesin, using cyanide, Krebs solution equilibrated with CO_2 or P_i solutions, which we had previously shown to selectively stimulate carotid chemoreceptor endings[18].

As well as the typical increase in rate and depth of respiration, these stimuli evoked pupillary dilatation, retraction of the nictitating membrane and piloerection, and the cardiovascular changes characteristic of the defense response[24]. Changes in blood pressure and heart rate were variable from one experiment to another, both in magnitude and direction, but in the fore- and hind limb muscles there was consistently a small vasoconstriction followed by a large dilatation of up to 150%. This dilatation still occurred in curarized animals which were artificially ventilated, and was not affected by vagotomy. There was an immediate decrease in mesenteric vascular conductance which always resulted in a substantial reduction in mesenteric flow. When the defense reaction was mild, as judged by the extent of the other autonomic effects, the renal conductance change was such that there was no change in renal flow. However, during a more powerful defense reaction there was a considerable decrease in both renal flow and conductance. These responses are like those produced during naturally-elicited alerting reactions in the conscious animal[6]. Furthermore, under althesin the same pattern of autonomic response is evoked by electrical stimulation of the radial nerve, a stimulus which would certainly elicit a defense reaction in a conscious animal.

The muscle vasodilatation in these reflexly-elicited responses was not the outcome of a single mechanism. In many experiments, it was sensitive to atropine and, hence, seemed mainly mediated by cholinergic fibers. In some, it was abolished by guanethidine, hence due most likely to inhibition of constrictor fiber activity. In others, it seemed to be some mixture of the two, often with a late vasodilatation which was abolished by propranolol and thus due to circulating adrenaline. All three factors doubtless contribute to some extent in any individual experiment.

These results indicate that the chemoreceptor input, in addition to a special effect on respiratory activity, can activate all parts of the brain stem defense area, including the region in the dorsal medulla which is known to inhibit sympathetic constrictor tone to skeletal muscle[8]. The full behavioral and autonomic response may be evoked by a powerful stimulus, while a mild stimulus may only lead to the cardio-vascular components of the reflex.

The Efferent Pathway for the Defense Reaction—Experiments on the Origin of Vasomotor Tone

Bilateral application of glycine to the ventral surface of the cat's medulla was recently shown to cause a pronounced and prolonged fall of arterial blood pressure, by acting on a restricted site near the surface[12]. This led us to carry out experiments on cats under althesin to find out whether the drug thus applied acts by blocking synapses in the efferent pathway for the autonomic components of the defense reaction; for this pathway was long ago shown to descend in this region of the ventral medulla[1,25].

We found that, on bilateral application of glycine to the sensitive area, respiration ceases and, with the animal now artificially ventilated, arterial blood pressure falls to a low level, due mainly to a fall in total peripheral resistance caused largely by vasodilatation in the mesenteric bed, with a small fall in cardiac output[11]. Within five min, mean arterial pressure falls to around 70 mmHg, and the circulatory response elicited by stimulation of the defense area of the amygdala or hypothalamus is substantially reduced, particularly the rise in arterial pressure and mesenteric vasoconstriction.

Localized electrical stimulation at, or just below, the surface of the medulla in the glycine-sensitive area elicits all the autonomic components of the defense reaction, including muscle vasodilatation and mesenteric and renal vasoconstriction, together with increased rate and depth of respiration. This pattern can be elicited from a narrow longitudinal strip in the medulla, three to four mm each side of the midline. The strip becomes superficial within the glycine-sensitive area, where it runs less than 500 μm from the surface. After a unilateral lesion within the glycine-sensitive area, restricted to this strip, the response to stimulation of ipsilateral defense areas is reduced. Glycine then applied to the contralateral medullary area alone produces fully the changes which, without the lesion, would only be seen after bilateral application.

Several interesting proposals can be made on the basis of these results. Firstly, the glycine-sensitive neurons on, or near, the ventral surface of the medulla may be the origin of the final common path for the visceral components of the defense reaction. Secondly, insofar as the "resting" blood pressure level is of central nervous origin, it results largely from continuing activity in the brain stem defense areas, relayed through the ventral medulla, and exerted chiefly on the resistance vessels of the gastrointestinal tract. Thirdly, since striking effects on ventilation can be obtained on localized stimulation or inactivation of the pathway for the defense reaction, the chemical sensitivity of the ventral surface of the medulla may not be related specifically to respiratory control, as has been assumed since the work of Mitchell, Loeschcke and their colleagues[23].

CONCLUSIONS

These three examples illustrate, each in its own way, how fruitful it has proved to adopt the general thesis that the brain organizes patterns of response, and to proceed therefrom by attempting to recognize biologically significant patterns and by identifying those regions of the brain stem which must act together to initiate them. It then becomes possible to study the afferent pathways involved, their relative effectiveness in facilitating or inhibiting each pattern and the connections by which their effects are achieved. Equally, the identification of efferent pathways is given a new impetus, particularly with the realization of the degree of integration for which they must be responsible. The traditional ideas of separate brain stem centers for single cardiovascular functions are no longer useful, let alone tenable.

REFERENCES

1   Abrahams, V. C., Hilton, S. M. and Zbrożyna, A. W., Reflex activation of vasodilator nerve fibres to skeletal muscle in decerebrate and intact cats, *J. Physiol.* (Lond.), 152 (1960) 54 P–55 P.
2   Abrahams, V. C., Hilton, S. M. and Zbrożyna, A. W., The role of active muscle vasodilatation in the alerting stage of the defence reaction, *J. Physiol.* (Lond.), 171 (1964) 189–202.
3   Bard, P., A diencephalic mechanism for the expression of rage with special reference to the sympathetic nervous system, *Amer. J. Physiol.*, 84 (1928) 490–515.
4   Cannon, W. B., *Bodily Changes in Pain, Hunger, Fear and Rage*, 2nd ed., D. Appleton & Co., New York and London, 1929.
5   Cannon, W. B. and Britton, S. W., Studies on the conditions of activity in endocrine glands. XV. Pseudaffective medulli-adrenal secretion, *Amer. J. Physiol.*, 72 (1925) 283–294.
6   Caraffa-Braga, E., Granata, L. and Pinotti, O., Changes in blood flow distribution during acute emotional stress in dogs, *Pflügers Arch.*, 339 (1973) 203–216.
7   Clarke, N. P., Smith, O. A. and Shearn, D. W., Topographical representation of vascular smooth muscle of limbs in primate motor cortex, *Amer. J. Physiol.*, 214 (1968) 122–129.
8   Coote, J. H., Hilton, S. M. and Zbrożyna, A. W., The pontomedullary area integrating the defence reaction in the cat and its influence on muscle blood flow, *J. Physiol.* (Lond.), 229 (1973) 257–274.
9   Eliasson, S., Lindgren, P. and Uvnäs, B., Representation in the hypothalamus and motor cortex in the dog of the sympathetic vasodilator outflow to the skeletal muscle, *Acta physiol. scand.*, 27 (1952) 18–37.
10 Green, H. D. and Hoff, E. C., Effects of faradic stimulation of cerebral cortex on limb and renal volumes in the cat and monkey, *Amer. J. Physiol.*, 118 (1937) 641–658.
11 Guertzenstein, P. G., Hilton, S. M., Marshall, J. M. and Timms, R. J., Experiments on the origin of vasomotor tone, *J. Physiol.* (Lond.), 275 (1978) 78 P–79 P.
12 Guertzenstein, P. G. and Silver, A., Fall in blood pressure produced from discrete regions of the ventral surface of the medulla by glycine and lesions, *J. Physiol.* (Lond.), 242 (1974) 489–503.
13 Hess, W. R. and Brugger, M., Das subkortikal Zentrum der affektiven abwehrreaktion, *Helv. physiol. Acta*, 1 (1943) 33–52.
14 Hilton, S. M., Hypothalamic control of the cardiovascular responses in fear and rage. In: *The Scientific Basis of Medicine Annual Reviews*, Athlone Press, London, 1965, pp. 217–238.
15 Hilton, S. M., The role of the hypothalamus in the organization of patterns of cardio-

vascular response. In: K. Lederis and K. E. Cooper (Eds.), *Recent Studies of Hypothalamic Function*, (Int. Symp. Calgary 1973), S. Kager, Basel, 1974, pp. 306–314.

16 Hilton, S. M., Ways of viewing the central nervous control of the circulation—Old and new, *Brain Res.*, 87 (1975) 213–219.

17 Hilton, S. M. and Joels, N., Facilitation of chemoreceptor reflexes during the defence reaction, *J. Physiol.* (Lond.), 176 (1965) 20 P–22 P.

18 Hilton, S. M., Spyer, K. M. and Timms, R. J., Stimulating action of inorganic phosphate on chemoreceptor afferent fibres of the carotid body, *J. Physiol.* (Lond.), 226 (1972) 61 P–62 P.

19 Hilton, S. M., Spyer, K. M. and Timms, R. J., Hind limb vasodilatation evoked by stimulation of the motor cortex, *J. Physiol.* (Lond.), 252 (1975) 22 P–23 P.

20 Hilton, S. M., Spyer, K. M. and Timms, R. J., The origin of the hind limb vasodilation evoked by stimulation of the motor cortex in the cat, *J. Physiol.* (Lond.), 287 (1979) 545–557.

21 Hoff, E. C., Kell, J. F., Jr. and Carrol, M. N., Jr., Effects of cortical stimulation and lesions on cardiovascular function, *Physiol. Rev.*, 43 (1963) 68–114.

22 Kennard, M. A., Focal autonomic representation in the cortex and its relation to sham rage, *J. Neuropath. exp. Neurol.*, 4 (1945) 295–304.

23 Loeschcke, H. H., Central nervous chemoreceptors. In: J. G. Widdicombe (Ed.), *International Review of Science, Physiology Series One, Vol. 2, Respiratory Physiology*, Butterworths, London, 1974, pp. 167–196.

24 Marshall, J. M., The cardiovascular response to stimulation of carotid chemoreceptors, *J. Physiol.* (Lond.), 266 (1977) 48 P–49 P.

25 Schramm, L. P. and Bignall, K. E., Central neural pathways mediating active sympathetic muscle vasodilation in cats, *Amer. J. Physiol.*, 221 (1971) 754–767.

26 Timms, R. J., The use of anaesthetic steroids alphaxalone and alphadalone in studies of the forebrain in the cat, *J. Physiol.* (Lond.), 256 (1976) 71 P–72 P.

27 Timms, R. J., Influences of the frontal cerebral cortex and corticospinal tract on the cardiovascular system, *Ph. D. Thesis*, University of Birmingham, 1977.

28 Timms, R. J., Cortical inhibition and facilitation of the defence reaction, *J. Physiol.* (Lond.), 266 (1977) 98 P–99 P.

29 Zwirn, P. and Corriol, J., Fibres corticopyramidales dilatrices des membres, *Archs. Sci. physiol.*, 16 (1962) 325–345.

CHAPTER 35

CLASSICAL AND CONTEMPORARY MODELS OF BEHAVIORAL INFLUENCES ON AUTONOMIC ACTIVITY

Joseph V. Brady

The Johns Hopkins University, School of Medicine, Baltimore, Maryland, USA

INTRODUCTION

The observation that autonomic functions can be influenced, sometimes in profound ways, by environmental circumstances and behavioral activities has been repeatedly confirmed in both the laboratory and the clinic[12,43]. While the mechanisms whereby these effects are produced remain, for the most part, obscure, traditional views continue to emphasize the prominent role of antecedent or concurrent environmental-behavioral events conceptualized as eliciting such autonomic reactions. Indeed, the enduring contributions of Pavlov[44], Sherrington[51] and Cannon[14] early in the present century, as well as the extensive literature of subsequent decades on the physiological effects of learning and conditioning[30] have all provided strong support for this classical model of behavioral influences upon the integrated functions of the autonomic nervous system. Experimental reports of recent vintage[42] have as well called attention to autonomic-behavioral interactions of a somewhat different sort based upon the influence exerted by environmental events which follow, and are contingent upon, previous visceral and glandular responses. The essential features of this more contemporary model emphasize interactions between antecedent autonomic changes and environmental consequences which bear a close temporal relationship to such responses, and suggest a provocative alternative to classical "stress" models of behavioral influences on autonomic activity.

RESULTS AND DISCUSSION

In our laboratory at Johns Hopkins, among others, studies within the framework of both these models continue to provide a vigorous and productive point of departure for experimental analysis, and the present report will attempt to highlight some of the comparative and interactive features of these two approaches as they are reflected in the magnitude, duration and specificity of such behaviorally-induced autonomic influences. For the purposes of this paper, the dependent measures will focus upon the cardiovascular effects of such behavioral interventions in a representative sample of mongrels, monkeys and humans. While the very contents of this volume provide abundant evidence to support the integrative nature of autonomic functions and the obvious need for a "total organism" view of such processes, technological and methodological developments in the monitoring and experimental manipulation of the circulation can nonetheless be seen to have paced the emergence of a scientifically operational laboratory psychophysiology.

The pioneering work of Pavlov, Sherrington and Cannon has been extended over the past half-century or more and elaborated in numerous volumes which document the effects of classical behavioral conditioning procedures upon physiological processes in general[7,46,47] and autonomic responses in particular[1,17,30]. In the past decade alone for example, a veritable tidal wave of classical cardiac conditioning studies have all but inundated the literature in this once arid area of experimental inquiry[30]. Though lacking the long-standing and prestigious background enjoyed by these classical conditioning studies, an active and productive research interest in the measurement of performance-related concurrent learning and conditioning effects has as well emerged over the past several decades. As reviewed initially by Brady[10] and more recently by Brady and Harris[12], several groups of laboratory studies in this area have focused upon the experimental production of altered physiological states emphasizing, for the most part, endocrine, cardiovascular and gastrointestinal changes. Significantly, there has also been an increasing emphasis upon enduringly chronic preparations[9,22,24,35], and aversive control procedures of established effectiveness, including conditioned suppression[20] and free-operant avoidance[52], continue to receive close psychophysiological attention as progressively more refined analysis of observed relationships is reflected in a range of concurrent autonomic learning and conditioning studies.

A recent series of studies, for example, on cardiovascular changes associated with operant avoidance procedures[2] provides evidence which bears upon the dynamic interplay between cardiac output and peripheral resistance in the behavioral control of blood pressure. The focus of these studies with dogs has been upon continuous monitoring of blood pressure and heart rate during free-operant (panel press) shock avoidance as illustrated in Fig. 1, and, significantly, during a fixed-interval pre-avoidance period systematically programmed to precede the required avoidance performance. Under these conditions, a unique divergence between heart rate and blood pressure changes was observed during pre-avoidance intervals up to 15 hr in length as shown in Fig. 2, with virtually all animals showing a characteristic systolic and diastolic increase accompanied by either a decrease or no change in heart rate[5]. Comparison involving similar performance requirements on a variable interval food reinforcement schedule revealed a markedly different preperformance cardiovascular pattern characterized by systematic increases in both heart rate and blood pressure[3]. And this differential "preparatory" pattern was confirmed both between individual animals maintained separately on each of the procedures (Fig. 3) and "within" the same animal alternately performing on the avoidance and food reinforcement schedule (Fig. 4). Moreover, direct measurements of cardiac output in dogs prepared with aortic flow probes during exposure to the avoidance program[6] confirmed that the pre-avoidance pressure changes were attributable to increased peripheral resistance, while

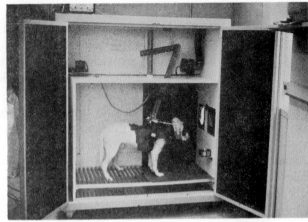

Fig. 1. Continuous cardiovascular monitoring during behavioral conditioning with a
harness-restrained dog.

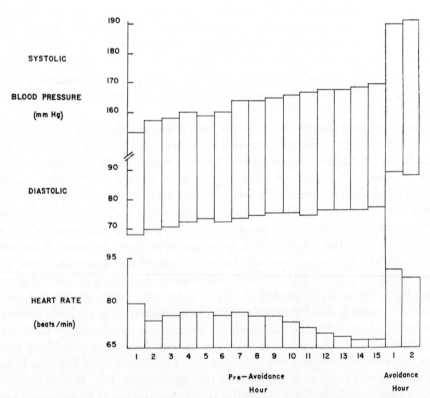

Fig. 2. Concurrent changes in blood pressure and heart rate during 15-hr pre-avoidance
intervals followed by two-hr avoidance periods. The data is presented in the form of
averages for 28 terminal experimental sessions with four dogs (seven sessions for
each dog).

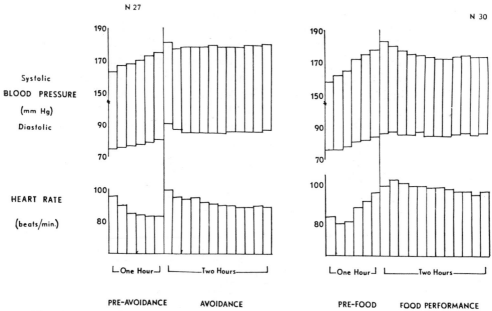

Fig. 3.   Concurrent changes in blood pressure and heart rate during consecutive 10-min
preperformance and performance intervals averaged over 27 "avoidance" sessions
(left panel) and 30 "food" sessions (right panel) for three dogs in each group.

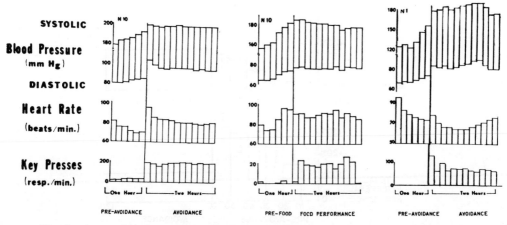

Fig. 4.   Average blood pressure, heart rate and panel response rate during consecutive 10-
min preperformance and performance intervals for 10 "avoidance" sessions (left
panel), 10 "food" sessions (middle panel) and one additional "avoidance" session
(right panel) following exposure to the 10 "food" sessions (middle panel) with the
same dog (Simon).

the pressure increases during the avoidance performance per se occurred as the peripheral resistance was actually observed to decrease and the cardiac output increased markedly, as shown in Fig. 5. Additional studies involving β-adrenergic blockade with the drug propranolol during the same experimental procedure, however, clearly showed that peripheral resistance levels do increase to maintain elevated pressure levels during avoidance when drug-induced heart rate reductions produce decrease in cardiac output[4].

    These recent extensions of classical or concurrent models of behavioral influences upon autonomic activity have been complemented over the past decade by laboratory studies within the framework of a more contemporary instrumental learning analysis of autonomic functions. The systematic series of investigations undertaken at Yale in the mid-1960's by Miller and his colleagues[41], for example, can be seen to have

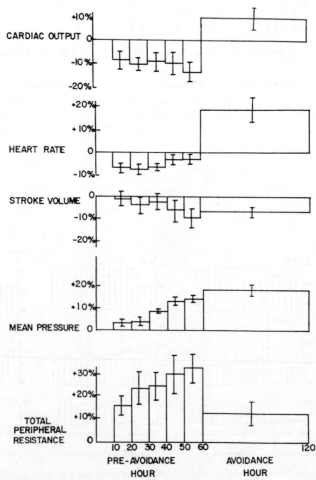

Fig. 5. Average levels of cardiac output, heart rate, stroke volume, mean arterial pressure and total peripheral resistance over successive 10-min intervals of pre-avoidance hour and for avoidance hour, as a whole, for a total of 20 experimental sessions for a group of four dogs.

activated a productive decade of "operant" learning research involving visceral and autonomic processes. There were, of course, notable precedents established in the earlier human experimental literature[38], and many reports had previously appeared on the "voluntary" control of physiological responses by yoga and related meditative techniques[55]. But the significant recent advances of laboratory animal research in this area would seem to be attributable, at least in part, to the prominent experimental focus upon explicit contingency relationships between specific antecedent physiological events on the one hand, and programmed environmental consequences on the other.

A prominent focus for such instrumental autonomic learning experiments has been provided by the behavioral control of cardiovascular functions, with the results of several studies demonstrating that both heart rate[19,21,32,54] and blood pressure[8,45,48,49,50] can be modified systematically by conditioning procedures which involve contingent programming of environmental consequences. Impressive large magnitude blood pressure elevations have been reported with the dog-faced baboon (*Papio* sp.) for example, under conditions which involved the application of operant "shaping" procedures"[31]. Both the amplitude and duration of the pressure change required to avoid shock and obtain food were gradually increased in small progressive steps to diastolic levels 50 to 60 mmHg above resting levels. More chronic studies of instrumentally-learned blood pressure changes with the baboon have emphasized the analysis of such procedures under conditions which provide for enduring elevations of 25 to 30 mmHg above baseline during daily 12-hr "conditioning" sessions alternating with 12-hr "rest" periods[33].

As part of these operant conditioning procedures, the experimental subjects are provided with two "feedback" lights: a white light which is associated with cardiovascular levels above a prespecified criterion, and in the presence of which food pellet rewards are delivered; and a red light which is associated with cardiovascular levels below that of a prespecified criterion, and in the presence of which aversive electric shocks are programmed. Under these conditions, a shock-free, food-abundant environment is made contingent upon the maintenance of effective control over selected circulatory functions. The conditioning procedures, diagrammed in Fig. 6, for example,

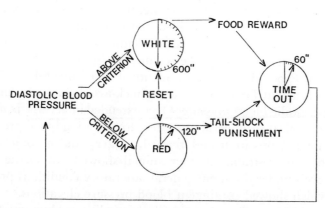

Fig. 6. Diagrammatic representation of blood pressure conditioning procedure as described in text.

required the animals to maintain prespecified diastolic blood pressure levels in order to obtain food and avoid shock. Five one-g pellets were delivered to the animal for every 10 min of accumulated time that the diastolic pressure exceeded criterion, as indicated by the white light. Conversely, the animal received a single, eight ma, 0.25 sec electrical shock through stainless steel electrodes applied to a shaved portion of the animal's tail for every 120 sec of accumulated time that the diastolic pressure was below criterion, as indicated by the red light. Additionally, each food delivery reset the shock timer postponing the delivery of shocks for an additional 120 sec, and each occurrence of an electric shock reset the food timer, postponing the delivery of food for at least an additional 10 min. A one min "time out" from stimuli and contingencies followed each food or shock delivery.

At the beginning of the training period, the criterion pressure levels were determined by the animal's preconditioning, resting, baseline diastolic pressure (approximately 75 mmHg). Increases in the criterion occurred at a gradual, progressive rate of about one to two mmHg per week over a period of two to three months. Conditioning sessions occurred daily during a 12-hr period from noon to midnight ("conditioning on") alternating with a 12-hr period from midnight to noon during which no programmed contingencies were in effect ("conditioning off"). In the course of a two to three month training interval, seven baboons attained diastolic blood pressure levels during the conditioning sessions which were elevated by at least 25 mmHg (approximately 33%) over baseline values, and they maintained these elevated pressures for more than 90% of each 12-hr session, as illustrated in Fig. 7. This figure shows consecutive 40-min interval averages, and summarizes, in the right-hand panel, the stable response pattern which developed after the baboons had been exposed to at least 40 daily 12-hr conditioning sessions. During these daily conditioning sessions, the animals received on the average about two shocks (currently<1) and 25 pellets per hr. Characteristically, sustained elevations of 30 mmHg or more in both systolic and diastolic blood pressure were maintained throughout the 12-hr "conditioning on" period accompanied by elevated but progressively decreasing heart rate over the course of the 12-hr interval. During the ensuing 12-hr "conditioning off" recovery period, heart rate continued to fall somewhat precipitiously, and blood pressure returned to approximately basal levels (or slightly above) within six to eight hours.

That these large magnitude, sustained elevations in blood pressure are related directly and specifically to the programmed contingency requirements of the instrumental conditioning procedure is further confirmed by the results obtained with two additional baboons exposed to virtually identical experimental conditions with the exception that concurrent food-reward and shock-avoidance were made contingent upon decreasing diastolic blood pressure. Over extended intervals (six months or more) of daily exposure to this instrumental procedure for lowering blood pressure (involving electric shocks, food deprivation and reward, surgery and chronic catheterization, confinement and chair restraint) neither animal showed any change from baseline cardiovascular levels under the same general laboratory conditions prevailing for the seven baboons which showed contingent blood pressure elevations.

Two additional baboons have been similarly conditioned but with the contingency directed at heart rate increases. Specifically, the conditioning procedure required

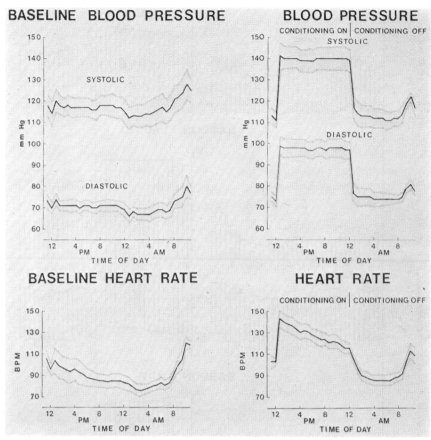

Fig. 7. Average blood pressure and heart rate values ($\pm$S. E.) for seven baboons over consecutive 40-min intervals during 28 pre-experimental baseline determinations (left panels), compared with 28 12-hr conditioning on, 12-hr conditioning off sessions (right panels).

the animals to maintain prespecified heart rate levels in order to obtain food and avoid shock. Initially, the criterion heart rate was set 10–15 bpm above the animal's pre-experimental resting baseline levels, with progressive increases programmed to occur at a rate approximating seven bpm per week over a period of eight to 10 weeks. Within this two to three month interval, heart rate doubled, reaching levels maintained above 165 bpm for more than 95% of each daily 12-hr conditioning session. During these conditioning sessions, the animal received, on the average, less than one electric shock and more than 20 food pellets per hr.

Figure 8 compares the concurrent changes in blood pressure and heart rate during the 12-hr conditioning on, 12-hr conditioning off periods with the changes in blood pressure and heart rate during the preconditioning baseline period. The data plot in Fig. 8 is in the form of averages for four consecutive 24-hr experimental conditioning sessions (right panel) for each of the two baboons and four consecutive 24-hr pre-experimental baseline sessions (left panel) for the same two animals before conditioning.

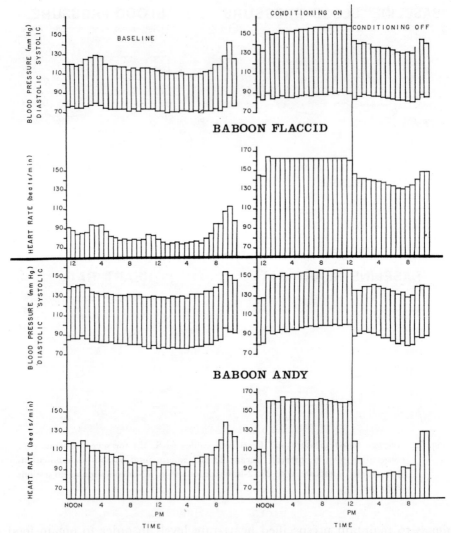

Fig. 8.   Heart rate and blood pressure values for baboons Flaccid (top) and Andy (bottom)
averaged over 40-min intervals during four consecutive pre-experimental baseline
days (left panels) compared with four consecutive days during the 12-hr conditioning on and 12-hr conditioning off heart rate conditioning program (right panels).

This figure shows consecutive 40-min interval averages, and summarizes in the right-
hand panel the response pattern which developed after the baboons had been exposed
to at least 40 daily 12-hr conditioning sessions.

Characteristically, the onset of the 12-hr conditioning sessions occasioned a rapid
rise in heart rate which was sustained at levels approximating 165 bpm throughout
the 12-hr conditioning on periods for both animals. For baboon Andy, heart rate rose
from a forenoon level of about 110 bpm to a sustained level (afternoon) of approximately 162 bpm. At midnight, when the 12-hr conditioning sessions terminated, heart

rate rapidly returned to baseline levels below 100 bpm. Conditioning on heart rate levels of similar magnitude were observed with baboon Flaccid, though it is noteworthy that the cardiac rate did not return to pre-experimental baseline levels for this animal. As shown in Fig. 8, Flaccid's conditioning off heart rate remained elevated above 130 bpm (compared to a pre-experimental baseline approximating 80 bpm) and the conditioning on levels approximating 165 bpm represented an increase of 20 to 30 bpm. For both subjects, blood pressure (both systolic and diastolic) showed a progressive rise of about 12 mmHg during the course of the 12-hr conditioning on period and returned to baseline levels during the 12-hr conditioning off interval.

These results show that marked and durable increases in heart rate can be produced in the baboon through the application of concurrent food reward and shock avoidance conditioning procedures. These heart rate elevations were sustained during daily 12-hr conditioning sessions and were accompanied by modest but progressive increases in blood pressure. Significantly, the heart rate increases generated in the animals under the heart rate contingency were at least 200% greater than the heart rate increases in the animals trained under the blood pressure contingency, while the blood pressure increase in the former was less than half as large as the pressure increase in the latter.

Although the physiological mechanisms that mediate these acute and chronic operant conditioning effects upon the circulation remain largely unexplored, it is conceptually obvious that alterations in cardiac output and total peripheral resistance must be involved, and preliminary studies with two baboons have confirmed the potential value of such hemodynamic analysis. The dye-dilution technique has been readily adapted for use with the catheterized, chair-restrained baboon, and the use of a cardiac output computer (Waters Instrument, Inc., Model DCR-701) facilitated the calculations.

The results of studies to determine the extent to which cardiac output changes are associated with such operant cardiovascular conditioning procedures suggest a close parallel to the heart rate pattern observed during these experimental periods. During the early portions of the blood pressure conditioning sessions, cardiac output is elevated, but is progressively reduced as the 12-hr conditioning on period continues.

Figure 9, for example, compares the average changes in diastolic blood pressure, cardiac output levels (measured by dye dilution method) and total peripheral resistance at selected intervals (i.e., 15, 30, 60, 120, and 180 min) over the first three hr of five daily 12-hr conditioning on sessions for baboon Flip maintaining continuously elevated arterial pressure levels in accordance with the procedures and results described above. The cardiac output levels measured 15 min after the beginning of the experimental session (at noon) were significantly elevated ($p < .02$) above presession control levels (the "zero" reference line in Fig. 9) recorded one hr before the start of the conditioning session. Thereafter, however, cardiac output levels can be seen to have declined over the first hr of the conditioning on period to approximate control levels throughout the remainder of the observation period. In contrast, peripheral resistance levels remained at or below control values during the first 15 min of the conditioning on periods, but increased progressively within the first hr to elevated levels that persisted throughout the remainder of the experimental observation period. This pattern of

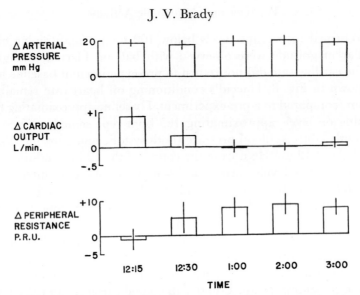

Fig. 9. Average changes in diastolic blood pressure, cardiac output and total peripheral
resistance for baboon Flip over the course of the first three hr of five daily 12-hr
operant blood pressure conditioning sessions.

cardiovascular changes (i.e., sustained pressure elevations accompanied by progressively decreasing heart rate and cardiac output) strongly suggests that alterations in
total peripheral resistance may play a prominent role in sustained control of the
circulation and is in accordance with the findings of Forsyth[25].

Experiments have also been completed on the effects of autonomic blockade upon
the circulatory change associated with operant cardiovascular conditioning of blood
pressure and heart rate in the baboon[28]. Of particular interest in these studies has been
the differential pattern of heart rate and blood pressure change observed in the course
of the 12-hr conditioning sessions suggesting that an increase in cardiac output and
heart rate may sustain the pressor response early in the session while peripheral vasoconstriction may contribute more markedly to the blood pressure elevations maintained during the later phases of the 12-hr conditioning on session. The effect of β-
blockade under such conditions appears to be a reduction in the heart rate increase
consistently observed during the initial phase of the 12-hr conditioning on period without affecting either the onset or maintenance of the conditioned diastolic hypertension.
Figure 10, for example, illustrates with baboon Kingfish the effect of propranolol
(0.5 mg/kg administered intravenously 15 min before the start of the session) in
attenuating the heart rate increase that normally accompanied onset of the 12-hr
conditioning on session (at arrow). Significantly, the operantly conditioned blood
pressure elevation can be seen to occur as rapidly and as effectively under the influence
of propranolol (lower section of Fig. 10) as under non-drug-control conditions (upper
section of Fig. 10). Similarly, α-blockade has been found to have little effect upon the
blood pressure elevations produced during the 12-hr conditioning on sessions, though
augmented tachycardias have been observed during the initial phase of the conditioning on period following phentolamine (0.3 mg/kg) administration. Significantly,

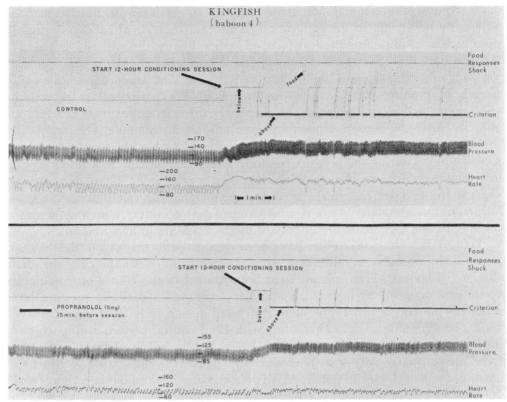

Fig. 10.   Polygraph records for baboon Kingfish showing the heart rate and blood pressure
response to the conditioning session onset at noon, before (top record) and after
(bottom record) β-adrenergic blockade. Note the elimination of the heart rate
increase that usually accompanied the blood pressure increase.

however, combined administration of both phentolamine (0.3 mg/kg) and propranolol
(0.3 mg/kg) does produce an attenuation (but not an elimination) of the instrumentally
conditioned blood pressure elevation both at onset and for extended intervals during
the 12-hr conditioning on maintenance period. These preliminary findings suggest
that under conditions of α-blockade, the instrumentally conditioned blood pressure
elevation is mediated by increases in cardiac output, while under β-blockade conditions, increases in peripheral resistance account for the conditioned pressure increase.
Similar studies have been initiated with two baboons maintaining instrumentally
conditioned heart rate elevations, and preliminary findings suggest that propranolol
administration (β-blockade) markedly reduces the animal's ability to produce and
sustain the required heart rate increases in order to avoid shock and obtain food.

Among the many feedback control systems regulating cardiovascular function,
the baroreceptor reflex assumes particular importance for understanding the physiological mechanisms mediating environmental-behavioral influences upon the circulation. Smyth, Sleight and Pickering[53] have proposed a technique for assessing
"baroreceptor sensitivity" in intact subjects. This technique is especially attractive

since it requires only minimal interference with the subject's normal functioning, and has recently been adapted for application to the chair-restrained baboon during the cardiovascular conditioning studies described earlier. Briefly, the method is based upon the observation that the baroreceptors respond to transient increases in blood pressure by, among other things, inducing a reflex bradycardia. The extent of this bradycardia per unit of pressure increase following injection of a peripheral vasoconstrictor (which exerts no direct action on the heart) may be taken as a measure of baroreceptor sensitivity. After angiotensin or phenylephrine infusion, for example, a linear relationship between heart rate and blood pressure was observed when the systolic pressure of successive pulses during the pressure rise were plotted against the R-R interval of the succeeding beat. Bristow, Honour, Pickering, Sleight and Smyth[13] have demonstrated a four- to five-fold decrease in the average slope defining this relationship in a group of hypertensives as compared to a control group of normotensives, a finding they interpret as reflecting a decreased sensitivity of the baroreflexes in hypertension.

Using this technique, studies have been conducted to investigate the effects of operant cardiovascular conditioning upon baroreceptor reflex function in chair-restrained baboons[29]. Five animals have been studied in the course of conditioning experiments designed to maintain sustained elevations in diastolic pressure levels (above 100 mmHg) or heart rate (above 150 bpm) during daily 12-hr operant cardiovascular conditioning sessions alternating with 12-hr control periods during which no programmed contingencies were in effect. Baroreflex "gain" (as defined by the slope of the pressure-rate plot) was determined by measuring the extent of heart rate change per unit of change in systolic blood pressure after intravenous injection of either a peripheral vasoconstrictor (phenylephrine) or vasodilator (nitroglycerine). Once each week, over a 13-week period, such determinations were made on seven separate occasions before, during, and after the daily 12-hr conditioning on session.

The upper section of Fig. 11 shows a typical polygraph recording of the changes in blood pressure and heart rate observed following phenylephrine infusion, and illustrates the systematic heart rate decrease associated with the pressure rise. The lower section in Fig. 11 shows a plot of the relationship between systolic pressure (plotted beat by beat) and heart rate over the eight-beat pressor response illustrated in the upper section of the figure. Using a negative correlation criterion with a chance probability level of 0.05 or less, better than 95% (75 of 79 infusion experiments) of the observed relationships were determined to be statistically reliable. Results obtained using this procedure have shown that significant decreases in baroreflex gain occur during the conditioning procedure. Determinations made 15 min after the start of the 12-hr conditioning on period reflected mean decreases in baroreceptor gain on the order of 30% to 40% in comparison with determinations made 1 hr before the daily conditioning on session was initiated. These changes are illustrated in Fig. 12 and indicate that alterations in baroreflex gain (though of lesser magnitude) were also observed in determinations made 15 min before (as compared to determinations made one hr before) initiation of the daily 12-hr conditioning on session (and in the absence of blood pressure elevations), suggesting the possibility of "anticipatory" changes in baroreflex function in preparation for the required blood pressure increase during the conditioning period. Additional experiments with animals maintaining operantly

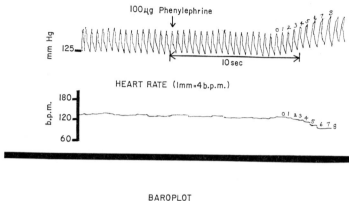

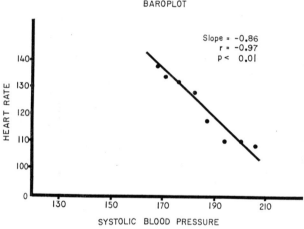

Fig. 11. Polygraph recording (upper section) and baroplot (lower section) showing the relationship between heart rate and systolic blood pressure following phenylephrine infusion.

conditioned heart rate increases of 60 to 80 beats per min (absolute level exceeding 165 bpm) failed to show such decreases in baroreflex gain. And nitroglycerine injections (administered under conditions identical to the phenylephrine infusions) reflected an increase in baroreflex gain with the "blood pressure increase" baboons, and either no change or a decrease in baroreflex gain with the "heart rate increase" baboons.

These preliminary findings raise provocative questions regarding the role of baroreceptor reflex changes in the establishment and maintenance of hypertensive pressure levels, and suggest the possibility that such baroreflex alterations can actually occur independently of the indicated blood pressure increases. Recent reports[16,27,36,37] have also provided evidence of baroreflex modulation by hypothalamic centers long associated with the control of "emotional" behavior, and Korner[39] has suggested that such mechanisms may be directly involved in cardiovascular reflex adaptations to environmental-behavioral interactions. Under any circumstances, and despite the

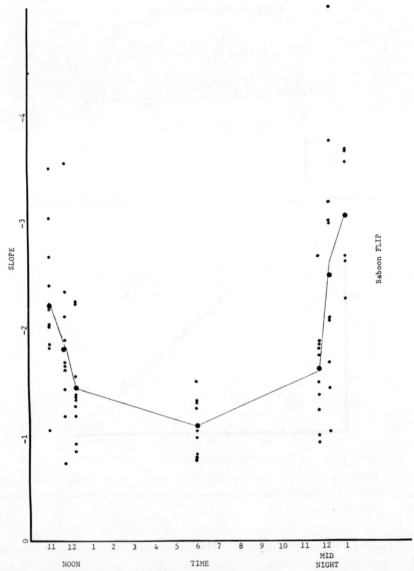

Fig. 12.   Slope of the baroplot (see Fig. 11) as a function of time during the 12-hr "on",
12-hr "off" blood pressure conditioning procedure. The large black data points
represent means of 10 determinations (six determinations at 1:00 A.M.) at each
selected temporal location.

complications introduced by the possibility of closed-loop effects (e.g., bradycardia
secondary to phenylephrine-induced hypertension producing lowered pressure due
to decreased cardiac output), continuing studies of the time course and reversibility
of such baroreflex sensitivity changes associated with the cardiovascular effects of
behavioral conditioning procedures promise to provide important insights into the
physiological and environmental interactions that, in concert, determine the acute and
chronic adjustments of the systemic circulation.

Both clinical[18,26] and experimental[15,34] accounts of the progressive alterations of the systemic circulation associated with chronically maintained blood pressure elevations have emphasized the potential contribution of repeated exposure to environmental-behavioral conditions which produce transient, frequently labile, pressor episodes as precursors of a more enduring change. Much of the behavioral evidence for this formulation has been developed over the past decade in studies by Forsyth[24] and others[11,35] emphasizing aversive behavioral control procedures, principally shock avoidance conditioning. Exposure to such aversive behavioral control procedures, and particularly to required shock avoidance performances, is consistently accompanied by significant elevations in blood pressure as compared to baseline values. During acute experiments, these pressure elevations tend to persist even after termination of the conditioning sessions, and long-term exposure to repeated daily avoidance conditioning sessions (up to 12 hr in length) have been observed to result in chronically elevated pressures developing only after several normotensive months on the procedure. Such findings are, of course, consistent with related observations on the cumulative effects of repeated hypothalamic stimulation[23] and subpressor doses of angiotensin[40].

Observations in our own laboratories over the past several years have indicated that continued exposure to recurrent cardiovascular conditioning sessions involving operant control of large magnitude increases in blood pressure and heart rate can be

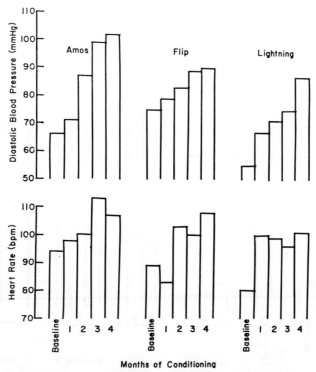

Fig. 13. Average heart rate and diastolic blood pressure for each of three baboons during conditioning off (rest) intervals, for pre-experimental baseline conditions, and over four consecutive months of operant diastolic blood pressure conditioning.

associated with significant and persistent effects upon the "resting" circulation. In the course of repeated daily exposures to a 12-hr "on", 12-hr "off" operant cardiovascular conditioning procedure, gradual but progressive increases in diastolic blood pressure during the daily 12-hr conditioning off or rest periods (i.e., no cardiovascular feedback and no food or shock contingencies in effect) were observed to develop over the successive months of the program in virtually all animals. Figure 13, for example, shows the mean diastolic pressure and heart rate levels for three animals during the conditioning off period averaged over four successive monthly intervals in the course of daily 12-hr exposures to the operant cardiovascular conditioning on procedure. Pre-experimental baseline values are shown for each animal, and the progressive pressure increases occurred under conditions that involved no feedback stimuli, food or shock delivery, and during intervals when direct observation of the animals usually revealed that they were sleeping.

In addition to the gradual but persistent increases in diastolic blood pressure during the daily 12-hr conditioning off or rest period, more chronic observations have been made with an animal followed for two years during which prolonged rest intervals (e.g., "vacations" of weeks to months during which no operant cardiovascular conditioning sessions were programmed, no feedback stimuli or shock ever occurred and food was freely available) have punctuated the otherwise continuous exposure to daily 12-hr "on", 12-hr "off" operant cardiovascular control schedules. Recovery of

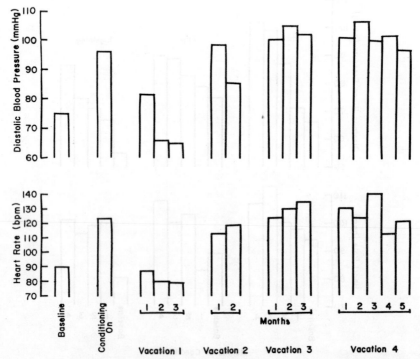

Fig. 14. Average heart rate and diastolic blood pressure for baboon Flip during conditioning off (rest) intervals, for baseline conditions, conditioning on, and consecutive months of four separate "vacation" periods.

baseline blood pressure and heart rate levels occurred rapidly (within seven to 10 days) during the early "vacation" cycles and became progressively retarded (several months or longer) as more extended exposures to the 12-hr "on", 12-hr "off" operant cardiovascular control schedule were repeated. Figure 14, for example, illustrates this progressive retardation of the heart rate and blood pressure recovery cycle for baboon Flip over successive "vacation" months following intermittent exposure to the daily operant blood pressure conditioning procedure. After the initial months of operant training, during which elevations in diastolic pressure of at least 20 mmHg were attained and consistently maintained during the daily 12-hr conditioning on sessions, recovery was relatively rapid and more than complete over the three-month "vacation" period (designated "Vacation 1" on the left-hand side of Fig. 14) which intervened before the next conditioning cycle. As the recurrent "vacation" cycles (i.e., Vacation 2, 3 and 4) were repeated (with intervening exposures to the 12-hr "on", 12-hr "off" conditioning procedure indicated by the spaces between "vacations"), sustained elevations in both blood pressure and heart rate were observed to persist, extending over a five-month period in the case of "Vacation 4" shown on the right-hand side of Fig. 14.

CONCLUSIONS

The results of these studies provide clear evidence that behavioral influences, whether mediated in accordance with classical or contemporary models, can exert orderly and specifiable effects upon the functional properties of the autonomic nervous system. Further, the systematic analysis of such interactive processes would seem to hold considerable promise for the enrichment of both clinical and experimental approaches to the understanding and amelioration of autonomically-mediated health disorders. Of perhaps even greater significance however, is the importance of such basic behavior science contributions to a comprehensive physiology of the intact, unanesthetized conscious organism. Increasing emphasis upon such long-term psychophysiological investigations provides tangible recognition of this developing frontier. Indeed, the identification and operational analysis of such behavioral interactions must be of central importance in delineating a research domain which has long acknowledged the critical role of environmental influences upon the integrative function of the autonomic nervous system.

The research reported in this paper is supported in part by National Heart, Lung and Blood Institute grants HL 17958 and HL 17970.

REFERENCES

1 Adam, G., *Interoception and Behavior*, Akademiai Kiado Publishing House of the Hungarian Academy of Sciences, Budapest, 1967, 152 pp.
2 Anderson, D. E. and Brady, J. V., Pre-avoidance blood pressure elevations accompanied by heart rate decreases in the dog, *Science*, 172 (1971) 595–597.
3 Anderson, D. E. and Brady, J. V., Differential preparatory cardiovascular responses to aversive and appetitive behavioral conditioning, *Cond. Reflex*, 7 (1972) 82–96.

4   Anderson, D. E. and Brady, J. V., Effects of beta blockade on cardiovascular responses to avoidance performances in dogs, *Psychosom. Med.*, 35 (1973) 84.

5   Anderson, D. E. and Brady, J. V., Prolonged pre-avoidance effects upon blood pressure and heart rate in the dog, *Psychosom. Med.*, 35 (1973) 4–12.

6   Anderson, D. E. and Tosheff, J., Cardiac output and total peripheral resistance changes during pre-avoidance periods in the dog, *J. appl. Physiol.*, 34 (1973) 650–654.

7   Beecroft, R. S., *Classical Conditioning*, Psychonomic Press, Goleta, California, 1966, 198 pp.

8   Benson, H., Herd, J. A., Morse, W. H. and Kelleher, R. T., Behavioral inductions of arterial hypertension and its reversal, *Amer. J. Physiol.*, 217 (1969) 30–34.

9   Brady, J. V., Experimental studies of psychophysiological responses to stressful situations. In: *Symposium on Medical Aspects of Stress in Military Climate*, Walter Reed Army Institute of Research., Government Printing Office, Washington, D. C., 1965, pp. 271–289.

10 Brady, J. V., Operant methodology and the production of a altered physiological states. In: W. Honig (Ed.), *Operant Behavior: Areas of Research and Application*, Appleton-Century-Crofts, New York 1966, pp. 609–633.

11 Brady, J. V., Endocrine and autonomic correlates of emotional behavior. In: P. Black (Ed.), *Physiological Correlates of Emotion*, Academic Press, New York, 1970, pp. 95–125.

12 Brady, J. V. and Harris, A. H., The experimental production of altered physiological states. In: W. K. Honig and J. E. R. Staddon (Eds.), *Handbook of Operant Behavior*, Prentice-Hall, Inc., New Jersey, 1976, pp. 596–618.

13 Bristow, J. D., Honour, A., Pickering, G., Sleight, P. and Smyth, H., Diminished baroreflex sensitivity in high blood pressure, *Circulation*, 39 (1969) 48.

14 Cannon, W. B., *Bodily Changes in Pain, Hunger, Fear and Rage*, Appleton, New York, 1915.

15 Charvat, J. P., Dell, B. and Folkow, B., Mental factors and cardiovascular diseases, *Cardiologia*, 44 (1964) 125–141.

16 Djojosuigto, A., Folkow, B., Klystra, B., Lisander, B. and Tuttle, R., Differential interaction between the hypothalamic defense reaction and baroreceptor reflexes, *Acta physiol. scand.*, 78 (1970) 376.

17 Dykman, R. A., On the nature of classical conditioning. In: C. C. Brown (Ed.), *Methods in Psychophysiology*, Williams & Wilkins, Baltimore, 1967, pp. 234–290.

18 Eich, R. H., Cuddy, R. P., Smulyan, H. and Lyons, R. H., Hemodynamics in labile hypertension. A follow-up study, *Circulation*, 34 (1966) 299–307.

19 Engel, B. T. and Gottlieb, S. H., Differential operant conditioning of heart rate in the restrained monkey, *J. comp. physiol. psychol.*, 73 (1970) 217–225.

20 Estes, W. K. and Skinner, B. F., Some quantitative properties of anxiety, *J. exp. Psychol.*, 29 (1941) 390–400.

21 Fields, C., Instrumental conditioning of the rat cardiac control systems, *Proc. nat. Acad. Sci. USA*, 65 (1970) 293–299.

22 Findley, J. D., Brady, J. V., Robinson, W. W. and Gilliam, W., Continuous cardiovascular monitoring in the baboon during long-term behavioral performances, *Commun. behav. Biol.*, 6 (1971) 49–58.

23 Folkow, B. and Rubinstein, E. H., Cardiovascular effects of acute and chronic stimulations of the hypothalamic defense area in the rat, *Acta physiol. scand.*, 68 (1966) 48.

24 Forsyth, R. P., Blood pressure responses to long-term avoidance schedules in the restrained rhesus monkey, *Psychosom. Med.*, 31 (1969) 300–309.

25 Forsyth, R. P., Regional blood flow changes during 72-hour avoidance schedules in the monkey, *Science*, 173 (1971) 546–548.

26 Frohlich, E. D., Kozul, V. J., Tarazi, R. C. and Dunstan, H. P., Physiological comparison of labile and essential hypertension, *Circulation Res.*, 26 & 27 (1970) I-55–I-69.

27 Gebber, G. L. and Snyder, D. W., Hypothalamic control of baroreceptor reflexes, *Amer. J. Physiol.*, 218 (1969) 124.

28 Goldstein, D. S., Harris, A. H. and Brady, J. V., Sympathetic adrenergic blockade effects upon operantly conditioned blood pressure elevations in baboons, *Biofeedback & Self-Regulation*, 2 (1977) 93–105.

29 Goldstein, D. S., Harris, A. H. and Brady, J. V., Baroreflex sensitivity during operant blood pressure conditioning, *Biofeedback & Self-Regulation*, 2 (1977) 127–138.

30 Harris, A. H. and Brady, J. V., Animal learning: Visceral and autonomic conditioning, *Ann. Rev. Psychol.*, 25 (1974) 107–133.

31 Harris, A. H., Findley, J. D. and Brady, J. V., Instrumental conditioning of blood pressure elevations in the baboon, *Cond. Reflex*, 6 (1971) 215–226.

32 Harris, A. H., Gilliam, W. J. and Brady, J. V., Operant conditioning of large magnitude 12-hour heart rate elevation in the baboon, *Pavlovian J. biol. Sci.*, 11 (1976) 86–92.

33 Harris, A. H., Gilliam, W. J., Findley, J. D. and Brady, J. V., Instrumental conditioning of large magnitude daily 12-hour blood pressure elevations in the baboon, *Science*, 183 (1973) 175.

34 Henry, J. P. and Cassel, J. C., Psychosocial factors in essential hypertension: Recent epidemiologic and animal experimental evidence, *Amer. J. Epidem.*, 90 (1969) 171–200.

35 Herd, J. A., Morse, W. H., Kelleher, R. T. and Jones, L. G., Arterial hypertension in the squirrel monkey during behavioral experiments, *Amer. J. Physiol.*, 217 (1969) 24–29.

36 Hilton, S. M., Hypothalamic regulation of the cardiovascular system, *Brit. med. Bull.*, 22 (1966) 243.

37 Humphreys, P. and Joels, N., The vasomotor component of the carotid sinus baroreceptor reflexes in the cat during stimulation of the hypothalamic defense area, *J. Physiol.* (Lond.), 226 (1972) 57.

38 Kimmel, H. D., Instrumental conditioning of autonomically mediated behavior, *Psychol. Bull.*, 67 (1967) 337–345.

39 Korner, P. I., Central nervous system control of autonomic function—possible implications in the pathogenesis of hypertension, *Circulation Res.*, 27 (1970) II-159.

40 McCubbin, J. W., DeMoura, R. S., Page, I. H. and Olmsted, F., Arterial hypertension elicited by subpressor amounts of angiotensin, *Science*, 149 (1965) 1394.

41 Miller, N. E., Learning of visceral and glandular responses, *Science*, 163 (1969) 434–445.

42 Miller, N. E., Biofeedback and visceral learning, *Ann. Rev. Psychol.*, 29 (1978) 373–404.

43 Mostofsky, D. I. (Ed.), *Behavior Control and Modification of Physiological Activity*. Prentice-Hall, Inc., Englewood, New Jersey, 1976, 504 pp.

44 Pavlov, I. P., *Conditioned Reflexes*. Translation, G. V. Anrep. Oxford University Press, London, 1927, 430 pp.

45 Plumlee, L. A., Operant conditioning of increases in blood pressure, *Psychophysiol.*, 6 (1969) 283–290.

46 Prokasy, W. F. (Ed.), *Classical Conditioning: A Symposium*, Appleton-Century-Crofts, New York, 1965, 421 pp.

47 Razran, G., The observable unconscious and the inferable conscious in current Soviet psychophysiology: Interoceptive conditioning, semantic conditioning, and the orienting reflex, *Psychol. Rev.*, 68 (1961) 81–147.

48 Shapiro, D., Schwartz, G. and Tursky, B., Control of diastolic blood pressure in man by feedback and reinforcement, *Psychophysiol.*, 8 (1971) 262.

49 Shapiro, D., Tursky, B., Gerson, E., et al., Effects of feedback and reinforcement on the control of human systolic blood pressure, *Science*, 163 (1969) 588–590.

50 Shapiro, D., Tursky, B. and Schwartz, G., Differentiation of heart rate and systolic

blood pressure in man by operant conditioning, *Psychosom. Med.*, 32 (1970) 417–423.

51 Sherrington, C. S., *The integrative Action of the Nervous System*, Cambridge University Press, Cambridge, England, 1906 (1947 edition).

52 Sidman, M., Avoidance conditioning with brief shock and no exteroceptive warning signal, *Science*, 118 (1953) 157–158.

53 Smyth, H. S., Sleight, P. and Pickering, G. W., Reflex regulation of arterial pressure during sleep in man: A quantitative method of assessing baroreflex sensitivity, *Circulation Res.*, 24 (1969) 109.

54 Stephens, J., Harris, A. H. and Brady, J. V., Large magnitude heart rate changes in subjects instructed to change their heart rates and given exteroceptive feedback, *Psychophysiol.*, 9 (1972) 283–285.

55 Wenger, M. A. and Bagchi, K., Studies of autonomic functions in practitioners of Yoga in India, *Behav. Sci.*, 6 (1961) 312–323.

SECTION VIII

HISTORY: PAST, PRESENT AND FUTURE RELATIVE TO STUDIES OF AUTONOMIC NERVOUS SYSTEM FUNCTIONS

The following sections were included in this symposium for two reasons. First, perspective is gained from consideration of history and some appreciation of new knowledge is acquired. It is also of interest that some of our modern studies are revivals or rediscoveries of ancient problems which our predecessors had to abandon because they did not possess the techniques which we can now apply. Knowledge evolves, develops from previously procured information and thought. Review and evaluation of our present state requires some reference to the past and a consideration of where we might be going.

The second reason for this section is that this symposium was sponsored by a Japan-U.S. Cooperative Science Program. It seemed appropriate that the history of scientific accomplishment in this field in our two nations be reviewed and compared. This has revealed more parallelism than one might have expected.

It is rather pedantic to say that the past and the present, to a high degree, determine what will occur tomorrow. It may be somewhat unsafe to predict what may happen in the future, but curiosity and the ability to formulate hypotheses do characterize the scientist.

CHAPTER 36

THE DEVELOPMENT OF OUR KNOWLEDGE OF THE
AUTONOMIC NERVOUS SYSTEM

Chandler McC. Brooks*
with the collaboration of
Koji Uchizono** and Masanori Uono***

*State University of New York, Downstate Medical Center, Brooklyn, New York, USA,
**National Institute of Physiology, Okazaki, Aichi, Japan, and
***Tokyo Metropolitan Hospital of Fuchu, Tokyo, Japan

INTRODUCTION

In concluding this review of the autonomic nervous system and its functions it is appropriate that the background of recent progress be considered. In doing so the following subjects will be reviewed:

The Evolution of Studies of the Autonomic Nervous System.

The Development of Autonomic System Studies in Japan and the USA:

1. The origin and development of interest in the autonomic nervous system in Japan;
2. American contributions to knowledge of the autonomic system.

New Advances and the Predictable Future.

THE EVOLUTION OF STUDIES OF THE AUTONOMIC NERVOUS SYSTEM

Numerous accounts of the history of discovery of the autonomic nervous system and its functions have already been published[3,4] and another is definitely not needed. There are, however, several reasons for considering past accomplishments in attempts to assay the significance of new ideas, new findings and to identify those leads which give the greatest promise for future investigations. A study of the history of a subject or field enables one to perceive how progress occurs and why it became possible in the past. It is obvious that certain special conditions are essential to scientific accomplishment. Secondly, one learns that scientists frequently again pick up an old discarded idea and develop it in a new fashion made possible by technological developments. Finally, a survey of past studies of the autonomic system reveals that many years often pass before a new discovery or concept is accepted and fully developed. Chart 1 lists some of the major contributions made in studies of the autonomic system. A definite acceleration of progress is obvious. Galen (129–199 A.D.) is generally considered to have been the first to dissect and identify parts of the autonomic system, but fourteen hundred years elapsed before the gross morphology of the system was known. Galen spoke of concurrent responses of muscles as connoting sympathetic action. He also believed that chemical materials, "humors", flowed through the body to determine its state or responses, but an even longer time elapsed before these latter precursors of ideas were developed into modern thought. Other Greeks and Romans made significant contributions to medicine and other branches of science before Rome fell (576 A.D.), but the confusion in Western Europe between then and the fifteenth century permitted no significant accomplishments in medically related science. The Eastern Empire lasted from 395 until 1453. There were Byzantine scholars and en-

Chart 1. Evolution of knowledge of the autonomic nervous system

Galen of Pergamon	A.D. 129–199	First dissection of autonomic system
Bartholomaeo Eustachio	1552	Ultimate dissection
Thomas Willis	1664	"Involuntary system" vs. voluntary
Joacque Benigne Winslow	1698	"Nervi sympathetici"—ganglia "little brains"
Francois Pourfour du Petit	1727	Sympathetic trunks origin in rami communicanti, not cranial nerves; "tonic activity"
Marie Francois Xavier Bichet	1771–1802	"La vie organique" (autonomic) "La vie animale" (somatic)
J. C. Reil	1807	"Vegetative" nervous system
C. G. Ehrenberg, 1833; R. Remak	1838	Microanatomy—myelinated and unmyelinated fibers
E. and E. H. Weber	1845	Inhibitory action—vagi
Johannes Müller	1848	Smooth muscle—autonomic innervation
Claude Bernard	1852–1877	Central control of autonomics—constancy of milieu interiur
E. Cyon and C. Ludwig	1866	Depressor reflex—feedback control
E. Du Bois-Reymond	1866	Cardiac accelerator fibers
M. Schiff	1870	Piloerectors, salivary nerves
F. L. Goetz	1875	Sudomotor fibers
S. L. Schenk and W. R. Birdsall	1880	Embryonic origin of autonomic system
G. Oliver and E. A. Schafer	1895	Active extracts from adrenal medulla
J. J. Abel	1898	Epinephrine—pure form
J. N. Langley	1898	Autonomic: parasympathetic and sympathetic
J. Takamine	1901	Crystalized adrenalin
T. R. Elliott	1904	Suggested chemical transmission
J. N. Langley	1907	Receptor substance
Reid Hunt	1911	Active choline derivatives
H. H. Dale	1914	Acetylcholine
O. Loewi	1921	"Vagusstoff" from vagal action
W. B. Cannon and Z. Bocq	1931	Active compound from sympathetics—sympathin
H. H. Dale	1933	"Cholinergic" and "adrenergic" transmitters
C. M. Greer, J. O. Pinkston, J. H. Baxter and E. S. Brannon	1938	Norepinephrine is sympathetic transmitter

cyclopedists who preserved the Hippocratic and Galenic codas and added a few original findings of their own. Progress was not stopped by absence of scholars or men of
ability. They were, however, preoccupied by debates of ecclesiastical doctrine, concern
for survival under attack by the Moslem world and subdued by authoritarianism.
They were Greek but had lost the curiosity, the democracy and the concepts of their
ancestors who laid the foundation of Western culture.

The Byzantines did protect the West until it could be stabilized again and with
the capture of Constantinople in 1453 their scholars moved westward and helped
precipitate the Renaissance[2]. The spirit of the Renaissance led men to explore and
discover Japan and the Americas. The Reformation was responsible in part for
settlement of America by the Pilgrims. Almost 1400 years thus elapsed before the dissection of the autonomic system was completed and the first phase—that during which
the gross morphology of the autonomic system was investigated—was completed. In
a plate published by Andreas Vesalius in 1555, the sympathetic trunks and vagi are
clearly shown. Bartholomaeo Eustachio produced plates of a splendid dissection in
1552 but they were buried in the papal library and were not published until 1714.
In the meantime, Thomas Willis in 1664 had published comparable work including
description of the rami communicates.

The next phase of development can be said to have extended from the time of
Joacque Benigne Winslow, a Swedish anatomist working in Paris at the start of the
18th century, to the end of the 19th century when the British physiologists Gaskell and
Langley were dominating the study of autonomic system function. During this period
anatomical knowledge was refined; earlier mistakes, such as the thought that the
sympathetic chains were cranial nerves, were corrected. Nomenclatures were agreed
upon and the objective was to determine function. Winslow in 1698 used the term
"sympathetic system"; Bichet and Reil used the terms "organique" and "vegetative"
to emphasize another aspect of the system's function. Francois Pourfous du Petit in
1727 showed that the "intercostal nerves" originated not from the brain but from the
spinal cord through the rami. He should be given credit along with Claude Bernard
and Brown-Séquard for discovery of the tonic activity of autonomic nerves. In 1764
Johnstone championed an idea held by Winslow, that the ganglia are "little brains"
—an idea soon discarded but recently resurrected to some degree. Johnstone knew,
as did Francois du Petit, that there were more postganglionic than preganglionic fibers
and that the postganglionic neurons formed tissue plexuses.

After invention of the microscope a new phase of anatomical study began which
has expanded and continued into the present. Ehrenberg in 1833 described the fiber
types we know as myelinated and unmyelinated. Remak in 1838 saw these fibers
originating from cell bodies and improved their descriptions. Jahannes Müller (1848)
described smooth muscle, finding it to be innervated by autonomic fibers. In 1852
Claude Bernard began his studies which led to our concepts of vasomotor control,
constancy of the milieu interieur and neural control of carbohydrate mobilization. In
1845 the Weber brothers discovered the inhibitory action of nerves (the vagi). Du Bois-
Reymond discovered the cardiac accelerators in 1866, the same year in which Cyon
and Ludwig not only discovered the depressor nerve but also "feed-back action" operating through the autonomic system. Others had discovered sudomotor fibers and pilo-

motor nerves by 1870 when Americans and Japanese began to study in Germany.

This era, in which modern experimental medicine is said to have been started by William Harvey, Magendie and their successors, concluded with the work of Gaskell and Langley. Using blocking agents and stimulation, they completed the analysis of where autonomic fibers went and what actions they had on peripheral tissues. Langley proposed the terminology now used and advanced the concept of "receptors". In 1895 Oliver and Schafer extracted active materials from the adrenal medulla. In 1904, at the turn of the century, Elliott suggested chemical transmission, a theme of study which occupied the attention of physiologists during the first quarter of the 20th century and introduced the modern age of refined chemical and anatomical analyses. Otto Löewi in 1921 discovered Vagusstoff; Cannon and Bocq in 1931 obtained evidence of the existence of the "sympathins" (sympathetic nerve transmitter); Dale in 1933 spoke of cholinergic and adrenergic transmission[1].

REFERENCES

1 Garrison, F. H., *History of Medicine*, 4th Ed., W. B. Saunders Co., Philadelphia, 1929.
2 Jenkins, R., *Byzantium, The Imperial Centuries*, Random House, New York, 1966.
3 Pick, J., *The Autonomic Nervous System*, J. B. Lippincott Co., Philadelphia, 1970.
4 Sheehan, D., The discovery of the autonomic nervous system, *Arch. Neurol. Psychiat.*, 35 (1936) 1081.

THE DEVELOPMENT OF AUTONOMIC SYSTEM STUDIES IN JAPAN AND THE USA

The symposium held to collect the information and concepts published here, though international in scope, was sponsored by a U.S.-Japan Cooperative Science Program. Some emphasis is thereby placed on the contributions of the scientists from these two nations as well as on how these link with those of representatives from other parts of the world. It is interesting that there have been numerous parallels in the development of medicine and science in Japan and the USA but the backgrounds from which present similarities and common interests have developed were vastly different.

Western medicine was introduced to Japan long before the first European successfully settled in North America in 1620. This continent was inhabited by native peoples who were displaced by Europeans who brought with them and imposed the culture of Europe. Japan, on the other hand, assimilated the science and medicine of the West. Japan had developed a rather sophisticated medicine and a medical literature based upon Chinese and Korean foundations several centuries before the first Westerners, Portuguese traders, reached Japan in 1542 and before St. Francis Xavier brought Christianity and Western medicine to Kyushu in 1549[1,2,5,6]. The oldest extant Japanese medical text, the *Ishimpo*, was written in 982 A.D. Two other books, the *Ton-i-sho* and the *Man-anpo*, were written in 1303 and 1315, respectively. They actually had separate sections for anatomy and physiology. Despite their established practices, the Japanese welcomed foreign physicians and a Portuguese by the name of

Louis de Almeida actually began the practice of Western medicine and built a hospital in Kyushu in 1556. Dutch and English trade was established with Japan in 1609 and 1613. The Dutch were particularly active in introducing their medical practices and literature. Western medicine was being adopted in Japan before it became certain that the first American settlements at Jamestown (1607) and Plymouth (1620) would survive. For a number of reasons the Westerners and their books were banned in 1638, but this ban was lifted in 1720. It is generally stated[2] that by 1772 the practice of westernized Japanese medicine and science had begun. It is somewhat difficult to determine why that date was chosen. Dutch influence again became paramount about then and the Japanese began to do autopsies and publish anatomical drawings and notes. In 1772 Shinto Kawaguchi and Gengai Ogino published the *Kaishi-hen* (anatomical notes) based on autopsies done in Kyoto. This date corresponds well with that of American independence, but like America nothing much happened until the mid 1800's. In 1857 the Dutch founded a medical school in Edo which was taken over by the Japanese government in 1860 and became Tokyo University. With the beginning of the Meiji period in 1868, as in America, Germanic medicine attained dominance. Young Japanese began to study alongside Americans at Leipzig and other German schools.

The Meiji government invited several Westerners to come to Japan to aid in medical and educational development. One of these was Dr. David Murray of Rutgers University. He went to Japan in 1873 as "Superintendant of Educational Affairs" and tried to find men to fill new University posts. In 1877 when a professor of zoology was needed for Tokyo University, no Japanese was available, so an American student of Louis Agassiz, Edward S. Morse of the Peabody Museum of Salem, was chosen and served from 1877 to 1879. He was succeeded by Charles Otio Whitman who had been studying in Leipzig. He served until 1881 before returning to the USA to begin a distinguished career. These Americans sent three students to study abroad who became the first three Japanese Professors of Zoology: K. Mitsukuri, I. Iijima and S. Watosé. They studied in Germany but two of them obtained their doctoral degrees under W. K. Brooks at the Johns Hopkins University in Maryland[3]. The point to be made is that during the latter part of the 19th century science and medicine in Japan and the USA were developing rapidly. Research had begun and contributions were soon to be made.

Japanese initial contacts with the West paralleled rather closely in time those occurring in Mexico and South America. It is known that Cortez built a hospital in Mexico in 1524 and that universities were founded in Lima, Peru by 1553 and Cordoba, Argentina by 1613. It is said that Sir Walter Raleigh brought curare from Guiana and the potato to Europe in 1584[2]. Cinchona bark from Peru was used in Europe for treatment of fever by 1630. In the part of North America now the USA, the first settlements were not made until 1607 (Jamestown, Virginia) and 1620 (Plymouth, Massachusetts). Harvard College was founded in 1636 and North America's first medical school in 1765 (University of Pennsylvania); the first medical degree given was conferred in 1770 on a Robert Tucker by Kings College, N.Y., which became Columbia University in 1784. The Declaration of Independence was signed in 1776 and the USA became an entity and began to assume full responsibility for the development of its own medicine and science.

Little of scientific importance happened during the first century of the USA's independence. Marked professional progress did occur and many universities were founded[4]. Reliance for advanced training of physicians and medical scientists was placed first on Great Britain, after 1800 upon the French and finally in the late 1800's young men went to Germany to study just as did the Japanese in that era. There were some academic achievements: Benjamin Franklin invented bifocal lenses (1780), Peter Middleton published the first American book on the history of medicine (1769), William Brown published the first American pharmacopoeia (1778), the American Academy of Arts and Sciences was founded in Boston (1780), Harvard Medical School was started (1782), a Board of Health with Paul Revere as its Chairman was established in Boston (1798), the Library of Congress was founded (1800). More to the point is the fact that America's first major contribution to physiology was made in 1833 when William Beaumont published his observations on gastric secretion[2,4]. Morton introduced ether anesthesia in 1846. In 1847 the American Medical Association was founded. It was not until the end of the 19th century that Americans began to make significant contributions and, surprisingly enough, some of the earliest had bearing on autonomic system function.

REFERENCES

1 Fujikawa, Y., *Nihon-igakushi* (Japanese Medical History) *1904, Standard Ed.* Nisshin-shoin, Tokyo, 1941.
2 Garrison, F. G., *History of Medicine*, 4th ed. W. B. Saunders Co., Philadelphia, 1929.
3 Gorbman, A., The development of academic zoology in Japan, *The Biologist*, 46 (1964) 49–72.
4 Shryock, H., *The Growth of Medical Research in America*. State University of New York (Printed by the Research Foundation), New York, 1956.
5 Uchiyama, K., The history of physiology in Japan before the Meiji period. In: *History of Medicine in Japan, Vol. 2*. Nihon Gakushi-in, 1955.
6 Uchiyama, K., Hayashi, T., Kinoshita, H., Natori, R., Shimazono, N., Brooks, C. McC. and Koizumi, K., *Japanese Physiology Past and Present*. Published for the XXIII Internat. Cong. Physiol. Sci., Tokyo, 1965.

1.   The Origin and Development of Interest in the Autonomic Nervous System in Japan

Specific interest in the autonomic system in Japan, as well as elsewhere, gradually emerged principally from a dominant concern with nerves and the central nervous system, but also from studies of cardiovascular function, the salivary glands and salivation, body temperature regulation and sweating and from observation of other organ system activities and their control. In illustrating early Japanese participation in this type of development the following examples have been selected from a listing of Japanese scientific contributions between 1873 and 1930, published in 1932 by a committee appointed to survey publication by Japanese physiologists[15] and from contributions listed in the *Japanese Handbook of Physiology*, published in 1967[4].

The eye and lacrimation.   The autonomic innervation of the eye is important to accommodation not only related to intensities of light but also to focus of the eye. The contributions of the Japanese to ophthalmology, studies of color vision, etc., are well known but there were also some early studies of autonomic control of the eye listed in the survey. S. Ishihara in 1919 published a paper on the accommodating power of the Japanese. In the same year A. Sakamoto wrote an article on pupillary phenomena in vagotonia. K. Yamada in 1922 published, in the *British J. Ophth.*, a paper on accommodation. Some other publications during the first quarter of this century were by K. Miyata (1923) on pupillary size; Y. Nakamura (1925) on the cervical sympathetic nerve and the pupillary reflex; U. Sunaga (1926) on the autonomic innervation of eye muscles; M. Okuyama (1928) on pupillary reactions.

The control of lacrimation did not receive the attention of many investigators but in 1925 H. Ichihara did study the parasympathetic control of these glands.

The salivary glands and salivation. The salivary glands have been studied principally by those concerned with their role in digestion, in control of thirst and in the phenomenon of conditioning. It has been known for many years that secretory processes in these glands are influenced by both parasympathetic and sympathetic innervation.

Tomosaburo Ogata in 1944 received the Gakushi-in-sho for his studies of salivary gland secretory activity[17]. He had suggested as early as 1935 that the salivary ducts might play an important role in salivary production and composition. We now know that autonomic nerves regulate acinar and duct cell roles in saliva formation (chap. 1, 2, this book, and Yoshida, et al., 1967—chap. 2, ref. 37). There are contractile elements in the ducts which are also affected by nerve action, but this was not recognized in early studies.

Action of autonomic nerves on muscle. There never was any question as to the ability of autonomic nerves to affect smooth muscle, but action on skeletal muscle has been controversial. The Japanese, like the Russians, early concluded that sympathetic nerves actually affected skeletal muscle in addition to controlling its blood supply. The Americans until recent years have tended to reject this thought. In 1926 T. Imagawa claimed to have observed effects on the muscle from stimulating sympathetic trunks. From 1927 to 1932 M. Nakanishi published six papers dealing with sympathetic innervation of skeletal muscle and actions thereon. The most vocal of proponents of autonomic control of muscle, however, was Ken Kure who, between 1914 and 1927, published six papers dealing with: "Parasympathetic nerves and diaphragm tonus"; "Nutritive effects of parasympathetic nerves on muscle"; "Parasympathetic innervation of skeletal muscle and its effect on tone and its trophic actions". Others studying the peripheral vascular system also mentioned direct autonomic nerve effects on muscle.

Control of the gastrointestinal tract and associated organs. Japanese interest in digestive system control has been extensive. In 1906 M. Ishihara reported studies of the swallowing reflex which, though not dependent on the autonomic system, is associated with autonomic activity. J. Yanase (1907) studied the origin of fetal peristalsis, publishing two papers in *Pflüger's Archives*. M. Takahashi (1916) published a number of papers dealing with intestinal motility and effects of nerves, bile and other chemicals thereon. S. Iwai between 1921 and 1923 reported three studies of the action of the vagi on stomach tone and motility. In 1922 S. Yamaguchi described his studies of the control of gastric secretion which we know now is affected by autonomic nerves. T. Shiraki

(1924) published work on vagotonia and intra-intestinal pressure. T. Saito from 1925 to 1926 published four papers on the effects of vestibular stimulation on intestinal motility. In 1925 and 1926 H. Ishikawa published a number of papers not only on neural control of the motility of the gut but also on function of cardiac nerves. Between 1927 and 1929 N. Mizuta reported (three papers) studies of oesophageal reflexes; H. Akiyama published (five papers) between 1928 and 1930 on parasympathetic control of the intestine and salivary glands. S. Matsue in 1929 studied gut motility in vagotomized rabbits. G. Usami (1928–1929) published three papers dealing with the role of the sacral parasympathetic in control of intestinal motility and absorption. These contributions dealt rather exclusively with control of motor activity.

In the 1930's interest in motility continued and from 1931–1936 T. Hukuhara published extensively (seven papers in *Pflüger's Arch.*) on the innervation and motility of the small intestine. A. Aiba (1933–1935) reported on neural control of the large intestine, as did K. Masuda in 1937 (two papers). M. Kawasaki in 1939 discussed innervation of the stomach.

Interest was not confined to motor activity and its control. N. Fujii in 1929 published a paper on gastric digestion and control of gastric secretion. H. Akiyama in addition to considering motility (1928–1930) also studied secretin liberation and its action. S. Okada in 1929 published studies of the humoral-neural regulation of pancreatic function. Bile liberation and action was considered by others about this time. S. Ochi (1927–1929) studied hormones of the G. I. tract. Fifteen years earlier Y. Shibata (1924) had reported his studies of neuroendocrine control of gastric function.

In addition to studies of the control of pancreatic exocrine secretion during the 1920's, numerous papers appeared relative to control of the liver: I. Matsuo (1923–1924) three papers on control of the gall bladder and, incidentally, the urinary bladder; E. Sakurai (1925) three papers on neural control of sphincter of Oddi; T. Kosaka (1929) the effect of adrenalin on liver temperature and function.

Some of the earlier studies of urinary bladder control by the autonomic system were chiefly anatomical. H. Tagami (1928—two papers), K. Arimoto and, also, O. Fujitani in 1929 published conclusions concerning the innervation of the bladder. In 1938 M. Kuru began to study bladder control. His interest was primarily clinical: the effects of cordotomies and various brain lesions. In 1966 he wrote an article for *Physiological Reviews* in which he described his own very extensive work as well as that of many earlier Japanese physicians and physiologists.

In conclusion, it can be said that there was parity with what was occurring elsewhere in this field, but no unique developments occurred during the early decades of this century.

Neural control of the endocrine secretions. Endocrinology has been a popular and productive study in Japan during the last half of this century. There also were some early contributions during the 1910's to 1920's when it was considered possible that the autonomic nerves might control secretory activity of the endocrine glands. The analysis at hand gives no clue as to whether the Japanese were involved in the early considerations of possible neural control of the thyroid or hypophysis, but they certainly were in studies of the endocrine pancreas and the adrenals.

Y. Tokumitsu in 1918 studied carbohydrate metabolism and the role of the adrenals and pancreas. From 1921 to 1925 T. Kumagai published three papers describing his studies of pancreatic endocrine secretory activity; Z. Katsura at the same time was paying particular attention to neural control of this gland. O. Nagasue (1925–1926) studied the effects of insulin on blood sugar; Y. Ohara determined its action on isolated intestinal motility; H. Akiyama (1930) repeated Banting's experiment of tying the pancreatic duct and observing effects on blood glucose levels and hunger. The most direct approach to the role of nerves in control of internal secretions of the pancreas was made by T. Hoshi. From 1924 to 1926 he conducted experiments and published five papers dealing with the role of the vagus nerves in the control of secretion of hormones from the pancreatic islets.

Early studies of the neural control of the adrenal medulla will be discussed later since they relate more to autonomic system function than to endocrinology in the usual sense. There is one matter of importance, however, which should be mentioned here; T. Iino and others showed (1930) that thyroid hormone potentiates the effects of adrenalin. This indicates some appreciation of gland interactions and hormone effects on autonomic system-induced reactions.

Reproductive endocrinology was studied extensively in the early 1900's. Then, as now, it was not considered that the autonomic nerves play a very important role. However, in 1920 M. Tanimoto published a paper on pregnancy and the autonomic nervous system and in 1930 K. Minamikawa published a discussion of the nervous system and reproduction. M. Wakimoto (1926–1928) studied dilator functions of the sacral parasympathetic nerves.

Autonomic nervous systems and temperature regulation. One of the most prominent Japanese physiologists of the first half of this century was Yas Kuno[5]. Although he studied other autonomic-controlled reactions such as the effects of hot baths, alcohol and other stressful influences on heart rate and blood pressure (ten papers between 1909–1925), he became known chiefly because of his work on body temperature regulation and the functions of sweat glands. A large number of papers were published from his laboratory in Manchuria reporting results he and his students obtained by recording qualitative and quantitative sweat output from individual sweat glands. They distinguished between temperature-induced sweating and psychologically- or tension-produced sweating of the hands and feet. Two members of this group, T. Kosaka in 1929 and M. Kaku, in 1931, published papers dealing particularly with neural control. Between the years 1920–1934 Yas Kuno published some ten papers on this subject but most important of all was his book on "The Physiology of Human Perspiration"[5], published in 1934, which became a classic. He also published another book on "Human Perspiration" in 1956[6] and a final paper in 1965.

Others who made significant contributions at a relatively early date were: Kiichiro Muto, who wrote between 1915–1917 about sweat gland innervation; K. Ogata, who dealt with influence of body posture, temperature and mental state on sweating; G. Usami, who in 1928 studied effects of section of parasympathetic nerves on sweating; Muto was particularly interested in the comparative physiology of sweating and showed that adrenalin injections produced sweating in some species (horses, sheep) but not in others (humans, cattle, cats). Adrenalin caused secretion from skin glands in frogs and toads. Pilocarpine caused sweating also in horses and sheep. This was blocked by atropine but atropine caused sweating in some other forms. Kuno, Yamada and Ohara in 1962 were still studying the effects of adrenalin on human sweat secretion. Physiological and pharmacological studies such as these eventually led to an appreciation of humoral transmission and Dale's discovery of cholinergic mediation of sweat production.

The sympatho-adrenal responses to cold exposure were also tested (S. Saito, 1928). Additional contributions will be mentioned in discussions of the development of work on adrenal gland functions.

Studies of reactions to heat and cold involved vasomotor change and cardiac adjustments. However, the history of this might better be discussed under the heading of cardiovascular reactions produced by the autonomic system.

Autonomic system involvement in cardiovascular functions: Control of the peripheral vascular system.   Possibly because of Takamine's work on adrenalin[16] and its actions, many Japanese experimented with this compound and compared its various actions with that of autonomic nerves. Yas Kuno (1924–1925) observed that an injection of adrenalin not only produced cardiovascular reactions but also influenced respiratory function and even caused apnea. S. Kajiwara (1925) published two papers on the action of adrenalin on renal blood vessels. T. En (1930) reported paradoxical effects of adrenalin on rabbit intestine and frog limb blood vessels. K. Nishimaru (1928) studied vasomotor nerves to vessels of the gastrointestinal tract, the pancreas and kidney. In other papers he described vasomotor nerves to hind limb vessels (1922) and to the lung (1923–1924). M. Ishihara had already in 1907 reported vagus effects on lung volume. T. Matsuda (1927) reported that the vagi as well as the sympathetic system affected the spleen. T. Kosaka (1929) showed that stimulating cervical sympathetics affected the cerebral circulation.

Not only did the Japanese participate in the analysis of actions of autonomic nerves in the vasomotor system, but they also studied vasomotor and related respiratory reflexes. H. Sato observed effects of warming and cooling the carotid blood on respiration (1929) and K. Endo observed the vasomotor and respiratory effects of stimulating carotid (baroreceptor) afferents (1938).

Control of the heart.   One of the early Japanese contributions to knowledge of the cardiovascular system was Sunao Tawara's 1906–1907 studies of the atrioventricular node. A less well-known early study, but one more related to autonomic system function, was that of K. Sassa and H. Miyazaki. In 1920 they observed, in confirmation of Bainbridge, that inflation of small balloons placed in the great veins and atria caused reflex acceleration of the heart. Miyazaki also published studies of the A-V conducting system (1916). M. Takino (1937) reported another cardiac reflex, a depressor response evoked by stimulating the pulmonary artery. This considerably antedates modern interests in such phenomena.

In 1925 K. Hukutake published a study of the histology and development of cardiac nerves; Y. Hata determined the effects of stimulating the accelerator nerves (sympathetics) on atrial conduction and H. Ishikawa studied the functions in general of the cardiac nerves. T. Hoshi (1926) published a study of nerve endings in cardiac muscle. At about this same time (1927) S. Oinuma wrote on the control of cardiac function and T. Okuno (1926–1928) studied the autoregulatory potential of isolated frog hearts (four papers). T. Suzuki studied the effects of denervating the heart. In 1929 C. Okamura reported the presence of ganglionic cells in heart muscle and H. Seto in 1935 published two papers on the anatomy of these ganglia.

These cardiovascular studies contributed to the analysis and understanding of the control of the cardiovascular system.

Studies primarily of autonomic system functions. Studies of neural control of tissue on organ functions are, of course, studies of the autonomic system but in surveying research done it is apparent that the interests of some individuals focused more directly on the nerves than on the organs. Examples of this have already been mentioned.

There were, of course, a number of somewhat isolated studies, for example, S. Asai from 1926 to 1928 published seven papers on the complexities of visceral afferents and K. Okamoto (1928–1929) produced a number of papers dealing not only with afferents but also centers involved in autonomic reflexes. There were a number of studies from 1925 to 1928 on innervation of muscle by the cervical sympathetics (T. Imagawa) and on the effects of section of this nerve on various entities such as cerebrospinal fluid composition (G. Usami). S. Matsue (1927–1928) published two papers dealing with effects of sectioning the vagi on renal glucose and NaCl secretion. S. Shiroki approached the interesting problem of the origin of autonomic system tonic activity by studying the effects of limiting movements of frogs and chickens on the parasympathetic system (two papers).

In retrospect it appears there were two direct lines or channels of development of Japanese interest in the autonomic nervous system and its functions. They were as follows:

The adrenal medulla and humoral transmission. Subsequent to the extraction of epinephrine from the adrenal medulla by Abel and production of crystalline adrenalin by Takamine in 1901[16] there was a continuing interest in the adrenal medulla, its control and the compounds it liberates. Walter B. Cannon mentions in his books Japanese studies carried on simultaneously with his own and, in particular, results obtained by Japanese physiologists using the cava pocket technique for obtaining blood and analyzing its adrenaline content. S. Kodama in 1923 and also T. Sugawara, M. Watanabe and S. Saito used this method to assay adrenal medulla activity under varied circumstances[1]. Quite a number of papers were published by Y. Satake, T. Sugawara, M. Watanabe and associates on the output of adrenaline and how it might be affected, from 1927 through 1955.

Evidently, at least 80 papers bearing the names of over 100 investigators were published between 1920 and 1940 relative to neurally (reflex or direct stimulation) induced adrenal medulla discharge and the effects of the compounds thus released. It is of interest that most of these were published in the *Tohoku Journal of Experimental Medicine* although a few appeared in foreign journals (*Quart. J. Exptl. Physiol.*, etc.) in English. The volume of studies in subsequent years has, of course, become much greater and the distribution much broader.

It is a little difficult to estimate the significance and influence of these contributions but the following summary does give some concepts of accomplishment.

1. The epinephrine content of the adrenals was assayed (I. Hujii, 1920; T. Kojima, 1932; S. Saito, H. Sato and T. Suzuki, 1932–).

2. The rate of accumulation or synthesis of epinephrine in the adrenal was examined by Y. Satow in 1938.

3. The nerve supply to the adrenals was studied by T. Hoshi, 1927 and Ken Kure, Y. Wada and S. Okinaka, 1932, to mention only a few. Others studied the effects on the gland of its denervation (Iino, 1930).

4. The release of epinephrine by reflex or direct stimulation of nerves was tested by S. Kodama, 1923; T. Aomura, 1928–1933; T. Kaiwa, 1931; E. Inaba, 1935.

5. T. Sugawara, 1925–1927; F. Watanabe, 1927–1935; and M. Wada, 1935–1940 with their associates were particulary active in testing the response of the adrenals to cold exposure, exercise (Wada) and a host of compounds. They determined the effects of strychnine, diphtheria toxin, caffein, nicotine, histamine, "peptone poisoning", epinephrine itself, pilocarpine, acetylcholine, physostigmine, etc. Such testing was carried on through the 1950's and 1960's by K. Yamashita. Others did similar studies at a relatively early date (E. Inaba, 1935; K. Saizyo, 1936; B. Hasama, 1937; H. Sato, et al., 1938; T. Hirano, 1939). Effects on the adrenal of tetrodotoxin were determined in 1930 (T. Aomura).

6. It was reported that epinephrine is liberated in insulin-induced hypoglycemia (K. Shimidzu, 1924; Y. Abe, 1924; T.-J. Yen, Aomura and Inaba, 1933).

7. Others studied effects of anesthetics, asphyxiation, hemorrhage, various stressor situations and agencies on epinephrine release (S. Kodama, 1923–1924; S. Saito, 1928–1929; H. Sato and T. Aomura, 1929–1933; F. Ohmi, 1933; H. Sato, H. Wada, et al., 1933–1935; M. Hatano, 1936).

8. Attempts were made to identify centers of the brain which might control epinephrine release (I. Hujii, 1920; T. Kaiwa and M. Wada, 1931).

Many other such studies were carried out later, culminating in the eventual study of receptors and blocking agents.

After Otto Loewi announced the liberation of "vagus stoff" from the heart following vagus nerve stimulation, there was much controversy over the validity of the claim. Among those who supported Loewi's conclusions were several Japanese physiologists. Y. Tsukiji in 1927 and O. Mochizuki in 1928 reported the production of "vagus stoff" by the frog heart. In 1928, also, K. Yasutake published three papers on "sympathetic stoff" and "vagus stoff". He also carried out a rather unique study: the effect of sympathetic nerves on cell permeability. Mention has already been made of the early use of sympatho- and parasympathomimetic drugs and blocking agents by Kiichiro Muto in 1916–1917 in studies of autonomic nerve actions. Interest in such drugs and in synaptic transmission and transmitters has been continuous.

Brief mention should be made of the fact that when in the late 1950's interest began to focus on central synapses and the possible action of amino acids as central synaptic transmitters, the Japanese physiologists were involved. For example, Takashi Hayashi[2,3] played an important role in demonstrating the actions of amino acids on central neuronal activity. With the advent of electron microscopy it became possible to determine in great detail the anatomical features of autonomic and other synaptic junctions and to see how transmitters were stored in neuron terminals. Technically and physiologically the Japanese have been at the forefront of such investigations (Uchizono[18]).

Studies of the autonomic system as a functional entity. Eventually in Japan, as in Europe and the USA, attention began to focus upon the autonomic system as a control unit and upon the special features of its subdivisions.

It is generally said that Ken Kure, a Professor of Medicine at the University of Tokyo who studied with H. E. Hering at Prague, was the first in Japan to inspire interest in the autonomic complex as a system of importance. In 1939 he received a special prize (Gakushi-in-sho) for his "study of spinal parasympathetic nerves". He was a very active but somewhat controversial figure who certainly did attract attention to both the autonomic system and Japanese physiology. He and others became particularly interested in the question of dorsal root vasodilator fibers. For example, S. Oinuma, between 1912 and 1924, published a number of papers on dorsal root vasodilator fibers and their possible role in vasomotor control. Ken Kure[7] called them a spinal parasympathetic system (1914–1927)[8]. Few agreed with his concepts but there is evidence of some effects from dorsal root efferent components.

Ken Kure's successor as the dominant figure in the field of autonomic system studies in Japan was Shigeo Okinaka. He wrote a number of books on the autonomic system[9,10,11] that significantly influenced interest in this field, particularly among clinicians. He began his work in association with Ken Kure in the 1930's and has published too much subsequently to list. However, in 1962, on the occasion of receipt of special recognition by the National Academy (Gakushiin Onshi-sho: Imperial Prize) he indicated the direction of his research from 1940 to 1961 as follows:

"1. The vagus nerve and its regulation of circulation; 2. autonomic nervous control of the coronary artery; 3. autonomic nervous system and pancreatic endocrine function; 4. neurohumoral control of the adrenal; 5. neurohumoral control of the thyroid; 6. stimulation of the posterior orbital surface and symptoms related to the autonomic nervous system; and 7. histochemical studies on the autonomic nervous system[12]".

In 1969 Dr. Okinaka delivered a lecture at the General Assemlby of the Japanese Society of Internal Medicine in which he described Professor Ken Kure's career and his own. He gave his view of the persons chiefly responsible for development of the neurosciences and the concept that the autonomic system acts through chemical mediators[13].

Professor Okinaka had an interest in clinical medicine, as the titles of his books and lectures indicate. This probably was responsible in part for the development of strong interests in the clinical aspects of autonomic system physiology in Japan.

Autonomic system dysfunction. Abnormalities of autonomic system function have long been known, but at the present time there is a very lively interest in these problems. At the international Congress of Neurovegetative Research held in Tokyo in 1977[14] numerous papers were presented from Japanese laboratories. For example:

Aging and pathological changes in human sympathetic ganglia: M. Tomonaga; Cyclic vomiting as autonomic seizure: E. Tamai, T. Hotta and T. Kimura; Autonomic and hemodynamic mechanisms of orthostatic hypotension in Shy-Dröger syndrome: N. Nakamura, M. Uchida, A. Kudo, T. Nomura and N. Tanaka; Vegetative dysfunction in Creutzfeldt-Jacob disease: M. Arai, T. Sata, S. Ono, H. Uchida, M. Kase and S. Katayama; and a case of familial dysautonomia without absent lacrimation seen in a Japanese girl: H. Shiihara, N. Kuromori, M. Okuni and I. Namba.

The history of the development of such interests is difficult to trace but at our request Professor Masanori Uono asked a number of clinicians to express their opinions of old and new Japanese contributions either made by clinicians to basic studies or to the resolution of clinical problems involving autonomic system dysfunction.

There were only a few clinical studies of significance published before the 1950's. In 1936 S. Katsunuma published a paper on disease and pathology of the diencephalon. T. Shinozaki in 1938 studied the physiology and pathology of the brain stem. In the 1930's to 1940's M. Takino reported studies of reflexes originating from within the pulmonary system and their clinical significance. Vasomotor reactions resulting from pulmonary emboli were also described by clinical investigators. In the early 1950's there were more numerous contributors. A book, *Function and Diseases of the Diencephalon*, was edited by Ishibashi in 1954; this contained many observations made by surgeons and others on human subjects. S. Katsuki in 1955 studied diseases of the brain stem and diencephalon. J. Murakami and E. Ando published an article on sympathectomy and its indication in the treatment of cerebral arteriosclerotic vascular disease (1955). In this same year studies on tumors of the pituitary gland were reported by G. Kusunoki. In the 1960's new aspects of clinical investigation began. I. Sano in 1960 reported reduction in the dopamine content of the brain in parkinsonism. Clinical neurochemistry had begun and the volume of research increased. Judging from the survey submitted, for every 50 papers published in this field in the 1950's, 100 were published in the 1960's and 150 in the 1970's.

It should be mentioned that in 1964 a jounal entitled *The Autonomic Nervous System* was started in Japan. It is now in its 16th volume; published in Japanese by the Japanese Society of the Autonomic Nervous System; S. Okinaka, President; M. Uono, Executive Secretary. Interest in the autonomic system is now very strong in Japan and several laboratories have attained distinction as centers of research in this field.

REFERENCES

1   Cannon, W. B., *Bodily Changes in Pain, Hunger, Fear and Rage*, D. Appleton and Co., New York, 1922.
2   Hayashi, T., Inhibition and excitation due to gamma-aminobutyric acid in the central nervous system, *Nature*, 182 (1958) 1076.
3   Hayashi, T., *Neurophysiology and Neurochemistry of Convulsion*, Dainihon-Tosho Co., Ltd., Tokyo, 1959.
4   *Japanese Handbook of Physiology*, Igaku Shoin Ltd., Tokyo, 1967.
5   Kuno, Y., *The Physiology of Human Perspiration*, Churchill, London, 1935.
6   Kuno, Y., *Human Perspiration*, Charles C. Thomas, Springfield, 1956.
7   Kure, K., Parasympathetic nerve fibers in spinal dorsal roots, *Tokyo Medical Journal (Tokyo I-shi)*, 42 (1928).
8   Kure, K., On the spinal parasympathetic outflow, *J. Neurol. (Shinkei-gaku Zasshi)*, 30 (1929).
9   Kure, K. and Okinaka, S., *The Autonomic Nervous System (General and Special Actions)*, Kanahara Publ. Co., Tokyo, 1931.

10 Okinaka, S., *The Autonomic Nervous System and its Clinical Application*, Igaku-Shoin, Tokyo, 1950.

11 Okinaka, S., *The Autonomic Nervous System and Clinical Studies*, Kyorin Shoin, Tokyo, 1956.

12 Okinaka, S., Study of the autonomic nervous system, *Tokyo Igaku Zasshi* (*Tokyo Medical Journal*), 70 (1962) 117–151.

13 Okinaka, S., My study and thought on internal medicine—experience in the study of the autonomic nervous system, *J. Jap. Assoc. Internal. Med.*, 58 (1969) 1147–1155.

14 *Proc. XVIII International Congress of Neurovegetative Research*, S. Okinaka (President), M. Yoshikawa (Vice-President) and M. Uono (Secretary), Tokyo, Japan, 1977.

15 *Publications in Japanese Physiology, 1873–1930*, Committee on Survey of the Publications in Japanese Physiology (Ed.), 1932.

16 Takamine, J., The isolation of the active principle of the suprarenal gland, *J. Physiol.* (Lond.), 27 (1901) 29–30P.

17 Uchiyama, K., Hayashi, T., Kinoshita, H., Natori, R., Shimazono, N., Wakabayashi, T., Brooks, C. McC. and Koizumi, K. (Eds.), *Japanese Physiology Past and Present*, For the XXIII International Congress of Physiological Sciences, Tokyo, Japan, 1965.

18 Uchizono, K., *Excitation and Inhibition—Synaptic Morphology*, Igaku Shoin Ltd., Tokyo, 1975.

2. American Contributions to the Advancement of Knowledge concerning Autonomic Nervous System Functions

The beginnings.   If one considers that U.S. history began in 1620 with the establishment of the Plymouth Colony in Massachusetts, it can be said that two and a half centuries of development were required before the USA began to make any major contributions to medicine and science. If one chooses to begin with 1776 when the USA attained political independence, only one century was required for attainment of medical and scientific independence[1,2].

Since knowledge of autonomic nervous system function has often come from studies of systems, it might be said that William Beaumont's 1833 study of Alexis St. Martin's gastric secretory and digestive processes[3] was an early contribution. Morton's introduction of ether anesthesia in 1846 was a helpful advance also. We can hardly claim Brown-Séquard as an American though he periodically held posts of importance in U.S. institutions. While in Philadelphia, about 1852[4], he did publish a paper describing experiments which, like those of Claude Bernard, demonstrated the function and tonic activity of sympathetic fibers[5]. It is of particular interest that 80 years later (1932) D. W. Bronk, another inhabitant of Philadelphia, made the first electrical recording of tonic activity in autonomic fibers[6].

It was not until the 1870's, when U.S. scientists began to return from studies in France and Germany and to establish research laboratories, that serious investigative work began. The required research laboratories were established at Harvard Medical School by Bowditch, at the Johns Hopkins University by Newell Martin, at the College of Physicians and Surgeons, N. Y. by Dalton and at Philadelphia by Weir Mitchel. Laboratories of physiological chemistry were established at Yale by Chittenden and at Michigan by Vaughan. Mention should also be made of Austin Flint of the Bellevue

Hospital Medical School. He wrote an extensive work on *The Physiology of Man* and studied, among other things, the glycogenic function of the liver and the physiology of muscular exercise. These were among the 28 physiologists who organized the American Physiological Society in 1887; it met first in New York on December 30 of that year. Several of the Society's first members did considerable research and a few studied reactions controlled at least to some degree by the autonomic nervous system[5]. For example, H. P. Bowditch and F. H. Ellis at Harvard published in 1885 and 1886 some papers on vasomotor reactions in muscle (*J. Physiol.*, 6 (1885) 437; 7 (1886) 309). Bowditch had studied with Carl Ludwig at Leipzig and published papers on the reactions of heart muscle from there. T. W. Mills, a Canadian working with Brooks of the Johns Hopkins at the Marine Laboratories, Beaufort, North Carolina in 1884, showed that he could inhibit the sea turtle's heart for six hours by alternate stimulation of the vagi. Henry Sewall of the University of Michigan published (*J. Physiol.*, 6 (1885) 162) extensive studies of the action of the depressor nerve on blood pressure and the heart. Isaac Ott in 1888 read a paper at the second meeting of the American Physiological Society on fever—he studied the role of the autonomic system. Samuel Meltzer of the Rockefeller Institute, in addition to founding the Society of Clinical Investigation and the *Journal of Proceedings of the Society of Experimental Biology and Medicine* and introducing the concept of a "safety factor" in physiological processes, also studied the action of adrenalin and nerves on blood vessels and the pupil (1904)[2].

Many other papers were published during the late 1800's by these and other early American physiologists which referred to actions of the autonomic system. Their focus of attention, however, was on the cardiovascular or digestive systems and not primarily intended to be contributions to autonomic system physiology. Thus, during this period when the British physiologists, Gaskell, Langley, Elliott and others, were so actively studying autonomic system function, no one considered contributions from the USA to be very significant to this field of interest. There was one exception and this might be considered the USA's first major contribution to the physiology of the autonomic system.

In 1898 John Jacob Abel, of the Johns Hopkins University Medical School, isolated epinephrine from the adrenal medulla. This was the first hormone or transmitter obtained in pure form and a new tool was placed in the hands of those studying the autonomic system. Elliott in 1904, observing that this compound could mimic the action of sympathetic nerves, suggested that these nerves might act by liberating epinephrine. This attainment by Abel was thus a precursor of the later discovery of chemical transmission of nerve action.

It is of particular interest that Jokichi Takamine, who had worked with Abel, succeeded in 1901 in obtaining epinephrine in crystalline form and it was introduced through Park Davis Company as Adrenalin. This latter name became most commonly used to describe products of the adrenal medulla (adrenaline and noradrenaline).

Another of Abel's students, Reid Hunt, who became Professor of Pharmacology and an associate of Walter B. Cannon at Harvard, in 1906 made a study of choline derivatives. Hunt and Taveau described the strong vasodilator effects of acetylcholine, likening its action to that of vasodilator nerves. In 1918 Hunt also showed that physostigmine or eserine, an alkaloid from the calabar bean of West Africa, greatly potentiates the action of acetylcholine. These observations were of great service to those who discovered cholinergic transmission of nerve action[7].

Walter B. Cannon and the contributions of his school of autonomic system physiology. Walter B. Cannon became interested initially in the autonomic system because of its action on the gastrointestinal system. In 1898 Cannon published his first paper dealing with mechanical action of the stomach as studied by means of X-rays, but it was not until 1905 that he mentioned the role of nerves, at least in the title of an article (*Med. News*, 86 (1905) 923–929). A year later he published a paper on the "Motor activities of the stomach and small intestine after section of the splanchnics and vagi", and in 1907 he studied the effects of vagotomies on esophageal peristalsis. In 1911 Cannon summarized his studies of this system in a book entitled *The Mechanical Factors of Digestion* (Edward Arnold, London). He never completely lost interest in gastrointestinal physiology although by 1909 his interest had started to shift toward consideration of functions of the autonomic system[8].

A survey of Cannon's publications[7] shows that in 1909 he began to publish his observations of "The influence of emotional states on functions of the alimentary canal". The role of the adrenal medulla (he spoke of the sympatho-adrenal system as a functional unity) in emotional excitement attracted his attention first and by 1914 "The emergency function of the adrenal medulla in pain and major emotions" (*Amer. J. Physiol.*, 33 (1914) 356–372) was one of his major concerns. He later applied this concept to the entire sympatho-adrenal complex. In 1915 he summarized his conclusions concerning this aspect of autonomic system function in a monograph entitled "*Bodily Changes in Pain, Hunger, Fear and Rage*" (D. Appleton Co., N. Y. and London).

Cannon's interests in emotions and emotional theory continued. He worked in this field with one of his early students, Philip Bard. Bard's role was to study central control of the emotions and the autonomic system. He eventually identified the caudal hypothalamus as being the portion of the brain essential to emotional expression and to the emergency or total discharge of the sympatho-adrenal system in sham rage and reaction to nociceptive stimuli. Cannon and Bard published a number of papers contributing to the theory of emotions[9].

It seems quite natural that Cannon's interest in the control of one endocrine gland, the adrenal, should lead him to a study of possible neural control of other glands. In 1915 he began to study with C. A. L. Binger, R. Fitz, later with McK. Cattell and others, possible neural control of the thyroid and possible neurogenic cause of hyperthyroidism. Cannon eventually felt that he wasted some valuable time over a ten-year period trying to demonstrate control of the thyroid by the autonomic system. Certainly, neural control of the thyroid gland is not like that of the adrenal medulla and he found nothing generally accepted as significant. Others about that same time were studying neural control of the pancreas, but that work too, was ignored with the discovery of humoral control of the endocrines. At the present time, however, U.S. physiologists and endocrinologists again recognize the role of the autonomic in control of both thyroids and the pancreas.

During World War I (1917–1919) Cannon was in Europe working on shock. He published numerous papers in which the role of the sympatho-adrenal system was considered. He continued his research on this subject for some time after returning from Europe and, as was his custom, he eventually summarized his conclusions in a monograph on traumatic shock and the effects of hemorrhage, "*Traumatic Shock*", 1923 (D. Appleton Co., New York and London). This experience contributed to his interest in balance of body states and what he later termed homeostasis.

It was in 1921 that Cannon began the work which showed that stimulation of sympathetic nerves to one organ could produce a response in a distant and denervated tissue. Incidentally, he discovered "denervation sensitization" while he was participating in the discovery of the chemical transmission of nerve action. This was a natural consequence of his interest in the adrenal medulla and the autonomic system. Cannon's last publication (1949) was "*Supersensitivity of Denervated Structures: A Law of Denervation*" (MacMillan Co., New York). He eventually obtained evidence in studies with Z. M. Bacq of Belgium and later with A. Rosenblueth that sympathetic nerves do liberate a compound which can act at a distance. He called the compound "sympathin" and had some concept of a determinant action of receptors in determing whether excitation or inhibition would result. He never received, for various reasons, adequate credit for his contribution to the discovery of chemical transmission[8].

Cannon was the first to study the effects of complete ablation of the sympatho-adrenal system as well as section of parasympathetic nerves. In 1927 he wrote a letter to the *Boston Med. & Surg. J.* describing the "dispensability of the sympathetic division of the autonomic nervous system". He soon published a fuller report with J. T. Lewis and S. W. Britton in that same journal. Cannon was aware that sympathectomy in the male produced sterility and of other undesirable consequences of complete sympathectomy. He was not supportive of the "heroic" sympathectomies done in an effort to cure hypertension.

Cannon was much interested in thirst, water balance, and the maintenance of blood sugar levels. In 1929 this new emphasis in his interests was indicated by two papers: One was entitled "Organization for physiological homeostasis", and the other "Functions of the sympathetic system in maintaining the stability of the organism". This interest culminated in a book entitled "*The Wisdom of the Body*" (W. W. Norton, New York, 1932).

During Cannon's career some 347 junior and senior scientists were members of his department and worked under his supervision. Approximately 20% of these were from foreign countries. His contributions were not all facts and ideas; he contributed a philosophy expressed in a book written in 1945, the year of his death, and republished and distributed to all participants in the International Congress of Physiological Sciences held in Washington, D. C. in 1968, "*The Way of an Investigator*" (W. W. Norton, New York).

The following chart (Chart 2) lists Cannon's major concepts concerning autonomic system function; these ideas dominate thought even today. They have been extended and added to of recent years, but they are still accepted in principle.

American contributions. Walter B. Cannon, his students and associates were not the only Americans who made significant contributions to knowledge of the autonomic nervous system. Albert Kuntz (1879–1957) was a contemporary of Cannon. He began his studies of the autonomic system in 1908, publishing a paper on the "Histogenesis of the sympathetic division" in 1909. His chief contribution was a book, "*The Autonom-*

activates, but most important of all—it integrates. Thus, two additional concepts have developed.

2) *The supportive function of the autonomic system.* It acts to adjust visceral functions to support somatic behavior. In doing this it affects sensory receptors[10], activates endocrine glands, shunts blood, affects heart pumping action, releases nutrients from stores and participates in organizing emotional support of behavior and in promoting anticipatory, preparatory action.

3) *The integrative action of the autonomic system* is related to the concept of supportive function but emphasizes the fact that the autonomic system has primary functions and often acts in advance of somatic behavior. It innervates all tissues of the body, is involved in all reactions of the body and by imposing patterns of inhibition and excitation produces the totality of response essential to effective behavior. It actually seems as much or more retentive of past stimulation experience than is the somatic and thus it integrates the new with the past. Although many autonomic patterns of response are built into the primitive basal automaton, the system is also controlled by higher centers. Control of the autonomic system is built into each level of the hierarchy of central nervous system centers which control all types of body behavior[16].

Advances in our knowledge of the autonomic system confirm its involvement in the functions of all systems and in the control not only of individuals but also in the intercommunications of society and reactions to the total environment.

REFERENCES

1 Björklund, A. and Nobin, A., Fluorescent histochemical and microspectrofluorometric mapping of dopamine and noradrenaline cell groups in rat diencephalon, *Brain Res.*, 51 (1973) 193–205.

2 Bohus, B., The influence of pituitary peptides on brain centers controlling autonomic responses. In: *Integrative Hypothalamic Activity, Progress in Brain Research, Vol. 41,* Elsevier, Amsterdam, 1974, pp. 175–183.

3 Brooks, C. McC., The autonomic system's involvement in behavior and homeostasis, *Proc. XVIII Internat. Congress of Neurovegetative Research,* Tokyo, 1977.

4 Brooks, C. McC. and Lange, G., The interactions of myogenic and neurogenic mechanisms that control heart rate, *Proc. nat. Acad. Sci. USA,* 74 (1977) 1761–1762.

5 Bunge, R. and Johnson, M., Nature and nurture in development of the autonomic neuron, *Science,* 199 (1978) 1409–1415.

6 Burnstock, G., Do some nerve cells release more than one transmitter? *Neuroscience,* 1 (1976) 239–248.

7 Burnstock, G. and Bell, C., Peripheral autonomic transmission. In: J. I. Hubbard (Ed.), *The Peripheral Nervous System,* Plenum Press, New York, 1974, pp. 277–317.

8 Carlsson, A., Flack, B. and Hillarp, N.-Å., Cellular localization of brain monamines, *Acta physiol. scand.,* 56, Suppl. 196 (1962) 1–28.

9 Koizumi, K. and Brooks, C. McC., Integration of autonomic system reactions, *Ergebn. Physiol.,* 67 (1972) 1–68.

10 Krnjevic, K., Chemical nature of synaptic transmission in vertebrates, *Physiol. Rev.,* 54 (1974) 418–440.

11 Ling, G. and Gerard, R. W., The normal membrane potential of frog sartorius muscle, *J. cell. comp. Physiol.,* 34 (1949) 383–396.

12   Schwartz, G. E., Biofeedback, self-regulation, and the patterning of physiological processes, *Amer. Scientist*, 63 (1975) 314–324.

13   Selye, H., Homeostasis and the reactions to stress. In: C. McC. Brooks, K. Koizumi and J. O. Pinkston (Eds.), *The Life and Contributions of Walter Bradford Cannon*, State Univ. of New York Press, Albany, 1975.

14   Slangen, J. L., The role of hypothalamic noradrenergic neurons in food intake regulation. In: *Integrative Hypothalamic Activity, Progress in Brain Research, Vol. 41*, Elsevier, Amsterdam, 1974, pp. 395–407.

15   Usdin, E., Homburg, D. A. and Barchas, J. D., *Neuroregulators and Psychiatric Disorders*, Oxford Univ. Press, New York, 1977.

16   Yalow, R. S., Radioimmunoassay: A probe for the fine structure of biologic systems, *Science*, 200 (1978) 1236–1245.

AUTHOR INDEX

SUBJECT INDEX